Core Topics in Cardiothoracic Critical Care

Core Topics in Cardiothoracic Critical Care

Second Edition

Edited by

Kamen Valchanov
Papworth Hospital

Nicola Jones
Papworth Hospital

Charles W Hogue
Northwestern University in Chicago

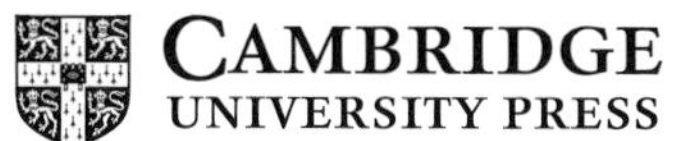

CAMBRIDGE
UNIVERSITY PRESS

University Printing House, Cambridge CB2 8BS, United Kingdom

One Liberty Plaza, 20th Floor, New York, NY 10006, USA

477 Williamstown Road, Port Melbourne, VIC 3207, Australia

314–321, 3rd Floor, Plot 3, Splendor Forum, Jasola District Centre, New Delhi – 110025, India

79 Anson Road, #06-04/06, Singapore 079906

Cambridge University Press is part of the University of Cambridge.

It furthers the University's mission by disseminating knowledge in the pursuit of education, learning, and research at the highest international levels of excellence.

www.cambridge.org
Information on this title: www.cambridge.org/9781107131637
DOI: 10.1017/9781316443415

First published 2008
Reprinted 2008
Second edition 2018

Printed in the United Kingdom by TJ International Ltd. Padstow Cornwall

A catalogue record for this publication is available from the British Library.

ISBN 978-1-107-13163-7 Hardback

Additional resources for this publication at www.cambridge.org/CardiothoracicMCQ

Contents

Section 7 – Disease Management in the Cardiothoracic Intensive Care Unit: Incidence; Aetiology; Diagnosis; Prognosis; Treatment

Section 8 – Provision and Delivery of Cardiothoracic Intensive Care

Colour plates are to be found between pages 230 and 231.

Contributors

Darryl Abrams
Department of Medicine, Columbia University College of Physicians and Surgeons, New York, NY, USA

Yasir Abu-Omar
Department of Surgery, Papworth Hospital, Cambridge, UK

Jason M Ali
Department of Surgery, Papworth Hospital, Cambridge, UK

Olly Allen
Department of Pathology, Papworth Hospital, Cambridge, UK

Joseph E Arrowsmith
Department of Anaesthesia and Intensive Care, Papworth Hospital, Cambridge, UK

Adam Baddeley
Department of Physiotherapy, Papworth Hospital, Cambridge, UK

Rubia Baldassarri
Department of Anaesthesia and Critical Care Medicine, Azienda Ospedaliero Universitaria Pisana, Pisa, Italy

Allanah Barker
Department of Surgery, Papworth Hospital, Cambridge, UK

Sérgio Barra
Department of Cardiology, Papworth Hospital, Cambridge, UK

Nicholas A Barrett
Department of Intensive Care, Guy's and St Thomas' NHS Foundation Trust, London, UK

Peter A Barry
Department of Surgery, Royal Marsden Hospital, London, UK

David Begley
Department of Cardiology, Papworth Hospital, Cambridge, UK

Marius Berman
Department of Surgery, Papworth Hospital, Cambridge, UK

Martin Besser
Department of Pathology, Papworth Hospital, Cambridge, UK

Paolo Bosco
Department of Surgery, Papworth Hospital, Cambridge, UK

Daniel Brodie
Department of Medicine, Columbia University College of Physicians and Surgeons, New York, NY, USA

Simon JA Buczacki
Department of Surgery, Addenbrooke's Hospital, Cambridge, UK

Christiana Burt
Department of Anaesthesia and Intensive Care, Papworth Hospital, Cambridge, UK

Lidia Casanueva
Great Ormond Street Hospital, London, UK

Pedro Catarino
Department of Surgery, Papworth Hospital, Cambridge, UK

Sumit Chatterji
Department of Medicine, Addenbrooke's Hospital, Cambridge, UK

Oana Cole
Department of Anaesthesia and Intensive Care, Papworth Hospital, Cambridge, UK

Max S Damian
Department of Neurology, Addenbrooke's Hospital, Cambridge, UK

Justin Davies
Department of Surgery, Addenbrooke's Hospital, Cambridge, UK

Michael G Davies
Department of Respiratory Medicine, Papworth Hospital, Cambridge, UK

Will Davies
Department of Cardiology, Papworth Hospital, Cambridge, UK

Ajay Desai
Department of Paediatric Intensive Care, Royal Brompton and Harefield NHS Foundation Trust, London, UK

Harikrishna M Doshi
Department of Surgery, Papworth Hospital, Cambridge, UK

Ghislaine Douflé
University Health Network, University of Toronto, Toronto, Ontario, Canada

Allaina Eden
Department of Physiotherapy, Papworth Hospital, Cambridge, UK

Ari Ercole
Department of Anaesthesia, Addenbrooke's Hospital, Cambridge, UK

Peter Faber
Department of Anaesthesia, Aberdeen Royal Infirmary, Aberdeen, UK

Shakil Farid
Department of Surgery, Papworth Hospital, Cambridge, UK

Simon J Finney
Department of Intensive Care, Barts Heart Central, St Bartholomew's Hospital, London, UK

Sophia Fisher
Department of Anaesthesia, Flinders Medical Centre, Adelaide, South Australia, Australia

Jo-anne Fowles
Department of Anaesthesia and Intensive Care, Papworth Hospital, Cambridge, UK

Kamrouz Ghadimi
Department of Anesthesiology, Duke University Hospital, Durham, NC, USA

S Ghosh
Department of Anaesthesia and Intensive Care, Papworth Hospital, Cambridge, UK

Margaret I Gillham
Department of Pathology, Papworth Hospital, Cambridge, UK

Stuart A Gillon
Department of Intensive Care, Guy's and St Thomas' NHS Foundation Trust, London, UK

Deepa Gopalan
Department of Radiology, Imperial College, London, UK

Fabio Guarracino
Department of Anaesthesia and Critical Care Medicine, Azienda Ospedaliero Universitaria Pisana, Pisa, Italy

Patrick Heck
Department of Cardiology, Papworth Hospital, Cambridge, UK

Joseph G Hobelmann
Department of Psychiatry, Johns Hopkins University School of Medicine, Baltimore, MD, USA

Lisen Hockings
Department of Intensive Care, The Alfred Hospital, Melbourne, Victoria, Australia

Charles W Hogue
Department of Anesthesiology, Northwestern University Feinberg School of Medicine, Chicago, USA

Stephen P Hoole
Department of Cardiology, Papworth Hospital, Cambridge, UK

J Irons
Department of Anaesthesia and Intensive Care, Papworth Hospital, Cambridge, UK

Swetha Iyer
Department of Surgery, Papworth Hospital, Cambridge, UK

David P Jenkins
Department of Surgery, Papworth Hospital, Cambridge, UK

Martin John
Department of Anaesthesia and Intensive Care, Papworth Hospital, Cambridge, UK

Matthew Jones
Judge Business School, University of Cambridge, Cambridge, UK

Nicola Jones
Deptartment of Anesthesia and Intensive Care, Papworth Hospital, Cambridge, UK

A Ruth M Kappeler
Department of Pathology, Papworth Hospital, Cambridge, UK

Andrew Klein
Department of Anaesthesia and Intensive Care, Papworth Hospital, Cambridge, UK

Gabriel Kleinman
Department of Anesthesiology, Northwestern University, Chicago, IL, USA

Makeida B Koyi
Department of Psychiatry, Johns Hopkins University School of Medicine, Baltimore, MD, USA

Unni Krishnan
Department of Cardiology, Papworth Hospital, Cambridge, UK

Anna Kydd
Department of Transplantation, Papworth Hospital, Cambridge, UK

Jerrold H Levy
Department of Anesthesiology, Critical Care and Surgery, Duke University School of Medicine, Durham, NC, USA

Jonathan H Mackay
Department of Anaesthesia and Intensive Care, Papworth Hospital, Cambridge, UK

Duncan Macrae
Department of Paediatric Intensive Care, Royal Brompton and Harefield NHS Foundation Trust, London, UK

Guillermo Martinez
Department of Anaesthesia and Intensive Care, Papworth Hospital, Cambridge, UK

Christopher IS Meadows
Department of Intensive Care, Guy's and St Thomas' NHS Foundation Trust, London, UK

James Moore
Department of Anaesthesia and Intensive Care, Papworth Hospital, Cambridge, UK

Kristian H Mortensen
Department of Radiology, Great Ormond Street Hospital, London, UK

Lachlan Miles
Department of Anaesthesia and Intensive Care, Papworth Hospital, Cambridge, UK

Sam Nashef
Department of Surgery, Papworth Hospital, Cambridge, UK

Amy Needham
Department of Anaesthesia and Intensive Care, Papworth Hospital, Cambridge, UK

Karin J Neufeld
Department of Psychiatry, Johns Hopkins University School of Medicine, Baltimore, MD, USA

Choo Yen Ng
Department of Surgery, Papworth Hospital, Cambridge, UK

Alia Noorani
Department of Surgery, Papworth Hospital, Cambridge, UK

Erik Ortmann
Department of Anesthesia and Intensive Care, Kerckhoff-Klinic, Heart and Lung Centre, Bad Nauheim, Germany

Marlies Ostermann
Department of Intensive Care, Guy's and St Thomas' NHS Foundation Trust, London, UK

Chinmay Padvardthan
Department of Anaesthesia and Intensive Care, Papworth Hospital, Cambridge, UK

Jayan Parameshwar
Department of Transplantation, Papworth Hospital, Cambridge, UK

Ken Kuljit Parhar
Department of Critical Care Medicine, University of Calgary, Calgary, Alberta, Canada

Barbora Parizkova
Department of Anaesthesia and Intensive Care, Papworth Hospital, Cambridge, UK

Js Parmar
Department of Transplantation, Papworth Hospital, Cambridge, UK

Evgeny Pavlushkov
Department of Surgery, Papworth Hospital, Cambridge, UK

Joanna Pepke-Zaba
Department of Respiratory Medicine, Papworth Hospital, Cambridge, UK

Stephen J Pettit
Department of Transplantation, Papworth Hospital, Cambridge, UK

Jonah Powell-Tuck
Department of Intensive Care, Guy's and St Thomas' NHS Foundation Trust, London, UK

Susanna Price
Department of Intensive Care, Royal Brompton and Harefield NHS Foundation Trust, London, UK

Lara Prisco
Department of Anaesthesia, Addenbrooke's Hospital, Cambridge, UK

Alastair Proudfoot
Department of Perioperative Medicine, St. Bartholomew's Hospital, London, UK

Andrew Roscoe
Department of Anaesthesia and Intensive Care, Papworth Hospital, Cambridge, UK

Antonio Rubino
Department of Anaesthesia and Intensive Care, Papworth Hospital, Cambridge, UK

Kiran Salaunkey
Department of Anaesthesia and Intensive Care, Papworth Hospital, Cambridge, UK

Anja Schneider
Zentrum für Akute und Postakute Intensivmedizin Kreisklinik Jugenheim, Seeheim-Jugenheim, Germany

Shahzad Shaefi
Department of Anesthesiology, Northwestern University, Chicago, IL, USA

Charles Shayan
Department of Anesthesiology, Northwestern University, Chicago, IL, USA

Ravi J De Silva
Department of Surgery, Papworth Hospital, Cambridge, UK

Pasupathy Sivasothy
Department of Medicine, Addenbrooke's Hospital, Cambridge, UK

Tom P Sullivan
Department of Anaesthesia and Intensive Care, Papworth Hospital, Cambridge, UK

Charlotte Summers
University of Cambridge School of Clinical Medicine, Cambridge, UK

Susan Stevenson
Department of Anaesthesia and Intensive Care, Papworth Hospital, Cambridge, UK

Mark Toshner
Department of Respiratory Medicine, Papworth Hospital, Cambridge, UK

Steven SL Tsui
Department of Surgery, Papworth Hospital, Cambridge, UK

Kamen Valchanov
Deptartment of Anesthesia and Intensive Care, Papworth Hospital, Cambridge, UK

Matt Varrier
Department of Intensive Care, Guy's and St Thomas' NHS Foundation Trust, London, UK

Alain Vuylsteke
Department of Anaesthesia and Intensive Care, Papworth Hospital, Cambridge, UK

Niki Walker
Department of Intensive Care, Royal Brompton and Harefield NHS Foundation Trust, London, UK

Ian Welsby
Department of Anesthesiology, Duke University Hospital, Durham, NC, USA

Vasileios Zochios
Department of Anaesthesia and Intensive Care, Papworth Hospital, Cambridge, UK

Foreword

I am very pleased to be able to provide a brief introduction to the owner, borrower or reader of this text. This book is an update of the successful 2008 *Core Topics in Cardiothoracic Care* text. When that book was published, it was the first to provide a detailed insight into the cardiothoracic critical care unit and was widely read and appreciated. Since then other authors have produced texts that explore this fascinating area of practice, but none have quite replicated that originality and quality... until now!

Cardiac critical care evolved quite separately from general intensive care. It essentially originated as a side room on the cardiac surgical ward in the 1950s where the patient who struggled after cardiac surgery was ventilated and cared for by the cardiac anaesthetist and surgeon. Today we have large multidisciplinary teams in large technology dominated purpose-built tertiary units. This has been a rapid and hugely successful evolution. Cardiothoracic critical care is now a full blooded and highly influential subspecialty in the ever expanding critical care field. Indeed I firmly believe that where cardiac intensivists tread today, general intensivists will follow tomorrow. This evolution has been accompanied by a vast expansion in research and regulation. No branch of medicine is so scrutinised and yet so open to new thinking and new solutions. The link between cardiothoracic anaesthesia and cardiothoracic critical care is vital in the joined up care of these complex patients, as is the close link with all the related specialties such as the surgeon, the cardiologist, the echocardiographer and so many more.

We are fortunate that the new generation of critical care doctors and authors from Papworth have stepped up and, combined with a very eminent US academic, revisited, reorganised and rewritten the problems and solutions in this area of practice. Kamen Valchanov and Nicola Jones have taken over the authorship from their mentors at the world leading Papworth Hospital and have produced a book that retains the vision and wisdom of the original and added the significant advances in knowledge, technology and practice. A significant positive change is the addition of Professor Charles Hogue of Johns-Hopkins, Baltimore and Northwestern University, Chicago for a North American perspective. Knowing them all, it is not in the least surprising that they have produced a book of such scope and such high quality. The contributing authors are all experts in their fields and are drawn from a wide international base.

This book will prove invaluable to the critical care nurse, the trainee anaesthetist, surgeon and intensivist. It will also be of value to the new and established consultants who are involved with patients with cardiothoracic disease, which extends well beyond the bounds of surgery now. I feel proud to have been invited to write this foreword and I am proud to fully recommend this work.

Nick Fletcher
Consultant in Cardiothoracic and Vascular Critical Care
St George's University Hospital, London UK

Past President of the Association for Cardiothoracic Anaesthesia and Critical Care (UK)

Preface to the Second Edition

Why the second edition of *Core Topics in Cardiothoracic Critical Care*? The first edition of *Core Topics in Cardiothoracic Critical Care* was published in 2008. It has been a great success, providing a comprehensive text for the specialty and selling so many paper copies that Cambridge University Press had to reprint the book to meet the demands of the market. The first editors Dr Alain Vuylsteke, Dr Andrew Klein, and Mr Sam Nashef laid the foundation stone. However, a lot has happened in the world of medicine since 2008, not least in cardiothoracic critical care. Indeed practice has expanded so much that cardiothoracic critical care has been recognised as a separate sub-specialty by the Faculty of Intensive Care Medicine in the UK. Therefore, the current editors were tasked with providing an updated version of this textbook, which will hopefully offer to the reader state-of-the-art information on the current practice in cardiothoracic critical care.

A Few Notes from the Editors

Different sources point to different events as the birth of our specialty of intensive care medicine. Most revolve around mechanical ventilation with some believing intensive care started in Boston in 1912 when a girl suffering from poliomyelitis received mechanical ventilation. Others feel that it is the organised care for polio victims in need of invasive ventilation that laid the foundations of the specialty. It is probably a little easier to define the birth of cardiothoracic critical care medicine as this was born when cardiac surgeons needed to leave patients who had undergone heroic operations in a place where they could recover. Similarly to general intensive care medicine we do not have a specific disease to treat, rather we have very sick patients with complex disorders of the cardiorespiratory system to care for.

How do we practise in this specialty? We provide organ support to patients who have undergone cardiothoracic surgery or who have failing cardiac or respiratory function, with the hope that they will respond to treatment and survive. However, these days with modern advances in life support technology, such as extracorporeal membrane oxygenation, death is no longer a binary phenomenon. As guardians of this technology we must be ever mindful of our patients' quality of life and the long-term outcome from our interventions. Importantly we must guard against sustaining life at all costs and offer patients and their loved ones, care which makes them happy, or at least acts in their best interests.

In 2018 a vast amount of evidence exists to guide this practice. However, it can be challenging to apply evidence from trials to the heterogeneous group of patients we treat in Cardiothoracic Critical Care each with unique, rapidly changing derangements of cardiorespiratory function. The world of evidence-based medicine is also riddled with problems of spurious evidence, and an ever-increasing number of articles describing scientific trials are being retracted by the publishers. In the end among a myriad of scientific and less scientific articles, guidelines and protocols, based on expert opinion, the patient has to be supported through their critical illness and recovery after surgery. In most cases good doctors, nurses and allied healthcare professionals use patient tailored approaches in their daily work to provide patients with the best possible care. We hope that the following text will offer ample and unbiased information to help us work in the best interest of each individual patient.

Kamen Valchanov
Nicola Jones
Charles W Hogue

Link between Cardiothoracic Anaesthesia and Intensive Care: Which Patients are Admitted to Critical Care?

Andrew Klein

Introduction

Admission to an intensive care area is undertaken for the diagnosis, management and monitoring of patients with conditions that require close or constant attention by a group of specially trained health professionals. Critical care encompasses all areas that provide level 2 and/or level 3 care as defined by the Intensive Care Society document 'Levels of Critical Care for Adult Patients, 2009' (Table 1). All level 2 and level 3 areas have higher staffing levels, specialist monitoring and more advanced treatment options available. Level 2 areas are commonly referred to as High Dependency Units (HDUs), while level 3 areas are Intensive Care Units (ICUs), and we will make this distinction in our text. In some hospitals, the two are separated geographically, whilst in others they coexist in one area.

It is extremely common for patients undergoing cardiothoracic interventions under anaesthesia to be admitted to an ICU or HDU afterwards and this can often be a preplanned decision based on the potential for the patient to become more critically unwell or unstable. However, given the current pressures placed on the health service, in terms of both bed occupancy and finances, each individual case should be considered and a decision made as to whether such an admission will be necessary. These decisions can often be very difficult and must take into consideration a number of factors.

Patient Related Factors

A patient's comorbidities, physiological reserve, prognosis and wishes should all be taken into account when planning their most appropriate postoperative destination. Prioritisation of patients for critical care beds should highlight only those patients likely to gain from an increased level of care and thus not those that are either too well or too sick to benefit.

It is clear that for some high-risk patients, such as those with known chronic organ failure undergoing cardiac surgery, admission to an ICU will be mandatory after anaesthesia. It is reasonable to expect their condition to worsen following a period of cardiopulmonary bypass, and preparations should be made for any necessary organ support, for example use of inotropes or haemofiltration.

Consideration must also be taken as to whether the patient is appropriate for long-term management on an ICU. An example of this might be a palliative thoracic oncology patient undergoing a procedure for symptom relief; such a patient might be more appropriately placed in an HDU with a limit on the medical interventions that would be appropriate. This management plan should be discussed and formulated with the patient and relatives prior to the procedure itself.

Diagnostic and Surgical Related Factors

A diagnostic model can be utilised in order to provide guidelines for admission, which identifies specific conditions and diseases where it is felt a higher level of care is always warranted. With respect to cardiothoracic intensive care, the majority of such conditions will fall under the umbrellas of the cardiac and/or respiratory systems. However, it is also possible for a patient to require admission on the basis of an additional diagnosis, such as sepsis or a neurological complication of surgery.

All patients undergoing sternotomy will mandate admission to either an ICU or cardiac recovery environment after their procedure. The differentiation between the two is discussed below. A number of cardiothoracic surgical procedures will always warrant ICU admission, due to the complex nature of the intervention and often long procedural times. Examples of these are repair of aortic dissection, or multiple valve procedures.

The majority of patients undergoing thoracic surgery will either be admitted to an HDU or discharged back to the ward following a period of close

Table 1 Levels of critical care

Level of care		Criteria for admission	Examples
0	General ward	• Requires hospitalisation but needs can be met through normal ward care	Intraveous drug administration Observations needed less than 4 hourly
1	Coronary care unit	• Recently discharged from higher level care • In need of additional monitoring/intervention, clinical input or advice • Requiring critical care outreach service support	Minimal 4 hourly observations Continuous oxygen therapy, management of epidural, chest drain in situ Risk of clinical deterioration, high early warning score
2	High dependency unit	• Requiring preoperative optimisation • Requiring extended postoperative care • Stepping down to level 2 from level 3 care • Requiring single organ support • Requiring basic respiratory plus basic cardiovascular support	Invasive monitoring to optimise fluid balance Major elective surgery, emergency surgery in unstable patient Minimal hourly observations Non-invasive ventilation, single intravenous vasoactive drug Continuous oxygen therapy and intra-aortic balloon pump
3	Intensive care unit	• Requiring advanced respiratory support alone • Requiring a minimum of two organ systems supported (except basic respiratory plus basic cardiovascular – level 2, as above)	Invasive mechanical ventilator support via endotracheal tube or tracheostomy Acute renal replacement therapy and vasoactive medication

monitoring in recovery after surgery. An HDU bed may often be requested to ensure vigilance in the immediate postoperative period, and also to allow optimisation of pain control.

Alternative Resources

Each individual institution will have slightly different facilities available for the care of their patients and these must be taken into consideration when planning postprocedural care. Early goal-directed therapy and utilisation of a 'fast-track' approach has been adopted successfully in many cardiothoracic centres and this may allow lower risk patients to be admitted to a cardiac recovery area as a temporary measure postoperatively, before being discharged back to a 'stepdown' unit or ward. For such systems to work and ensure safe patient care, there must be immediate access to critical care and adequate numbers of trained nursing staff. This model has been proven to be successful in some hospitals and can potentially improve patient flow. However, for many institutions the safest option remains to admit all cardiac surgical patients to the ICU postoperatively. The priority in such institutions is then to discharge out into a stepdown unit as soon as possible after extubation and a period of stability.

Admission to an ICU may also depend on the availability of a required specific treatment for an individual patient. Some centres provide specialised advanced organ support, such as extracorporeal membrane oxygenation. Also, cardiothoracic surgery is a high-risk specialty fraught with potential complications, some of which might require transfer out to an alternative centre, for example to access neurosurgical intervention.

Time of Admission

A well-organised cardiothoracic surgical centre should incorporate a robust system of communication with both its ICU and HDU with respect to the daily admission requirements and bed availability. The majority of patients undergoing anaesthesia will require elective admission and surgical activity will be planned according to such requirements.

However, the ICU and HDU must also always take into account the potential for unplanned emergency admissions, either transferred in for surgical intervention, or due to unexpected complications intraoperatively. Patients should be admitted to the required higher level of care before their condition reaches a point from which recovery may be extremely difficult. In reality, it is often much better practice to assume a bed will be needed for your patient, than be left in a situation where the availability is not there and the patient is unstable. This could potentially lead to a worsened patient outcome, and may also put unnecessary pressure on the relevant intensive care unit to discharge prematurely.

Conclusion

It is often assumed that all patients undergoing cardiothoracic surgery will warrant admission to either an ICU or HDU postoperatively and in many instances that remains the case. Cardiothoracic anaesthesia is a high-risk specialty and it is imperative that the postoperative care system in place in each institution is safe and robust.

However, variety in admission indications and rates does exist. In recent years there have been advances in providing 'fast-track' surgery, and cardiac recovery units have become increasingly popular. In addition, thoracic surgery does not always necessitate an HDU bed and often an adequate level of care can be provided on general wards with critical care outreach support. Requirements for a higher level of care are by no means well defined and clinical practice will continue to evolve with time.

Given the current climate in the health care system, with a constant pressure for beds and a drive to improve patient flow, it is extremely important that each case undergoing cardiothoracic anaesthesia is considered individually and the safest care for that patient determined. Such planning will take into consideration patient related factors, their diagnosis and required surgery and the resources available in the institution.

Scoring Systems and Prognosis

Allanah Barker and Sam Nashef

Crystal Balls

Knowing the likelihood of survival after cardiac surgery is useful for multiple reasons including for weighing the potential risks versus benefits of surgery. Further, accurate predicting of outcome allows for comparison with the actual outcome and thus insight into the overall performance of the cardiac surgical unit. Knowledge of who is likely to develop major morbidity also has an impact on the use of valuable resources and may allow for sensible planning of operating lists. In addition, some believe that being able to predict mortality with some certitude may help clinicians to determine when further efforts are futile. Unfortunately, the perfect predictor – a crystal ball to foresee the future – has not yet been fully developed.

Risk Models or Scoring Systems

Scoring systems allow reasonable prediction of outcome after cardiac surgery. Many models have been devised to work out the likelihood of survival, and these and others have also been shown to predict major morbidity, long-term survival and resource use with some accuracy. Models can be broadly divided into two groups:

- *Preoperative models*, applied before the operation, with no knowledge of intraoperative events; and
- *Postoperative models*, applied immediately after the operation on admission into the critical care unit, taking some account of what the operation did to the patient.

Preoperative Models

These are most useful for

- Establishing the risk of surgery as an adjunct to surgical decision making (determining the indication to operate on the basis of risk-to-benefit assessment);
- Providing the patient with information, which is helpful in obtaining consent;
- Helping to measure the performance of the service by comparing actual and predicted outcomes; and
- Comparing the performance of different institutions, surgeons and anaesthetists by correcting for risk when outcomes are assessed.

Preoperative models take no account of what happens in the operating theatre and are therefore less useful in predicting which of a number of postoperative patients with complications are likely to emerge intact from the critical care unit.

There are probably more risk models in cardiac surgery than in any other branch of medicine. Most rely on a combination of risk factors, each of which is given a numerical 'weight'. Weights are added, multiplied or otherwise mathematically processed to come up with a percentage figure to predict mortality or survival. In additive models, the weights given to the risk factors are simply summed to give the predicted risk. They are easy to use and can be calculated mentally or 'on the back of an envelope'. They are less accurate than more sophisticated systems and have a tendency to overscore slightly in low-risk patients and to underscore considerably in very high-risk patients. Examples of such models are the Parsonnet (the pioneering heart surgery risk model) and the original additive EuroSCORE for cardiac surgery overall. Other models deal specifically with cardiac surgical subsets, like coronary surgery and valve surgery. Sophisticated models use Bayesian analysis, logistic regression or even computer neural networks. They do not allow easy bedside calculation, necessitating a computer for determining risk. They are, however, more stable than additive models across the risk range and slightly more accurate in exact risk prediction. Examples of such models are the Society of Thoracic Surgeons (STS) model, the logistic EuroSCORE and EuroSCORE II for overall cardiac surgery.

The widespread application of scoring systems in heart surgery has allowed robust performance measurement and probably contributed to the dramatic drop in cardiac surgical mortality seen in the last 15 years.

Preoperative Model Risk Factors

Not surprisingly, several common risk factors are included in all models (age, gender and left ventricular (LV) function). Other risk factors are included in some models but not in others, such as hypertension, diabetes and obesity. Models also differ depending on whether they deal with all cardiac surgeries or a specific subset, such as coronary surgery or valvular surgery. They share many risk factors and it would be repetitive to list them all here, but the models are easily accessible and there are interactive calculators available online: www.euroscore.org and http://riskcalc.sts.org/stswebriskcalc/. EuroSCORE II also offers a smartphone 'app' for use at the bedside.

Age

There is an increased risk above the age of 60 years.

Gender

Females have a higher operative mortality than males, possibly because of smaller coronary artery size, smaller blood volume predisposing to risks associated with perioperative anaemia and transfusion, although the definitive reason for the difference is unknown.

Left Ventricular Function

As estimated by echocardiography or angiography, LV function is a good measure of cardiac status, but determination can be operator dependent and it is difficult to produce an accurate and reproducible percentage ejection fraction. Thus, LV function is generally classified as 'good', 'moderate' or 'poor'; EuroSCORE II has an additional category of 'very poor'.

Type of Surgery

General cardiac risk models take into account patients that undergo different surgeries – the risk for coronary artery bypass graft (CABG) surgery is less than for valve surgery, which in turn is less than that for surgery of the thoracic aorta. Combined procedures like valve with CABG carry a higher risk than single procedures.

Extent of Cardiac Disease

The severity of coronary disease is subjective and therefore not included in surgical risk scores. The Syntax score allows for a measure of the severity of disease, but is time consuming and partly subjective. Left main stem disease may be associated with more risk. Objective measures of cardiac disease include recent myocardial infarction (MI), unstable angina and mechanical complications of MI such as acute rupture of the mitral valve or ventricular septum.

Repeat Operation

Previous cardiac surgery (or previous sternotomy) increases difficulty of access and prolongs operative time. These patients therefore carry an increased risk of bleeding as well as possibly having more advanced disease than those undergoing their first cardiac procedure.

Lung Disease

The presence of chronic pulmonary disease such as chronic obstructive pulmonary disease (COPD) has a large impact on how a patient is managed in anaesthetic and ventilatory terms. After cardiac surgery, patients with concurrent lung disease are more likely to require extended ventilation and to develop pulmonary complications, such as chest infections. Lung function is difficult to quantify with a single test and severity is based partly on subjective judgements. However, chronic pulmonary disease is taken into account in the EuroSCORE and STS.

Renal Disease

Renal dysfunction, as evidenced by dependence on dialysis, increases mortality by as much as 40%, but the spectrum of renal failure is wide and difficult to quantify. Creatinine levels are easy to measure, but are not always an accurate measure of true kidney function. The original EuroSCORE uses grossly deranged serum creatinine (>200 μmol/l) as a measure of significant renal impairment. Other scores use dialysis dependence. The best measure is probably creatinine clearance (CC), and this now features in EuroSCORE II, where the categories of renal dysfunction have expanded into four: normal function (CC > 85 ml/minute), moderate (CC 50–85 ml/minute), severe (CC <50 ml/minute) and on dialysis (regardless of CC). Interestingly, patients with severe dysfunction but not on dialysis yet fare worst.

Other Risk Factors

These include peripheral vascular disease, neurological dysfunction, degree of urgency, diabetes, hypertension and degree of pulmonary hypertension. In addition, various scoring systems give weight to the type of operation performed.

Postoperative Models

These models benefit from information that is only available after the completion of the operation, such as the physiological parameters on admission to critical care. Many have been devised for critically ill patients outside the cardiac surgical specialty, but have been used and validated in cardiac surgery. The most well-known models are the Acute Physiology and Chronic Health Evaluation (APACHE) and the Sequential Organ Failure Assessment (SOFA) (Table 1). The APACHE score is used on admission to critical care to assess the risk of in-hospital death, whereas the SOFA was developed to quantify the severity of a patient's illness using the degree of organ dysfunction at any one time. The BRiSc score is specifically aimed at predicting patients likely to bleed excessively after heart surgery.

Postoperative Model Risk Factors

Postoperative risk scores look at each organ system systematically and score according to derangement of function. Basically, the more organ dysfunction, the poorer the prognosis.

Respiratory

Oxygenation and the requirement for ventilatory support are used as measures of respiratory function.

Circulatory

Most scores which are applied postoperatively use mean arterial pressure as an easily measured and monitored parameter. However, whereas APACHE concentrates on derangement of normal physiology, SOFA concentrates on the need for (and level of) inotropic support.

Neurological

Trends are more useful than a snapshot at a particular point in time, but the Glasgow Coma Scale is easily measured and provides an easily reproducible measure of neurological status.

Renal

As preoperatively, the mainstay of renal function is serum creatinine level as it is easily measured and a relatively inexpensive test; this variable can be used to monitor changes in renal function and to compare current with preoperative function.

Gastrointestinal/Hepatic

Both APACHE and SOFA use bilirubin levels as a measure of liver function. APACHE is used more widely in general critical care units and includes many more variables, such as amylase, albumin (as a rough measure of nutritional status) and other liver function tests. The APACHE score also contains variables to measure metabolic function and septic status. These criteria are less relevant in cardiac surgery.

Thoracic Surgery

Risk modelling is not as developed in thoracic surgery, although recently some attempts have been made to produce models for predicting mortality after lung resection. The most important risk factors associated with a poor outcome are age (older people do less well) and how much functioning lung remains long after the resection (the more, the better).

Learning Points

- Many models help to predict the outcome of cardiac surgery, and these can be applied before or after the operation.
- Preoperative models help in the decision making, consent and assessment of clinical performance.
- Postoperative models can help to plan resource use and provide information to relatives.
- Models devised specifically for mortality have also been found to be useful in predicting major morbidity, resource use and long-term outcomes.
- No amount of risk modelling can predict with certainty which patient will live and which will die and they should be used as an adjunct rather than as a replacement for sound clinical judgement.

Table 1 Postoperative cardiac surgery risk assessment scores

Organ system	SOFA	APACHE
Respiratory	Oxygenation (PaO_2/FiO_2)	Respiratory rate non-ventilated
	Respiratory support	PaO_2 with FiO_2 1.0
		$PaCO_2$
Coagulation/haematological	WCC	WCC
		Haematocrit
		Platelet count
		Prothrombin time
Circulatory	Mean arterial pressure	Mean arterial pressure
	Dopamine dose	Heart rate ventricular response
	Adrenaline dose	Central venous pressure
	Norepinephrine dose	Evidence of acute MI
	Dobutamine use	Arrhythmia
		Serum lactate
		Arterial pH
Neurological	Glasgow Coma Scale	Glasgow Coma Scale
Renal	Creatinine	Creatinine
	Urine ouput/24 hour	Urine output/24 hour
		Blood urea nitrogen
Gastrointestinal/hepatic	Bilirubin	Amylase
		Albumin
		Bilirubin
		Alkaline phosphatase
		Liver enzymes
		Anergy by skin testing
Septic		Cerebrospinal fluid positive culture
		Blood culture positive
		Fungal culture positive
		Rectal temperature
Metabolic		Calcium level
		Glucose
		Sodium
		Potassium
		Bicarbonate
		Serum osmolarity

Abbreviations: APACHE, Acute Physiology and Chronic Health Evaluation; FiO_2, fraction of inspired oxygen; MI, myocardial infarction; $PaCO_2$, partial pressure of carbon dioxide in arterial blood; PaO_2, partial pressure of oxygen in arterial blood; SOFA, Sequential Organ Failure Assessment; WCC, white cell count.

Further Reading

Arts D, de Keizer NF, Vroom MB, et al. Reliability and accuracy of sequential organ failure assessment. *Critical Care Medicine*. 2005; 33: 1988–1993.

Knaus WA, Draper EA, Wagner DP, et al. APACHE II: a severity of disease classification system. *Critical Care Medicine*. 1985; 13: 818–829.

Nashef S. *The Naked Surgeon. The Power and Peril of Transparency in Medicine*. London: Scribe, 2015.

Nashef SAM, Roques F, Michel PR, et al. European system for cardiac operative risk evaluation (EuroSCORE). *European Journal of Cardio-Thoracic Surgery*. 1999; 16: 9–13.

Nashef, SAM, Roques F, Sharples LD, et al. EuroSCORE II. *European Journal of Cardio-Thoracic Surgery*. 2012; 41: 1–12.

Parsonnet V, Dean D, Bernstein AD. A method of uniform stratification of risk for evaluating the results of surgery in acquired adult heart disease. *Circulation*. 1989; 79: 3–12.

Vuylsteke A, Pagel C, Gerrard C, et al. The Papworth Bleeding Risk Score: a stratification scheme for identifying cardiac surgery patients at risk of excessive early postoperative bleeding. *European Journal of Cardio-Thoracic Surgery*. 2011; 39: 924–930.

Abbreviations

AC	Assist-Control ventilation
ACBT	Active Cycle of Breathing Technique
ACEI	Angiotensin Converting Enzyme Inhibitor
ACLS	Advanced Cardiac Life Support
ACT	Activated Clotting Time
AD	Advanced Directive
AEDs	Automated External Defibrillators
AEG	Atrial Electrocardiogram
AEP	Auditory Evoked Potentials
AF	Atrial Fibrillation
AFE	Amniotic Fluid Embolism
AKI	Acute Kidney Injury
ALG	Anti-human Lymphocyte Globulin
ALS	Advanced Life Support
AMP	Adenosine Monophosphate
APACHE	Acute Physiology and Chronic Health Evaluation
APRV	Airway Pressure Release Ventilation
aPTT	Activated Partial Thromboplastin Time
AR	Aortic Regurgitation
ARB	Angiotensin Receptor Blockers
ARDS	Acute Respiratory Distress Syndrome
ARF	Acute Respiratory Failure
ASD	Atrial Septal Defect
ATG	Anti-human Thymocyte Globulin
ATLS	Advanced Trauma Life Support
AVNRT	Atrioventricular Node Re-entrant Tachycardia
AVSD	Atrioventricular Septal Defect
BAL	Bronchoalveolar Lavage
BALF	Bronchoalveolar Lavage Fluid
BIPAP	Biphasic or Bilevel Positive Airway Pressure
BIPDs	Bilateral Independent PDs
BIS	Bispectral Index
BiVAD	Bilateral Ventricular Assist Device
BLS	Basic Life Support
BLUE	Bedside Lung Ultrasound in Emergency
BNP	B-type Natriuretic Peptide
BPF	Bronchopleural Fistula
BPS	Behavioural Pain Scale
BTC	Bridge to Candidacy
BTS	British Thoracic Society
BTT	Bridge to Transplant
BURP	Backwards, Upwards and Rightward Pressure on the thyroid cartilage
CABG	Coronary Artery Bypass Grafting
CAM-ICU	Confusion Assessment Method for the ICU
CAP	Community Acquired Pneumonia
CC	Creatinine Clearance
CCA	Critical Care Area
CCS	Canadian Cardiovascular Society
ccTGA	Congenitally Corrected Transposition of the Great Arteries
CCU	Coronary Care Unit
CDC	Centers for Disease Control
cEEG	Continuous Electroencephalography
CF	Cystic Fibrosis
CHD	Congenital Heart Disease
CHF	Congestive Heart Failure
CICO	'Can't Intubate, Can't Oxygenate'
CIN	Contrast Induced Nephropathy
CI	Cardiac Index
CIS	Clinical Information Systems
CK	Creatinine Kinase
CKD	Chronic Kidney Disease
CLABSI	Central Line Associated Bloodstream Infections
CLAD	Chronic Lung Allograft Dysfunction
CMR	Cardiac Magnetic Resonance
CMV	Continuous Mandatory Ventilation
CMV	Cytomegalovirus
CNI	Calcineurin Inhibitors
CO	Cardiac Output

COAD	Chronic Obstructive Airways Disease, same as COPD
COPD	Chronic Obstructive Pulmonary Disease
CP	Constrictive Pericarditis
CPAP	Constant Positive Airway Pressure
CPAx	Chelsea Critical Care Physical Assessment Tool
CPB	Cardiopulmonary Bypass
CPE	Carbapenemase Producing Enterobacteriaceae
CPOT	Critical Care Pain Observation Tool
CPP	Cerebral Perfusion Pressure
CRP	C-Reactive Protein
CT	Computerised Tomography
CTCA	Computerised Tomography Coronary Angiogram
CTEPH	Chronic Thromboembolic Pulmonary Hypertension
CV	Stroke Volume
CVC	Central Venous Catheter
CVD	Cardiovascular Disease
CVP	Central Venous Pressure
CXR	Chest X-Ray
DAG	1,2-Diacylglycerol
DBD	Donation after Brain Death
DBexs	Deep Breathing Exercises
DCD	Donation after Circulatory Death
DD	Diastolic Dysfunction
DNAR	Do Not Attempt Resuscitation Order
DOLS	Deprivation of Liberty Safeguards
DSI	Daily Sedation Interruption
DT	Destination Therapy
DTI	Direct Thrombin Inhibitor
DVT	Deep Venous Thrombosis
EACA	Epsilon Aminocaproic Acid
ECC	Emergency Cardiovascular Care
$ECCO_2R$	Extracorporeal Carbon Dioxide Removal
ECG	Electrocardiography
ECLS	Extracorporeal Life Support
ECMO	Extracorporeal Membrane Oxygenation
ECPR	Extracorporeal Cardiopulmonary Resuscitation
EDA	End-Diastolic Area
EEG	Electroencephalography
EF	Ejection Fraction
ELISA	Enzyme-Linked Immunosorbent Assay
ELSO	Extracorporeal Life Support Organisation
EMR	Electronic Medical Records
ERP	Enhanced Recovery Programmes
ESBL	Extended Spectrum Beta-Lactamases
ESG	Endovascular stent graft
ETT	Endotracheal Tube
EVLWI	Extravascular Lung Water Index
EWMA	Exponentially Weighted Moving Average
EWS	Early Warning Scores
FAC	Fractional Area Change
FALLS	Fluid Administration Limited by Lung Sonography
FAM	Functional Assessment Measure
FB	Flexible Bronchoscopy
FBC	Full Blood Count
FDO_2	Fraction of Oxygen Delivered
FEV1	Forced Expiratory Volume for 1 second
FFP	Fresh Frozen Plasma
FIM	Functional Independence Measure
FIRDA	Frontal IRDA
FOUR	Full Outline of Unresponsiveness
FRC	Function of Residual Capacity
FS	Fraction of Shortening
FVC	Forced Vital Capacity
GBS	Guillain–Barré Syndrome
GCS	Glasgow Coma Score
GEDVI	Global End-Diastolic Volume Index
GICS	Gastrointestinal Complication Score
GPCR	G Protein Coupled Receptors
GUCH	Grown-Up Congenital Heart disease
HD	Haemodialysis
HDF	Haemodiafiltration
HDU	High Dependency Unit
HES	Hydroxyethil Starch
HF	Haemofiltration
HFV	High Frequency Ventilation
HIT	Heparin Induced Thrombocytopenia
HIV	Human Immunodeficiency Virus
HLHS	Hypoplastic Left Heart Syndrome
HOCM	Hypertrophic Obstructive Cardiomyopathy
HSV	Herpes Simplex Virus
HTEA	High Thoracic Epidural Analgesia
IABP	Intra-aortic Balloon Pump
ICD	Implantable Cardioverter-Defibrillators
ICP	Intracranial Pressure

ICSD	Intensive Care Delirium Screening Checklist
ICU-AW	Intensive Care Unit Acquired Weakness
IE	Infective Endocarditis
IJV	Internal Jugular Vein
IMCA	Independent Mental Capacity Advocate
IMV	Invasive Mechanical Ventilation
INR	International Normalised Ratio
INTERMACS	Interagency Registry for Mechanically Assisted Circulatory Support
IPF	Idiopathic Pulmonary Fibrosis
IR	Interventional Radiology
IRDA	Intermittent Rhythmic Delta Activity
IRV	Inversed Ratio Ventilation
IS	Incentive Spirometry
ISHLT	International Society for Heart and Lung Transplantation
ITBVI	Intrathoracic Blood Volume Index
IUGR	Intrauterine Growth Retardation
IVC	Inferior Vena Cava
IVS	Interventricular Septum
JET	Junctional Ectopic Tachycardia
LAD	Left Anterior Descending artery
LAS	Lateral Amiotrophic Sclerosis
LBBB	Left Bundle Branch Block
LCx	Left Circumflex Artery
LMA	Laryngeal Mask Airway
LMCA	Left Main Coronary Artery
LMWH	Low Molecular Weight Heparin
LTACH	Long-Term Acute Care Hospitals
LV	Left Ventricle
LVAD	Left Ventricular Assist Device
LVEDV	Left Ventricular End-Diastolic Volume
LVESV	Left Ventricular End-Systolic Volume
LVOT	Left Ventricular Outflow Tract
LVOTO	Left Ventricular Outflow Tract Obstruction
LVSF	Left Ventricular Systolic Function
MACE	Major Adverse Cardiac Events
MALDI TOF MS	Matrix Assisted Laser Desorption/Ionisation Time-of-Flight Mass Spectrometry
MAO	Monoamine Oxydase
MAP	Mean Arterial Pressure
MCCD	Mechanical Chest Compression Devices
MCFP	Mean Circulatory Filling Pressure
MDR	Multidrug Resistance
MDT	Multidisciplinary Team
MET	Medical Emergency Teams
MHI	Manual Hyperinflation
MI	Myocardial Infarction
MIC	Minimum Inhibitory Concentration
MMF	Mycophenolate Mofetil
MMV	Mandatory Minute Ventilation
mPAP	Mean Pulmonary Arterial Pressure
MR	Mitral Regurgitation
MRSA	Methicillin Resistant *Staphylococcus aureus*
MSE	Myoclonic Status Epilepticus
MSSA	Methicillin-Sensitive *Staphylococcus aureus*
mTOR	Mammalian Target of Rapamicin Inhibitors
MUST	Malnutrition Universal Screening Tool
MV	Mitral Valve
NAAT	Nucleic Acid-Based Amplification Technologies
NAP4	Fourth National Audit Project
NAVA	Neurally Adjusted Ventilatory Assist
NCS	Non-convulsive Seizures
NCSE	Non-convulsive Status Epilepticus
NHSBT	National Health Service Blood and Transfusion
NI	Narcotrend Index
NICE	National Institute for Clinical Excellence
NIPPV	Non-invasive Positive Pressure Ventilation
NIRS	Near Infrared Spectroscopy
NIV	Non-invasive Ventilation
NMDA	*N*-Acetyl-D-Aspartate receptor
NOAC	Newer Oral Anticoagulants
NRS	Nutritional Risk Screening
NVE	Native Valve Endocarditis
NYHA	New York Heart Association
OD	Optical Density
OHCA	Out-of-Hospital Cardiac Arrest
OIRDA	Occipital IRDA
OpCAB	Off pump Coronary Artery Bypass
PAC	Pulmonary Artery Catheter
PAH	Pulmonary Arterial Hypertension
PAP	Pulmonary Arterial Pressure
PAWP	Pulmonary Arterial Wedge Pressure
PBM	Patient Blood Management
PBW	Predicted Body Weight
PCAS	Post-Cardiac Arrest Syndrome
PCI	Percutaneous Coronary Intervention

PCP	*Pneumocystis jirovecii Carinii Pneumonia*
PCR	Polymerase Chain Reaction
PCT	Procalcitonin
PCWP	Pulmonary Capillary Wedge Pressure
PD	Peritoneal Dialysis
PDA	Posterior Descending Artery
PDE	Phosphodiesterase Inhibitors
PDR	Posterior Dominant Rhythm
PDs	Periodic Discharges
PE	Pulmonary Embolism
PEA	Pulmonary Endarterectomy
PEEP	Positive End Expiratory Pressure
PF	Pulmonary Fibrosis
PF4	Platelet Factor 4
PFIT	Physical Functional Intensive Care Test
PGD	Primary Graft Dysfunction
PH	Pulmonary Hypertension, same as PAH
PKC	Protein Kinase C
PLC	Phospholipase C
PPCs	Postoperative Pulmonary Complications
PPCI	Primary Percutaneous Coronary Intervention
PPCM	Peripartum Cardiomyopathy
PPHN	Persistent Pulmonary Hypertension of the Newborn
PPV	Pulse Pressure Variation
PRC	Post-resuscitation Care
PRES	Posterior Reversible Encephalopathy Syndrome
PRVC	Pressure Regulated Volume Controlled Ventilation
PSI	Patient State Index
PT	Prothrombin Time
PTE	Pulmonary Thromboendarterectomy, same as PEA
PTLD	Post-transplantation Lymphoproliferative Disorder
PVE	Prosthetic Valve Endocarditis
PVR	Pulmonary Vascular Resistance
RAP	Right Atrial Pressure
RASS	Richmond Agitation Sedation Scale
RBBB	Right Bundle Branch Block
RCM	Restrictive Cardiomyopathy
RCT	Randomised Controlled Trial
ROC	Receiver Operating Characteristic
ROSC	Return of Spontaneous Circulation
ROTEM	Rotational Thromboelastometry
RRT	Renal Replacement Therapy
RV	Right Ventricle
RVP	Right Ventricular Pressure
RVAD	Right Ventricular Assist Device
RWMA	Regional Wall Motion Abnormalities
SACP	Selective Antegrade Cerebral Perfusion
SAH	Subarachnoid Haemorrhage
SAM	Systolic Anterior Motion
SAS	Sedation Agitation Scale
SDD	Selective Digestive Decontamination
SE	Status Epilepticus
SGA	Subjective Global Assessment
SIMV	Synchronised Intermittent Mandatory Ventilation
SLED	Slow Low-Efficiency Dialysis
SMR	Standardised Mortality Ratio
SOFA	Sepsis Related Organ Failure Assessment
SR	Sarcoplasmic Reticulum
SRA	Serotonin Release Assay
SSEP	Somatosensory Evoked Potentials
SSRI	Selective Serotonin Reuptake Inhibitor
SVC	Superior Vena Cava
SVCS	Superior Vena Cava Syndrome
SVR	Systemic Vascular Resistance
TAA	Thoracic Aortic Aneurysm
TAH	Total Artificial Heart
TAPSE	Tricuspid Annular Plane Systolic Excursion
TAPVD	Total Anomalous Pulmonary Venous Drainage
TCPC	Total Cavopulmonary Connection
TEG	Thromboelastography
TETS	Transcutaneous Energy Transfer Systems
TEVAR	Thoracic Endovascular Aortic Repair
TGA	Transposition of the Great Arteries
TnC	Troponin C
TNF	Tumour Necrosis Factor
TOE	Transoesophageal Echocardiography
TOF	Tetralogy of Fallot
TPG	Transpulmonary Gradient
TR	Tricuspid Regurgitation
TRALI	Transfusion Related Lung Injury
TTE	Transthoracic Echocardiography or Thoracic Expansion Exercises as TTEs
TTM	Targeted Temperature Management
TXA	Tranexamic Acid

URR	Urea Reduction Ratio
VALI	Ventilator Associated Lung Injury
VAP	Ventilator Associated Pneumonia
VATS	Video Assisted Thoracic Surgery
VF	Ventricular Fibrillation
VHI	Ventilator Hyperinflation
VRE	Vancomycin Resistant Enterococci
VSD	Ventricular Septal Defect
VT	Ventricular Tachycardia
VTI	Velocity-Time Integral
VTM	Viral Transport Media
vWF	von Willebrand Factor
WCRS	Withdrawal of Cardiorespiratory Supports
WOB	Work of Breathing
WPW	Wolff–Parkinson–White syndrome

Chapter 1

History and Examination

Lachlan Miles and Joseph E Arrowsmith

The first rule of diagnosis, gentlemen!
Eyes: first and most; hands: next and least; tongue: not at all!

Sir Lancelot Spratt – as played by James Robertson Justice

In: Doctor in the House (1954, The J. Arthur Rank Organisation)

Introduction

Patients may be admitted to the specialist cardiothoracic critical care unit from a variety of sources (Figure 1.1). In all elective admissions, and in the majority of emergency admissions, a clinical history will already have been elicited and a physical examination performed – often more than once. Most patients will already have undergone extensive investigation or therapeutic intervention, and the underlying diagnosis or diagnoses will have been established. Despite this seemingly ideal situation, the cardiothoracic intensivist should adopt an inquisitive attitude and use the so-called 'history and physical examination' to confirm previous findings, assess disease progression and exclude new pathology. Contrary to popular belief, this is often the most efficient and effective means of predicting and detecting significant comorbid conditions. Clinical investigations should therefore be considered an adjunct to, rather than a substitute for, basic medical assessment.

In the critical care setting, particularly when a patient is physiologically unstable or has reduced consciousness, the conventional stepwise approach to the history and physical examination will usually require modification (Table 1.1). Indeed it may have to be conducted *during* or *after* initial resuscitation.

History

The Conscious Patient

All available sources of information should be drawn upon to construct as detailed a history as possible. Where the patient is conscious and able to respond to direct questioning, this important primary source of information should not be overlooked. Rather than using 'open' questions and expecting them to recount their entire current and past medical history in a concise fashion and in chronological order, it is often easier to ask the patient to confirm previously documented information and append newly acquired information as necessary. When faced with an acutely unwell and possibly deteriorating patient, the skilled intensivist needs to be able to quickly gather sufficient information to aid diagnosis and guide management. Of particular importance is the patient's understanding of their medical condition, their insight into treatment options and prognosis, and their expectations. Corroborative history from family and carers is also invaluable, especially in the setting of acute delirium or dementia, where the patient's own account may be unreliable. This information should be solicited and documented whenever possible.

Symptoms of cardiorespiratory disease (e.g. angina pectoris, dyspnoea, orthopnoea, syncope, palpitations, ankle swelling, etc.) (Table 1.2) should be actively sought, as should any recent progression in symptom severity. Symptoms should be described in terms of their nature (using the patient's own words), onset, duration, progression, modifying factors and associations. The impact of symptoms on functional status should be documented using the New York Heart Association (NYHA) classification and the Canadian Cardiovascular Society (CCS) angina scale.

Table 1.1 Modification of conventional history and physical for use in critical care

	Conventional	Critical care
History	History of presenting complaint Past medical history Past surgical/anaesthetic history Drug history, allergies, sensitivities Recreational substance (mis)use Educational level/native language Social/employment history Religious/cultural beliefs Family history Systematic enquiry Sensory impairments Review of medical notes	Handover information Review of medical notes Information from family members
Physical	Patient supine – reclining at 45° Cardiovascular Respiratory Gastrointestinal Genitourinary Neurological Integument	Patient supine, lateral or prone ABC (Airway, Breathing, Circulation) Lines, tubes, drains and catheters Drug and fluid infusions Ongoing physiological monitoring Anatomical examination

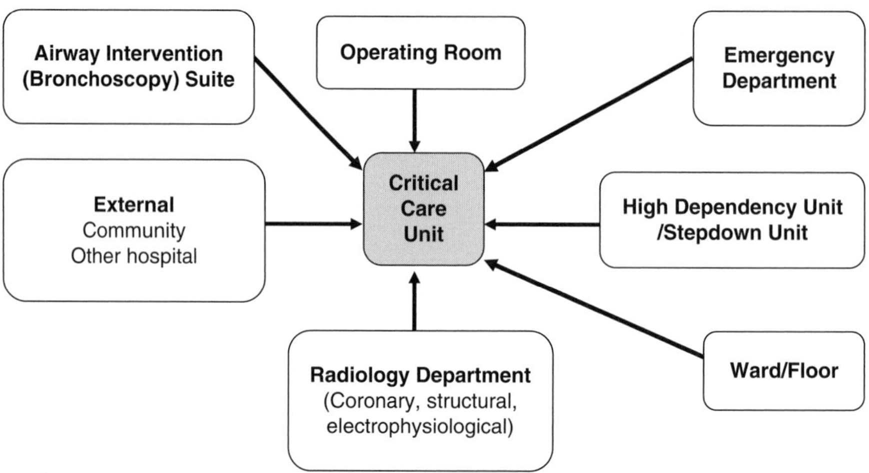

Figure 1.1 Cardiothoracic critical care admission sources.

Enquiry into the patient's past medical history should include coexisting conditions, previous hospital admissions, surgical procedures and complications, prolonged hospitalisation and unplanned admissions to a critical care unit. It is important to note the indication for any surgical procedure or therapeutic intervention (e.g. splenectomy, permanent pacemaker, angioplasty), the outcome of the procedure and any anaesthetic related morbidity. A history of difficult tracheal intubation is of particular note, both with respect to the unintubated patient who may require intervention during their stay, and the patient who is already intubated who will require extubation before discharge to the ward. Factors known to be associated with increased mortality and morbidity (e.g. congestive cardiac failure, peripheral vascular disease, renal insufficiency, arterial hypertension, pulmonary hypertension, diabetes mellitus, chronic pulmonary disease, neurological disease and previous cardiovascular surgery) should be documented.

Table 1.2 Common symptoms associated with cardiorespiratory conditions

Cardiovascular	Respiratory
Syncope	Recent overseas travel
Chest pain	Fever and/or rigors
Fatigue or exercise intolerance	Facial or sinus pain
Exertional dyspnoea	Chest pain
Paroxysmal nocturnal dyspnoea	Cough
Orthopnoea	Sputum production (volume, time course, purulence)
Palpitations	Haemoptysis
Intermittent claudication or ischaemic rest pain	Dyspnoea
Stroke or transient ischaemic attack	Exercise intolerance
Cough or sputum production	History of bird keeping, asbestos exposure, or other sources of occupational lung disease
Peripheral oedema	

Where the patient has been admitted following a diagnostic or therapeutic intervention (e.g. coronary angiography or angioplasty), a comprehensive medical and nursing 'handover' is essential. This is particularly important when the patient has been brought to hospital by emergency ambulance and taken directly to the angiography suite. Similarly, when a patient is transferred from another hospital for specialist cardiothoracic care (e.g. surgical repair of acute type A aortic dissection), a formal handover of clinical information and documentation is an absolute prerequisite for the transfer of clinical responsibility and for safe ongoing care. In many areas a formal handover document or aide memoire is used both to guide and to document the comprehensive handover of clinically relevant information.

It is essential to record current and recent prescription drug administration, including formulation, dosage and route of administration. In addition, the medication history should include drugs taken 'as required', proprietary or 'over-the-counter' medicines, complimentary or alternative therapies, and recreational drugs. This latter category should include alcohol and tobacco products. A history of allergic or other idiosyncratic reaction to a specific drug (e.g. suxamethonium) or class of drugs (e.g. penicillins) should be sought and documented.

Where adherence to a particular cultural or religious belief system (e.g. Jehovah's Witnesses) has the potential to influence any aspect of critical care management, this should be comprehensively documented. In some instances it may be appropriate to explore and document a patient's specific wishes in a number of hypothetical clinical scenarios, including limits of care. It is often preferable that limits of care be discussed with the patient and family early on in the critical care stay, rather than late in the course of the illness when the patient is in extremis. It is important that both the patient and the family have a realistic understanding of what intensive care can offer, rather than relying on preconceived ideas.

The Unconscious Patient

The unconscious, critically unwell patient represents a special challenge for any clinician. From a cardiothoracic point of view, such patients cover a wide range of potential presentations, including, but not limited to the following:

- A patient transferred from the operating theatre or catheter laboratory following an invasive procedure;
- A patient admitted following out-of-hospital cardiac arrest, via either the catheter laboratory or the emergency department;
- A patient requiring ongoing organ support following an interventional cardiology or bronchoscopic intervention; and
- A ward patient who has physiologically deteriorated and requires more advanced treatment modalities or resuscitation.

When reviewing an obtunded patient the clinician is deprived of many of the usual visual and auditory clues that guide patient assessment, forcing the use of alternative sources of information. Family members and carers are often the key source of information regarding recent symptoms, and it is often possible to establish the temporal course of the presenting complaint with thorough questioning. In many respects, it is often possible to obtain a full history, provided that the right questions are asked, and an open mind maintained.

A thorough review of the medical record is also invaluable when the patient is not able to speak for him or herself. Written correspondence from other clinicians (e.g. surgeons, cardiologists, respiratory physicians, general practitioners) will answer many questions regarding the course of illness leading up to admission. Where questions remain unanswered regarding the previous clinical course, direct communication with these sources is encouraged, not only to obtain further information, but as a matter of courtesy regarding the condition of their patient.

Physical Examination

The Conscious Patient

Whilst a comprehensive physical examination is sometimes not possible given the limitations that reception and resuscitation of the critically ill patient places on assessment, a full physical examination should nevertheless be attempted. There is also a frequent temptation for the clinician to rely on the battery of monitors that an intensive care admission entails, especially during daily review of the patient, or to perform an investigation rather than seek clinical findings. This is a fallacy, as even an abbreviated physical examination during a ward round may reveal a finding (e.g. bronchial breathing) that may take hours to manifest as worsening hypoxia or increasing oxygen requirement, permitting early investigation and intervention.

General Inspection

This should initially be undertaken from the end of the bed, so as to better appreciate the overall Gestalt. The initial focus should be on the patient. Central or peripheral cyanosis may be evident in the setting of hypoxaemia or shunting. The patient posture provides many important clues, especially when assessing respiratory effort. Pursed lip breathing to increase end-expiratory pressure and a 'tripod' position with the shoulders rotated forward and the hands on the lower extremity to engage the accessory muscles are evidence of respiratory distress. Attention should then be turned to the various drug infusions being administered, the relevant concentration, rate and route of administration. Peripheral and central venous access should be noted and recorded including available lumens for other medications and the size of each catheter if the administration of volume is required. Invasive monitoring (e.g. arterial line, pulmonary artery catheter), circulatory support devices (intra-aortic balloon pump, ventricular assist device and extracorporeal circuits) and renal replacement therapy should also be evaluated. An indwelling urinary catheter may be present, and if so, the volume and concentration of urine in the drainage bag should be noted.

The postoperative cardiac or thoracic surgical patient will have a variable number of mediastinal and pleural drains in situ. The volume of blood in these should be recorded so that an accurate estimation of any ongoing blood loss can be made. An air leak may also be present when pleural drains are on suction, and the magnitude and respiratory phase of this should be judged. Where epicardial pacing wires are present, their function should be confirmed. If in use, external pacing should be converted from fixed rate mode to demand mode, with an appropriate backup rate.

The Hands and Arms

Examination of the hands reveals much about the circulatory state of the patient. Cold and shut down extremities with delayed capillary return may suggest a high degree of systemic vascular resistance, usually because of hypovolaemia or low cardiac output state, or alternatively, an acutely ischaemic limb. In contrast, warm peripheries suggest a normal or high cardiac output state. Finger clubbing may be indicative of chronic cardiorespiratory disease, notably congenital, cyanotic heart disease, non-small-cell lung cancer and suppurative lung conditions such as cystic fibrosis or bronchiectasis.

The peripheral pulses can give clues to the presence of significant valvulopathy (e.g. the 'water hammer' pulse of severe aortic regurgitation) and regional perfusion abnormalities, particularly in aortic dissection (i.e. radioradial and radiofemoral delay). Inspection of the palmar creases was popularised for the estimation of plasma haemoglobin concentration, but has subsequently proven to be unreliable. Rarely, the immunological and embolic phenomena of infective endocarditis (Janeway lesions and Osler's nodes) may be evident.

The Neck

Neck examination in the critical care environment is often difficult, due to the presence of indwelling jugular venous catheters. In the event that the neck is unencumbered, examination of the jugular venous waveform can be used to assess right atrial filling and compliance, atrioventricular dissociation (cannon a-waves) and torrential tricuspid regurgitation (massive cv-waves). These abnormalities are also visible on the central venous waveform if invasive monitoring is present.

If pericardial tamponade is suspected, an early sign of compromise is an increase in right atrial pressure on deep inspiration (Kussmaul's sign). If the patient's trachea is not intubated, it is wise to conduct an airway assessment at this juncture if not already performed. Auscultation of the carotid arteries may reveal bruits consistent with turbulent flow if there is a substantial atheroma burden, or the referred murmur of aortic stenosis.

The Praecordium

As for other parts of the body, and as alluded to in the starting quotation, examination of the chest should follow the traditional route of observation, palpation, percussion and auscultation. Ideally, both the anterior and posterior chest should be examined, as the lower lobes of the lung (particularly on the left) can take up much of the posterior aspect, preventing examination of the other lobes if the anterior chest is not examined. The often high volume of ambient noise in the critical care environment may make ausculation challenging. Subtle abnormalities may be missed, and seemingly positive findings may be misinterpreted. It is wise to correlate findings not consistent with the overall condition of the patient with appropriate investigation. Radiological investigation and bedside modalities such as ultrasound and transthoracic echocardiography are valuable for this purpose.

The Abdomen

Initially, at least, the abdomen is rarely a focus in the cardiothoracic critical care unit. Interest in this region is limited largely to distension and the presence of bowel sounds or the absence thereof. However, small or large bowel ischaemia is a not uncommon phenomenon following cardiac surgery, as a result of a low cardiac output state, embolic phenomenon or use of intra-aortic balloon counterpulsation. A high index of suspicion is required for this condition, particularly in the setting of an unexplained lactataemia and worsening acidosis, despite the presence of a seemingly adequate cardiac output. The opportunity should be taken at this point to assess the back of the patient for sacral oedema, as this is the most dependent point in the semirecumbent patient, and is an important finding when assessing volume status.

The Legs

An assessment of the legs completes the examination. Like the hands, the lower extremities reveal much about perfusion status, thus capillary refill and skin temperature should be assessed. The posterior tibial and dorsalis pedis pulses should be sought, particularly if the femoral vessels have been used for arterial access. Whilst a rare event, acute lower limb ischaemia is a recognised complication of a wide range of invasive devices, in particular peripheral venoarterial ECMO cannulae and the intra-aortic balloon pump. It is important to note that even if a distal reperfusion line is incorporated into an ECMO circuit, distal pulses may be absent. However, the limb should feel warm and well perfused or, at the very least, similar to its counterpart.

Deep venous thrombosis is a common complication in many postoperative patients, and whilst at least half of these are completely asymptomatic, the remainder may exhibit the classical signs of calf tenderness, swelling, distended superficial veins and warmth. The traditional test for this condition, Homan's sign (rapid passive dorsiflexion of the ankle with the aim of causing pain in the calf), is no longer recommended because of the risk of clot fragmentation and acute pulmonary embolism.

Finally, the presence and extent of any peripheral oedema should be assessed. Oedema is, by definition, an excess of interstitial fluid, and therefore must be the result of a derangement of the Starling forces across the microcirculation (increased capillary hydrostatic pressure, decreased plasma colloid oncotic pressure, increased capillary permeability or deranged lymphatic drainage).

The Unconscious Patient

As for history, the physical examination of the unconscious individual is hindered by the lack of patient participation. Nevertheless, such an examination should always be undertaken with the same care as if the patient were awake and fully conscious. The presence of the mechanical ventilator at the bedside increases the ambient noise level, further impairing the ability of the clinician to auscultate. Heavy sedation or neuromuscular blockade naturally prevents patient movement, and simple tasks such as leaning the patient forward to auscultate the chest are impossible. Nevertheless, an attempt should be made, as much valuable information can still be gained, particularly with respect to tissue perfusion.

As for physical examination in the conscious patient, assessment of the unconscious patient should follow in the same stepwise fashion. Many of the same clinical features may be found on careful inspection.

Caution should be taken during joint manipulation and palpation. The patient will not be able to report discomfort or resist painful movements, and tissue damage may result if the examiner is overly rough. Examination of the abdomen in the unconscious patient is considerably confounded, especially in the setting of neuromuscular blockade. This is because the early features of gut ischaemia or peritonism will be absent, partly because the patient is unable to report discomfort, but also because of a lack of abdominal muscle tone. As a result, the early features of guarding and tenderness to percussion (formerly tested as 'rebound tenderness') are absent. Consequently, abdominal distension, free gas under the diaphragm and a rising lactate in the setting of apparently adequate cardiac output may be the only features of a major intra-abdominal pathology. A high index of suspicion must be maintained as a result.

Daily assessment of the unconscious patient should also include a brief neurological examination. Naturally, a full assessment of muscle power cannot be undertaken, but a brief examination for features of an upper motor neurone lesion such as hypertonia, hyperreflexia and clonus (in the absence of neuromuscular blockade) can be quickly and easily performed. As described in detail in Chapter 16, on sedation and analgesia, the indications for deep sedation and neuromuscular blockade are becoming fewer as cardiothoracic critical care evolves, and targeted sedation and sedation breaks are increasingly de rigueur. Conscious state can be graded with any number of specialist sedation scores, which are beyond the scope of this chapter – however, response to approach, voice and pain should be assessed. A variety of different techniques have been described to evaluate response to painful stimulus. However, firm pressure over the superior orbital notch is usually the most unambiguous means of assessing global response, as peripheral stimulation may not give an accurate assessment of localisation if a hemiplegia is present. Likewise, withdrawal to stimulation, decerebrate and decorticate posturing can be difficult to assess when the focus point is on the hand or foot.

Conclusions

The presence of advanced monitoring modalities and ready access to bedside investigations, combined with difficult examination conditions, are all powerful motivators to de-emphasise the traditional focus on history and examination. Whilst cardiothoracic critical care requires a different skill set to that of the emergency department or ward, the temptation to forgo the basic diagnostic process must be resisted, as history and examination findings serve to clarify the clinical scenario and highlight evolving problems that monitoring may not detect for some time. Furthermore, history and physical examination allow appropriate targeting of investigations, minimising patient discomfort and unnecessary cost to the health system.

Learning Points

- The cardiothoracic intensivist should adopt an inquisitive approach to history and physical examination so as to confirm previous findings, assess disease progression and exclude new pathology.
- It can be challenging to elicit a history and undertake a physical examination in the critically ill patient and it may be necessary to modify the conventional stepwise approach.
- Advanced monitoring modalities are prone to artefact and incorrect interpretation and should not be seen as a substitute for a thorough history and physical examination.
- On admission/discharge from cardiothoracic critical care a formal handover of clinical information is an absolute prerequisite for continuity of care.
- It may be necessary to explore and document a patient's specific wishes in a number of hypothetical clinical scenarios so as to inform decision making should the patient deteriorate.

Further Reading

Arrowsmith JE. Symptoms and signs of cardiac disease. In: Mackay JH, Arrowsmith JE (Eds). *Core Topics in Cardiac Anesthesia*, 2nd Edition. Cambridge: Cambridge University Press, 2012, pp. 75–80.

Campeau L. Grading of angina pectoris. *Circulation*. 1976; 54: 522–523.

Criteria Committee of the New York Heart Association. *Nomenclature and Criteria for Diagnosis of Diseases of the Heart and Great Vessels*, 9th Edition. Boston, MA: Little Brown & Co, 1994, pp. 253–256.

Glynn M, Drake WM (Eds). *Hutchison's Clinical Methods: An Integrated Approach to Clinical Practice*. Oxford: Saunders, 2012.

Chapter 2

Electrocardiography

David Begley

Introduction

Electrocardiography (ECG) has been the main heart investigation method for most of the twentieth century and still plays a pivotal role in diagnostics. ECGs can provide a wealth of information about cardiac function and can often show early signs of systemic abnormalities as well. In order to accurately interpret an ECG it is important to first ensure its correct acquisition. The process involves recording small electrical changes on the skin that occur as a result of cardiac muscle depolarisation. Ten electrodes are used to record the heart's electrical activity in 12 different orientations, which encompass the 12 'leads' of the ECG. It is important therefore to ensure that these 10 electrodes are consistently applied in order to accurately assess for any abnormalities. In addition, account must be made of sources of interference.

Recording the ECG

As posture may affect the appearance of the ECG it is preferably performed in the supine position where practicable. Skin preparation is important to reduce artefacts and may include hair removal and/or skin cleansing.

Limb Electrodes

Moving the limb electrodes away from the distal limbs may affect the ECG appearance and it is therefore preferable that these are placed just proximal to the wrists and ankles in order to produce consistent results. Limb electrodes are often colour coded to aid placement.

- Right arm (RA, red) proximal to right wrist
- Left arm (LA, yellow) proximal to left wrist
- Left leg (LL, green) proximal to left ankle
- Right leg (RL, black) proximal to right ankle

Precordial (Chest) Electrodes

Most errors occur in placement of the chest electrodes, especially V_1 and V_2, which may be placed too high. This can have a significant effect on the resultant ECG. Correct anatomical positioning must be adhered to, with the centre of the electrode aligned with the correct location.

- V_1 (C_1) fourth intercostal space, right sternal edge
- V_2 (C_2) fourth intercostal space, left sternal edge
- V_3 (C_3) midway between V_2 and V_4
- V_4 (C_4) fifth intercostal space, midclavicular line
- V_5 (C_5) horizontal level with V_4, anterior axillary line
- V_6 (C_6) horizontal level with V_4, midaxillary line

After placement of V_1 and V_2, V_4 is located in the fifth intercostal space, midclavicular line. V_3 is then placed directly in between V_2 and V_4. V_5 and V_6 are located at the same horizontal level as V_4, perpendicular to the midclavicular line.

Filter Settings and Calibration

Most filter settings are set by default but it is recommended that the low frequency filter is set on or below 0.05 Hz. This filter will account for respiration. If it is set too high, it will distort the ST segment. This may also reduce the accuracy of detecting myocardial ischaemia based on ST segment shifts. The high filter setting should be set on or above 100 Hz. This filter setting should account for the artefact created by muscle tremor. The mains filter (50 Hz) is normally set to 'Off'.

A standard ECG has a voltage calibration of 10 mm/mV and is recorded with a paper speed of

25 mm/s. This results in 10 second recording. Each small square is equal to 40 ms and each large square (5 small squares) is equal to 200 ms.

The 12 'Lead' ECG

The 12 'leads' of an ECG correspond to 12 vectors along which depolarisation of cardiac tissue is recorded. Each is created by measuring the electrical potential between two points. In each case one of the ten electrodes is the positive pole. There are three bipolar limb leads where another electrode is the negative pole. The negative pole for the unipolar limb leads and the precordial leads is a composite pole (V_W) called Wilson's central terminus, which is created by averaging the potential recorded by RA, LA and LL electrodes:

$$V_W = {}^1/_3\,(RA + LA + LL).$$

The six limb leads view the heart in the coronal (vertical) plane while the six precordial leads view the heart in a perpendicular transverse (horizontal) plane.

Bipolar Limb Leads

- Lead I is the potential difference between LA and RA,

  I = LA – RA.

- Lead II is the potential difference between LL and RA,

  II = LL – RA.

- Lead III is the potential difference between LL and LA,

  III = LL – LA.

Unipolar Augmented Limb Leads

- Lead aVR is the potential difference between RA and V_W,

  $aVR = {}^3/_2\,(RA - V_W)$.

- Lead aVL is the potential difference between LA and V_W,

  $aVL = {}^3/_2\,(LA - V_W)$.

- Lead aVF is the potential difference between LL and V_W,

  $aVF = {}^3/_2\,(LL - V_W)$.

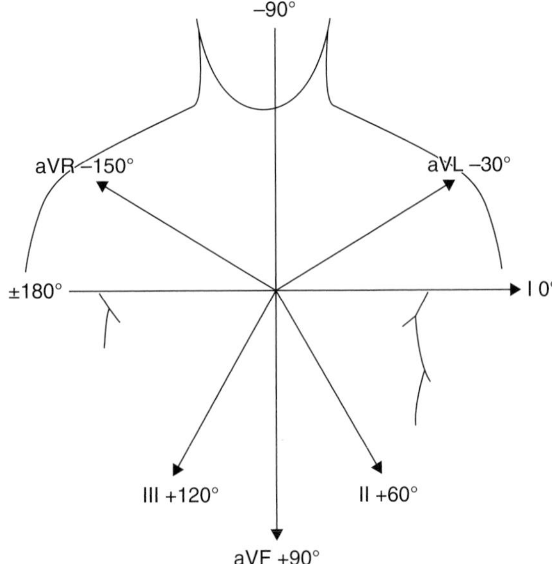

Figure 2.1 Hexaxial reference system.

The vectors created by the bipolar and augmented limb leads together form the hexaxial reference system (see Figure 2.1).

Precordial Leads

For each of the precordial leads the positive pole is the corresponding electrode and the negative pole is V_W.

ECG Arrangement

A standard ECG records a 2.5 second tracing of each lead arranged in a grid of four columns and three rows. A marker depicts the change from one lead to the next in each row and can be confused with part of the ECG. The first column contains leads I, II and III, the second column aVR, aVL and aVF, the third column V_1, V_2 and V_3 and the final column contains leads V_4, V_5 and V_6. A fourth row is often provided as a continuous tracing to aid determination of rhythm.

Although each lead records electrical activity of the heart from a different angle, contiguous leads are associated with different anatomical regions.

- Inferior leads — II, III and aVF
- Anterior leads — V_3 and V_4
- Septal leads — V_1 and V_2
- Lateral leads — I, aVL, V_5 and V_6

Interpretation of the ECG

Waves and Intervals

P Wave

The P wave (see Figure 2.2) represents depolarisation of the right and left atria. In normal sinus rhythm, its origins are from the sinus node, which is normally located posteriorly high in the right atrium. Therefore, the P wave is positive (upright) in all leads except aVR, and can be positive or biphasic in V_1. It typically has duration <80 ms.

In right atrial enlargement, the P wave is tall and peaked, and is prolonged and bifid in left atrial enlargement.

PR Interval

The PR interval is measured from the beginning of the P wave to the beginning of the QRS complex and represents the time taken for atrial depolarisation and conduction through the AV node. A normal PR interval varies between 120 and 200 ms.

If the PR interval is shorter than 120 ms then conduction is bypassing the AV node (see Wolf–Parkinson–White syndrome). Prolongation of the PR interval indicates 1° AV block. Depression of the short isoelectric segment between the end of the P wave and the beginning of the QRS complex can indicate pericarditis.

QRS Complex

Q, R and S waves form the QRS complex, which represents ventricular depolarisation. If the first deflection is negative it is termed the Q wave, otherwise an initial positive deflection is an R wave. A final negative deflection is the S wave. Normally the whole QRS complex is <120 ms in duration. Q waves represent left to right depolarisation of the interventricular septum and are typically seen in left sided leads (I, aVL, V_5 and V_6). Small Q waves can be seen in most leads except V_1, V_2 and V_3.

Large Q waves are pathological if >40 ms wide, and >2 mm deep or >25% of the height of the QRS complex. This can represent myocardial infarction, cardiomyopathy or electrode malposition.

If the QRS complex is particularly tall this may indicate left ventricular hypertrophy. A number of criteria have been developed to aid diagnosis, none of which are perfect. Most commonly used is the Sokolow–Lyon index:

- S wave in V_1 + R wave in V_5 or V_6 (whichever largest) > 3.5 mV.

There is a large S wave in lead V_1, which gradually becomes smaller (absent) by lead V_6. Its presence or absence is rarely of clinical significance.

J Point

The J point is the junction between the QRS complex and the subsequent ST segment. Elevation or abnormalities of the J point are frequently seen and their significance is debated. Elevation of the J point is observed in hypothermia.

ST Segment

The ST segment is the section between the end of the QRS complex (J point) and the T wave. It is typically isoelectric and represents the period of time when the ventricles remain depolarised prior to repolarisation. If the ST segment is down sloping or depressed, this may indicate myocardial ischaemia. ST segment elevation, taken as more than 1 mm, 80 ms following the J point, may indicate myocardial infarction but has a false positive rate between 15 and 20% (even slightly higher in women). Abnormalities of the ST segment can also occur in pericarditis and left ventricular hypertrophy.

T Wave

The T wave represents ventricular repolarisation. It is typically positive in all leads except aVR and V_1. A variety of situations can result in T wave abnormalities, which are often non-specific. Myocardial ischaemia and left ventricular hypertrophy can result in T wave inversion. Metabolic abnormalities can also manifest as T wave abnormalities.

U Wave

The U wave is poorly understood but may represent repolarisation of the interventricular septum or papillary muscles and therefore can be observed on the normal ECG, although their absence is not pathological. Prominent U waves are observed in hypokalaemia and hypothyroidism.

QT Interval

The QT interval is measured from the beginning of the QRS complex to the end of the T wave. There are

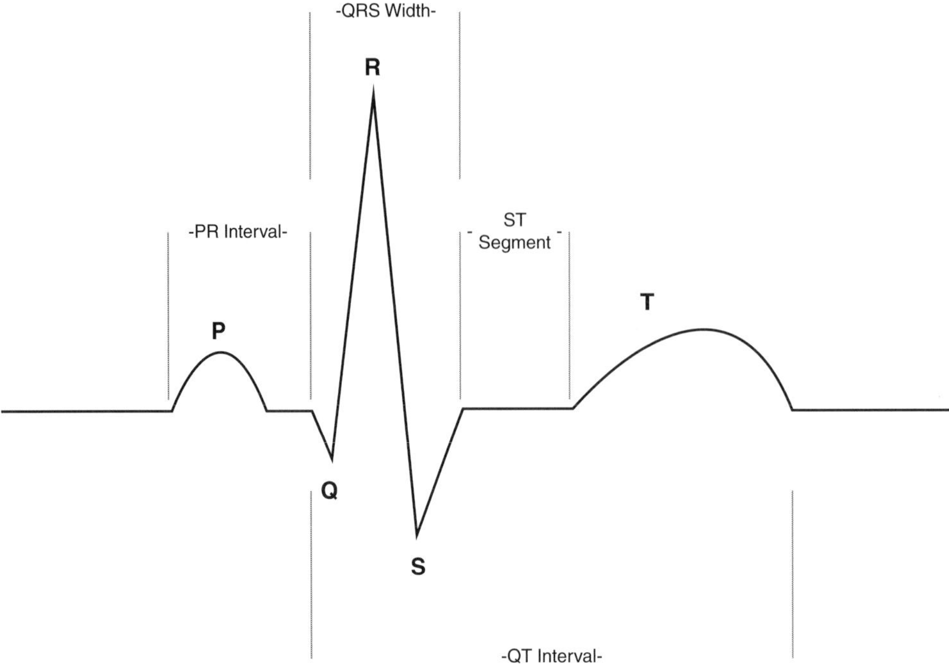

Figure 2.2 PQRST intervals.

several issues regarding its measurement, not least determining where the T wave ends. The best lead to measure the QT interval is lead V_3 or II. Several consecutive beats should be measured with the longest value taken. Prominent U waves are not normally included in the calculation and the end of the T wave is then assumed to be where the downslope of the T wave would cross the isoelectric line. If depolarisation is prolonged, the difference between the measured QRS complex and 120 ms should be subtracted from the measured QT interval.

Because of the close relationship of the QT interval and heart rate (the QT shortens with increasing heart rate), a correction factor must be applied. Although many methods have been developed to calculate a corrected QT (QT_c), the one most widely used is Bazett's formula:

$QT_c = QT / \sqrt{RR}$ interval.

The RR interval is measured in seconds such that at a heart rate of 60 bpm the RR interval is 1, and $QT_c = QT$. The QT_c is typically less than 440 ms. Gender, however, also has an effect on QT_c and therefore a value of less than 460 ms is acceptable for women.

An abnormally prolonged QT_c can predispose to malignant ventricular arrhythmias. A long QT can be the result of a genetic abnormality or due to a variety of medications.

Rate and Rhythm

Heart Rate

The heart rate is most accurately obtained by dividing the cycle length (RR interval) into 60,000. However, this is more easily achieved by dividing the number of large squares on a standard ECG between successive QRS complexes into 300. These formulae work well provided the rhythm is regular. However, if the rhythm is irregular then we can take advantage of the fact that the ECG is recorded over 10 seconds. Counting the number of QRS complexes across the ECG and multiplying by 6 will give an estimate of the heart rate.

Rhythm

The presence of P waves on their own does not indicate sinus rhythm. It is important to ensure that their morphology (as discussed earlier) is consistent with an origin from the sinus node. A disparate morphology might indicate an ectopic atrial origin and prompt closer scrutiny. If the P wave is not clear on the surface ECG then, post cardiac surgery, the temporary atrial

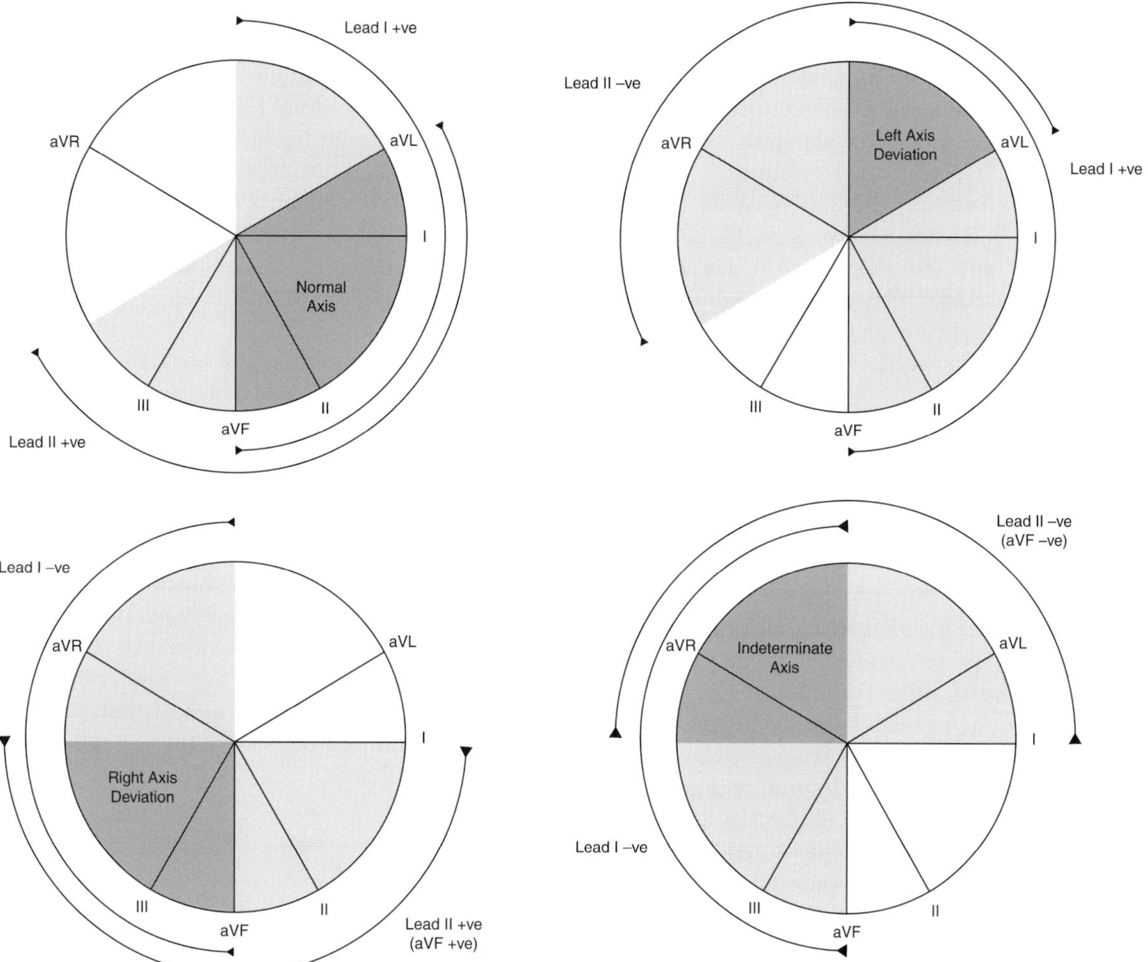

Figure 2.3 Mean frontal axis.

pacemaker wires can be used to create an atrial electrocardiogram (AEG). This is recorded by connecting the atrial pacing wires to the left and right arm leads, or to one of the precordial chest leads, and may be useful in differentiating various tachy and brady arrhythmias.

Axis and QRS Transition

The **mean frontal axis** (Figure 2.3) of the heart provides an average electrical axis (vector) of ventricular depolarisation. Any deviation from a normal axis may indicate pathology. This may be in the form of structural abnormalities (i.e. increased muscle mass – left ventricular hypertrophy or loss of muscle mass – following myocardial infarction) or electrical abnormalities (i.e. accessory AV connections or bundle branch block). A normal QRS axis is usually between –30° and +90°.

The mean frontal axis provides a mean electrical ventricular depolarisation vector in two dimensions only. The **QRS transition** provides an indication of the ventricular depolarisation in the third dimension (z axis). The QRS transition is determined from the precordial leads. The QRS complex in lead V_1 is usually negative and gradually becomes more positive through V_6. The transition zone is where the QRS changes from being predominantly negative to being predominantly positive. This usually occurs at V_3 or V_4.

Calculating the QRS Axis

To estimate the QRS axis we focus solely on the limb leads (not V_1–V_6) and use the fact that depolarisation towards any lead will provide a positive deflection in that lead.

If lead I is positive, the axis must lie between −90° and +90°. If lead II is negative, then the axis is between −30° and −240°. Together the axis must be between −30° and −90°. This is **left axis deviation**.

If lead I is negative, the axis must lie between −90° and −270°. If lead aVF is positive, the axis must be between 0° and 180°. Together the axis must be between −90° and 180°. This is **right axis deviation**.

If lead I is negative and lead aVF is negative, then the axis lies between −90° and 180°. This is an **indeterminate axis**.

Arrhythmias

Conduction Abnormalities

Bundle Branch Block

Electrical impulses transmitted through the AV node and bundle of His are conducted to the ventricular myocytes via the left and right bundles.

The right bundle remains sheathed in connective tissue within the septum until it reaches the base of the papillary muscle when it divides into multiple fibres connecting with the Purkinje fibres. The left bundle however divides immediately into anterior and posterior fascicles supplying Purkinje fibres within the left ventricle.

Right bundle branch block (RBBB) occurs when there is loss of conduction through the right bundle branch. The left ventricle is excited normally by the left bundle branch but the right ventricle is depolarised via conduction through the myocardium from the left ventricle. As a result, ventricular depolarisation is prolonged and there is an extra deflection indicated by rapid left ventricular depolarisation followed by slower right ventricular depolarisation. A QRS duration >100 ms indicates incomplete block and a duration >120 ms indicates complete block. A terminal R wave is observed in lead V_1 (rsR′) and a slurred S wave in leads I and V_6. The T wave should be deflected opposite the terminal deflection of the QRS complex. Right bundle branch block can be observed in normal individuals without cardiac disease.

Left bundle branch block (LBBB) is demonstrated by a QRS >120 ms, a QS or rS complex in lead V_1 and a notched R wave in lead V_6. Involvement of only the left anterior fascicle results in left axis deviation and less marked widening of the QRS complex. This is called **left anterior hemiblock** (LAHB). A qR complex is observed in lateral leads I and aVL, and rS pattern in the inferior leads II, III and aVF. Due to its broad nature and dual blood supply, **left posterior hemiblock** (LPHB) is much less common. It is characterised by right axis deviation, a rS complex in lateral leads and qR complex in inferior leads.

AV Block

When conduction between the atria and ventricles is impaired, AV block is said to be present. If the PR interval is prolonged beyond 200 ms but each P wave remains associated with a single QRS complex, **1° AV block** is present.

Progressive beat-to-beat prolongation of the PR interval with the final beat not conducting to the ventricles is **Mobitz 1 2° AV block** (Wenckebach phenomenon). However, if the PR interval remains unchanged prior to loss of conduction to the ventricles then **Mobitz 2 2° AV block** is present.

When there is complete dissociation between atrial and ventricular depolarisation (i.e. no association between P waves and QRS complexes) **3° AV block** is present.

Tachyarrhythmias

Supraventricular Arrhythmias

Atrial flutter: Atrial flutter refers to any macro re-entrant rhythm within the atria. Typical atrial flutter is a right atrial rhythm where depolarisation occurs continuously, usually in a counterclockwise fashion, around the tricuspid valve. The AV node will conduct at a variable rate depending on other factors such as concomitant medication etc. The resultant ECG demonstrates a continuously cycling baseline between QRS complexes. These 'flutter' waves have a slow phase and a fast phase, are negative in the inferior leads, positive in lead V_1 and isoelectric in lead I which is perpendicular to the re-entrant circuit.

Atrial fibrillation (AF): Although theories regarding the exact mechanisms responsible for atrial fibrillation abound, it is still poorly understood. In essence, however, there are multiple re-entrant circuits and wavelets that are constantly colliding and interrupting each other. The AV node is continuously receiving impulse, which again will be conducted at a variable rate. The ECG will demonstrate a chaotic baseline, constantly changing in frequency and amplitude.

AV node re-entrant tachycardia (AVNRT): The AV node receives multiple inputs within the transition zone around the compact AV node. These inputs may have different properties with regards to conduction velocities and refractory periods. This discordance can result in a re-entrant rhythm between the different connections. The ECG depicts a regular narrow complex tachycardia with no discernable P waves as both atria and ventricles are depolarised simultaneously.

AV re-entrant tachycardia (AVRT): Additional accessory electrical connections between the atria and ventricles can result in pre-excitation. The relatively quick conduction over the accessory connection results in the ventricle beginning to depolarise from an area other than those directly supplied by the bundle branches. This ventricular depolarisation is fused with depolarisation from the normal conduction system as signals catch up through the AV node. The slurred onset of the resultant QRS complex is termed a 'delta' wave and represents pre-excitation.

Under certain circumstances, impulse can continuously cycle between the AV node and accessory connection. If the AV node is the anterograde limb of the circuit, the resultant arrhythmia is orthodromic AVRT. Rarely, the accessory connection is the anterograde limb and the resultant arrhythmia is antidromic AVRT. The ECG of orthodromic AVRT will show a narrow complex tachycardia (no pre-excitation evident) with inverted P wave discernible shortly after the QRS complex. Antidromic AVRT will show a maximally pre-excited QRS complex.

Subjects with pre-excitation and symptoms that may be related to it (palpitations, breathlessness, presyncope and syncope) are said to have Wolff–Parkinson–White syndrome (WPW).

Ventricular Arrhythmias

A broad complex tachycardia is ventricular tachycardia (VT) until proved otherwise. Patients should be assessed and treated promptly within current guidelines. Distinguishing between ventricular tachycardia and supraventricular tachycardia with aberrant ventricular depolarisation can be difficult. Clearly dissociated P waves, fusion beats (partial ventricular depolarisation over the AV node) and capture beats (complete ventricular depolarisation over the AV node) are all good indicators of VT but are frequently absent. Other features, which are suggestive of VT are:

- Absence of typical LBBB or RBBB
- Indeterminate axis
- Very broad QRS >160 ms
- Positive/negative concordance
- R wave > R′ in V_1.

Learning Points

- Accurate electrode placement is essential to ECG interpretation.
- Care should be taken to examine all leads when making measurements.
- QRS axis and transition can be used together to indicate underlying ventricular abnormalities.
- Narrow complex tachycardias can often be distinguished by their ECG features.
- Broad complex tachycardias should be considered to be ventricular tachycardia until proved otherwise.

Further Reading

Bazett HC. An analysis of the time-relations of electrocardiograms. *Heart*. 1920; 7: 353–370.

Eldridge J, Richley D. Recording a standard 12-lead electrocardiogram. An Approved Methodology by the Society for Cardiological Science & Technology (SCST), 2014.

Sokolow M, Lyon TP. The ventricular complex in left ventricular hypertrophy as obtained by unipolar precordial and limb leads. *American Heart Journal*. 1949; 37: 161–186.

MCQs

1. **Electrode V_2 is positioned at the following position:**
   (a) Right sternal edge, 3rd intercostal space
   (b) Right sternal edge, 4th intercostal space
   (c) Left sternal edge, 3rd intercostal space
   (d) Left sternal edge, 4th intercostal space
   (e) Left sternal edge, 5th intercostal space

2. **The QT_c attempts to correct the QT interval to a heart rate of:**
   (a) 50
   (b) 55
   (c) 60
   (d) 70
   (e) 75
3. **A normal QRS axis lies between:**
   (a) −90° and +90°
   (b) −30° and +90°
   (c) −30° and +120°
   (d) 0° and +90°
   (e) 0° and +120°
4. **A gradual beat-to-beat lengthening of the PR interval followed by a dropped beat is known as:**
   (a) 1° AV block
   (b) Mobitz 1 2° AV block
   (c) Mobitz 2 2° AV block
   (d) Complete AV block
   (e) Normal
5. **An ECG with a continuously cycling regular baseline between QRS complexes is likely to be showing:**
   (a) Atrial flutter
   (b) Atrial fibrillation
   (c) AVNRT
   (d) Orthodromic AVRT
   (e) Antidromic AVRT

Exercise answers are available on p.467. Alternatively, take the test online at www.cambridge.org/CardiothoracicMCQ

Chapter 3

Echocardiography in the Cardiothoracic Intensive Care Unit

Ghislaine Douflé and Andrew Roscoe

Introduction

Since its introduction into the intensive care environment in the early 1980s, echocardiography has been recognised as an invaluable tool. Transthoracic echocardiography (TTE) provides a non-invasive, portable imaging modality, which allows for rapid diagnosis and cardiovascular monitoring in the critically ill. Transoesophageal echocardiography (TOE) produces better resolution images and is often utilised as an adjunct, or when TTE image quality is inadequate.

Focused echocardiography provides a goal directed ultrasound examination to address specific diagnostic and monitoring questions.

Indications for Echocardiography

In the critically ill patient echocardiography has been shown to provide supplemental information to physical examination and other monitoring modalities. It may be performed for diagnostic reasons, as a haemodynamic monitor, to assess volaemic status, or for procedural guidance.

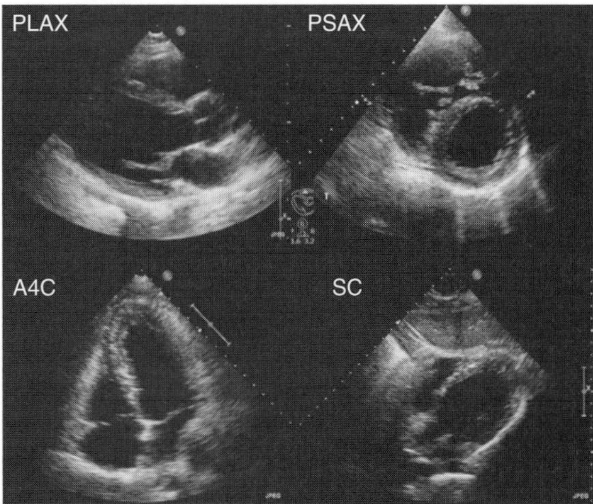

Figure 3.1 Basic focused transthoracic echocardiography views. PLAX, parasternal long-axis; PSAX, parasternal short-axis; A4C, apical four-chamber; SC, subcostal.

Focused Scanning

A focused TTE evaluation comprises four views of the heart: parasternal long-axis and short-axis, apical four-chamber and subcostal views (Figure 3.1). Each view provides basic information on biventricular function, volaemic status, valvular function, and the presence of pleural or pericardial collections. When integrated with clinical examination and other haemodynamic parameters, point-of-care echocardiography provides a bedside tool for diagnosis and monitoring of cardiovascular pathophysiology. Multiple focused cardiac scanning protocols are now in use across the globe (e.g. FICE, FEEL, FATE) and extended algorithms have been developed to allow basic assessment of valvular pathology and quantification of ventricular function. Focused scanning requires not only the development of skills to obtain adequate ultrasound images, but also the knowledge to interpret the findings and the experience to request a comprehensive study when indicated. Consequently, training and accreditation programmes are now established to ensure competency and focused echo is a skill to be possessed by all critical care physicians.

Left Ventricle

Left ventricular (LV) systolic function (LVSF) is frequently altered in the critically ill, either as a cause of decompensation, or as a consequence of critical illness: the incidence of LVSF in septic shock, for example, may be as high as 60%.

Advances in perioperative management and myocardial protection have seen a reduction in the incidence of postcardiotomy cardiogenic shock, but it may still occur in up to 6% of cardiac surgical procedures, and is associated with high mortality. Early

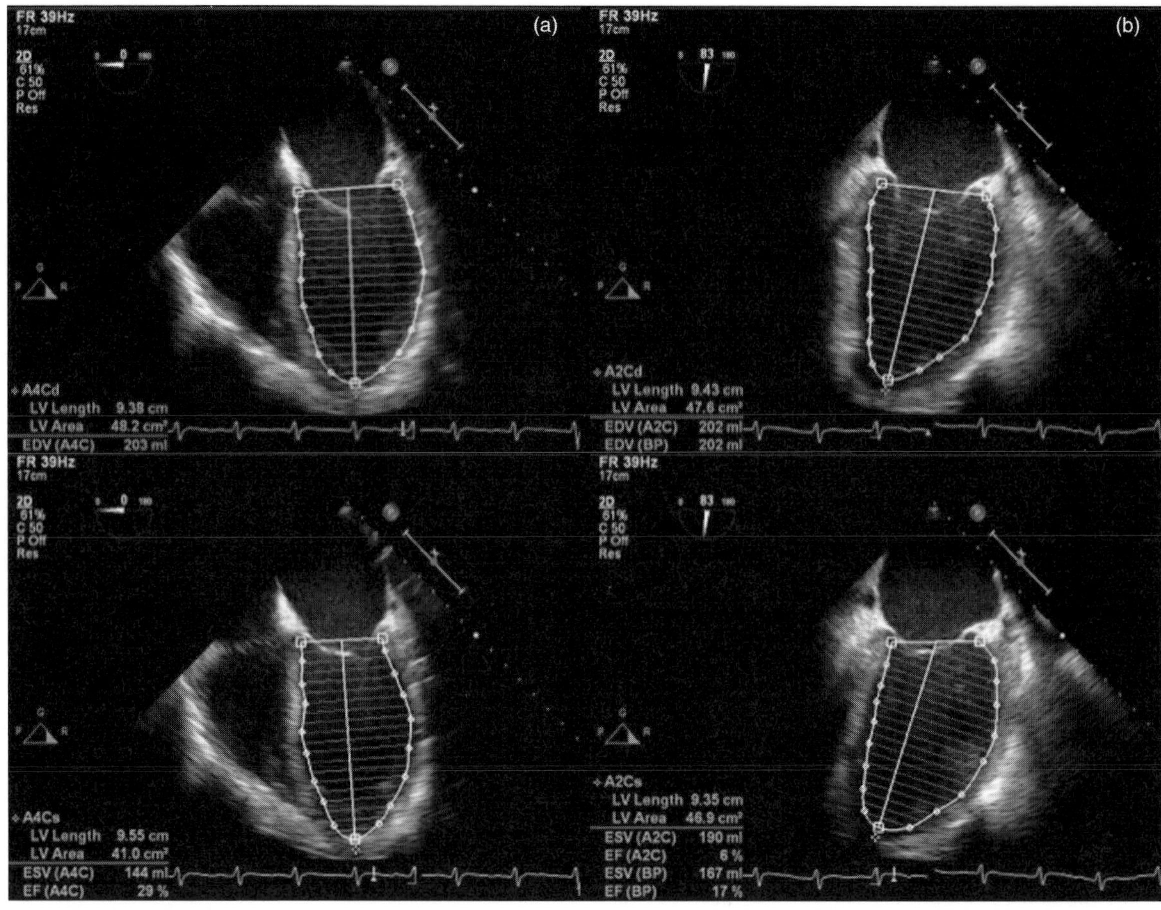

Figure 3.2 TOE midoesophageal four-chamber (a) and two-chamber (b) views, showing biplane method (modified Simpson's rule) to derive left ventricular ejection fraction.

postoperative detection or exclusion of LV dysfunction is paramount to initiate prompt and appropriate therapy.

Although some studies have reported good correlation between qualitative and quantitative assessment, objective quantification of LVSF is recommended and allows for interobserver comparisons.

Fractional shortening (FS), derived from M-mode linear measurements, is a quick and reproducible measure of LVSF. However, it is only representative of a single dimension, and in the presence of regional wall motion abnormalities (RWMA) may give an inaccurate measure of global LVSF.

Ejection fraction (EF) is calculated from estimates of LV end-diastolic volume (LVEDV) and end-systolic volume (LVESV). EF derived from the FS, using the Teichholz method, is limited by its assumptions of the geometric LV shape, and is no longer recommended. The modified Simpson rule involves tracing the LV cavity in the four-chamber and two-chamber views at end-diastole and end-systole to estimate LVEDV and LVESV (Figure 3.2). Three-dimensional echocardiography has also been shown to produce accurate and reproducible measures of LV volumes. EF is calculated as:

$$EF = (LVEDV - LVESV) / LVEDV.$$

The presence of RWMA before and after cardiac surgery is not uncommon, but the detection of new defects warrants further investigation. After coronary artery bypass grafting (CABG) surgery, a new RWMA suggests myocardial ischaemia or possibly infarction from multiple causes including a compromised coronary artery bypass graft occlusion, coronary vasospasm, inadvertent left circumflex artery ligation during mitral valve (MV) surgery (presenting with LV lateral wall akinesia), coronary ostial compromise after aortic root surgery and others. The 17-segment LV model is typically used and each segment is scored as follows:

1 normokinesia, normal regional wall motion
2 hypokinesia, reduced regional wall motion
3 akinesia, no movement of one or more segments
4 dyskinesia, paradoxical movement of one or more segments in relation to other LV areas.

However, RWMA may occur in the absence of significant coronary artery disease: postoperative epicardial pacing induces abnormal motion of the interventricular septum (IVS) and posterior LV; stress induced (Takotsubo) cardiomyopathy classically presents with apical akinesia and ballooning; the inferior and inferolateral LV walls are most often affected in myocarditis.

The assessment of LV diastolic function should form an integral part of a routine examination, especially in patients presenting with heart failure. In fact, up to 50% of patients with CHF have isolated LV diastolic dysfunction (DD) in the presence of a normal LVEF. In addition, LVDD may play an important role in a subset of patients difficult to wean from mechanical ventilation.

Patients with dynamic LV outflow tract (LVOT) obstruction exhibit hypotension, a low cardiac index and high LV filling pressures, but deteriorate with inotropic administration. Typically seen in hypertrophic obstructive cardiomyopathy (HOCM) and post-MV repair surgery, it may also occur in severe hypovolaemia. Echocardiography is indispensable in making the correct diagnosis, allowing expeditious treatment revision to vasopressor therapy, volume loading and cessation of inotropic support. Echocardiography findings include the presence of a significant gradient in the LVOT, systolic anterior motion (SAM) of the MV and mitral regurgitation (MR).

Right Ventricle

Acute right ventricular (RV) failure after cardiac surgery carries a poor prognosis. It occurs frequently after heart transplantation and LV assist device (LVAD) implantation. RV dysfunction is a well-recognised complication of acute respiratory distress syndrome (ARDS) and RV-protective ventilation strategies have emerged to impact on RV function.

In the presence of tricuspid regurgitation (TR), RV systolic pressure can be reliably estimated by applying the simplified Bernoulli equation to the peak TR jet velocity.

Due to its geometry, echocardiographic quantification of RV systolic function is challenging. Longitudinal measures of function, such as tricuspid annular plane systolic excursion (TAPSE) and tissue Doppler derived tricuspid lateral annular systolic velocity (S′), provide excellent measures of RV function. They are easily obtainable by TTE, but with TOE, values can be underestimated due to linear malalignment. Their use in the perioperative setting is less robust: opening of the pericardium is accompanied by a significant decline in TAPSE and S′ without an associated decrease in global RV function. This makes preoperative and early postoperative comparisons unreliable. RV fractional area change (FAC) provides an accurate measure of global RV function (Figure 3.3), correlates with RVEF derived from magnetic resonance imaging and is an independent predictor of mortality. Global longitudinal strain and three-dimensional imaging offer alternative measures of RV performance.

Valvular Heart Disease

In the early postoperative period, echocardiography is used to assess adequacy of valve repair, competence of valve replacement, detection of significant paravalvular leaks, recognition of patient-prosthesis mismatch, and iatrogenic valve injury.

Valvulopathies responsible for acute deterioration can be postischaemic, infective and traumatic in origin. Acute myocardial infarction (MI) may be complicated by papillary muscle rupture and severe MR. Infective endocarditis (IE) is a life threatening condition. TOE is recommended in patients with high clinical suspicion of IE. It is essential to determine the size and precise location of vegetations, extent of leaflet destruction and valvular dysfunction, the presence of abscess cavities or fistulae, and dehiscence of prosthetic valves (Figure 3.4). Echocardiography findings are crucial in predicting embolic risk and establishing the timing of surgical intervention.

Pericardium

Cardiac tamponade is a clinical diagnosis comprising haemodynamic instability associated with equalisation of diastolic filling pressures and large respiratory

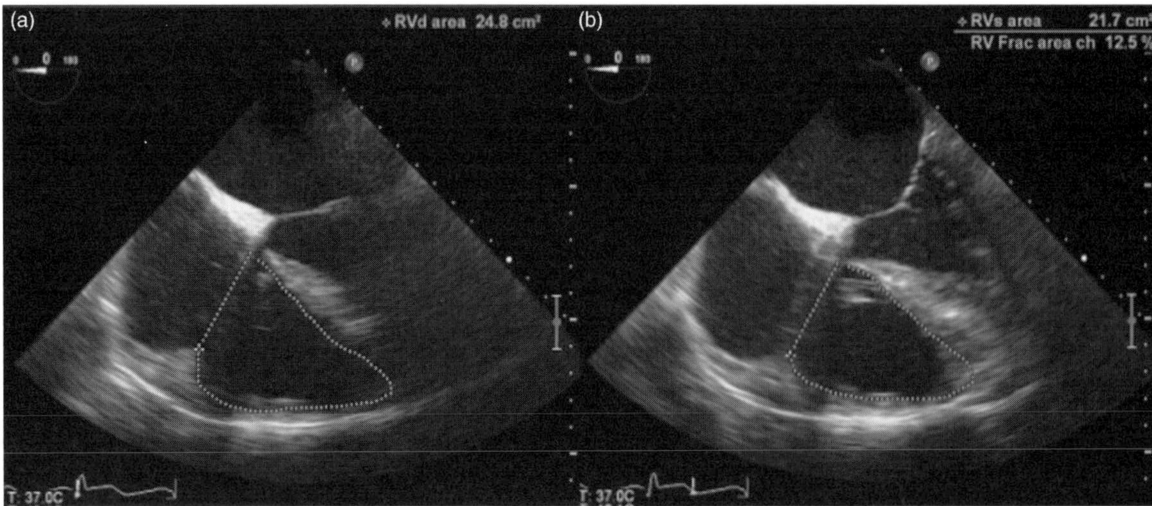

Figure 3.3 TOE midoesophageal four-chamber right ventricular views in end-diastole (a) and end-systole (b), used to calculate right ventricular fractional area change.

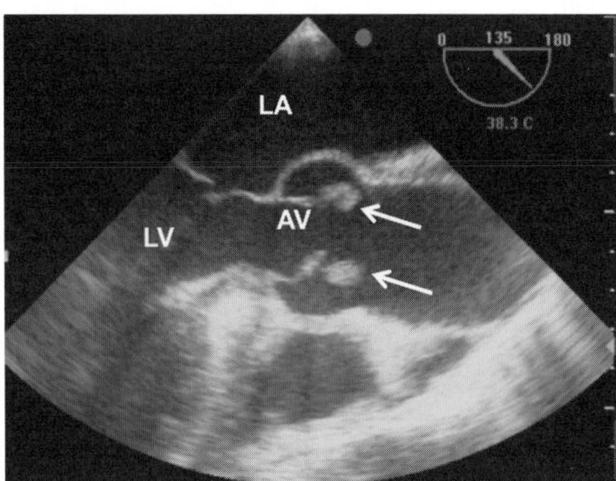

Figure 3.4 TOE midoesophageal long axis view, showing vegetations (arrows) on the aortic valve (AV). LA, left atrium; LV, left ventricle.

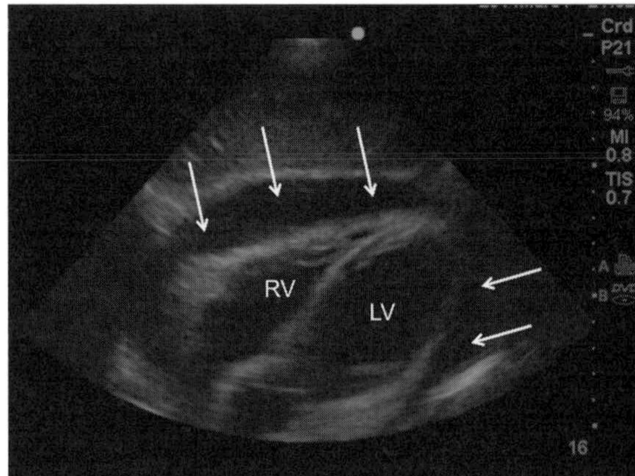

Figure 3.5 TTE subcostal view, showing a large pericardial effusion (arrows). LV, left ventricle; RV, right ventricle.

fluctuation in arterial pressure (pulsus paradoxus). After cardiac surgery, however, classic signs of cardiac tamponade are often mild and atypical presentations are not uncommon. Localised pericardial collections and thrombus formation may cause isolated left-sided compression, with normal right-sided pressures. A high index of suspicion is required postcardiac surgery and TTE or TOE often provides rapid confirmation of diagnosis (Figure 3.5). Loculated and posterior collections may necessitate TOE. In patients with significant pulmonary hypertension, RV diastolic collapse may be absent. In haemodynamically stable patients, echocardiography may be utilised to monitor the progression of a pericardial effusion.

Constrictive pericarditis (CP) results in impaired diastolic filling due to a rigid, non-compliant pericardium. Patients present with chest pain, dyspnoea and peripheral oedema. Although usually idiopathic in origin, it can occur post-MI and postcardiac surgery. It is important to differentiate it from restrictive cardiomyopathy (RCM).

Echocardiographic features to distinguish CP from RCM include a hyperechogenic pericardium, dynamic changes in LV diastolic filling velocity with respiration and preservation of myocardial relaxation velocities.

Aorta

Aortic dissection typically presents with chest pain and symptomology overlaps that of acute MI, however, it may be asymptomatic perioperatively. Contrast computed tomography (CT) and cardiac magnetic resonance (CMR) usually confirms the diagnosis, but TOE may assist in demonstrating complications, including aortic regurgitation (AR), pericardial effusion, pleural effusion and RWMA secondary to coronary involvement of the dissection flap. In particular, TOE examination of the mechanism of AR is essential to determine the surgical plan.

In the haemodynamically unstable postoperative patient, an echocardiographic study must include assessment of the aorta: the incidence of intraoperative iatrogenic type A dissection is approximately 0.2%.

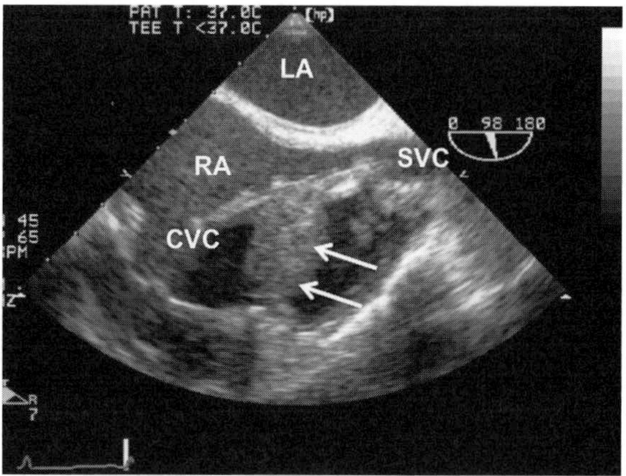

Figure 3.6 TOE midoesophageal bicaval view, showing thrombus (arrows) attached to a central venous catheter (CVC), in the right atrium (RA). LA, left atrium; SVC, superior vena cava.

Intracardiac Shunts

Previously undiagnosed interatrial shunts may present with hypoxaemia or paradoxical emboli, particularly in patients subjected to increased positive airway pressures. Right-to-left shunting via a persistent foramen ovale is observed in up to 20% of patients with ARDS and refractory hypoxaemia.

Post-MI cardiogenic shock may be precipitated by ventricular septal defect that often requires placement of an intra-aortic balloon pump and urgent surgical correction. Echocardiographic examination must exclude this rare but life threatening complication in patients with haemodynamic instability after an MI involving the interventricular septum.

Intracardiac Masses

Cardioembolism accounts for 15–30% of ischaemic strokes. Echocardiography represents the mainstay in evaluation for left-sided cardiac masses. In atrial fibrillation, thrombus typically develops in the left atrial appendage; thrombus also occurs in areas of LV akinaesia or aneurysm, and on pacemaker wires or indwelling catheters in the right side of the heart (Figure 3.6). Other potential embolic sources include tumours and vegetations.

Pulmonary Embolism

Although CT remains the gold standard for the diagnosis of pulmonary embolism (PE), echocardiography may be of value for the patient too unstable to transfer to the radiology suite. RV dilatation, RV dysfunction (McConnell's sign), peak TR jet velocity >2.7 m/s and pulmonary artery acceleration time <80 ms all support the diagnosis of PE.

Cardiac Arrest

A focused TTE exam may be of value in the rapid identification of reversible causes of cardiac arrest. To avoid interruptions in chest compressions, a subcostal view is obtained during the 10-second pulse check. Readily detectable reversible causes include hypovolaemia, tamponade, tension pneumothorax, myocardial ischaemia and signs of PE.

Trauma

Chest wall trauma usually precludes the acquisition of adequate TTE views. TOE, as the preferred modality, aids in the diagnosis of myocardial contusion, pericardial effusion, and valvular and aortic injuries.

Haemodynamic Monitoring

Inferior vena cava (IVC) diameter and its respiratory variation as a marker of fluid responsiveness has been well characterised. Initially described in spontaneously breathing patients, its extension to the ventilated population remains debatable. The effect of positive pressure tidal volumes and pulmonary compliance on IVC variability makes interpretation problematic. Even with spontaneous ventilation, increased work of breathing with the generation of extreme negative intrathoracic pressures IVC collapsibility can be misleading. IVC collapsibility and distensibility indices have been developed to improve reliability in determining fluid responsiveness. The superior vena cava (SVC), an intrathoracic structure, offers a more reliable parameter of fluid responsiveness in the ventilated patient, but requires TOE for visualisation.

LV end-diastolic area (EDA) can be easily measured in short-axis views of the heart. Reduced LVEDA is suggestive of hypovolaemia and may predict fluid responsiveness. However, in the presence of RV failure, the LV will appear underfilled, and inspection of the LV in isolation may result in inappropriate fluid administration. Measurement of LVOT velocity-time integral (VTI) provides a surrogate for LV stroke volume. Respiratory variation in LVOT VTI has been used to guide fluid responsiveness and to calculate the cardiac output.

Procedural Guidance

Ultrasound plays a pivotal role in the field of mechanical circulatory support. Intra-aortic balloon pump insertion and positioning can be optimised by TOE, and immediate aortic complications readily detected. Echocardiography can be used to guide cannulation of extracorporeal life support (ECLS), to manage patients on ECLS and to assess suitability for weaning from support. Pericardiocentesis should be performed under echocardiography guidance.

Summary

The role of echocardiography in the critical care setting is expanding. As with any monitoring tool, physicians need to be aware of its limitations and integrate the findings with the clinical context. Comprehensive training, accreditation and maintenance of skills are essential to ensure appropriate use and interpretation.

Learning Points

- Echocardiography is pivotal in the evaluation of the unstable patient.
- Focused echo is a skill to be possessed by all critical care physicians.
- Comprehensive training is essential to ensure appropriate use.
- Objective quantification of ventricular function is recommended.
- Echocardiography has an increasing role to play in patients on ECLS.

Further Reading

Charron C, Caille V, Jardin F, et al. Echocardiographic measurement of fluid responsiveness. *Current Opinion in Critical Care*. 2006; 12: 249–254.

Chockalingam A, Mehra A, Dorairajan S, Dellsperger KC. Acute left ventricular dysfunction in the critically ill. *Chest*. 2010; 138: 198–207.

Doufle G, Roscoe A, Billia F, et al. Echocardiography for adult patients supported with extracorporeal membrane oxygenation. *Critical Care*. 2015; 19: 326.

Douglas PS, Garcia MJ, Haines DE, et al. ACCF/ASE/AHA/ASNC/HFSA/HRS/SCAI/SCCM/SCCT/SCMR 2011 Appropriate use criteria for echocardiography. *Journal of the American Society of Echocardiography*. 2011; 24: 229–267.

Expert Round Table on Echocardiography in ICU. International consensus statement on training standards for advanced critical care echocardiography. *Intensive Care Medicine*. 2014; 40: 654–666.

Krishnan S, Schmidt GA. Acute right ventricular dysfunction: real-time management with echocardiography. *Chest*. 2015; 147: 835–846.

Lang RM, Badano LP, Mor-Avi V, et al. Recommendations for cardiac chamber quantification by echocardiography in adults: an update from the American Society of Echocardiography and the European Association of Cardiovascular Imaging. *Journal of the American Society of Echocardiography*. 2015; 28: 1–39.

Vignon P. Ventricular diastolic abnormalities in the critically ill. *Current Opinion in Critical Care*. 2013; 19: 242–249.

Walley PE, Walley KR, Goodgame B, et al. A practical approach to goal-directed echocardiography in the critical care setting. *Critical Care*. 2014; 18: 681.

Zafiropoulos A, Asrress K, Redwood S, et al. Critical care echo rounds: Echo in cardiac arrest. *Echo Research Practice*. 2014; 1: D15–D21.

MCQs

True or False

1. **Regarding left ventricular systolic dysfunction:**
   (a) The incidence in septic shock is up to 60%
   (b) Occurs in 20% of patients after cardiac surgery
   (c) Can be accurately quantified by fractional shortening in patients with regional wall motion abnormalities
   (d) Can be accurately quantified by modified Simpson's biplane method in patients with regional wall motion abnormalities
   (e) Septal wall akinesia after mitral valve surgery suggests injury to the left circumflex coronary artery

2. **Tricuspid annular systolic plane excursion (TAPSE):**
   (a) Can easily be measured with transthoracic echocardiography
   (b) Is a measure of the longitudinal function of the left ventricle
   (c) A value >20 mm suggests right ventricular dysfunction
   (d) Allows for calculation of the estimated right ventricular systolic pressure
   (e) Typically increases in value after pericardial incision

3. **Regarding fluid responsiveness:**
   (a) Inferior vena cava (IVC) collapsibility >50% always indicates hypovolaemia
   (b) Superior vena cava collapsibility index is a more reliable parameter of fluid responsiveness than IVC
   (c) Left ventricular outflow tract (LVOT) VTI variation can be used to guide fluid administration
   (d) Left ventricular end-diastolic area (LVEDA) is measured in the long-axis views of the heart
   (e) Reduced LVEDA is suggestive of hypovolaemia

4. **Features of left ventricular outflow tract (LVOT) obstruction include:**
   (a) Systolic anterior motion of the anterior mitral valve leaflet
   (b) Pressure gradient in the LVOT
   (c) Worsening hypotension with adrenaline administration
   (d) Mitral valve regurgitation
   (e) Clinical improvement with administration of fluids and vasopressors

5. **Cardiac tamponade:**
   (a) Remains a clinical diagnosis
   (b) Can present with atypical features after cardiac surgery
   (c) Always presents with right ventricular diastolic collapse
   (d) Can be diagnosed by focused transthoracic echocardiography
   (e) May be caused by a small loculated collection

Exercise answers are available on p.467. Alternatively, take the test online at www.cambridge.org/CardiothoracicMCQ

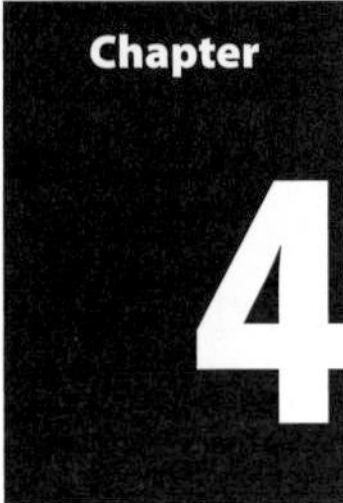

Coronary Angiography

Unni Krishnan and Stephen P Hoole

Definition

Coronary angiography uses radio-opaque contrast agent to delineate the anatomy of the coronary circulation. This may be performed either invasively using specially designed intra-arterial catheters or non-invasively by computerised tomography (CT) imaging. This chapter will focus on invasive coronary angiography and its role in current clinical practice.

Historical Perspective

The Nobel Laureate Werner Forssmann is credited with the first cardiac catheterisation in 1929 although this was exclusively right heart catheterisation via the left antecubital vein. Various reports of non-selective coronary angiography in human subjects followed in the 1940s and 1950s, culminating in the first selective (albeit serendipitous) coronary angiogram performed in 1958 by Frank Mason Sones in his basement laboratory at the Cleveland Clinic. Melvin P Judkins and Kurt Amplatz made significant modifications to the technique in the 1960s. They designed catheters specifically for selective coronary cannulation, developing J-tipped guidewires that were introduced via the catheter lumen, and popularised the Seldinger technique of percutaneous arterial access via the femoral route. Eponymously named catheters designed by Judkins and Amplatz are still routinely used for coronary angiography today.

Indications

Invasive coronary angiography remains the gold standard investigation for the assessment of coronary anatomy. The indications for coronary angiography in the assessment of ischaemic heart disease are described in detail in joint ESC, ACCF, ACC and AHA guidelines for the diagnosis and management of patients with stable ischaemic heart disease, acute coronary syndromes including STEMI, heart failure, sudden cardiac death, valvular heart disease, preoperative evaluation for non-cardiac surgery and major organ transplantation. These are summarised in Table 4.1. A detailed report listing the appropriate use criteria for coronary angiography was published in 2012. Appropriate use of invasive coronary angiography to investigate stable angina is also discussed in section 1.5 of the NICE guidance on the management of stable angina.

Preprocedural Assessment

Route of Arterial Access

The latest available annual report of the British Coronary Interventional Society indicates a steady increase in the use of radial access and a corresponding decline in femoral access for percutaneous coronary intervention (PCI). Diagnostic angiography has also followed a similar trend over the last decade. With multiple clinical trials suggesting a net reduction in adverse clinical events with radial access for PCI, this trend is likely to continue.

Assessment of the peripheral arterial supply is important before deciding the route of access for invasive coronary angiography. Symptomatic lower limb peripheral arterial disease, abdominal aortic aneurysms with thrombus in situ or previous vascular surgery (peripheral arterial bypass and/or grafts) may preclude a femoral approach although femoral access can be gained if necessary through Gore-Tex™ grafts. Increasingly, radial arterial access is utilised, as the hand has a dual arterial blood supply. Confirmation of ulnar artery patency (and/or radial artery patency in patients that have had this artery cannulated previously) is recommended by performing a modified Allen's (or reverse Allen's) test, plethysmography or pulse oximetry.

Table 4.1 Indications for invasive coronary angiography

Indicated	Rationale
ACS (STEMI/NSTEMI/UA) Stable CAD Prior to non-cardiac surgery Pretransplant assessment	High pretest probability of CAD and/or symptoms despite two antianginal medications and/or a positive non-invasive function test and/or in cases where revascularisation may improve prognosis
New diagnosis of heart failure Survivor following sudden cardiac death/ventricular arrhythmia	To delineate coronary anatomy and rule out or confirm significant CAD
Prior to heart value surgery	If age >35 years or postmenopausal at any age
Not indicated	
Preoperative evaluation Pretransplant	'Routine' angiography in the absence of clinical suspicion or where non-invasive tests indicate low pretest probability

Angiography of coronary artery bypass graft conduits is traditionally performed from a femoral arterial access although the left radial artery is also an appropriate route of access for left internal mammary grafts. In patients awaiting assessment for haemodialysis, it is prudent to avoid radial access as this is a commonly used site for arteriovenous fistulae.

History of Adverse Reaction/Allergy

Any prior history of allergy to contrast agents is an important consideration. The onset and severity of the reaction should be explored as well as the indication for invasive coronary angiography before deciding whether further contrast exposure is justified. Although a history of seafood allergy is often documented, there is no evidence to suggest that this increases the likelihood of adverse reaction to iodinated contrast media. The risk of a serious allergic reaction is reported as 0.02–0.5%. It is routine practice to administer systemic steroids several hours before the procedure and antihistamines 1–2 hours prior to angiography in patients with a history of suspected or confirmed adverse reactions.

Consent

Written informed consent by a competent operator following discussion of potential complications is mandatory prior to the procedure (see Complications section).

Access Site Preparation

The area of skin around the access site (radial artery or femoral artery) may need to be prepared according to standard aseptic surgical practice.

Premedication

An anxiolytic is useful in allaying anxiety and to avoid spasm of the radial artery. This is usually achieved by appropriately timed oral or parenteral benzodiazepines after consent has been obtained.

Prehydration

Acute kidney injury is rare following diagnostic coronary angiography, which typically uses <100 ml of contrast agent. Contrast induced nephropathy (CIN) is a form of acute kidney injury following administration of an iodinated contrast agent and is usually reversible. A 25% rise in serum creatinine levels from baseline at 48 hours after administration of the contrast agent is often set as a threshold for diagnosis of CIN in clinical trials. International guidelines recommend the use of isoosmolar contrast agents to reduce the risk of CIN. Prehydration with isotonic saline has been shown to be effective in preventing CIN especially in women, diabetics and in those requiring high volumes of contrast agent (>250 ml). Trials comparing intravenous saline versus bicarbonate prehydration have failed to demonstrate any advantage of one agent over the other. We recommend the use of 0.9% saline for periprocedural hydration in patients at risk of CIN. Patients are encouraged to drink clear fluids freely in the periprocedural period. A risk score based on eight clinical variables proposed by Mehran et al. more than a decade ago has been validated in a recent study as a reliable tool in predicting the risk of CIN in ACS patients undergoing coronary angiography.

Anticoagulation

A careful review of the indication for anticoagulation and the risk of thrombosis from interruption of anticoagulant therapy should be made in all cases. In an elective setting the anticoagulant is temporarily suspended where possible, although coronary angiography may be performed via the radial route in anticoagulated patients if necessary. Such cases should be discussed with the operator and planned on an individual patient basis. A meta-analysis of studies that compared uninterrupted anticoagulation with interruption ± heparin bridging suggests that coronary angiography may be safely performed by continuing warfarin therapy with a target INR of 2.0–2.5.

Antiplatelet Agents

There is no reason to discontinue antiplatelet therapy prior to diagnostic angiography. In instances where angiography may proceed to PCI it is mandatory to treat the patient with loading doses of antiplatelets according to local protocols.

Many of these preprocedural checks are confirmed with a World Health Organisation (WHO) surgical check list.

Coronary Angiography

Image Acquisition, Analysis and Interpretation

Invasive coronary angiography is an accurate imaging modality to delineate luminal anatomy although, unlike non-invasive CTCA, it cannot comment on the arterial wall. Multiple views (projections) are acquired by radiography by injecting iodinated contrast into the coronary arteries whilst being mindful of minimising contrast and radiation exposure to the patient, as a stenosis in the 'lumenogram' may be eccentric or foreshortened and could otherwise be missed. This is especially true in bifurcation lesions.

The right and left coronary arteries arise from the corresponding coronary sinuses immediately above the aortic valve. The right coronary artery runs in the right atrioventricular (AV) groove until the crux (the anatomical intersection of the right and left AV grooves and the posterior interventricular groove). Along its course the RCA supplies the sinoatrial and atrioventricular nodes, the right atrium and right ventricle and frequently the inferoposterior wall of the left ventricle as it enters the posterior interventricular groove as the posterior descending artery (PDA) in over 80% of cases. This is referred to as a right dominant circulation.

The left main coronary artery (LMCA) runs a short course (usually 5–10 mm) before bifurcating into the left anterior descending artery (LAD) that runs in the anterior interventricular groove and the left circumflex artery (LCx) which mirrors the course of the right coronary artery in the left AV groove. The LAD supplies most of the interventricular septum through its septal perforating branches and the anterolateral wall of the left ventricle from two or more diagonal branches. Obtuse marginal branches arise from the LCx and supply the posterolateral LV myocardium. In 10% of cases the LCx continues as the PDA (left dominant circulation) in the posterior interventricular groove, while in the remaining 10% of cases both the RCA and the LCx provide branches to the posterior interventricular groove (codominant circulation). Typical coronary angiographic images are represented in Figure 4.1.

Haemostasis and Postprocedural Care of Access Site

Manual compression may be employed to gain haemostasis at the site of arterial puncture. The radial artery is more superficial and readily compressed by a band applied around the wrist. Femoral punctures can be compressed by a FemoStop device if manual compression is not sufficient to achieve haemostasis. Intravascular or extravascular closure devices (such as the AngioSeal™ or Proglide™ devices) are also used routinely following femoral puncture and can help to achieve haemostasis earlier when compared to manual compression. The AngioSeal™ device was noted to be more expensive and resulted in a slight delay in the patient leaving the catheter suite,

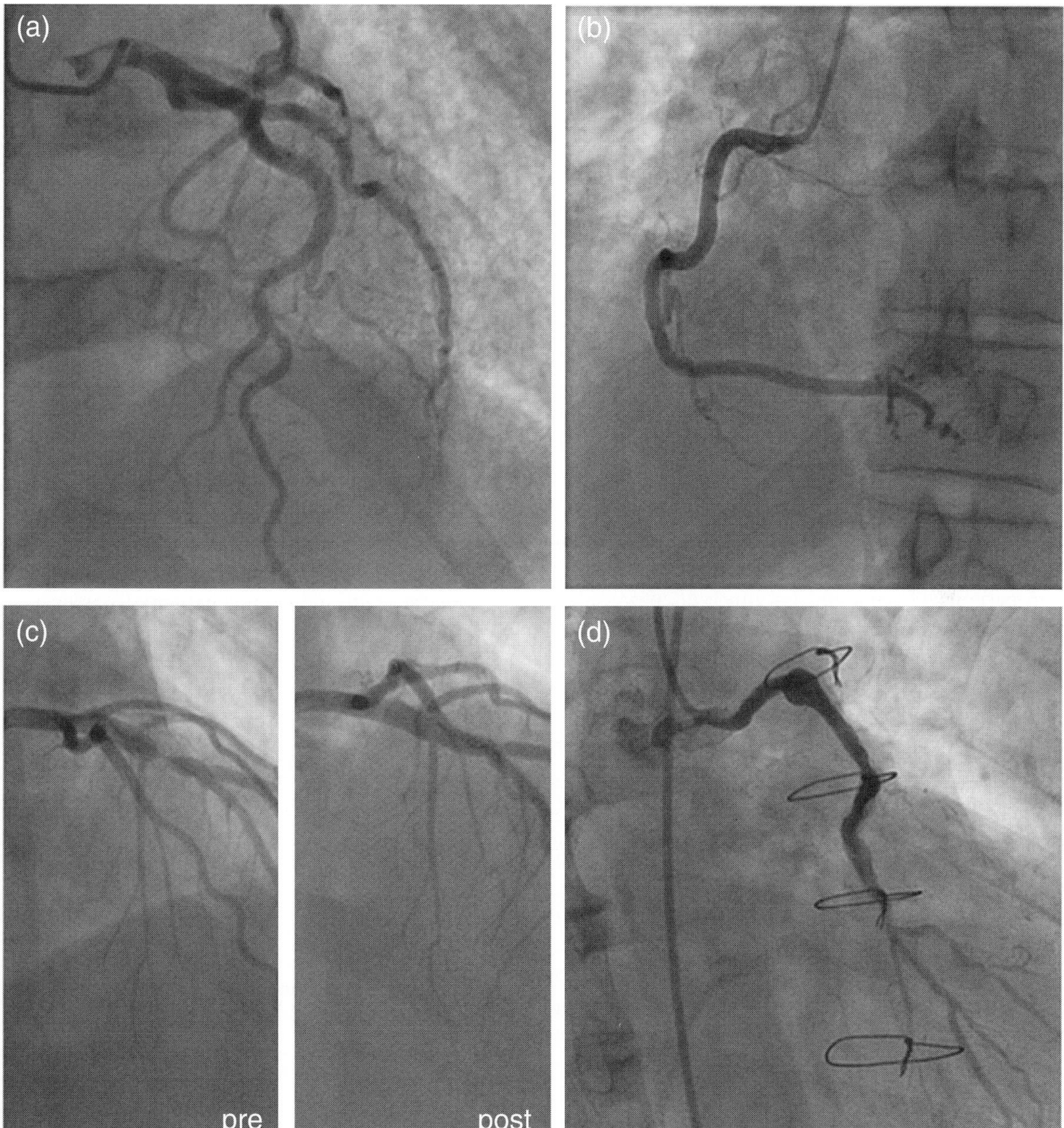

Figure 4.1 Diagnostic angiograms of (a) normal left coronary artery, (b) normal right coronary artery, (c) prepercutaneous and postpercutaneous coronary intervention to left anterior descending artery and (d) a saphenous vein graft.

but facilitated early patient ambulation and caused less patient discomfort compared to the FemoStop device.

Patency of the radial artery following angiography has been shown to be increased by the use of 5F versus 6F sheaths, administration of 5000 units of heparin via the side port of the arterial sheath and a technique of 'patent' haemostasis using specially designed compression bands.

Complications

These may occur during or after the procedure. Serious complications are rare with a reported cumulative incidence of <0.5%.

Major Adverse Cardiac Events (MACE)

Death is rare after coronary angiography and has been consistently noted to be around 0.1% in large registries, whilst the rate of myocardial infarction ranges from 0.06% to 0.17% depending on the location of atherosclerotic disease. Emergency coronary artery bypass surgery is rarely indicated (<0.1%). Ischaemic stroke rates of 0.05–0.1% have been reported and can arise from catheter manipulation in an atherosclerotic ascending aorta, catheter related thrombosis and embolism, air embolism or vessel dissection.

Access Site Complications

These occur more frequently following femoral arterial access and include local haematoma (with or without retroperitoneal extension in 0.15%), pseudoaneurysm, iatrogenic arteriovenous (AV) fistula and rarely arterial thrombosis or embolisation. Sudden haemodynamic collapse may be the first indicator of a retroperitoneal haematoma but this is often preceded by persistent tachycardia with or without hypotension and flank pain. A tender, pulsatile mass with a systolic bruit is commonly noted in pseudoaneurysm while a continuous bruit may be audible in cases of AV fistula. Clinical suspicion should prompt urgent Doppler ultrasound and/or CT imaging to establish the diagnosis. Urgent referral to a vascular surgical unit is often indicated in such cases.

Benign vasovagal episodes precipitated by femoral sheath removal are reported in 5–6% of patients, especially if the patient is dehydrated, but rapidly respond to intravenous fluid and atropine.

Local complications are less common following radial access but include pseudoaneurysm and sterile granuloma caused by deposition and hypersensitivity reaction to the hydrophilic coating on the surface of radial sheaths. The more serious complication of compartment syndrome caused by local tissue compression from a radial haematoma occurs in <0.01% of cases but can be limb threatening if not rapidly decompressed. It is heralded by the six Ps in the affected limb: pulseless, painful, pale, paraesthesia, paralysis and perishing cold.

Contrast Complications

Complications related to the contrast agent include CIN and allergic reaction to the iodinated compounds (discussed above). Allergic manifestations may range from skin rash to sudden unexplained haemodynamic collapse during or after the procedure.

Learning Points

- Invasive angiography is the gold standard test for delineation of coronary lumen anatomy.
- Written informed consent by a competent operator following discussion of potential complications is mandatory prior to the procedure.
- Coronary angiography is an extremely safe procedure in experienced hands with an overall complication rate of 0.1–0.5%.
- The use of radial arterial access for coronary angiography has steadily increased and may confer a net clinical benefit by reducing the risk of vascular complications.
- Contrast induced nephropathy can be avoided by appropriate prehydration and use of isoosmolar contrast agents in high risk patients.

Further Reading

Abellas-Sequeiros RA, Raposeiras-Roubin S, Abu-Assi E, et al. Mehran contrast nephropathy risk score: Is it still useful 10 years later? *Journal of Cardiology*. 2015; 67: 262–267.

Barbeau GR, Arsenault F, Dugas L, Simard S, Lariviere MM. Evaluation of the ulnopalmar arterial arches with pulse oximetry and plethysmography: comparison with the Allen's test in 1010 patients. *American Heart Journal*. 2004; 147: 489–493.

Delaney A, Carter A, Fisher M. The prevention of anaphylactoid reactions to iodinated radiological contrast media: a systematic review. *BMC Medical Imaging*. 2006; 6: 2.

Fleisher LA, Fleischmann KE, Auerbach AD, et al. ACC/AHA guideline on perioperative cardiovascular evaluation and management of patients undergoing noncardiac surgery. *Circulation*. 2014; 130: 2215–2245.

Krone RJ, Johnson L, Noto T. Five year trends in cardiac catheterization: a report from the Registry of the Society for Cardiac Angiography and Interventions. *Catheterization and Cardiovascular Diagnosis*. 1996; 39: 31–35.

NICE. Management of Stable Angina. NICE Guidelines CG 126. July 2011.

Patel MR, Bailey SR, Bonow RO, et al. ACCF/SCAI/AATS/AHA/ASE/ASNC/HFSA/HRS/SCCM/SCCT/SCMR/STS 2012 Appropriate use criteria for diagnostic catheterization. *Journal of the American College of Cardiology*. 2012; 59: 1995–2027.

Ryan TJ. The coronary angiogram and its seminal contributions to cardiovascular medicine over five decades. *Circulation*. 2002; 106: 752–756.

Schabelman E, Witting M. The relationship of radiocontrast, iodine, and seafood allergies: a medical myth exposed. *Journal of Emergency Medicine*. 2010; 39: 701–707.

Valgimigli M, Gagnor A, Calabro P, et al. Radial versus femoral access in patients with acute coronary syndromes undergoing invasive management: a randomised multicentre trial. *Lancet*. 2015; 385: 2465–2476.

MCQs

1. **Coronary angiography is indicated in the following scenarios EXCEPT:**
   (a) Prior to aortic valve surgery in a 48 year old male with bicuspid aortic valve
   (b) In a 56 year old male with exertional angina
   (c) New onset heart failure with severe global LV impairment on echocardiography
   (d) Prior to balloon mitral valvuloplasty in a 29 year old female with mitral stenosis
   (e) Following out of hospital cardiac arrest and good neurological recovery

2. **Which of the following is most useful in reducing the risk of contrast induced nephropathy?**
   (a) 0.45% saline by intravenous infusion
   (b) 0.9% saline prehydration is most useful at preventing CN
   (c) 10% sodium bicarbonate by intravenous infusion
   (d) Intravenous furosemide infusion at a rate of 20 mg/hour
   (e) Use of hyperosmolar contrast agents

3. **The advantages of radial access for coronary angiography include all except:**
   (a) Lower rate of access site bleeding
   (b) Lower rate of bleeding requiring transfusion
   (c) Early ambulation post procedure
   (d) Shorter fluoroscopic screening time during angiography
   (e) Lower rate of pain and discomfort post procedure

4. **Which of the following is FALSE?**
   (a) The circumflex artery may supply the proximal interventricular septum
   (b) The PDA usually arises from the RCA
   (c) Diagonal branches usually supply the posterolateral LV myocardium
   (d) The SA nodal artery arises from the proximal RCA
   (e) The AV nodal artery is usually the last branch of the RCA before it enters the posterior interventricular groove

5. **A 55 year old man is recovering on ITU following a witnessed cardiac arrest. New onset atrial fibrillation is noted on the ECG and a bedside echocardiogram suggests moderate–severe LV systolic impairment with pronounced anteroseptal hypokinaesia. Further evaluation is planned with invasive coronary angiography. Which of the following is the most appropriate step before the procedure?**
   (a) Administer regular dose of diuretics
   (b) Load with aspirin and clopidogrel orally
   (c) Start loading dose of warfarin
   (d) Administer intravenous prehydration with 1 l 0.9% saline over 2 hours
   (e) (b) and (d)

Exercise answers are available on p.467. Alternatively, take the test online at www.cambridge.org/CardiothoracicMCQ

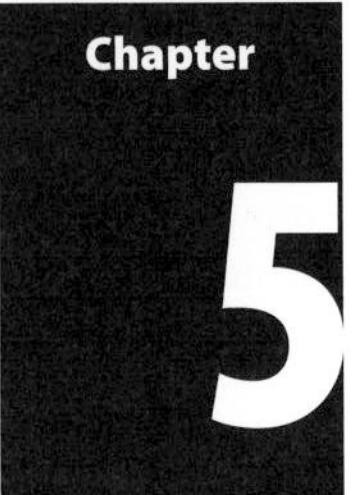

Bronchoscopy in the Cardiothoracic Intensive Care Unit

Sumit Chatterji and Pasupathy Sivasothy

Introduction

In 1897 Gustav Killian, a German laryngologist, performed the first airway examination in a human, with a rigid oesophagoscope, to remove a piece of bone lodged in a mainstem bronchus. The next milestone occurred with Shigeto Ikeda in 1964 and the development of the first flexible bronchoscope capable of examining the airways down to subsegmental bronchi. Flexible bronchoscopy (FB) has been used clinically since 1966 and has largely replaced rigid bronchoscopy as the technique of choice for airway examination and intervention. It can be of significant help in the diagnosis and management of pulmonary pathology in severely ill patients in the cardiothoracic intensive care unit (CICU). Intensivists, interventional pulmonologists and cardiothoracic surgeons are typical operators in this setting. Given its widespread use, it may be surprising that its role, efficacy and safety in critically ill patients has largely been limited in the published literature to small case series and expert opinions. A few meta-analyses have attempted to evaluate its role, particularly in the context of ventilator acquired pneumonia.

Patients in a CICU are typically selected for predominantly cardiac or respiratory support, with over 40% on mechanical ventilation. Patients are varied and include recipients of heart/lung transplants, immunocompromised established transplant recipients, those receiving anticoagulation or multiple antiplatelet agents, and those with chronic cardiac or respiratory disease. Polypharmacy is common, with the potential for multiple drug interactions adding to issues facing the bronchoscopist, which need to be carefully evaluated before deciding to proceed. Determining the appropriateness of the procedure, then optimising the patient and environment to ensure a safe and effective intervention, depends on a multidisciplinary approach with the physician/surgeon, intensivists, interventional pulmonologist and nurses all involved.

In this chapter, the role of bronchoscopy in the CICU, contraindications, preparation, procedural considerations and potential complications will be discussed.

Indications for Bronchoscopy

One can generally group the indications for bronchoscopy into diagnostic and therapeutic reasons, though there is often overlap. Examples of this include haemoptysis, foreign body removal, central airway obstruction, tracheo-oesophageal fistula and removal of proximal sputum plugs. Studies suggest 65% to 79% of bronchoscopies performed in the ICU setting are conducted on patients being mechanically ventilated, and of these 47% to 75% have a therapeutic indication. In one review of bronchoscopies performed in critically ill patients on an ICU, 45% were performed to remove bronchial secretions, 35% for collecting samples from the lower respiratory tract, 7% for airway assessment, 2% for haemoptysis, 0.5% for assisting difficult tracheal intubation and 0.5% for removing foreign bodies.

Indications for bronchoscopy in a CICU are summarised in Table 5.1.

Orotracheal Intubation

Difficult Intubation

FB can be useful to facilitate difficult endotracheal intubations in patients with a Cormack–Lehane score of 3 or more, limited mobility of head and neck, cervical spine fractures, or where severe coagulopathy or excessive secretions might make intubation with a layngoscope inadvisable. Despite its advantages in these situations, it is typically only used in a small proportion (0.07–3.4%) of patients in the ICU setting. The oral route is preferred as a larger diameter endotracheal tube (ETT) can be passed. Adult bronchoscopes have a diameter of approximately 6 mm,

Table 5.1 Indications for bronchoscopy in a CICU

Primarily diagnostic

- Pneumonia (nosocomial, ventilator associated, immunocompromised host)
- Acute inhalational injury or burns
- Assessment for airway trauma (post blunt or penetrating thoracic injury)
- Localised wheeze or stridor
- Diffuse or focal lung disease (infiltrates or mass lesions)
- Assessment of bronchial stump or anastomosis
- Assessment of graft rejection (transbronchial lung biopsies)

Primarily therapeutic

- Airway management (difficult intubation, double lumen endotracheal tube placement, endotracheal tube replacement)
- Atelectasis (lobar or whole lung) due to proximal mucus plug
- Airway foreign bodies
- Massive haemoptysis
- Strictures and stenoses (balloon dilatation and stents)
- Central airway obstruction due to tumour (cryodebulking, electrosurgery, laser)
- Tracheo-oesophageal fistula (stenting)
- Bronchopleural fistula (fibrin glue, endobronchial valve insertion)
- Percutaneous dilational tracheostomy insertion

able to pass through a size 7.5 ETT or larger – typical sizes used in adult patients. To prevent damage to the bronchoscope, a bite block is advised. As four minutes or more must be allowed to accomplish intubation, this technique is not recommended for apnoeic or near apnoeic patients.

Double Lumen Endotracheal Tubes

FB can be used to assist placement of a double lumen ETT used for differential ventilation or management of massive haemoptysis. A thin 4 mm diameter bronchoscope can pass through a 35F double lumen tube; the smallest size used in adults.

Changing Endotracheal Tubes

Occasionally an ETT may need to be changed due to cuff leakage or to facilitate a bronchoscopic intervention. If endotracheal reintubation is expected to be difficult, a flexible bronchoscope may be used to facilitate the exchange as an alternative to a bougie. The stomach contents are aspirated via a nasogastric tube, following which the new ETT is inserted over the bronchoscope and inserted into the posterior pharynx, whilst suctioning secretions. The existing ETT cuff is deflated and the bronchoscope/new ETT passed through the vocal cords alongside the old ETT. The old ETT is then withdrawn and the new tube adjusted accurately under direct vision prior to cuff inflation.

Controlled Extubation

Patients with suspected upper airway obstruction are ideal candidates for FB directed extubation. Examples include bilateral vocal cord paralysis, tracheomalacia or tracheal stenosis due to causes such as multiple intubation attempts, prolonged intubation or airway injury. The bronchoscope is inserted into the ETT just beyond the tip, the cuff deflated and the bronchoscope/ETT slowly removed en bloc. During withdrawal, if there is endoscopic evidence of significant subglottic or glottic obstruction, the ETT can be safely reinserted under direct vision.

Diagnosis of Respiratory Infection in Ventilated Patients

Ventilator Associated Pneumonia (VAP)

Pneumonia is the most common infection in the CICU. The overall incidence of VAP ranges from 9% to 25% in the general ICU population, with rates up to 70% in those with acute respiratory distress syndrome (ARDS). The risk increases over the first 10 days and can affect two thirds of patients who have been ventilated for more than 30 days. Mortality ranges from 35% to 90%. Bronchoscopically directed lavage, protected brushing and occasionally deep lung biopsies (transbronchial lung biopsies) are often used to determine the cause of infection. Qualitative or quantitative (number of colony forming units, or number of intracellular organisms) techniques can be used to analyse the samples obtained. This results in a wide range of reported sensitivities of bronchoscopic techniques (51–100%) with the overall impression that bronchial lavage and brushing are safe techniques for microbiological diagnosis in ventilated patients. However, well-conducted systematic reviews looking at bronchoscopic versus 'non-invasive' techniques (tracheal suctioning, blind catheter brushing) in reducing mortality and ICU stay in clinically diagnosed VAP patients have shown no statistically significant differences in mortality, duration on mechanical ventilation, length of ICU stay or antibiotic change. The British Thoracic Society therefore recommends directed non-invasive diagnostic strategies in preference to bronchoscopy in ventilated patients suspected to have VAP.

Immunocompromised Patients

Patients with solid organ transplants receiving immunosuppressive medications in the CICU are at higher risk of developing opportunistic fungal infections, including *Pneumocystis jirovecii*, invasive aspergillosis, candidiasis, cryptococcus, bacterial infections and viral infections such as cytomegalovirus. In areas of high prevalence in the UK, or in patients from endemic areas worldwide (Sub-Saharan Africa, Far East, Southeast Asia, parts of Eastern Europe and South America), tuberculosis must also be excluded.

Bronchoalveolar lavage (BAL) with 120–200 ml of instilled 0.9% saline can be performed via the bronchoscope into an affected lobe. If diffuse changes are present, bilateral BAL (preferentially of the upper lobes) appears to provide the highest sensitivity. BAL is reported to have sensitivity for *P. jirovecii* of 90–98% and is considered the gold standard. Diagnostic sensitivity for pulmonary tuberculosis can be increased from up to 30% based on microscopy alone to 86% with rapid PCR techniques, and is preferable to transbronchial lung biopsies in the majority of ICU patients due to the potential risk of pneumothorax or bleeding. For patients with suspected invasive aspergillosis, BAL galactomannan testing has shown superiority to fungal staining and culture, with sensitivity of 94% and specificity of 79% and should be considered if available.

Managing Lobar or Whole Lung Atelectasis

FB has been used in ventilated patients with lobar or whole lung atelectasis who have failed to respond to treatments such as physiotherapy, nebulised saline, mucolytics or repositioning (including prone ventilation). In several small case series it has been shown to be effective in immediate reversal of lobar atelectasis. Physiotherapy and conventional non-invasive measures are still recommended first line treatment with bronchoscopy reserved for the following situations:

- Life threatening whole or near-whole lung collapse;
- Lobar atelectasis due to proximal sputum plug with a lack of visible air bronchograms on radiology;
- Failure to respond to chest physiotherapy and other measures;
- Where physiotherapy or repositioning is not feasible (e.g. thoracic trauma, spinal fractures)
- Patients with neuromuscular disorders and impaired cough;
- Cystic fibrosis patients (copious inspissated secretions);
- Lung transplant patients with tenacious plug composed of necrotic tissue and mucus.

Diagnosis and Management of Haemoptysis

Bronchoscopy in conjunction with CT can be useful to identify the endobronchial source of haemoptysis in intubated patients with persistent or excessive bleeding from the ETT. It is also typically employed (usually through an ETT) for diagnosis and control of massive haemoptysis, defined as 400 ml in 24 hours, or 200 ml in any one event. Through the bronchoscope, iced saline, fibrin precursors or topical adrenaline 1/10,000 can be instilled to attempt haemostasis in a bleeding segment. Alternatively, the bronchoscope can be used to facilitate the passage of specific endobronchial blockers (e.g. Cohen flexitip® or Arndt®) and a Fogarty or Swan-Ganz catheter to occlude the bleeding lobe or segment. Finally, an ETT can be directed bronchoscopically into the normal lung to isolate the bleeding side and avoid spillover of blood, or help direct a dual lumen ETT to achieve the same effect. Where facilities and expertise exist, rigid bronchoscopy may be preferable in cases of massive haemoptysis as it provides a secure airway, large volume suction capability and easy access to the airways with endobronchial blocking devices. All these measures attempt to secure the airway, ensure adequate oxygenation, prevent soiling of the normal lung and in some cases allow definitive airway intervention – or buy time for a surgical or interventional radiology solution.

Thoracic Trauma

Tracheobronchial injuries affect up to 2.8% of severe blunt chest trauma and accidental deaths. Sternal or upper rib fractures can indicate significant blunt force injury and likelihood of internal problems so bronchoscopic examination is mandatory. Physical and radiological signs include hypoxaemia, haemoptysis, pneumothorax, surgical emphysema, haemothorax, pneumomediastinum, flail chest and the so-called 'falling lung sign' on chest radiograph (pneumothorax with atelectatic lung collapsing *away* from the mediastinum) which is pathognomonic of rupture of a mainstem bronchus.

Persistent Bronchopleural Fistula (BPF)

The incidence of BPF after pulmonary resection varies between 4.5–20% after pneumonectomy and 0.5% after lobectomy. Risk factors for this serious complication include right-sided pneumonectomy, a long bronchial stump, residual cancer at the bronchial margin, devascularisation of the bronchial stump, prolonged ventilation and reintubation after resection. Many patients may not be fit enough to have repeat surgery where intercostal drainage and sometimes pleurodesis methods fail. The extent of the air leak may prevent lung reinflation and delay ambulation, even with Heimlich valves or portable suction devices (e.g. Thopaz®, Medela Switzerland). Bronchoscopy can be used in these patients to identify the predominant lobe/segment causing the air leak (by employing an endobronchial occluding balloon), followed by insertion of one-way valves preventing airflow into that segment. Examples of valves used for this purpose include Emphasys® (Pulmonx, Redwood, USA), Spiration IBV® (Olympus Medical, Japan) or Watanabe spigots® (Novotech, France). These devices require considerable expertise to deploy accurately and are usually inserted by interventional pulmonologists.

Physiological Effects of Bronchoscopy

In the non-intubated adult patient, a standard 5.7 mm diameter bronchoscope occupies only 10% of the cross-sectional area of the trachea. Therefore, in spontaneously breathing patients endotracheal pressures generated are similar to those in patients without bronchoscopy.

In an intubated, ventilated patient, the effect is quite different. The obstructive effect of the bronchoscope is added to that of the ETT, with the potential to cause quite dramatic changes in respiratory mechanics, gas exchange and haemodynamics. Indeed, a 5.7 mm bronchoscope occupies 40% of the cross-sectional area of a 9.0 mm inner diameter ETT, 51% of a 8.0 mm ETT and 66% of a 7.0 mm ETT.

Complicating the effect of the bronchoscope on the patient's physiology are patient-specific factors including the underlying diagnosis (for example, atelectasis, ARDS, central airway obstruction, obesity, hypotension), the effects of sedation and the procedure being undertaken (such as suctioning to clear airway debris).

All these factors need consideration prior to undertaking FB, and in intubated patients particular attention needs to be paid to ensuring an adequate sized airway and choosing an appropriately sized bronchoscope for the task (a thinner scope may be safer but will have less suctioning capacity and may not allow passage of certain instruments such as a cryoprobe).

Table 5.2 summarises the main physiological effects of bronchoscopy in intubated patients.

Procedures Performed with Bronchoscopy

Flexible bronchoscopes typically have working channels 2.0–3.2 mm in diameter, allowing varying suction capacity or ability to pass specialised instruments to perform interventions.

Additionally, linear endobronchial ultrasound scopes available today (with approximate external diameter 6.9 mm) can be used via larger ETTs to facilitate transbronchial needle aspiration of mediastinal lymph nodes or masses.

Advanced bronchoscopic interventions are generally the remit of the interventional pulmonologist or thoracic surgeon.

Procedures likely to be encountered in the CICU are detailed in Table 5.3.

Contraindications to Bronchoscopy

There are very few absolute contraindications to performing FB. Among these are non-cooperation or refusal by the awake patient, operator inexperience, lack of suitable equipment and the inability to maintain adequate oxygenation during the procedure.

The remainder are considered relative contraindications as they place the patient at risk of certain complications. FB in these settings should be weighed carefully against potential risks to the patient. Hypoxaemia defined as an inability to maintain SpO_2 > 90% can predispose to arrhythmias through myocardial ischaemia and recent acute coronary syndromes increase the risk of fatal myocardial ischaemia.

Relative contraindications include:

- Severe hypoxaemia with CPAP or FiO_2 >0.5 to achieve a PaO_2 >9.0 kPa;
- Acute coronary syndrome within 4 weeks;

Table 5.2 Effect of bronchoscopy on respiratory physiology in the ventilated patient

	Outcome	Additional notes
Respiratory mechanics	Increased • PEEP (10–15 cmH_20, up to 35 cmH_20) • Peak inflation pressures (up to 80–90 cmH_20) • FRC (30%) Reduced • V_T • FEV1 (40%, bronchospasm can exacerbate) • PEEP (with suction) • FRC (with suction)	V_T reduction 200–300 ml with suctioning Main determinants of effect are ETT internal diameter, bronchoscope external diameter and duration of suctioning Cough can further exacerbate peak airway pressures risking barotrauma Auto-PEEP can develop leading to raised FRC, reduced FEV1 and expiratory tidal volumes
Gas exchange	Increased • $PaCO_2$ (average 1 kPa) • PaO_2 (in some cases with secretion clearance or due to auto-PEEP recruitment) Reduced • PaO_2 (average 2.5 kPa) • SpO_2 (>5% desaturation in over 65% cases) • SpO_2 falls below 90% in at least 20% cases	Suction can reduce PaO_2 by 40%. Mechanisms include atelectasis, small airway collapse, reduced V_T, reduced FRC and increased V/Q mismatch Low FEV1, prior LTOT, raised BMI and significant comorbidities are risk factors for an exaggerated response
Haemodynamics	Increased • Heart rate • Mean arterial pressure • Cardiac output • Pulmonary artery pressure • Intracranial pressure (can increase >100%) Reduced • Mean arterial pressure (if significant auto-PEEP)	Sympathetic stimulation due to hypoxaemia, hypercapnia and mechanical irritation of the airways Raised ICP potentially caused by a combination of hypoxaemia, hypercapnia and cough with auto-PEEP. Is usually compensated by the raised mean arterial pressure during the procedure

- Uncontrolled arrhythmia;
- Systolic blood pressure <90 mmHg despite vasopressors;
- Uncontrolled bronchospasm;
- Auto-PEEP >15 cmH_20;
- Bleeding diathesis (thrombocytopenia <20–50 × 10^9/l, INR >1.5, clopidogrel, newer oral anticoagulants (NOAC), chronic renal failure);
- Severe pulmonary arterial hypertension;
- Intracranial hypertension.

The Bronchoscopy Procedure

Preparation

The Patient

Ensure the patient is correctly identified and consent obtained if feasible. Radiology must be reviewed to identify the reason for the procedure and a target area for sampling or intervention. The full blood count and coagulation parameters must be within safe limits. If on warfarin for a metallic heart valve, discuss with the cardiologist and typically discontinue and cover with low molecular weight heparin (LMWH) until the INR is below 1.5 (omitting the LMWH dose 24 hours prior to bronchoscopy). For other indications, warfarin may be stopped or partially reversed with vitamin K if a biopsy is planned. Clopidogrel should also be discontinued 7 days prior where possible as there is a significant risk of bleeding with biopsies. NOACs can be stopped 48 hours prior. Review the list of relative and absolute contraindications to consider whether the procedure can be safely deferred.

The Equipment

A working sterilised video bronchoscope of appropriate diameter and monitor/stack is required. It can be difficult to position the equipment around a bed space when there are other pieces of equipment in the vicinity. The best position involves the operator on one side of the bed, facing the monitor/stack on

Table 5.3 Bronchoscopic procedures performed in the CICU

Procedure	Basic or advanced	Indications	Requirements
Bronchial wash	Basic	Bronchial clearance and sampling	Platelet count >20
Bronchoalveolar lavage	Basic	Cytological and microbiological sampling	Platelet count >20
Bronchial brush	Basic	Cytological and microbiological sampling	Platelet count >50 INR <1.5
Bronchial biopsy	Basic	Histological and microbiological sampling	Platelet count >50 INR <1.5
Foreign body extraction	Basic/Advanced	Removal of airway foreign body	Platelet count >50 INR <1.5 Working channel diameter >2.6 mm (for larger forceps or retrieval baskets)
Transbronchial biopsy	Advanced	Histological and microbiological sampling	Platelet count >50 INR <1.5
Cryotherapy	Advanced	Freezing/extraction of endobronchial tissue or debris	Platelet count >50 INR <1.5 Working channel diameter >2.6 mm
Diathermy	Advanced	Tissue debridement Haemostasis	Platelet count >50 INR <1.5 Insulated scope Avoid FiO_2 >0.4 (risk of airway fire) Care with pacemakers Earth electrode pad
Balloon dilatation	Advanced	Intrinsic or mixed benign or malignant airway narrowing	Platelet count >50 INR <1.5
Stenting	Advanced	Malignant or benign airway stenosis	Platelet count >50 INR <1.5 Some operators prefer fluoroscopy
Endobronchial ultrasound	Advanced	Sampling mediastinal or hilar nodes/ mass	Platelet count >50 INR <1.5 Size 9.0 ETT if intubated
Endobronchial valves	Advanced	Persistent bronchopleural fistula	Platelet count >50 INR <1.5 Working channel diameter >2.6 mm

the other side. If fluoroscopy is needed, the patient will need to be transferred onto a screening trolley, which allows access to a 'C arm' imaging device. All bronchoscopic accessories required for the procedure should be assembled. For patients with an ETT (or tracheostomy) being ventilated, a 'swivel adaptor' is connected between the tube and ventilator tubing to allow bronchoscope access without losing ventilation pressure (see Figure 5.1). For those not being invasively ventilated, ensure an appropriate mode of delivery of ventilation or oxygen is established (e.g. a Venturi mask, CPAP or non-invasive ventilation full face mask, laryngeal mask airway). The patient's vital signs and electrocardiogram should be continuously monitored during and after the procedure. Consider end-tidal CO_2 monitoring in hypercapnic patients.

Personnel and Skills

Typically, in the CICU, a bronchoscopy requires the bronchoscopist, an anaesthetist (to separately monitor sedation and ventilation parameters), a nurse assisting the bronchoscopist and a further nurse to control the position of the ETT/tracheostomy or provide general support for the procedure. The bronchoscopist and their nursing assistant should have the requisite competency to perform the intended procedures and be

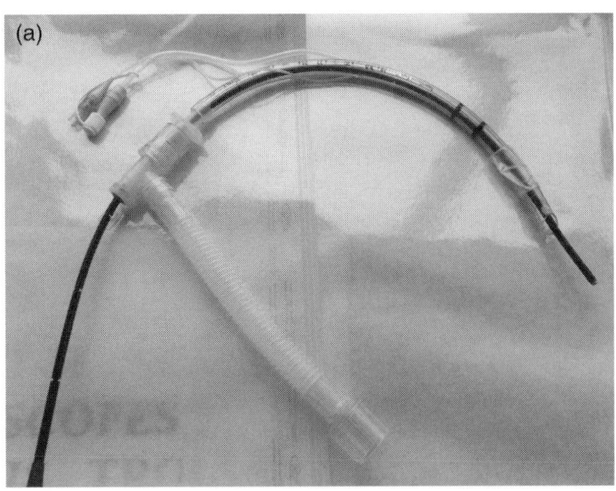

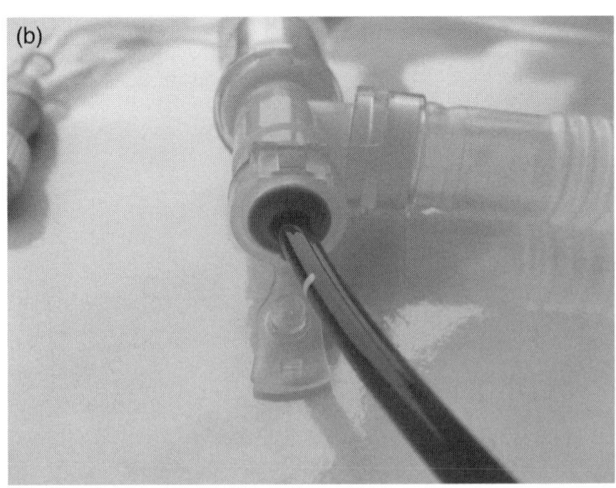

Figure 5.1 Bronchoscopy swivel catheter mount. (a) Close up image of the bronchoscope entering the catheter mount via a self-sealing soft rubber ring. This allows for reduced air leakage during bronchoscopy of an invasively ventilated patient. (b) Bronchoscope entering the catheter mount and passing via the endotracheal tube (ET). To ensure smooth passage down the ET tube, lubricant is applied to the outside of the bronchoscope. (A black and white version of this figure will appear in some formats. For the colour version, please refer to the plate section.)

familiar with the equipment and devices used. They must also be able to deal efficiently with potential complications.

Precautions

All staff should wear personal protective equipment. At the very least gloves, an apron, face mask and eye shield. For patients with potentially transmissable diseases through aerosolisation, an FFP3 or respirator face mask should be used and local infectious disease control guidance sought where needed.

The bronchoscope should be lubricated with sterile gel to facilitate easy passage and reduce the risk of damage.

Ventilation and Oxygenation Options

Adequate ventilation during bronchoscopy aims to achieve a consistent SpO_2 >90% with patient comfort and normal haemodynamics. If the procedure is likely to be complex and prolonged, or have significant risk of airway compromise, invasive ventilation or a laryngeal mask airway should be considered – or in some cases rigid broncoscopy in theatre. If invasively ventilated, the patient is preoxygenated with FiO_2 1.0 starting 10 minutes preprocedure.

With Conscious Sedation

- Self-ventilating with oxygen delivered by nasal cannulae or a face mask (Venturi or Hudson).
- Self-ventilating on CPAP or non-invasive ventilation (NIV) with oxygen. Studies have demonstrated this can be an effective option in patients in respiratory failure with PaO_2/FiO_2 <300 and can be well tolerated by patients. A full face mask or hood can be used with the bronchoscope accessing the mask through a swivel adaptor attached to the front of the mask (see Figure 5.2).

With General Anaesthesia

- Laryngeal mask airway. This can be useful for complex procedures (e.g. airway debridement, stenting) where the bronchoscope is withdrawn and reinserted repeatedly.
- ETT. Most patients in the CICU will be mechanically ventilated by ETT. The internal diameter of the ETT should be *at least 2 mm larger* than the external diameter of the bronchoscope to permit effective ventilation and prevent scope damage. The ETT should also be withdrawn as necessary to allow the bronchoscope easy access to both main bronchi.
- Tracheostomy. The internal diameter of the tube (usually quoted as the internal diameter of the outer tube if an inner tube is also present) must be 2 mm greater than the external diameter of the scope. A standard adult bronchoscope with external diameter 5.5–6.2 mm should safely fit in a size 8–10 tracheostomy tube. The inner tube should be removed if present and the 15 mm connector attached to a swivel adaptor. Special care should be taken during scope withdrawal

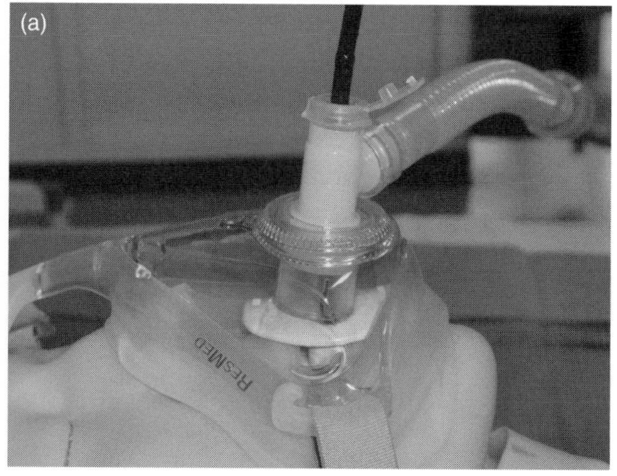

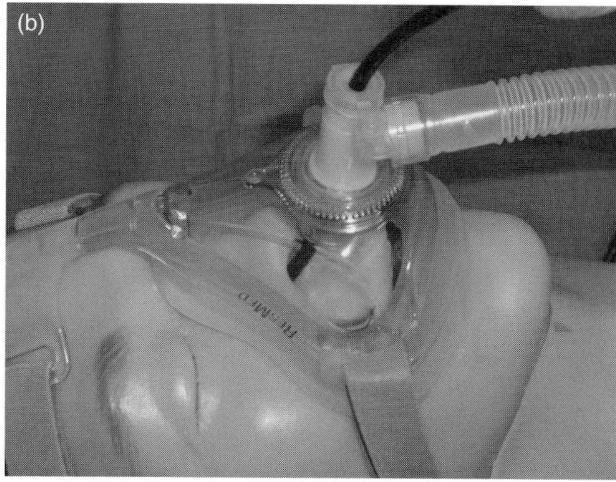

Figure 5.2 Bronchoscopy during non-invasive ventilation using modified full face masks (a) via the oral approach using a bite block and (b) via the nasal approach. (A black and white version of this figure will appear in some formats. For the colour version, please refer to the plate section.)

to prevent tube displacement or shearing of the scope on the distal end of the tracheostomy tube. Fenestrated tubes can pose particular risks in this regard.

The Procedure

In spontaneously breathing patients on oxygen, or CPAP/NIV, the upper airway is anaesthetised with lidocaine spray and the nostrils with lidocaine gel. Care must be taken with lidocaine dosing in the elderly and those with cardiac, hepatic or renal impairment. Although up to 15.4 mg/kg has been used without adverse effects, mild forms of lidocaine toxicity have also been reported with doses above 9.6 mg/kg. The British Thoracic Society recommends a dose not exceeding 8.2 mg/kg ideal body weight. Effective cough suppression can be associated with total lidocaine dose <160 mg and the aim should be to use the lowest dose to achieve the desired effect. The dose used must always be documented. The transnasal approach is contraindicated in patients with coagulopathy due to the risk of epistaxis. The oral approach requires a mouth guard to prevent biting of the bronchoscope. A summary of the process in ventilated patients is given in Table 5.4.

Complications of Bronchoscopy

Reported complications of FB in the ICU are less than 10% with a mortality rate 0.01–0.05%. Death from bleeding ranges from 0.03% to 0.05% and is usually confined to those undergoing biopsy (typically transbronchial lung biopsy) procedures. The risk of bleeding is increased in immunocompromised patients, lung transplant recipients, renal or hepatic disease, malnutrition, platelet dysfunction or those with acquired coagulopathies.

Other risks include pneumothorax (7–15% with lung biopsies), significant cardiac arrhythmia (3–5%), oxygen desaturation, which may persist for several hours postprocedure (especially in patients with ARDS), bronchospasm and haemodynamic instability. Postbronchoscopy fever occurs in 5–16% of patients due to release of inflammatory mediators a few hours after the procedure and is self-limiting. Finally, one must also be aware of the effect of medications used during the procedure. Lidocaine toxicity may present with tremulousness, shivering, dizziness and progress to sedation, unconsciousness, and convulsions followed by cardiorespiratory collapse. Blood concentrations after topical application may be 30% of that obtained by rapid intravenous administration. In the ventilated patient, early features may not be clinically apparent and therefore care must be exercised with dosing and the operator vigilant for signs of toxicity.

Learning Points

- Flexible bronchoscopes typically have an external diameter 5.5–6.2 mm with working channel 2.0–3.2 mm. Be familiar with local equipment. Some instruments require a larger working channel.
- The inner diameter of an ETT must be at least 2 mm larger than the external diameter of the bronchoscope. Replace the ETT or use a smaller bronchoscope if necessary.

Table 5.4 Summary of the bronchoscopy process in ventilated patients

1	Ensure ETT/tracheostomy internal diameter >2 mm larger than diameter of bronchoscope. Change if needed, or consider using a thin/paediatric scope if necessary.
2	Attach a swivel adaptor to the 15 mm connector.
3	Increase sedation and consider opiate antitussive or muscle relaxants.
4	FiO_2 increased to 1.0 starting 10 minutes prior to procedure. Unless life-saving, postpone bronchoscopy if SpO_2 remains <90%.
5	Mandatory ventilation mode used. Volume control may result in unacceptably high peak airway pressures. Pressure controlled modes require an increase in peak pressure setting.
6	Aim for tidal volume (TV) 6–8 ml/kg ideal body weight.
7	PEEP stopped or reduced by 50% during the procedure.
8	Lubricate the scope well with sterile gel and insert through the swivel adaptor into the airway. An assistant should hold the ETT throughout the procedure.
9	Instill 2 ml aliquots of 1–2% lidocaine to trachea, carina, right and left bronchial tree.
10	Use suction sparingly and no more than 3 seconds each time.
11	If using diathermy or laser in the airway, ensure the FiO_2 is < 0.4 to minimise the risk of airway fire.
12	Monitor blood pressure, pulse, electrocardiography, oximetry, end-tidal CO_2, sedation, VT and peak airway pressures throughout the procedure.
13	If oxygenation cannot be maintained, or there is haemodynamic instability, the procedure must be terminated and the patient stabilised.
14	Check the position of the ETT at the end of the procedure.
15	Wean FiO_2 and reinstate preprocedure ventilation parameters after the procedure.
16	A chest X-ray after bronchoscopy is important to exclude complications including pneumothorax and to assess the result of an intervention.

- Physiological effects are variable but generally include increased PEEP, FRC and airway pressures, with reduction in SpO_2, VT and FEV1. Parameters need continuous monitoring and ventilation settings adjusted where appropriate.
- Unless for life-saving intent, bronchoscopy must not be performed where SpO_2 cannot be maintained >90% with FiO_2 1.0.
- Be alert to signs of local anaesthetic toxicity. Use the lowest effective dose and no more than 8.2 mg/kg ideal body weight. Document the dose used.

Further Reading

Antonelli M, Conti G, Rocco M, et al. Noninvasive positive-pressure ventilation versus conventional oxygen supplementation in hypoxemic patients undergoing diagnostic fiberoptic bronchoscopy. *Chest.* 2002; 121: 1149–1154.

Bion JF, Barrett H; CoBaTrICE Collaboration, European Society of Intensive Care Medicine. Development of core competencies or an international training programme in intensive care medicine. *Intensive Care.* 2006; 32: 1371–1383.

British Thoracic Society Interventional Bronchoscopy Guideline Group. British Thoracic Society guideline for advanced diagnostic and therapeutic flexible bronchoscopy in adults. *Thorax.* 2011; 66: 1–21.

Chen A, Kollef MH. Bronchoscopy in the intensive care unit. In: Wang K-P, Mehta AC, Turner JF (Eds). *Flexible Bronchoscopy*, 3rd Edition. Oxford: Wiley-Blackwell, 2012. doi:10.1002/9781444346428.ch24

Du Rand IA, Blaikley J, Booton R, et al. British Thoracic Society guideline for diagnostic flexible bronchoscopy in adults. *Thorax.* 2013; 68: 1–44. doi:10.1136/thoraxjnl-2013-203618

Estella A. Bronchoscopy in mechanically ventilated patients. In: Haranath SP (Ed). *Global Perspectives on Bronchoscopy.* InTech, 2012. http: //cdn.intechopen.com/pdfs/37333/In Tech-Bronchoscopy-in_mechanically_ventilated_patients.pdf.

Khalil A, Soussan M, Mangiapan G, et al. Utility of high-resolution chest CT scan in the emergency management of haemoptysis in the intensive care unit: severity, localization and aetiology. *British Journal of Radiology.* 2007; 80: 21–25.

Kreider ME, Lipson DA. Bronchoscopy for atelectasis in the ICU. *Chest.* 2003; 124: 344–350.

Krell WS. Pulmonary diagnostic procedures in the critically ill. *Critical Care Clinics*. 1988; 4: 393–407.

Lindholm C, Ollmann B, Snyder J, Millen E, Grenvik A. Cardiorespiratory effects of flexible fiberoptic bronchoscopy in critically ill patients. *Chest*. 1978; 74: 362–367.

Olopade CS, Prakash UBS. Bronchoscopy in the critical care unit. *Mayo Clinic Proceedings*. 1989; 64: 1255–1263.

Raoof S, Mehrishi S, Prakash UB. Role of bronchoscopy in modern medical intensive care unit. *Clinics in Chest Medicine*. 2001; 22: 241–261.

Toma TP, Kon OM, Oldfield W, et al. Reduction of persistent air leak with endoscopic valve implants. *Thorax*. 2007; 62: 830–833.

MCQs

1. **Which of the following is true during bronchoscopy in a ventilated patient?**
   (a) Tidal volume is reduced
   (b) PEEP is reduced during suctioning
   (c) PaO_2 can rise in some scenarios
   (d) Mean arterial pressure can be reduced
   (e) All of the above

2. **Which of the following is NOT a relative contraindication for bronchoscopy?**
   (a) Tachyarrhythmia
   (b) PEEP >15 cmH_2O
   (c) Aspirin
   (d) INR >1.5 or platelets <20 × 10^9/l
   (e) Intracranial hypertension

3. **Which of the following will fit down a double lumen endotracheal tube?**
   (a) Linear EBUS (endobronchial ultrasound) scope
   (b) Standard bronchoscope with outer diameter of 5.7 mm
   (c) Interventional bronchoscope with outer diameter of 6.2 mm
   (d) Paediatric bronchoscope
   (e) Rigid bronchoscope

4. **When undertaking a bronchoscopy via a tracheostomy which one of the following is correct?**
   (a) The tracheostomy tube should have an internal diameter >2 mm compared to the bronchoscope
   (b) The inner tube should remain in situ
   (c) No additional considerations are needed if the tube is fenestrated
   (d) Additional sedation is routinely required in addition to topical local anaesthetic
   (e) A swivel adaptor is not required in this setting

5. **Which of the following cannot be done directly via the working channel of the flexible bronchoscope?**
   (a) Bronchial biopsy
   (b) Endobronchial valve placement for bronchopleural fistula
   (c) Cryotherapy
   (d) Bronchial stent placement
   (e) Foreign body extraction

Exercise answers are available on p.467. Alternatively, take the test online at www.cambridge.org/CardiothoracicMCQ

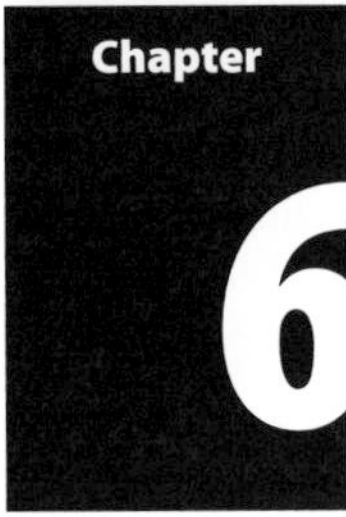

Microbiology Testing

A Ruth M Kappeler and Margaret I Gillham

Introduction

Infections in cardiothoracic intensive care units are common, either as the primary presenting illness as in the case of infective endocarditis or severe respiratory failure, or as a secondary complication of cardiothoracic procedures. Moreover, infectious complications are known to impact on morbidity and mortality. The sites of infection encountered include surgical site infections (including organ space), device related infections (prosthetic valve endocarditis, ventricular assist device infections), bloodstream infections, line related infections, respiratory tract, gastrointestinal tract and urinary tract infections.

The time taken to identify microorganisms in clinical samples can have an impact in the management of patients with sepsis. Best practice in collection and timely processing of microbiological samples is essential, not only to ensure optimal antimicrobial management and thereby outcome, but also to ensure optimal infection control management of patients within cardiothoracic units. The ability to culture organisms from clinical samples is affected by type and quality of the specimen, prior antibiotic therapy, transportation, storage conditions of samples and time to sample processing. Emerging technologies are enabling faster identification and quantification of pathogens, resulting in more rapid diagnostics. This has the potential not only to affect patient outcome but also to ensure better antimicrobial stewardship by enabling targeted antimicrobial therapy and avoidance of unnecessary antimicrobial use which can lead to adverse effects for patients and encourage development of resistance in bacteria. It is necessary to perform a systematic physical examination before requesting diagnostic tests as this will enable test selection and avoid unnecessary sampling.

The importance of microbiological diagnostics to cardiothoracic units cannot be underestimated and units need to ensure that processes are in place to enable appropriate sampling of patients and as short a time as possible to sample processing whether the unit has an on-site or off-site laboratory. There should be 24 hour access to the laboratory for handling urgent samples and for viewing results. Furthermore, round-the-clock accessibility to infection specialists is crucial to ensuring correct test selection, timely reporting, interpretation of microbiology results, infection control and antimicrobial advice.

Ordering of Tests

Most hospitals use an electronic ordering system for pathology requests, including those for microbiology. Testing protocols can be set up to ensure that the appropriate range of tests is ordered for different clinical scenarios. For example, patients admitted with severe respiratory failure for ECMO will require extensive testing on admission to critical care (see Table 6.1 for guidance on test selection for this scenario) whereas patients admitted for elective cardiac surgery, who have no complications, will only require preoperative screening samples. Electronic ordering systems can be set up as specimen or sample type based. It is important to ensure from the outset that the way the system is configured not only allows ease of ordering for the clinical user but also includes a degree of demand management to reduce inappropriate testing. Electronic test ordering also allows the development of testing sets whereby a standard protocol for microbiology testing can be agreed according to the patient's circumstances, and the same testing strategy can be followed each time. This can be beneficial in cases of severe respiratory failure on ECMO where an infective cause is suspected or for patients who develop postoperative sepsis.

Correct Sampling Procedures

General principles apply to collection of all microbiology samples. They should be collected at the correct

Table 6.1 Suggested testing set for patients with severe respiratory failure requiring ECMO

Baseline tests

Sample	Organism
Blood	Human immunodeficiency (HIV) virus Herpes simplex virus (HSV) IgG and PCR Cytomegalovirus (CMV) IgG and PCR *N. meningitidis* PCR Pneumococcal PCR Mycoplasma and chlamydia serology Blood cultures
Bronchoalveolar lavage	Respiratory virus PCR CMV, HSV, adenovirus PCR *Pneumocystis jirovecii* PCR Galactomannan *Legionella* culture and PCR *Mycoplasma pneumoniae* PCR *Chlamydophila pneumoniae* PCR Smear and culture for *Mycobacterium tuberculosis* Fungal culture Routine culture
Nose and throat viral swab	Respiratory virus PCR Consider pernasal swab for pertussis
Urine sample	Culture *Legionella* antigen Pneumococcal antigen

Additional tests

Risk factor/clinical feature	Organisms to consider
Immunocompromised	Cryptococcus
Exposure to rodents or contaminated fresh water	Leptospirosis Hantavirus
Rash	Varicella zoster virus HSV Measles
Toxic shock	*Staphylococcus aureus* and *Streptococcus pyogenes*
Travel	MERS, avian influenza, malaria
Animal contact	Anthrax, *Coxiella*

time, using the correct technique, the correct volume and in the correct specimen containers. Lids must be tightened securely as leakage may mean specimen rejection, and clinicians and laboratories must ensure that the correct procedures are followed so that samples are transported safely and in a timely manner to the laboratory. Samples requiring immediate attention for processing should be notified to the laboratory in advance and identified as urgent. All samples should be transported with completed information identifying the patient, time and date collected, tests required and antibiotic history. This may be in bar code format or with a physical request form. Samples with risk of infection should be identified by the clinical user and visible to the laboratory handling the sample. Where possible, samples should be collected prior to antibiotic therapy but this should not lead to delays in managing the patient or administering antibiotics.

Hand hygiene should be performed before and after specimen collection. Personal protective equipment (gloves, waterproof apron) is required during specimen collection when contact with bodily fluids is anticipated. Masks may be required for collection of respiratory samples, for example with sputum induction.

Blood cultures are taken when bacteraemia is suspected and should be taken via a dedicated venepuncture, peripherally, rather than through an existing line. Where endocarditis or device related infection is suspected, up to three sets can be taken at separate times over a 24 hour period. However, it is the actual volume of blood that is important, therefore inoculating one bottle with the correct volume of blood is of greater value than sharing the blood volume between multiple bottles. Local procedures should be followed when taking blood cultures to minimise the risk of contamination with skin flora. When using vacuum blood taking systems, care should be taken that blood cultures are inoculated first before filling other blood tubes. This is to prevent the possibility of bacterial contamination from blood tubes entering the blood culture bottles, resulting in a ‘pseudobacteraemia’ assigned to the patient.

Stool samples should only be sent for microbiology testing when an infective cause is suspected for patients with diarrhoea. The Bristol stool scale can be used to identify diarrhoea stools where types 5–7 indicate diarrhoea. *Clostridium difficile* should be considered as a cause of hospital acquired infective diarrhoea in cardiothoracic centres and requested as a specific test. Laboratory testing should follow national testing guidelines to ensure optimal diagnosis. In the

UK this amounts to a combination of tests looking for presence of the *C. difficile* organism and the presence of toxin.

Care should be taken when obtaining respiratory samples that sputum is collected rather than saliva. Physiotherapists can help with obtaining a good quality respiratory sample. Any respiratory sample obtained in a trap should be transported in a leak-proof CE marked specimen container. Lower respiratory tract samples can be obtained by directed or non-directed BAL. Respiratory samples in particular must reach the laboratory in a timely manner and should be processed within 2–3 hours to maximise the chance of culturing respiratory tract organisms.

Wound swabs are best obtained after first cleansing the wound. This reduces the risk of contamination of the sample with therapeutic agents that may be contained within the dressing material. Dry swabs should be moistened with sterile water (or saline) or transport media. Where possible the whole wound should be swabbed using a zigzag movement while rotating the swab.

Fluid from vesicular lesions can be aspirated or swabs used to collect the vesicular fluid and inoculated into viral transport media (VTM).

Urine samples are collected as a midstream sample after first cleaning the urethral meatus with soap and water or saline. Disinfectants should be avoided as they can irritate the urethral mucosa. However, the vast majority of patients in ICU will have a urinary catheter in situ. Catheter specimens of urine should only be taken where urosepsis is suspected. The correct local procedure should be followed and urine sampled through the catheter sampling port.

If urine samples cannot be examined within 2 hours then they should be refrigerated until they can be processed by the laboratory. Urine samples held at room temperature will allow overgrowth of bacteria, affecting the result. The addition of boric acid to urine containers will preserve the urine sample for longer where transport delays exist.

Surgical Samples

Any samples obtained at the time of surgery should be placed into a sterile pot for onward transportation to the laboratory. Samples may include native or prosthetic heart valves, sternal wound biopsies or samples of pus or fluid. These surgical samples are precious, unrepeatable specimens and should be notified to the laboratory ahead of the sample arriving to ensure as short a time as possible to sample processing. Microscopy performed on arrival in the laboratory can provide essential information on the presence of organisms and can aid antimicrobial management. In patients who have had previous cardiac surgery and who develop a deep infection or endocarditis where no pathogen is identified, mycobacterial infection should be considered.

Screening for Resistant Organisms

Screening for methicillin resistant *Staphylococcus aureus* (MRSA) prior to cardiac surgery and on admission to hospital is standard practice in UK hospitals. Persons carrying MRSA will be offered decolonisation treatment prior to surgery, where time allows. Some centres also screen for methicillin sensitive *Staphylococcus aureus* (MSSA) and offer decolonisation prior to cardiac surgery or insertion of ventricular assist devices (VAD). Screening for other resistant organisms is carried out according to local and national recommendations but may include vancomycin resistant enterococci (VRE), carbapenemase producing Enterobacteriaceae (CPE), multidrug resistant (MDR) *Acinetobacter spp*., Enterobacteriaceae producing extended spectrum β-lactamases (ESBL) or AmpC β-lactamases. The frequency and nature of who is screened depends on local resistance patterns, carriage rates, and healthcare associated infection rates within the local setting and those of referring hospitals. It is important to note that any screening programme should be monitored on a regular basis and action taken when carriage or clinical infection rates exceed those expected for a local unit. The implementation of an enhanced screening programme also depends on what action can be taken if patients are found to be positive. This may involve commencement of specific infection control precautions and/or alteration in prophylactic regimens for surgery, VAD insertion or transplantation to ensure that the antibiotic cover at the time of surgery covers the resistant organism. One very important factor in being able to action positive screening results within critical care units is the availability of side rooms.

Microscopy and Culture

Microscopy and culture of samples continues to be the mainstay of microbial diagnostics. Microscopy is a quick, useful test indicating the presence of organisms from normally sterile sites, for example blood, pericardial fluid or surgical samples, and also for determining smear positivity in the case of *Mycobacterium tuberculosis*. Microscopy is less useful at determining the presence of pathogens in samples from non-sterile sites, i.e. the respiratory tract. Urine microscopy can aid in the differentiation between infection or contamination of the sample by the presence of significant numbers of pus cells. Microscopy of urine samples is not helpful in catheterised patients. Culture of the sample is more informative than microscopy to enable organism identification and sensitivity testing. However, this takes time and is influenced by transport times, storage conditions and prior antibiotic use. Culture results from non-sterile sites require a degree of interpretation, taking into account the expected normal flora from the specific site. Furthermore, there are some organisms that by their very nature are difficult to culture, or cannot be cultured or present a danger to laboratory staff. Thereby other methods of organism identification are used.

Antibiotic Susceptibility Testing

Performing antimicrobial sensitivity testing is another important function of the microbiology laboratory. The aim is to inform antimicrobial treatment decisions and detect antimicrobial resistance. Sensitivity testing requires live organisms and is performed using a variety of testing methods. Manual disc diffusion assays are the mainstay of antimicrobial testing for most organisms in UK laboratories, alongside gradient diffusion methods (including E-tests). Disc testing provides a qualitative measurement, recording the organism as sensitive, intermediate or resistant. More qualitative methods that provide a more accurate minimum inhibitory concentration (MIC) are required for organisms that give borderline results with disc diffusion methods or where a more accurate measure is required, for example in management of endocarditis. In addition to manual methods, there are automated methods commercially available.

Therapeutic Drug Monitoring for Antimicrobials

This is another important function traditionally carried out in microbiology laboratories but now often performed in blood science laboratories. Drug monitoring is important in drugs with a narrow therapeutic window where it is important to ensure maximum drug dosing with minimum risk of toxicity, for example aminoglycosides and glycopeptides. Pharmacokinetics and dynamics of various antimicrobials vary in vivo, for poorly understood reasons, in many cardiothoracic critical care patients. This is especially true in patients on ECMO where maximum licensed drug dosing regimens may need to be used in drugs with a wide therapeutic window. The alternation of PK/PD is poorly understood in this set of patients but drugs may be sequestered or broken down as a result of the ECMO circuit. Dosing regimens may need to be adjusted based on levels informed by therapeutic drug monitoring.

New Technologies

Speed is an essential factor in the diagnosis of sepsis and in other acute organ dysfunction states, i.e. severe respiratory failure, where the appropriate management of infection affects outcome. One of the issues is that the diagnosis of sepsis can be difficult as clinical signs can overlap with other non-infectious systemic inflammatory states and blood culture results may take days to complete. New technologies being developed and introduced into clinical laboratories have the potential to speed up microbial diagnosis within cardiothoracic units.

Molecular Testing

The development of polymerase chain reaction (PCR) and other nucleic acid-based amplification technologies (NAATs) over the last 20 years has helped to address some of the downsides of culture. The introduction of such molecular techniques into routine clinical microbiology laboratories has revolutionised microbial diagnostics. These techniques are now used as the primary diagnostic method for HIV, hepatitis viruses and respiratory viruses. Amplifying and detecting microbial and genetic sequences within a prepared clinical sample improves speed, sensitivity and specificity of microbial testing and is not so affected by specimen transport times or prior antibiotic use. The range of organisms that molecular tests are routinely used for has expanded from HIV, hepatitis viruses and respiratory viruses into bacterial, fungal, parasitic and atypical agents. These techniques are not only used for the diagnosis of infectious disease but also in the detection of drug resistant genes. These methods, with the development of nanotechnology, are also now used for point-of-care testing.

Sequencing

Several sequence based methods have been used to identify microorganisms directly from clinical samples including blood cultures, biopsies and heart valves. The cost of these tests is high compared with conventional diagnostic methods and they are best used on samples from normally sterile sites. However, amplification and sequencing of 16S rRNA present within heart valve samples where no organism has been cultured has changed microbial diagnostics in culture-negative endocarditis. Amplification and sequencing of 18S rRNA is also of value in the identification of fungal pathogens from samples from normally sterile sites, for example pleural fluid, lung biopsy. These techniques are being researched and developed for use in samples from other sites, including the lower respiratory tract.

Mass Spectrometry

Matrix-assisted laser desorption/ionisation time-of-flight mass spectrometry (MALDI TOF MS) is being used currently for the routine identification of bacterial colonies from positive cultures. Although it requires culture of the organism and sensitivity testing by conventional means, it provides rapid turnaround of pathogen identification with a minimal amount of labour compared with traditional identification methods.

Microarrays

This 'test-all' approach allows identification of a large panel of microbial pathogens from a single sample on a single test card within one test run. Cards can be developed to cover a whole range of relevant pathogens based on a syndromic approach. This may prove useful in the infection diagnosis of patients with severe respiratory failure requiring ECMO. The cost of this test is comparable to the combined cost of running the PCR tests individually by conventional means, but has potential clinical benefit in terms of ease of requesting, sampling and turnaround times.

Interpretation of Results

The finding of an organism from a normally sterile site is usually diagnostic of infection with that pathogen. Some organisms are only ever present when causing an infection, therefore their detection implies infection, for example, *Mycobacterium tuberculosis*. Other organisms detected from non-sterile sites require a degree of interpretation of the result to consider when the organism is a pathogen, when it is normally found at that site or when it represents contamination of the sample. The diagnosis of infection in these circumstances needs to be taken into consideration with the clinical picture, inflammatory markers, presence of fever and localising signs. If the organism is repeatedly isolated and pus cells are seen on microscopy, the evidence points to the likelihood of the organism being pathogenic.

Liaison with Medical Microbiologists

Close liaison on a regular basis between clinical teams and infection specialists is essential to optimise infection prevention, diagnosis and management of cardiothoracic patients. Such specialist input will not only optimise appropriate use of antibiotics and infection control management, but will also assist with specimen requesting, provision of laboratory services, appropriate use of technologies, and rapid interpretation and communication of critical results.

Learning Points

- Infections in cardiothoracic intensive care units are common and antimicrobial drugs are used widely and sometimes unnecessarily.
- Correct diagnosis of infections requires careful physical examination of patients as well as appropriate microbiology testing.
- New technologies being developed and introduced into clinical laboratories have the potential to speed up microbial diagnosis within cardiothoracic units.
- Close liaison on a regular basis between clinical teams and infection specialists is essential.
- Such specialist input will not only optimise appropriate use of antibiotics and infection control management, but will also assist with specimen requesting, provision of laboratory services, appropriate use of technologies, and rapid interpretation and communication of critical results.

Further Reading

Caliendo AM, Gilbert DN, Ginocchio CC, et al. Better tests, better care: improved diagnostics for infectious diseases. *Clinical Infectious Diseases*. 2013; 57(Suppl 3): S139–S170.

Dellinger RP, Levy MM, Rhodes A, et al. Surviving sepsis campaign: international guidelines for management of severe sepsis and septic shock. *Intensive Care Medicine*. 2013; 39: 165–288.

Kohler P, Kuster SP, Bloemberg G, et al. Healthcare-associated prosthetic heart valve, aortic vascular graft, and disseminated *Mycobacterium chimaera* infections subsequent to open heart surgery. *European Heart Journal*. 2015; 36: 2745–2753.

Liesenfeld O, Lehman L, Hunfeld KP, et al. Molecular diagnosis of sepsis: new aspects and recent developments. *European Journal of Microbiology and Immunology*. 2014; 4: 1–25.

Robich MP, Sabik JF, Houghtaling PL, et al. Prolonged effect of postoperative infectious complications on survival after cardiac surgery. *Annals of Thoracic Surgery*. 2015; 99: 1591–1599.

Schweizer ML, Chiang HY, Septimus E, et al. Association of a bundled intervention with surgical site infections among patients undergoing cardiac, hip or knee surgery. *Journal of the American Medical Association*. 2015; 313: 2162–2171.

Tsai D, Lipman J, Roberts JA. Pharmacokinetic/pharmacodynamic considerations for the optimization of antimicrobial delivery in the critcally ill. *Current Opinion in Critical Care*. 2015; 21: 412–420.

Vondracek MI, Sartipy U, Aufwerber E, et al. 16S rDNA sequencing of valve tissue improves microbiological diagnosis in surgically treated patients with infective endocarditis. *Journal of Infection*. 2011; 62: 472–478.

Wolk DM, Dunne(Jr) WM. New technologies in clinical microbiology. *Journal of Clinical Microbiology*. 2011; 49(suppl 9): S62–S67.

MCQs

True or False

1. **Microscopy has been superseded as a method used in bacteriology laboratories.**
2. **Molecular testing can only be used for organism identification and not for detection of antimicrobial resistance.**
3. **Sequencing techniques are best used for samples from normally sterile sites.**
4. **The length of time a sample takes to get to the laboratory does not affect the ability to culture pathogens.**
5. **Finding an organism in a sample always indicates an infection.**

Exercise answers are available on p.467. Alternatively, take the test online at www.cambridge.org/CardiothoracicMCQ

Chapter 7

Radiology for Cardiothoracic Intensivists

Kristian H Mortensen, Peter A Barry and Deepa Gopalan

Introduction

Diagnostic imaging of patients in the cardiothoracic intensive care unit (ICU) can pose unique challenges. Where possible, the patient should be imaged in situ using mobile chest X-ray (CXR) and ultrasound, including transthoracic (TTE) and transoesophageal echocardiography (TOE), unless computed tomography (CT) is specifically required. An outline of the advantages and limitations of each imaging modality is followed by presentation of the optimal use and escalation of imaging to diagnose specific cardio-respiratory conditions in the context of this highly specialised setting.

Cardiothoracic Imaging Modalities

Chest X-ray

Chest X-ray (CXR) has a high diagnostic accuracy for the assessment of the position of lines, tubes and drains. When compared with this area and imaging of the lungs and pleural spaces, the accuracy of CXR is less impressive for cardiovascular disease, and hence CXR should never delay other definitive cardiovascular imaging in the ICU patient. In established cardiorespiratory disease, serial CXR has an additional role in the investigation of evolving respiratory compromise or non-response to treatment. Despite ease of use, daily routine bedside CXR is no longer encouraged because this does not appear to improve outcomes in ICU patients compared with a directed approach.

In the majority of ICU patients, the CXR is acquired bedside with the patient in the semi-erect or supine position. This has several effects: (a) This gives an anteroposterior (AP) projection, with apparent enlargement of cardiac and mediastinal structures compared to the posteroanterior (PA) projection obtained in the ambulatory setting; (b) An optimal full-inspiratory view is rarely attainable; (c) Distribution of fluid and air in the pleural space is altered, where a pneumothorax will locate to the anterior pleural space and pleural effusions settle posteriorly on supine CXR, albeit loculations may limit the free movement of pleural collections particularly. This may happen when there is longstanding pleural disease, prior malignancy or previous surgical intervention, and ultrasound or CT will often be preferable; (d) Forward slumping may obscure apical pulmonary disease or pneumothorax; (e) Rotation – as judged by medial clavicles not being equidistant from the midline relative to the spinous processes – may mimic mediastinal disease; and (f) Artefacts such as skin folds, hair braids, asymmetrical soft tissues, monitoring leads and other radio-opaque equipment overlying the field of interest, may degrade the diagnostic quality and should be minimised prior to imaging.

Ultrasound

Bedside thoracic ultrasound is predominantly used for assessment of pleural effusions, and to confirm CXR findings. Ultrasound may give clues to the nature of a pleural effusion, and has an important role in image-guided thoracic interventions. In experienced hands, ultrasound can also assess for pneumothorax, but emphysematous lung has the potential to cause misdiagnosis and ultrasound is of limited practical use. Extensive subcutaneous emphysema and severe obesity may limit adequate visualisation of the pleural spaces. Echocardiography is invaluable in the assessment of cardiac valves and chamber function as well as any pericardial disease, and has been dealt with in a dedicated chapter (see Chapter 3).

Computed Tomography

Thoracic CT is of immense value in the assessment of the ICU patient, particularly when CXR findings are equivocal or if complex disease processes are suspected. CT adds valuable information to CXR findings in up to 70%, changing management in 22%. The cross-sectional nature of CT allows more detailed interrogation of disease processes and can also provide image guidance for interventions. CT has a particular role when cardiac and great vessel disease such as pulmonary embolus (PE) and acute aortic syndrome are suspected, but is also a key diagnostic tool for the diagnosis of postoperative thoracic collections, pleural or pulmonary sepsis, malignancy, complications of mechanical ventilation, concurrent pulmonary pathologies, and in the assessment of life support device related complications. The diagnostic yield of CT must be weighed against the risks of transporting the ICU patient to the imaging department. Potentially nephrotoxic intravenous iodinated contrast medium should be used with caution, and where potential benefit outweighs risk, attention to pre-emptive renal protection and coordination of the timing of contrast administration with haemodialysis are helpful. Radiation constraints are less of an issue in this setting, however repeated CT imaging should be monitored.

Imaging for Cardiac Emergencies

Chest Pain

Chest pain in the ICU requires urgent appraisal. The differential diagnosis is varied, ranging from life threatening emergencies to more benign conditions. A clue to the aetiology can be gained by focused history, physical examination and electrocardiogram, with imaging playing a smaller role.

Acute Coronary Syndrome

A minority of patients, particularly elderly and females with risk factors for atherosclerosis such as hypertension, chronic renal disease or previous cerebrovascular events, may sustain an acute myocardial infarction while being hospitalised for another reason. The first step in its management is expeditious recognition to optimise myocardial salvage and reduce mortality by a prompt attempt of reperfusion therapy. Non-invasive imaging such as ECG-gated cardiac CT is not recommended as it will not only delay consideration for primary percutaneous coronary intervention (PCI) or fibrinolysis but also often will be non-diagnostic, particularly in patients with cardiogenic shock, heart failure or ventricular tachyarrhythmia.

Acute Aortic Syndrome

Aortic dissection, intramural haematoma and penetrating ulcer together comprise acute aortic syndrome (Figure 7.1), which is classically encountered in patients with systemic hypertension or those with predisposing factors such as connective tissue disease. However, it can also occur in healthy vessels as a consequence of iatrogenic injury following intra-arterial catheterisation and intra-aortic balloon pump insertion. Potentially devastating consequences of aortic dissection include extension into the aortic annulus leading to severe aortic regurgitation, rupture into the pericardium causing cardiac tamponade or multiorgan ischaemia (coronary, cerebral, spinal, and visceral).

CXR has limited value in diagnosing acute aortic syndrome, with a sensitivity of 64% and a specificity of 86%. Typical features are useful when present, such as upper mediastinal widening, double aortic contrast and discrepancy between the diameters of the ascending and descending aorta, displacement of the trachea and of the left main bronchus, ill definition of the aortopulmonary window, left apical cap, pleural effusion, haemothorax and widening of the left paravertebral sulcus, but their absence cannot exclude the diagnosis. The CXR may be completely normal in 11–15%. Echocardiography has immense value in unstable patients as it is portable, quick and can even be used in theatres to facilitate diagnosis. The aortic root, valve and proximal ascending aorta can all be assessed with relative ease using echocardiography, which also has the ability to document ancillary findings such as impairment of ventricular function and haemopericardium. A major limitation of the transthoracic approach, TTE, is the inability to clearly visualise beyond the proximal ascending aorta. The transoesophageal approach, TOE, has a much higher sensitivity of up to 98% for detecting entry tear sites, coronary and great vessel involvement and differential flow characteristics in the false lumen. TOE, however, requires sedation and also cannot image the entire thoracic aorta.

Multidetector CT has sensitivity and specificity of almost 100%. The high negative predictive value in combination with rapid image acquisition and wide availability has made CT the investigation of choice in an acute setting. Triple rule out is a new concept that can be used in the same study to evaluate the aorta, coronary arteries and pulmonary vasculature. It requires ECG-gating and should ideally be performed using a

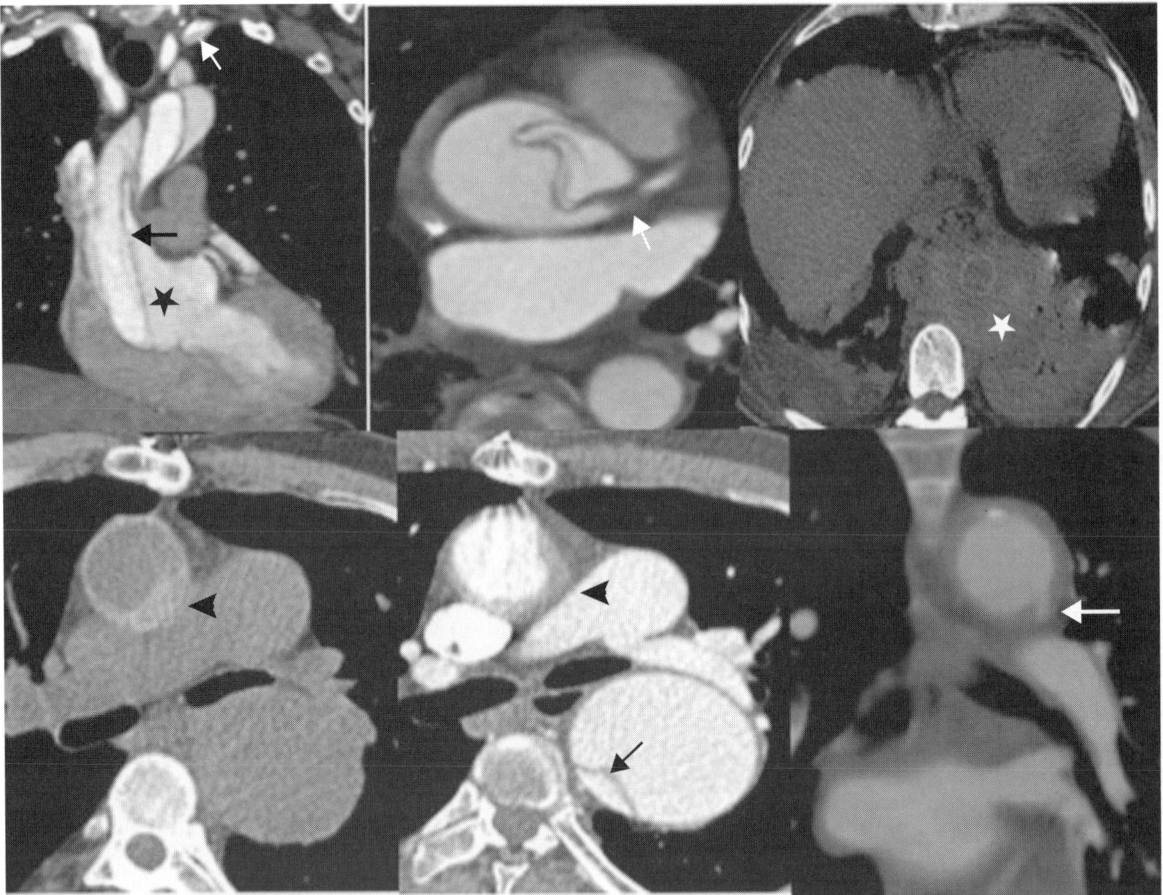

Figure 7.1 Acute aortic syndrome. Top panel, far left and middle images: ECG-gated CT in a 65 year old male with acute type A aortic dissection. The aortic root is dilated (black star) with a dissection flap (block black arrow) that extends into neck vessels (thin white arrow) and the ostium of the left main stem coronary artery (middle image, block white arrow). Top panel, far right image: rupture of descending thoracic aneurysm with high attenuation blood (white star) around the aorta. Bottom panel: different CT findings of acute aortic syndrome in different patients. Intramural haematoma with a rim of high attenuation material on the unenhanced CT (far left image); aneurysmal descending aorta with a dissection flap (middle image, thin black arrow); small penetrating ulcer in the descending thoracic aorta (far right image, notched arrow).

scanner with 64 slice or higher detector number. The need for simultaneous opacification of pulmonary and systemic circulation can be particularly challenging in haemodynamically unstable patients and in some circumstances it is better to do one focused examination rather than an all-in-one approach. Initial unenhanced data are useful to demonstrate crescentic foci of high attenuation in the aortic wall due to intramural haematoma or a thrombosed false lumen. On a contrast-enhanced examination, the classical feature of dissection is an intimal flap that separates the true lumen that is contiguous with the undissected vessel from the false lumen. The false lumen generally has a larger cross-sectional area, thin linear strands of low attenuation material representing the incompletely sheared media (cobweb sign) and a wedge of haematoma (beak sign) that forms to create a space for the development of the false lumen. Occasionally, circumferential dissection can be complicated by intimo-intimal intussusception (windsock sign). Secondary features of aortic dissection include displacement of intimal calcification, delayed enhancement or thrombosis of the false lumen and complications such as mediastinal and pericardial haematoma and compromise from coronary, neck vessel, mesenteric, renal and peripheral vascular involvement. Penetrating ulcers are shown as focal crater-like pouching of the aortic wall with irregular edges in the presence of extensive

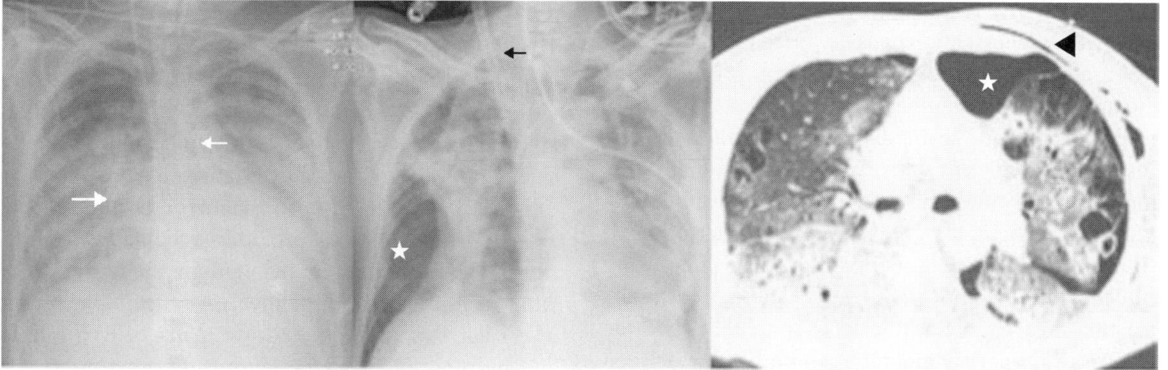

Figure 7.2 Pulmonary oedema and acute respiratory distress syndrome with pneumothorax. Far left image: CXR with pulmonary oedema in a 60 year old male in the aftermath of acute myocardial infarction. Note the intra-aortic balloon pump (block white arrow) and Swan–Ganz catheter (thin arrow). Middle image: CXR of a 45 year old male with acute respiratory distress syndrome on extracorporeal membrane oxygenation (black block arrow). There is a supine, right-sided pneumothorax (white star) with deepened costophrenic sulcus and contralateral mediastinal shift suggestive of tension pneumothorax. Far right image: axial CT thorax in a different patient with acute respiratory distress syndrome. Note the gravitational, dependent consolidation in the posterior lung segments with diffuse ground-glass opacification and fibrosis. There is a left pneumothorax (white star) and surgical emphysema (black arrow head).

aortic atheroma, which is most common in the middle and distal thirds of the thoracic aorta.

CT is the imaging modality of choice for suspected rupture. A peripheral hyperattenuation crescent within the thrombus of an aneurysm on an unenhanced CT is a sign of acute or impending rupture, as is the close apposition of the posterior aortic wall to the spine (draped aorta sign). Rupture into mediastinal, pericardial or pleural spaces gives rise to high attenuation haematoma in the respective anatomical space. Fistulous communication with the tracheobronchial tree or oesophagus is a recognised complication. CT may not show the communication, but development of haemoptysis/haematemesis and new onset of pulmonary haemorrhage/consolidation should raise the clinical suspicion.

Pulmonary Oedema

Pulmonary oedema may be hydrostatic as seen in cardiac disease, renal failure or overhydration. Alternatively, it may be non-cardiogenic due to increased permeability oedema as encountered in acute respiratory distress syndrome (ARDS) (Figure 7.2). Differentiating cardiogenic and non-cardiogenic pulmonary oedema is arduous, and most optimally would require measurement of pulmonary capillary wedge pressure. Image findings in hydrostatic pulmonary oedema depend on the degree of elevation of the pulmonary capillary wedge pressure: (a) no abnormality (<12 mmHg); (b) early oedema (12–15 mmHg) with vascular engorgement and peribronchovascular cuffing; (c) interstitial oedema (15–25 mmHg) with progressive blurring of the pulmonary vessels with engorgement of peribronchovascular spaces, Kerley lines and subpleural effusions; and (d) alveolar oedema (> 25 mmHg) with nodular or acinar areas of increased opacity that evolve into frank consolidation. CXR can detect the majority of these changes and is often adequate, particularly when the morphological findings are complemented by haemodynamic data. CT is reserved for cases where there is a need to distinguish hydrostatic oedema from other causes. The combination of upper lobe predominant ground-glass opacification with a central distribution and central airspace consolidation favours hydrostatic oedema. Conversely, ARDS classically gives rise to a gravitational anteroposterior density gradient within the lung due to dense consolidation in the dependent region and normal or hyperexpanded lung in the non-dependent regions, which merge into a background of diffuse ground-glass opacification. Additionally, ARDS persists for days to weeks, does not respond to diuretic therapy and may progress to a reticular pattern due to secondary fibrosis.

Cardiogenic Shock

Cardiogenic shock is characterised by systemic hypotension and tissue hypoxia secondary to decreased cardiac output. Diagnostic evaluation should be carried out in conjunction with resuscitative efforts. Ultrasonography and TTE are essential bedside imaging modalities, which allow rapid assessment of multiple organ systems including cardiac chambers for biventricular function, proximal aorta for aortic dissection, pleural and pericardial spaces for effusions, and the abdominal cavity for peritoneal fluid and organ appearances. A portable CXR is useful for the exclusion of pneumothorax, whilst targeted imaging such as thoracic CT should be considered in patients in whom the aetiology of the circulatory failure remains unclear despite initial bedside imaging. Coronary angiography should not be delayed in patients with suspected myocardial infarction who might be candidates for revascularisation.

Pericardial Tamponade

Tamponade can occur due to collection of fluid, blood, pus, air or soft tissue within the pericardial space (Figure 7.3). Although challenging, it is foremost a clinical diagnosis and must be considered in all patients with unexplained cardiogenic shock or pulseless electric activity. TTE is the most appropriate initial imaging modality as it facilitates assessment of the haemodynamic impact and may guide diagnostic and therapeutic pericardiocentesis. Progressively enlarging cardiac silhouette resulting in a globular featureless water-bottle appearance is a characteristic feature on serial CXRs. However, tamponade due to pneumopericardium can cause reduction in the size of the cardiac silhouette with sharp outlining of the pericardium by radiolucent air. CT is not routinely indicated for the diagnosis and should be reserved for cases where there is diagnostic uncertainty. The attenuation value of the collection on a precontrast scan can give a clue to its nature, with haemopericardium typically being of higher attenuation than simple fluid. Imaging features such as compression of the cardiac chambers and coronary sinus, straightening of the right heart border, interventricular septal bowing, distension of the systemic veins and reflux of contrast medium into the azygos vein may be seen even on non-ECG gated CT. Although the addition of gating will improve the anatomical and functional delineation, the need for prompt treatment should override any potential delays in image acquisition. Percutaneous drainage should be performed using image guidance, and echocardiography, fluoroscopy or CT have all been shown to be successful, with the relative use of each technique much depending on the institutional and individual preferences.

Right Ventricular Failure

The aetiology varies from worsening of compensated right ventricular failure, frequently seen in chronic left-sided heart or pre-existing lung disease such as emphysema, to acute right ventricular failure in massive pulmonary embolus, right-sided myocardial infarction, ARDS or sepsis (Figure 7.4). Pulmonary artery catheterisation provides reliable and continuous monitoring of haemodynamic parameters whilst echocardiography allows for bedside evaluation of cardiac function although estimates of RV systolic and pulmonary artery pressure can be inaccurate in patients with chronic lung disease and those undergoing IPPV. CXR is of limited value and can demonstrate generic features such as cardiomegaly and proximal pulmonary artery dilatation. It can be useful for tracking of lung parenchymal changes like atelectasis or consolidation and pleural effusions, and for the assessment of lines, tubes and drains. CT can be more useful in detailing this pathology.

Pulmonary Embolus

CT pulmonary angiography is the imaging modality of choice in suspected PE. With optimisation of contrast enhancement (Hounsfield unit >200 in the main pulmonary artery) and minimisation of motion artefact, the high spatial resolution of modern CT scanners allows for the detection of emboli down to 2–3 mm. Acute emboli can occlude the entire lumen, or form central filling defects surrounded by a rim of contrast, causing the 'polo mint' sign on images perpendicular to the long axis of a vessel and 'railway track' sign on longitudinal images. When peripheral, thrombi form an acute angle to the vessel wall as opposed to chronic thrombus that is eccentric with obtuse angle to the fibrosed arterial wall. The presence of stenosis, intravascular webs, bronchial collaterals and mosaic perfusion patterns implies chronic thromboembolic disease. Peripheral wedge-shaped areas of hyperattenuation representing infarcts can be seen in acute as well as chronic thromboembolic disease. Obstruction of more than 30% of the pulmonary circulation can raise the pulmonary vascular resistance sufficiently to produce significant pulmonary hypertension. CT signs of RV strain include a right-to-left ventricular diameter ratio >1.0, leftwards septal bowing, abrupt increase in size of the azygos vein, widening of the vascular pedicle, and reflux of contrast medium into a distended inferior vena cava and hepatic veins.

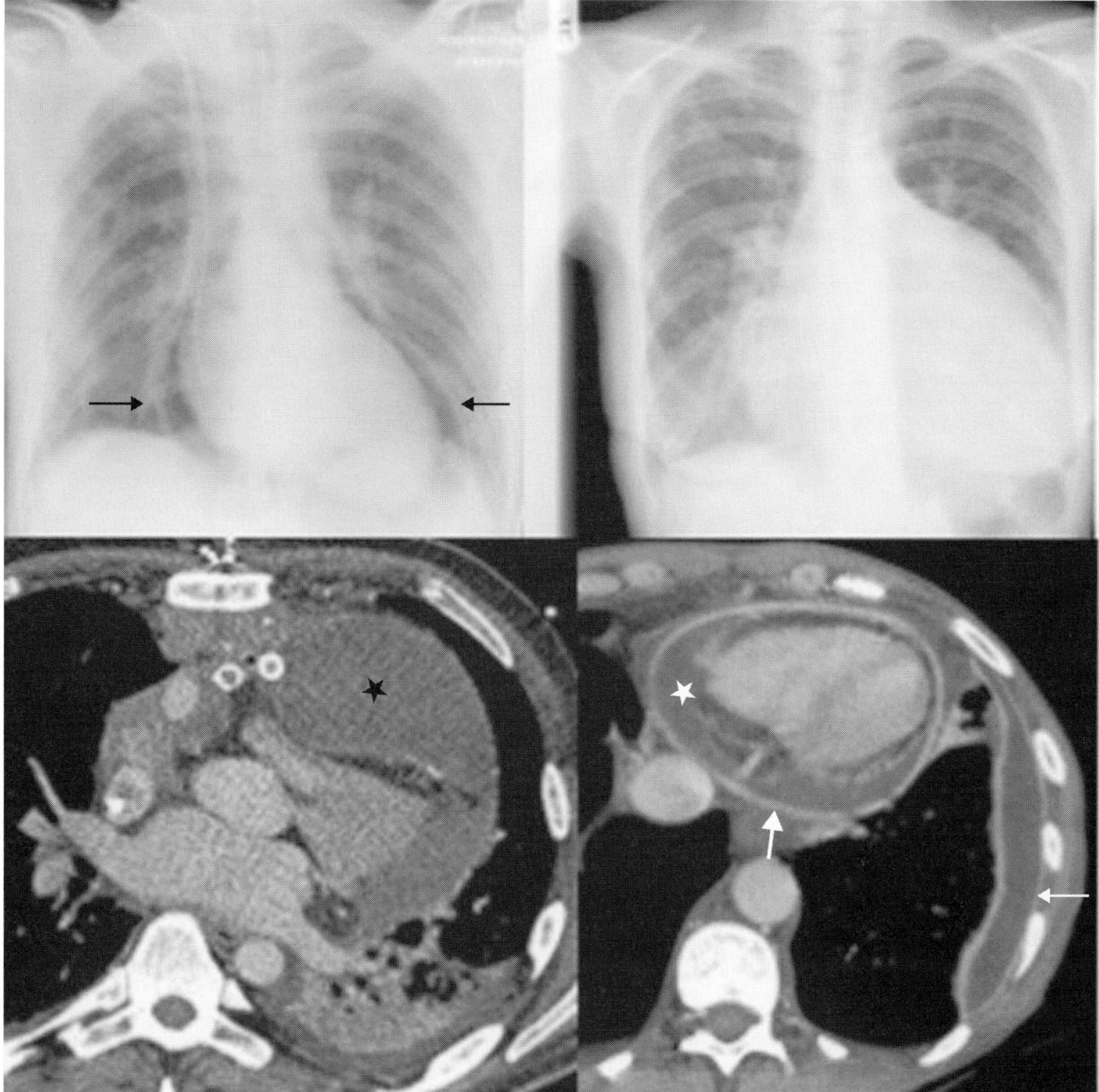

Figure 7.3 Pericardial tamponade. Top panel: pneumopericardium (left image, black arrows) and globular cardiac silhouette secondary to pericardial effusion (right image) on CXR. Lower panel: pericardial collections on CT. Haematoma (left image, black star) with compression of the underlying cardiac chambers, and ventricular assist device catheters in situ. Circumferential pericardial thickening and enhancement (right image, block white arrow) secondary to a purulent collection (white star) with an enhancing left pleural collection (thin white arrow).

Complications of Cardiac Surgery

The use of cardiopulmonary bypass during cardiac surgery results in a distinct group of postoperative complications. Unexplained hypotension, tachycardia and pulmonary oedema should raise the suspicion of post-surgical cardiac dysfunction. Coronary artery graft occlusion, prosthetic valve malfunction, pericardial tamponade and left ventricular outflow tract obstruction are some potential culprits. In addition to haemodynamic assessment and ECG, TTE is often the most useful initial imaging modality. CXR excludes non-cardiac complications such as pneumothorax, haemothorax, pneumonia, atelectasis, pleural effusions and diaphragmatic injury, and malposition of lines and

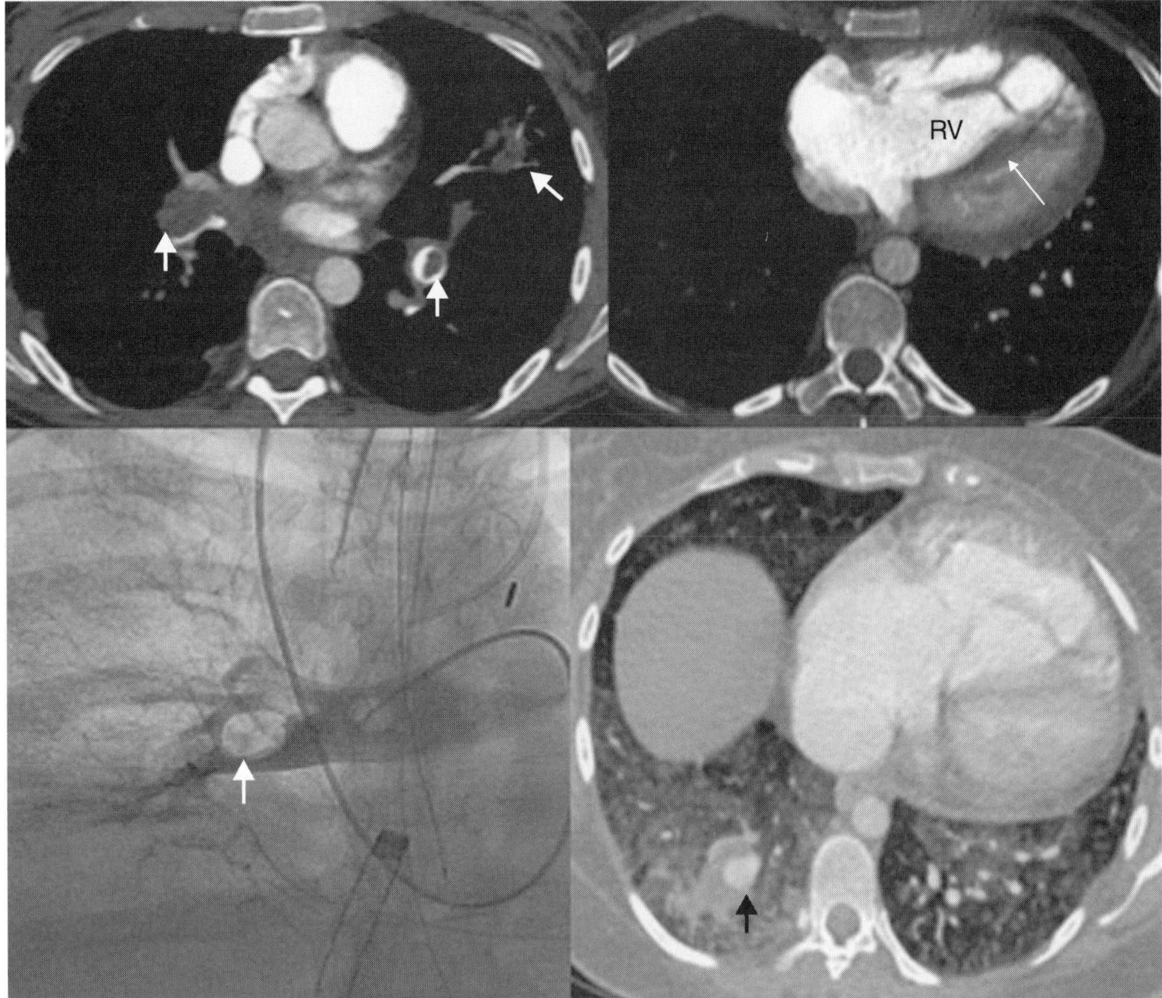

Figure 7.4 Right ventricular failure. Top panel: massive, acute pulmonary emboli (block white arrows) with right ventricular (RV) enlargement alongside interventricular septal bowing (thin white arrow) and a pulmonary infarction (notched arrow). Bottom panel: catheter angiography with thrombolysis for acute pulmonary embolus (left image, white arrow) and another patient with idiopathic pulmonary arterial hypertension with right-sided cardiac chamber dilatation and right ventricular hypertrophy (right image). The latter patient had acute decompensation with development of pneumonia in the right lower lobe complicated by formation of segmental pulmonary artery pseudo-aneurysm (right image, black block arrow).

tubes. Neurological complications such as ischaemic cardiovascular insults or intracranial haemorrhage will often require an unenhanced CT for confirmation. Bowel ischaemia can be precipitated by atheroembolism, intracardiac thrombus, atrial fibrillation, acute aortic syndrome and tissue hypoperfusion. Arterial and portal venous phase CT of the abdomen and pelvis is often needed but since up to 30% of patients who have undergone cardiac surgery can suffer from acute renal injury, iodinated contrast medium should be used with caution. Some abdominal conditions such as cholecystitis can be diagnosed by ultrasound, whilst persistent elevation of inflammatory markers and metabolic disturbances that require exclusion of intra-abdominal sepsis will require a CT for more comprehensive assessment.

Respiratory Emergencies

CXR is the first line imaging modality, in the setting of both de novo and persistent or worsening oxygenation levels. CT offers superior accuracy for the underlying cause, but serial bedside radiography may in many instances be sufficient.

Desaturation Associated with Pleural Abnormalities

Pneumothorax

Pneumothoraces are common in the ICU but their recognition is lacking with up to 30% missed on CXR. Even small pneumothoraces are important because they may rapidly become clinically significant during positive pressure ventilation. The volume of the pneumothorax dictates the associated pulmonary changes, which range from small areas of atelectasis to extensive collapse. Imaging of tension pneumothorax, with ensuing circulatory compromise, must not delay emergency decompression. If CXR has been obtained, signs of tension include extensive lucency of the hemithorax with contralateral mediastinal shift and ipsilateral diaphragmatic flattening.

Stereotypical CXR signs of pneumothorax include a medial position of the visceral pleural line, with absent bronchovascular markings lateral to this line. The air typically collects at the apex when erect or semi-erect but the movement of air may be impeded by loculations. The supine CXR is more challenging, with signs of pneumothorax including the following: (a) a deep, sometimes tongue-like, lateral costophrenic sulcus; (b) sharp demarcation of the diaphragm or cardiomediastinal silhouette; (c) gas outlining the costophrenic or cardiophrenic sulci; and (d) hyperlucent right upper quadrant. Skinfolds can be mistaken for a pneumothorax, but should be differentiated by noting continuation of the line beyond the thoracic cavity and the presence of vascular markings beyond the apparent line. Previous imaging may show the presence of a bulla in emphysematous patients. A lateral decubitus, horizontal shoot-through or expiratory CXR may help clarify the presence of a suspected pneumothorax when there is doubt. However, the sensitivity of CT and its ability to assess the underlying cause make it the diagnostic modality of choice in these situations. CT is also more sensitive to pneumomediastinum, which in the ventilated patient may be due to barotrauma, and CT may be preferred when extensive subcutaneous emphysema hinders the ability to diagnose underlying pneumothorax.

Pleural Effusion

Fluid in the pleural space is exceedingly common in the critically ill, and may be a transudate, exudate, pus, blood or chyle. Blunting of the costophrenic angles is a sine qua non on the erect or semi-erect CXR, and there may be associated volume loss of the adjacent lung. When the effusion accumulates in the subpulmonary space, the findings include: (a) a seemingly elevated hemidiaphragm with a lateral shift of the diaphragmatic apex and blunted costophrenic angle; and (b) increased density below the diaphragm with no bronchovascular markings and a gastric air bubble that is situated well below the apparent diaphragm. On supine CXR, the costophrenic angle may not be blunted but there may be: (a) a hazy 'veil-like' opacity, with bronchovascular markings visible, due to dependent layering of the fluid in the paravertebral gutters and posterior pleural space; and (b) an apical cap (when this is most dependent) and fissural thickening. The presence of gas locules and loculations should raise the possibility of empyema (Figure 7.5). CT better characterises the complex pleural collection, depicting pleural thickening, enhancement and separation in empyema, and can differentiate hypodense fluid and pus from hyperdense blood, especially important after recent surgery or trauma. The need for sampling is governed by clinical presentation.

On the erect CXR, blunting of a lateral costophrenic angle can be seen with as little as 200 ml but may be absent with as much as 500 ml. The semi-erect CXR is less sensitive to pleural fluid and may miss even moderate effusions. Bedside ultrasound is very useful with the pleural fluid demarcated by either the echogenic visceral pleura or by lung that may be hyperechoic when there is atelectasis, collapse or consolidation. The fluid can have internal echoes, layering and septations depending on its nature and duration. Even though some guidance can be taken from ultrasound appearances (e.g. most transudates are without internal echoes), ultrasound appearances should not be taken as specific to the nature of the fluid. Ultrasound can also aid sampling of pleural fluid and drain insertion, improving the safety of these procedures.

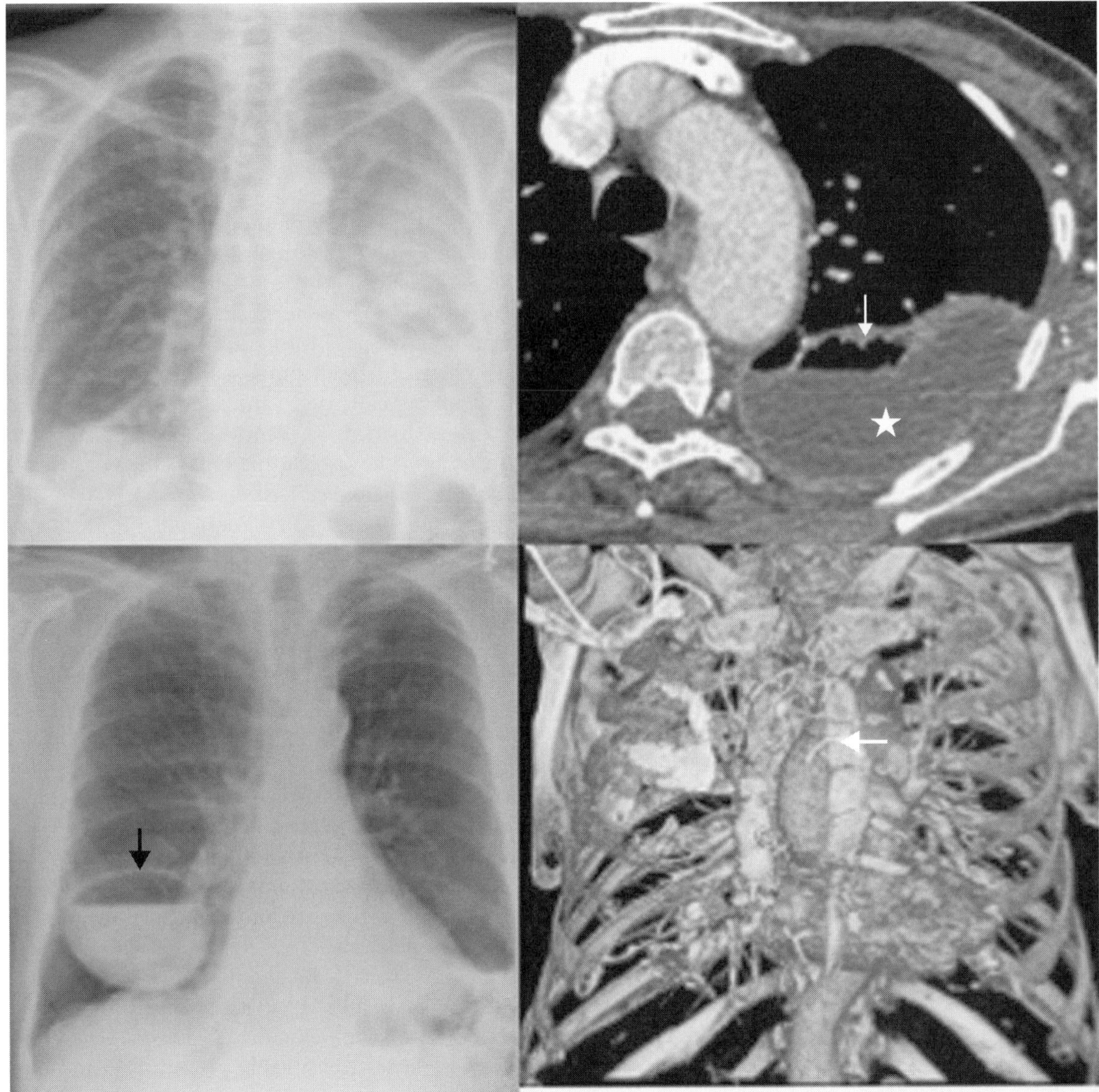

Figure 7.5 Empyema, lung abscess and sepsis. Top panel: CXR and CT demonstrate a loculated left pleural collection with (right image, white star) locules of free air secondary to empyema (right image, thin white arrow). Bottom panel: CXR of a cavitating lung abscess (left image, block black arrow) and left lower lobe collapse with a tiny effusion in an immunocompromised patient. Another profoundly septic patient with recent aortic valve replacement has sternal dehiscence due to osteomyelitis shown on CT (right image, block white arrow). (A black and white version of this figure will appear in some formats. For the colour version, please refer to the plate section.)

Desaturation Associated with Pulmonary Abnormality

Atelectasis and Collapse

Atelectasis and collapse represent pulmonary volume loss, with the latter implying more extensive, lobar involvement. Volume loss is the most common finding on CXR in the ICU setting, often present as subsegmental linear atelectasis in the dependent lower lobes, and resolves spontaneously. CXR findings in collapse and atelectasis will depend on the extent of volume loss but classically are those of increased opacity with (a) loss of contour of the diaphragm, heart or mediastinum, (b) shift of pulmonary fissures, hilar points, mediastinal structures or hemidiaphragm, (c) bronchovascular crowding or (d) hyperinflation of non-affected lung. With smaller atelectasis, for example due to scarring or a patchy area of insufficient surfactant with alveolar collapse, a linear opacity with little volume loss is more typical.

The distinction between obstructive atelectasis, due to endobronchial obstruction or compression, and passive atelectasis, caused by external compression of alveoli, is important. In the ventilated patient, endobronchial obstruction from mucus plugging is a common cause of acute segmental atelectasis or lobar collapse, which responds well to endobronchial intervention. Other causes of obstructive atelectasis include aspiration, inhaled foreign body, blood clots, endotracheal tube malposition and bronchial neoplasm. Passive atelectasis or collapse when air is forced out of the alveoli will necessitate therapeutic measures addressing the underlying cause. Air bronchograms favour an obstructive over a passive process and indicate higher likelihood of successful inflation following bronchoscopy. The differentiation from pneumonia may be difficult, especially on the supine CXR where volume loss is more difficult to assess. Here CT may help by showing relatively reduced enhancement in infective consolidation.

Pneumonia

Pneumonia is common in the ICU with aspiration and mechanical ventilation contributing as risk factors. The radiographic diagnosis of pneumonia can be particularly challenging in the ventilated patient, with as many as 62% with clinical diagnosis of pneumonia not recognised from CXR. Consolidation is the key radiographic finding, occurring when the airspaces have become filled with inflammatory material. The vessels are obscured and air bronchograms appear due to increased visibility of large airways. The increased density of the involved lung leads to effacement of the contours of the structures that it abuts (the diaphragm, mediastinum and heart), which aids in localising consolidation to specific lobes. In addition, a straight line indicates consolidation limited by a fissure. Pleural effusions are common ancillary findings, and in the septic patient the possibility of empyema must always be considered. Pneumonic consolidation may take the form of: (a) lobar pneumonia, classically with diffuse consolidation of a lobe; (b) bronchopneumonia, with more patchy involvement but also limited to a lobe; and (c) interstitial pneumonia, with initially more linear opacities that can have a nodular appearance. Appearances similar to infective consolidation can appear with fluid, blood, aspirate or tissue filling the alveoli, and correlation with markers of sepsis and clinical presentation are essential. Classically, the consolidation caused by pneumonia will take days to improve whereas for instance that due to pulmonary oedema resolves within hours.

In many cases of pneumonia there will be predisposing lung disease, with an acute or chronic insult causing hypoxia. It can be extremely helpful to compare with prior CXRs and to look for underlying pathology within areas of non-consolidated lung. Common associations of acute pneumonic exacerbations on chronic lung disease include emphysema, bronchiectasis and interstitial lung disease, which in the majority of cases will be recognised by CT or CXR. Disease progression can be rapid, and early CT can help diagnose occult disease in patients with persistent sepsis of unknown origin, with as many as 40% of CXRs in immunocompromised patients not demonstrating pneumonic consolidation. CT also has an important role when there is a suspicion of pneumonia related complications such as cavitation, empyema, abscess formation or bronchopleural fistulation. Mediastinal collections are also a differential diagnosis in septic patients, especially in the postoperative patient, and CT should be utilised when findings are inconsistent with pneumonia.

Aspiration

Risk factors include intubation, impaired cough or gag reflex, sedation and enteric tube feeding. Aspiration in the recumbent position most commonly affects the upper lobes (posterior segment) and lower lobes (superior segment). A rapid onset of ill-defined areas of ground-glass opacity, consolidation or nodularity represents acute airway plugging and surrounding inflammatory response, and can be seen on CXR and CT. The imaging findings often increase over the initial 24–48 hours and diminish thereafter. Progression or persistence indicates the development of complications. CT may depict the dependent changes in more detail but its main role is demonstration of suspected cavitation and abscess formation, which are increased in patients who aspirate non-sterile stomach contents.

Acute Respiratory Distress Syndrome

ARDS is a severe form of acute lung injury, where increased capillary permeability causes influx of fluid and protein into the interstitium and alveoli. ARDS may be caused by a whole range of both intrathoracic or extrathoracic disease. The radiological diagnosis of ARDS is, in the appropriate clinical context, made based on bilateral pulmonary opacities in the absence of heart failure. In its classical form, ARDS follows a triphasic pattern: (a) exudative phase (day 1–7), with an initially normal CXR followed by patchy, symmetrical bilateral consolidation; (b) proliferative phase (day 7–14), when the initial changes persist but may take on a more coarse and linear pattern; and (c) fibrotic phase (>15 days), when the changes begin to resolve and may completely resolve or leave the lungs fibrotic. In the exudative phase, appearances are similar to pulmonary oedema but ARDS is indicated when there is a more peripheral and dependent distribution with a lack of response to diuretics. In addition, the patient with ARDS without prior cardiac disease will have normal cardiac size with absence of upper lobe diversion, septal lines and pleural effusions. CT may aid the characterisation of ARDS, showing an anterior-posterior gradient, heterogeneous mixture of ground-glass opacity and consolidation, and bronchial dilation within affected areas. Decreased lung compliance increases the risk of complications of the required positive pressure ventilation, including pneumothorax, interstitial emphysema and pneumomediastinum. This may be surveyed with serial CXRs but when there is extensive disease, pneumothoraces may be extremely difficult to diagnose without the use of CT.

Desaturation Associated with Trauma and Surgery

CT diagnoses 20% more injuries than CXR, in particular pulmonary contusions, aortic injuries and osseous trauma. Many CXR-detected injuries are also upgraded in severity by CT. Nevertheless, bedside CXR maintains an important role for the immediate diagnosis of large pneumothoraces, flail chest, and malpositioned lines and tubes.

Pulmonary contusions are areas of alveolar haemorrhage that occur in intact lung parenchyma, and are most commonly seen in blunt trauma when tearing-shearing forces have been applied. Contusions may become apparent any time from the time of injury until 6 hours after, and can progress during the initial 24–48 hours whereafter they start to resolve over the following 7–10 days. Classically, contusions are ill-defined patchy areas of ground-glass opacity and consolidation that do not adhere to the bronchopulmonary segmental anatomy and often have subpleural sparing. If resolution within the expected timeframe does not occur, then compounding diseases such as pneumonitis from fat embolism, aspiration, ARDS and pneumonia need to be entertained. Lacerations are areas where the lung parenchyma has lost its integrity, which may appear as focal abnormalities on imaging that may be filled with air or blood (pneumatocele or haematoceles, respectively). In the patient with deteriorating oxygenation after initial stabilisation, undiagnosed haemothorax or pneumothorax will need to be excluded using bedside CXR initially. Tracheobronchial tears and bronchopleural fistulation (BPF) are often difficult to detect on initial imaging, and should be suspected with worsening pneumothorax, pneumomediastinum or pleural effusions. Most BPFs are, however, not traumatic but result from surgical intervention (pneumonectomy) or necrotising pneumonia, with other causes including neoplasia and radiotherapy. Radiological findings of BPF include a drop in the air-fluid level exceeding 2 cm during the postoperative period or the reappearance of an air-fluid level in a patient who has undergone pneumonectomy (Figure 7.6).

Postoperative lung torsion (Figure 7.7) can cause rapid clinical deterioration and is due to rotation of a lobe or the whole lung around the hilar structures resulting in compromise of the airways, vasculature and the lymphatic drainage. Rapid opacification of the lung or unusual position of a collapsed lobe on a radiograph should raise the suspicion. CT is often required prior to lung salvage and demonstrates obliteration of the proximal pulmonary artery and accompanying bronchus with poorly enhancing consolidation, ground-glass attenuation, interlobular septal thickening and intralobular linear attenuation with bulging of the neofissure. Traumatic phrenic nerve injury and diaphragmatic rupture may be concealed by positive pressure ventilation and may also need fluoroscopy or CT for confirmation.

Conclusion

The highly specialised setting of the cardiothoracic intensive care unit demands detailed knowledge of the natural history and treatment complications of

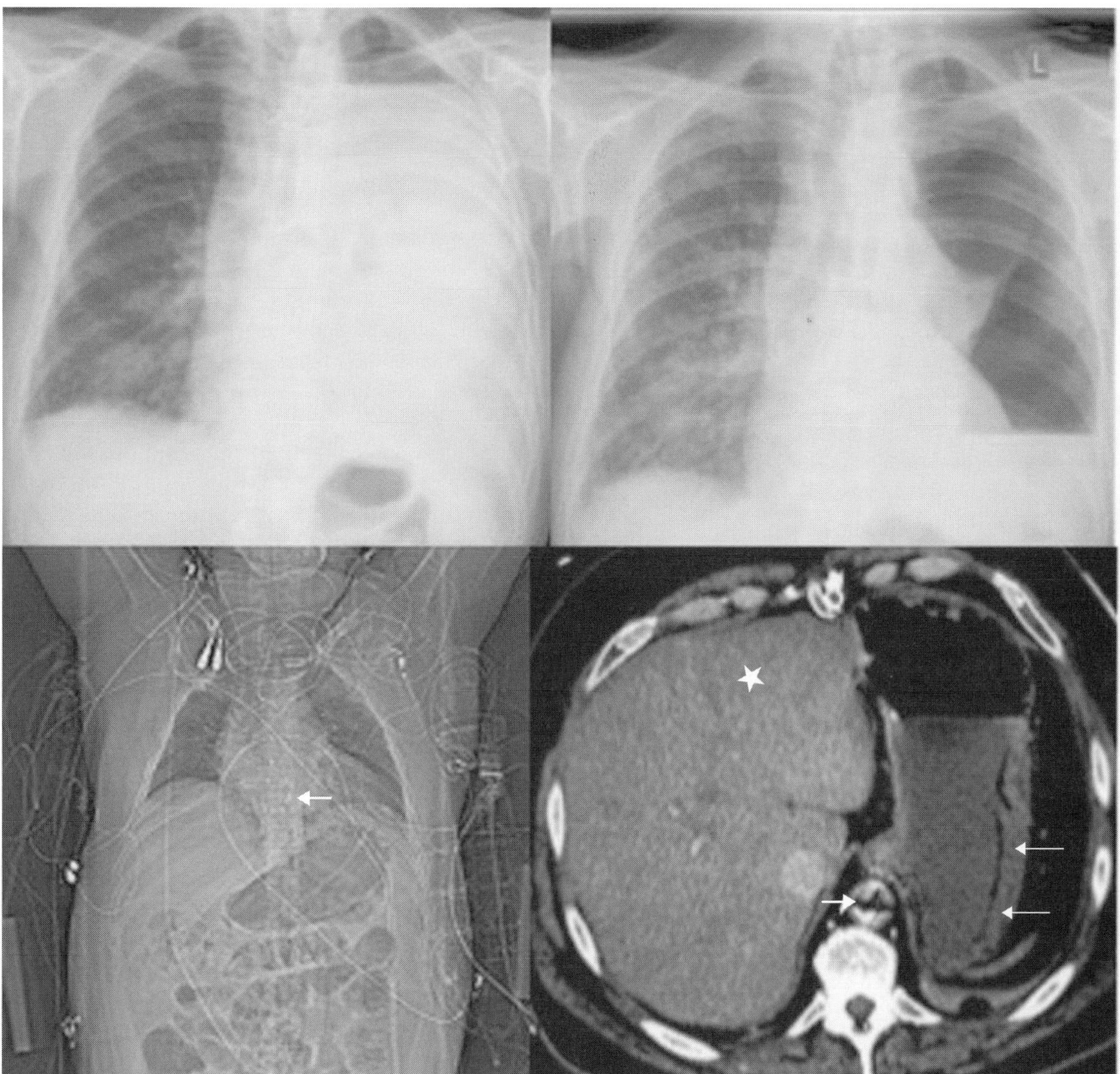

Figure 7.6 Bronchopleural fistula and abdominal ischaemia. Top panel: CXR performed on day 19 (left image) and day 23 (right image) after left pneumonectomy with the drop in the air-fluid level highly suspicious for bronchopleural fistula; this would require CT confirmation. Bottom panel: elderly patient with septic shock and an intra-aortic balloon pump (left image, notched arrow) in the distal descending thoracic aorta. There is multiorgan ischaemia as evidenced by heterogeneous liver attenuation (right image, white star), thickened stomach with intramural gas (right image, thin white arrows). Also note small bowel dilatation on the CT scout view (left image).

particular disease processes. The timely recognition of specific imaging findings necessitates close collaboration between specialised radiologists and clinicians. Serial imaging must, where available, be reviewed in light of ever changing clinical circumstances. In certain life threatening emergencies, lack of imaging should not delay prompt intervention.

Learning Points

- Systematic CXR evaluation is essential taking into account the positioning of the patient and mode of acquisition at the time of imaging.
- CXR should be undertaken to help answer a specific clinical question; routine CXR, as a part

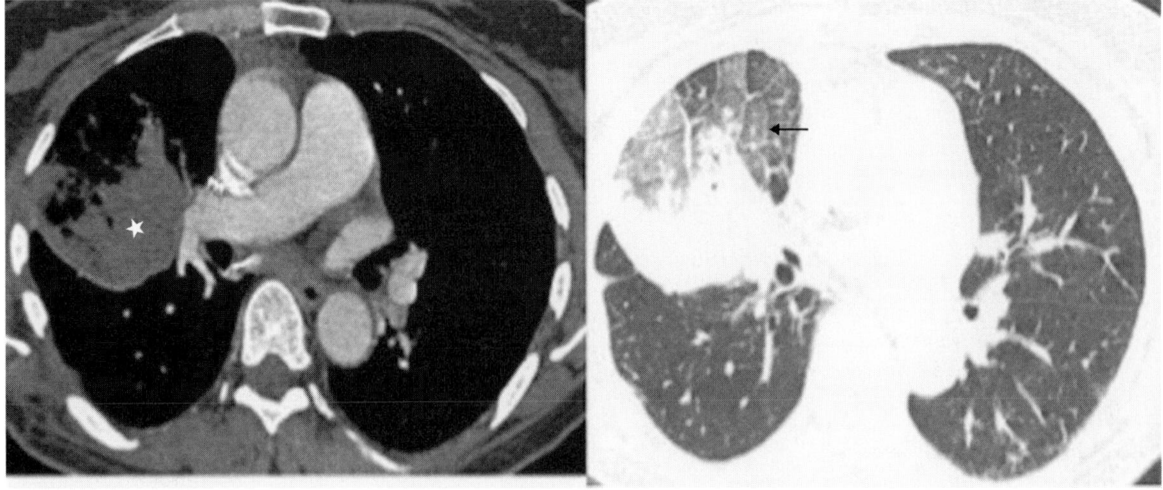

Figure 7.7 Pulmonary torsion.
Thoracic CT on mediastinal (left image) and lung (right image) windows in a patient with severe deterioration 2 days following right lobectomy. There is tapered obliteration of the proximal pulmonary artery and accompanying bronchus with poorly enhancing consolidation (left image, white star), diffuse ground-glass attenuation (right image) and interlobular septal thickening (right image, thin black arrow), which are all features in keeping with ischaemia and oedema due to lobar torsion.

of the daily assessment of patients in the intensive care unit, does not improve outcomes.

- Review of previous CXRs provides important diagnostic clues to the nature of thoracic disease and helps identify causes for acute clinical deteriorations by demonstrating the evolution over time.
- Bedside echocardiography should be the first line imaging for assessment of cardiac function, cardiac valves and the pericardium.
- CT should be reserved as a problem-solving tool, to be used only when the diagnosis is unclear even after careful review of portable imaging.

Further Reading

Amorosa JK, Bramwit MP, Mohammed TL, et al. ACR appropriateness criteria routine chest radiographs in intensive care unit patients. *Journal of the American College of Radiology*. 2013; 10: 170–174.

Ayres J, Gleeson F. Imaging of the pleura. *Seminars in Respiratory and Critical Care Medicine*. 2010; 31: 674–688.

Bentz MR, Primack SL. Intensive care unit imaging. *Clinics in Chest Medicine*. 2015; 36: 219–234, viii.

Eisenhuber E, Schaefer-Prokop CM, Prosch H, Schima W. Bedside chest radiography. *Respiratory Care*. 2012; 57: 427–443.

Franquet T, Gimenez A, Roson N, et al. Aspiration diseases: findings, pitfalls, and differential diagnosis. *Radiographics*. 2000; 20: 673–685.

McMahon MA, Squirrell CA. Multidetector CT of aortic dissection: a pictorial review. *Radiographics*. 2010; 30: 445–460.

Oikonomou A, Prassopoulos P. CT imaging of blunt chest trauma. *Insights into Imaging*. 2011; 2: 281–295.

Sheard S, Rao P, Devaraj A. Imaging of acute respiratory distress syndrome. *Respiratory Care*. 2012; 57: 607–612.

Trotman-Dickenson B. Radiology in the intensive care unit (Part I). *Journal of Intensive Care Medicine*. 2003; 18: 198–210.

MCQs

1. **Signs of right lower lobe collapse on CXR include:**
   (a) Inability to see the line of the right hemidiaphragm
   (b) Inability to see the line of the right heart border
   (c) High position of the left hilum
   (d) Decreased transradiance of the right upper lobe
   (e) High position of the right horizontal fissure

2. **Alveolar opacities in hydrostatic pulmonary oedema are seen on CXR:**
   (a) With a pulmonary capillary wedge pressure <25 mmHg
   (b) Immediately with an increase in intracapillary pressure
   (c) Prior to the development of pleural effusions
   (d) After blurring of the pulmonary vasculature
   (e) with a distinctive appearance from ARDS
3. **A peripheral crescent of high attenuation in the aortic wall in unenhanced CT is seen with the following:**
   (a) Penetrating ulcer
   (b) Intramural haematoma
   (c) Aortic aneurysm less than 6 cm
   (d) Atherosclerotic plaque
   (e) Aortic aneurysm greater than 6 cm
4. **CT pulmonary angiographic features of acute PE include:**
   (a) Central vascular filling defect
   (b) Eccentric vascular thrombus
   (c) Intravascular webs
   (d) Pulmonary stenosis
   (e) Thrombus forms obtuse angle with the vessel wall
5. **Echocardiographic indicators of haemodynamic compromise secondary to pericardial tamponade include:**
   (a) Inspiratory collapse of right-sided chambers
   (b) Early-systolic right ventricular inversion
   (c) Rightward septal shift
   (d) Reciprocal respiratory variation on Doppler transvalvular flow
   (e) Increase in inferior vena caval diameter during inspiration

Exercise answers are available on p.467. Alternatively, take the test online at www.cambridge.org/CardiothoracicMCQ

Chapter 8

Airway Management in Cardiothoracic Intensive Care: Intubation and Tracheostomy

Martin John and Christiana Burt

The ability to safely secure and manage a definitive airway on the cardiothoracic intensive care unit is an essential and challenging skill. Patients are frequently haemodynamically compromised with reduced cardiorespiratory reserve, resulting in poor tolerance of suboptimal ventilation.

Important airway competencies within cardiothoracic intensive care include endotracheal intubation and tracheostomy forming techniques, as well as a good working knowledge of how to rescue the airway should initial attempts fail.

Tracheal Intubation

The presence of a cuffed tube within the trachea represents a secure airway, providing protection from aspiration and facilitating positive pressure ventilation. Endotracheal tubes are made from polyvinyl chloride and are sized based on their internal diameter in millimetres. Since the internal diameter is inversely proportional to airflow resistance, it is appropriate to use the largest size that can be easily accommodated (usually 8–9 mm for males and 7–8 mm for females).

Many patients following cardiac surgery already have an endotracheal tube in place when admitted to the critical care unit. In these patients a period of haemodynamic stability may be required before preparations are made for discontinuation of sedation and extubation. It is important to document the endotracheal tube position, laryngoscopic grade and whether there were any difficulties with facemask ventilation and/or intubation following induction.

In contrast, the postoperative management of patients following thoracic surgery tends to focus on early extubation and the avoidance of positive pressure mechanical ventilation where possible. This is to avoid positive pressure stress on suture and staple sites, which may increase the risk of postoperative complications including persistent air leaks.

Patients who are breathing unsupported or receiving non-invasive ventilation may require intubation for a number of reasons (Table 8.1).

Airway Assessment

When planning any intubation, it is important to perform an initial airway assessment to gauge whether there may be any potential difficulties with facemask ventilation or laryngoscopy. A key finding from the 4th National Audit Project on major airway events in the UK found that poor airway assessment contributed to poor airway outcomes. The degree of harm from airway incidents was also found to be highest in intensive care patients.

Recognised predictors of difficult intubation are listed in Table 8.2. An absence of these signs however does not guarantee straightforward airway management.

Performing Endotracheal Intubation

The intubating environment on the intensive care unit can be very different from that of the elective operating room. Critically ill patients have less physiological reserve and often require intubation urgently to address cardiorespiratory collapse. They may not be fasted and often experience delayed gastric emptying, so a rapid sequence induction with cricoid pressure is often performed.

Preparation

Prior to intubation, it is necessary to prepare the patient, drugs, equipment and intubating team. Roles should be applied to appropriately skilled personnel and a backup plan for a failed intubation should be in place. Essential equipment required for emergency intubation, along with rescue equipment in case of difficulty, should be immediately available in the

Table 8.1 Indications for tracheal intubation on the critical care unit

Hypoxia
Hypercarbia
Reduced conscious level
Increased work of breathing
Cardiac arrest
Airway obstruction
To facilitate transfer

Table 8.2 Predictors of difficult intubation

Receding chin
Short neck
Thick neck
Limited neck extension/flexion
Long upper incisors
Prominent overbite
Inability to extend mandibular incisors anterior to the maxillary incisors
Less than 3 cm interincisor distance
High arched palate
Less than 3 finger breadth thyromental distance
Mallampati score greater than II
Non-compliant mandibular space

Adapted from American Society of Anesthesiologists Task Force on Management of the Difficult Airway (2013).

intensive care unit and moved to the patient's bedspace. A 'difficult airway' trolley containing basic and advanced equipment is an ideal way to organise this.

Patient

Critically ill patients requiring intubation should have standard monitoring (non-invasive blood pressure, electrocardiography, pulse oximetry) and working intravenous access as a minimum. Capnography to confirm correct tube position after intubation should be immediately available.

Head position should be gently manipulated (if it is safe to do so) into the 'sniffing the morning air position' which includes a mild amount of cervical flexion (a pillow is usually necessary behind the head to provide this) and mild atlanto-occipital extension in order to optimise direct laryngoscopic view. In obese patients extra pillows may be necessary behind the shoulders in order to allow atlanto-occipital extension.

Equipment

Basic airway equipment includes: a self-inflating bag, gum-elastic bougie, oropharyngeal airway, functioning laryngoscope (with a spare in case of failure) and at least two options of appropriately sized endotracheal tubes. A supraglottic airway device (laryngeal mask airway, LMA) should also be present in case of intubation difficulty, in order to assist with rescue oxygenation. A suitable device for emergency cricothyrotomy should also be available in case of failure to intubate or oxygenate.

It is necessary to be able to tilt the patient's bed in a head-down position in case of regurgitation during airway manipulation and to have working suction available. It is also prudent to ensure the ventilator to be used after intubation is fully operational and attached to a reliable oxygen source.

Occasionally it may be necessary to site a double-lumen endotracheal tube rather than a single-lumen tube, either to facilitate protection of one lung from soiling by secretions or blood from the other lung, or to enable differential ventilation of the lungs. Double-lumen tube placement requires additional experience and specific training.

Drugs

Rapid sequence induction involves the administration of a predetermined dose of intravenous induction agent followed immediately by a neuromuscular blocking drug to achieve rapid loss of consciousness and optimal intubating conditions with minimal patient apnoea time.

The haemodynamic side effects of the common induction agents at dosages used in anaesthetic practice are such that their administration in critically ill patients can cause catastrophic cardiovascular collapse. To reduce the amount of induction agent needed, operators often coadminister opioids and benzodiazepines. Despite coinduction, vasopressors are still frequently needed following induction and should be immediately available.

Suxamethonium has been the traditional neuromuscular blocking agent used to achieve paralysis due to its speed of onset and offset. Rocuronium is now an alternative option, since the recently developed sugammadex allows immediate block reversal in case of emergency.

The choice of drugs used should be tailored to the individual critical care patient based on an assessment

Table 8.3 Commonly used intubating drugs

Drug	Comments
Thiopentone	Fastest speed of onset
	Cardiovascular suppression
	Potential harm from extravasation
Propofol	Rapid speed of onset
	Suppresses laryngeal reflexes
	Cardiovascular suppression
Ketamine	Slower onset time
	Cardiovascular stability
	Bronchodilation
Etomidate	Rapid speed of onset
	Cardiovascular stability
	Possible adrenal suppression
Midazolam	Slower onset time
	Prolonged duration of action
	Reduces anaesthetic dose requirements
Opioids	Unreliable amnesic
	Limits sympathetic response to intubation
	Reduces anaesthetic dose requirements
Suxamethonium	Rapid onset and offset of paralysis
	Hyperkalaemia
	Risk of malignant hyperthermia
Rocuronium	Rapid onset of neuromuscular block
	Rapid reversal with sugammadex

of aspiration risk, physiological reserve and indication for intubation (Table 8.3).

Team

Clear roles matched to the skillset within the team need to be allocated prior to induction. The team leader is responsible for the overall running of the intubating process and ideally should not be performing any other tasks. The first intubator performs preoxygenation, laryngoscopy and intubation, with a second intubator on standby in case of failure. One team member is responsible for administering drugs and another should be competent at performing cricoid pressure.

Endotracheal Intubation: Sequence of Events

The salient sequence of events during an uncomplicated tracheal intubation on the intensive care unit is preoxygenation, cricoid pressure, anaesthetic induction, paralysis, laryngoscopy and confirmed endotracheal intubation.

Preoxygenation

Preoxygenation describes the process of replacing nitrogen with oxygen in the functional residual capacity (FRC) of the lungs to maximise oxygen stores. This allows for a longer apnoeic time to secure the airway before desaturation occurs, and should be performed where possible. Effective preoxygenation is performed by encouraging the patient to take tidal volume breaths of 100% oxygen through a tight fitting mask (to prevent entrainment of air) at flows above 10 l (to minimise rebreathing) for 3–5 minutes. Since FRC is lower in the supine position, adopting a head-up position can improve oxygen storage capacity. An expired oxygen concentration of 90% signifies effective preoxygenation. These ideal conditions for preoxygenation are not always possible, particularly in patients requiring intubation for respiratory failure who are deteriorating despite non-invasive respiratory support, or who are not able to cooperate with instructions. In these patients a careful attempt at preoxygenation can often be made, but care must be taken not to cause stomach inflation, which increases the risk of regurgitation and aspiration.

Cricoid

Cricoid pressure is a manoeuvre intended to reduce the risk of aspiration during induction. The circumferential cricoid cartilage is the most inferior laryngeal structure and can be pressed against the body of the fifth cervical vertebrae to compress the oesophageal lumen. The thumb and index finger are placed either side of the cartilage and a posterior force of 10 N is applied before induction, which is increased to 30 N following loss of consciousness. The assistant applying cricoid pressure needs to be experienced since incorrect technique can result in airway obstruction and a poor view on laryngoscopy.

Laryngoscopy

Laryngoscopy is most commonly performed with a curved Macintosh laryngoscope blade (sizes 3–5) to allow visualisation of the glottis and enable intubation under direct vision. The laryngoscope is held in the left hand and the blade is inserted into the oral cavity to the right side of the midline, which allows

Table 8.4 Cormack and Lehane classification of laryngoscopy view

Grade 1	Full view of vocal cords/glottis
Grade 2	Only posterior commissure/arytenoid cartilages visible
Grade 3	Only epiglottis visible
Grade 4	No glottic structure visible

distraction of the tongue to the left. The tip is then slowly advanced over the base of the tongue and into the valecula, where an anterior vector force is applied to remove the tongue from the line of sight. The laryngeal view is graded according to the Cormack and Lehane classification (Table 8.4). Poor views can often be improved by external laryngeal manipulation (BURP; backwards, upwards and rightward pressure on the thyroid cartilage) or a reduction in cricoid pressure. With grade 3 and 4 views, the glottic aperture is not visualised and advanced airway equipment such as videolaryngoscopes and fibreoptic scopes may be required to aid intubation.

Confirming Correct Positioning

It is crucial to confirm that the endotracheal tube is in the trachea as opposed to the oesophagus following intubation. The most reliable test confirming correct positioning is six successive carbon dioxide traces on the capnograph with a value for end-tidal carbon dioxide ($EtCO_2$) that corresponds to that expected for the patient. The absence of CO_2 on the capnograph trace should prompt immediate suspicion of incorrect tube position, with direct laryngoscopy or fibreoptic bronchoscopy to resite the tube into the trachea. Failure to recognise oesophageal intubation will result in severe hypoxia within minutes followed by cardiac arrest and death. Clinical signs such as chest wall movement and breath sounds on auscultation, and misting within the tube, as well as appropriate compliance of the inflating bag are of value, but can all occur and give false reassurance with oesophageal intubation. Extra care is needed to confirm correct tube placement in patients in cardiac arrest undergoing CPR, or patients who are on venoarterial extracorporeal membrane oxygenation (VA ECMO) support since the value for $EtCO_2$ on the capnograph trace will be lower than normal despite a correctly sited endotracheal tube (reduced pulmonary blood flow). If the value for $EtCO_2$ is <2 kPa, extra steps should be taken to ensure that tube placement is correct.

The endotracheal tube should be sited to roughly 2 cm above the carina. Once capnography has confirmed placement within the patient's airway, clinical examination can be used to avoid endobronchial intubation, but in difficult cases or where there is doubt, fibreoptic bronchoscopy can be used to ensure optimal placement above the carina. Too far in and flexion of the patient's neck may cause contact with the carina causing irritation and bronchospasm or right main bronchial intubation. If the tube is not advanced far enough into the trachea, extension of the neck can lead to inadvertent extubation.

Difficult Intubation

A difficult intubation is defined as an inability to secure the airway with an endotracheal tube following three attempts, and occurs more commonly in critically ill patients. Repeated intubation attempts (more than three) can lead to airway oedema or bleeding, which will worsen visualisation with subsequent attempts. Expert help needs to be sought early, and the priority is to oxygenate via bag-mask ventilation aided by airway manoeuvres (jaw thrust, head tilt–chin lift) and adjuncts (oropharyngeal, nasopharyngeal airways), or ventilation via a supraglottic device. Management should follow local and national protocols (see Further Reading).

If ventilation and oxygenation are satisfactory, a definitive airway is required by another technique. Allowing the patient to wake up (recommended in the elective setting) is unlikely to be an appropriate option in the critically ill patient.

Advanced airway options available to secure a definitive airway in the 'can't intubate, can ventilate' scenario include the following.

1. *Videolaryngoscopy* There are a number of videolaryngoscopes available to aid intubation. All contain a distal light source and camera to allow indirect visualisation of the glottis on a screen. These devices obviate the need for a direct line of sight in order to intubate.
2. *Asleep fibreoptic intubation* A fibrescope preloaded with an endotracheal tube can be passed either orally or nasally under direct vision into the trachea.
3. *Intubation through the existing laryngeal mask airway* An Aintree catheter (hollow bougie) can be loaded on to a fibrescope and the whole unit passed through the lumen of the ventilating

laryngeal mask airway and into the trachea under direct vision. Upon removal of the fibrescope, an endotracheal tube can then be passed over the Aintree catheter.

4. *Intubating laryngeal mask airway* The intubating laryngeal mask airway is specifically designed to allow an endotracheal tube to blindly pass through its lumen into the trachea.
5. *Tracheostomy* Tracheostomies are usually performed electively on intubated patients. However in the difficult intubation scenario in the critically ill, there may be a case for direct tracheostomy formation whilst ventilating with a laryngeal mask airway.

Failed Ventilation

Failure of ventilation is defined as the inability to maintain oxygen saturations above 90% (if initially above this value) whilst administering 100% oxygen using a facemask or laryngeal mask airway.

Failed ventilation with increasing hypoxaemia in the setting of a difficult intubation, the 'can't intubate, can't oxygenate' scenario, is a rare but life threatening emergency. The immediate priority is to achieve oxygenation and since the upper airway route has failed, an invasive approach via the cricothyroid membrane is recommended. The cricothyroid membrane lies inferior to the vocal cords, is relatively avascular and can normally be easily located below the thyroid cartilage and above the cricoid cartilage.

There are three types of cricothyroidotomy approach:

1. *Small cannula devices* (2–3 mm ID) Kink resistant cannulae can be directed caudally into the trachea and their position confirmed by aspirating air freely. The resistance through these narrow devices is large, so a high pressure (2–4 bar) oxygen source is needed to oxygenate. Some degree of upper airway patency is required to allow passive exhalation. This limits their use beyond short-term rescue oxygenation.
2. *Large-bore devices* (>4 mm ID) These devices are inserted using either the Seldinger or cannula-over-needle technique. The larger diameter accommodates a 15 mm standard breathing circuit, which allows the patient to be effectively low pressure ventilated.
3. *Surgical cricothyroidotomy* (>6 mm ID) The surgical approach involves making a horizontal scalpel incision through the cricothyroid membrane. Caudal traction on the membrane can then be applied from a tracheal hook to allow intubation with a size 6 mm ID cuffed tracheal or tracheostomy tube.

Managing the Intubated Patient

Attention to the endotracheal tube needs to be maintained following intubation in order to prevent airway related morbidity. Continuous waveform capnography should be used for every intubated patient to ensure correct tube positioning and allow surveillance against tube migration. Endobronchial intubation should be monitored for using auscultation, and chest X-ray. Checking the cuff pressure regularly is important since excessive pressures can cause tracheal mucosal damage, whereas an inadequate pressure can lead to microaspirates and ineffective ventilation. Cuff pressures between 20 and 30 cmH_2O are recommended.

To reduce the risk of inadvertent extubation, judicious use of sedation is required as well as care when moving patients.

Extubation

Tracheal extubation is the process of removing the endotracheal tube to allow the patient to protect and maintain their own airway. To increase the likelihood of a successful extubation on the intensive care unit, a number of criteria firstly need to be met:

1. Indication for intubation has been corrected,
2. Haemodynamic stability,
3. Adequate ability to cough and clear secretions,
4. Neurologically appropriate,
5. Adequate oxygenation without requiring high levels of PEEP/FiO_2,
6. Fully rewarmed (i.e. after cardiac surgery),
7. Minimal chest drain output.

A spontaneous breathing trial can then be performed using a T-piece or low-level pressure support and low PEEP to determine the likelihood of extubation success.

A backup reintubation plan should always be part of the extubation strategy as it may be more difficult than the original intubation. Tracheal extubation in the presence of a known difficult airway can be performed over an airway exchange catheter, which may be tolerated for up to 72 hours.

To perform an extubation in an uncomplicated airway, the patient should be given 100% oxygen for at least 3 minutes and the nasogastric tube (if present) should be suctioned. Gentle positive pressure should be applied followed by cuff deflation and controlled tube removal. Patients may initially be extubated onto a facemask and Waters circuit with 100% oxygen in order to assess adequacy of spontaneous ventilation.

Tracheostomy

Tracheostomy refers to the creation of a stoma at the skin surface, which is in continuity with the trachea. This procedure is commonly performed on the cardiothoracic intensive care unit and involves the insertion of a tracheostomy tube usually between the second and third tracheal rings. Despite being one of the oldest airway interventions, controversy still exists regarding the optimal timing, insertion technique and type of tracheostomy tube to use.

Advantages

Tracheostomy tubes offer a number of practical and clinical advantages over oral endotracheal tubes when managing the critically ill.

1. The work of breathing is reduced since the dead-space and airflow resistance is less than for equivalent sized endotracheal tubes.
2. Suctioning the tracheobronchial tree in patients with a high secretion burden is easier.
3. Tracheostomy tubes are well tolerated, which often allows the sedation and associated adverse effects to be reduced.
4. Mouth hygiene is easier to maintain and phonation as well as swallowing is possible.
5. Complications associated with prolonged translaryngeal intubation such as vocal cord damage and laryngeal ulceration are avoided.

Indications

The most common indication for tracheostomy in the intensive care setting is to facilitate prolonged mechanical ventilation and weaning. Recent estimates suggest that approximately 5% of patients following cardiac surgery require mechanical ventilation for at least 7 days due to perioperative complications, often on a background of underlying respiratory disease.

Other indications for tracheostomy include failure of protective airway reflexes, management of excessive secretions and relief of upper airway obstruction.

Tracheostomy Tubes

Tracheostomy tubes are made from either polyvinyl chloride, silicone or metal, and are available in a variety of shapes and sizes. When sizing tracheostomy tubes, important dimensions to consider include the diameter (inner and outer), length (proximal and distal) and curvature.

The optimal tracheostomy tube size provides the maximum internal diameter to facilitate airflow, whilst confining the outer diameter to roughly three quarters of the tracheal lumen. This minimises resistance across the tube and also allows adequate airflow around the tube during weaning and attempted phonation.

Since the trachea is essentially straight, the tip of an inappropriately long and curved tracheostomy tube can traumatise the anterior tracheal wall, whilst shorter tubes can abut posteriorly. To avoid these problems, angled tracheostomy tubes have a straight portion designed to lie more anatomically within the trachea.

Tracheostomy tube length is also an important consideration since patients with large necks often need a longer proximal portion, whereas patients with tracheal pathology (tracheomalacia) may need extra distal length to bypass disease.

Two different sizing systems exist, which can cause confusion since one is based on the length (and taper) of the outer tube, whilst the other refers to the internal diameter. As a reference for the clinician and to avoid sizing errors, the diameters and distinguishing features of tracheostomy tubes are marked on the flange.

Cuffed and Uncuffed Tubes

In the intensive care setting, most patients will initially require a cuffed tracheostomy tube to facilitate positive pressure ventilation and protect against aspiration. To reduce the risk of tracheal mucosal ischaemia and subsequent stenosis, a high volume/low pressure cuff inflated to a pressure of no more than 20–25 cmH_2O is recommended. Uncuffed tracheostomy tubes allow for airway clearance but do not protect from aspiration, so are usually reserved for patients with adequate bulbar function who are unable to clear secretions.

Single and Double Cannula Tubes

Tracheostomy tubes can be stand-alone single lumen devices or contain an accompanying inner cannula (double cannula tubes). Double cannula tubes are inherently safer since in the event of obstruction the inner cannula can be removed completely and independently from the outer lumen to manage the blockage. For this reason, and to facilitate cleaning, it is often the preferred choice of tube for patients discharged to a stepdown unit or ward. Many intensive care units now use double cannulas from the outset. It is however important to appreciate that the addition of an inner cannula reduces the functional internal diameter of the tracheostomy tube, which increases airflow resistance and the work of breathing. Furthermore, in some designs, attachment to the ventilator is only possible when the inner tube and its associated 15 mm connector is in place.

Fenestrated and Non-fenestrated Tubes

Fenestrated tracheostomy tubes have single or multiple openings located posteriorly and above the cuff. Following cuff deflation during spontaneous ventilation, the fenestrations encourage maximal airflow through the larynx to allow phonation and an assessment of native airway patency in preparation for decannulation. Fenestrated tracheostomy tubes are often used in conjunction with one-way speaking valves. These valves cap the tracheostomy tube and allow inspiration but close on expiration, which directs airflow through the larynx when the patient exhales. Non-fenestrated inner tubes should be used if positive pressure ventilation is required to avoid air leaks.

Insertion Technique

Tracheostomies can be performed as open surgical procedures, most commonly in the operating theatre or percutaneously at the bedside.

Both procedures carry low complication rates in experienced hands and individual unit practice is largely determined by resource and local preference.

The percutaneous approach is logistically easier and proponents suggest that peristomal bleeding and infection rates are lower. Surgical tracheostomies, however, are more appropriate in patients with difficult neck anatomy and in the emergency scenario.

Percutaneous Tracheostomy

Patients are in the supine position and often have a bolster placed between their shoulders to allow adequate neck extension and exposure. Preprocedural ultrasound scanning of the neck is now increasingly being used to assess the anterior neck landmarks. Sedation needs to be increased to anaesthetic levels and paralysis should be given. It is important to ventilate with 100% oxygen.

Capnography to confirm correct tube positioning is mandatory and bronchoscopy through the tracheal tube to guide tracheostomy placement is recommended. In order to accommodate the tracheostomy tube, the endotracheal tube needs to be withdrawn under bronchoscopic guidance so the tip lies at the level of the cricoid cartilage prior to needle puncture.

All percutaneous tracheostomy tube placements are based on the Seldinger technique, with initial needle aspiration and guidewire insertion midway between the cricoid cartilage and sternal notch. This usually correlates to the space between the second and third tracheal rings. Tract dilatation and tracheostomy railroading can be performed using single step or sequential dilators, balloon inflation, forceps dilatation, or by the retrograde translaryngeal approach.

Surgical Tracheostomy

This procedure is often performed in an operating room under general anaesthesia. A vertical incision below the cricoid cartilage is usually made and following blunt dissection down, the strap muscles and thyroid isthmus are retracted to expose the trachea for tracheostomy placement. Open-ended stay sutures can be sited either side of the tracheal stoma to facilitate postoperative tube reinsertion in case of displacement.

Timing

Controversy exists as to when the optimal time is to perform tracheostomy placement. The benefit of a tracheostomy over prolonged translaryngeal intubation needs to be balanced against the likelihood of the patient needing extended ventilation and the risks associated with the procedure.

The largest randomised controlled trial to date (Tracman) found no benefit in performing early tracheostomies within 4 days, and suggested delaying this procedure until day 10 of translaryngeal ventilation. The initial tracheostomy tube is usually cuffed, non-fenestrated and may be either single or double cannula in design. It is recommended that the first routine tube change should not be performed within 4 days after a surgical tracheostomy and 7–10 days after a percutaneous one to allow the stoma and tract to be established first. The decision to change the tracheostomy tube should be multidisciplinary, based on the weaning, swallowing and ventilatory needs of the patient. For the first tube change or if there are anticipated difficulties, the exchange is usually performed over a guide such as a gum-elastic bougie, exchange catheter or suction tubing. With well-established tracts a guide is not usually needed. During all tube exchanges, however, there needs to be the necessary equipment and personnel available to manage failure.

Tracheostomy Management

A large proportion of adverse airway events on the intensive care unit involve tracheostomies and can be fatal. To minimise the risk of accidental decannulation or migration, the tracheostomy tube should be safely secured with sutures or an approved tracheostomy tube holder. Sedation should be used judiciously and care taken upon patient rolling and moving. In case of accidental tracheostomy dislodgement or removal, the safest approach is oral reintubation of the trachea to stabilise the situation.

Humidified air should be given in order to prevent the formation of excessively viscous secretions, which can obstruct the tube. Heat and moisture exchangers can be used for this purpose in patients who are either self-ventilating or needing ventilator support. To help manage especially thick secretions, heated water baths may be needed. Intermittent suctioning and physiotherapy at intervals dependent on patient secretion burden is also beneficial. The management of suspected dislodgement should follow guidance from the National Tracheostomy Safety Project (Figure 8.1 and Chapter 26 Airway Emergencies).

Swallowing

Swallowing allows early establishment of oral feeding and contributes to the psychological well being of patients with tracheostomy tubes. However, these patients are at risk of aspiration since the tube and cuff can impede normal laryngeal movements during swallowing as well as cause oesophageal compression. Prior to allowing oral feeding, patients need to be able to tolerate cuff deflation and should have passed a bedside swallowing assessment by a speech therapist.

Weaning and Decannulation

There is no clear consensus on the optimal tracheostomy weaning protocol and different units vary in their practice. The overriding theme is to gradually reduce ventilatory support and encourage normal airflow patterns in the upper airways to such an extent that the patient can manage without the tracheostomy tube. This involves increasing periods of cuff deflation, changing to smaller diameter and fenestrated tubes, and using speaking valves or caps. A successful wean requires patient commitment and regular multidisciplinary input from nurses, physiotherapists, speech therapist, intensivists and surgeons.

Decannulation should occur as soon as the tracheostomy tube is no longer required and it is safe to do so. This occurs at the end of a successful wean, with multidisciplinary team agreement and when core criteria have been met (Table 8.5). It is advisable to decannulate during the morning when the patient is fasted and can be observed during the day with equipment and expertise to manage any complications to hand.

Summary

The establishment and maintenance of a patent airway with ventilation to the lungs is a critically important first step in the management of a patient on the cardiothoracic intensive care unit. Capnography is an essential adjunct for any patient receiving artificial

Table 8.5 Patient decannulation criteria

Able to maintain and protect their own airway
Adequate respiratory function, free from ventilator support
Haemodynamically stable
Absence of fever or active infection
Consistently alert
Strong cough
Competent swallow
Clinically stable
No forthcoming procedures requiring anaesthesia (within 7–10 days)

Adapted from the National Tracheostomy Patient Safety Manual 2013.

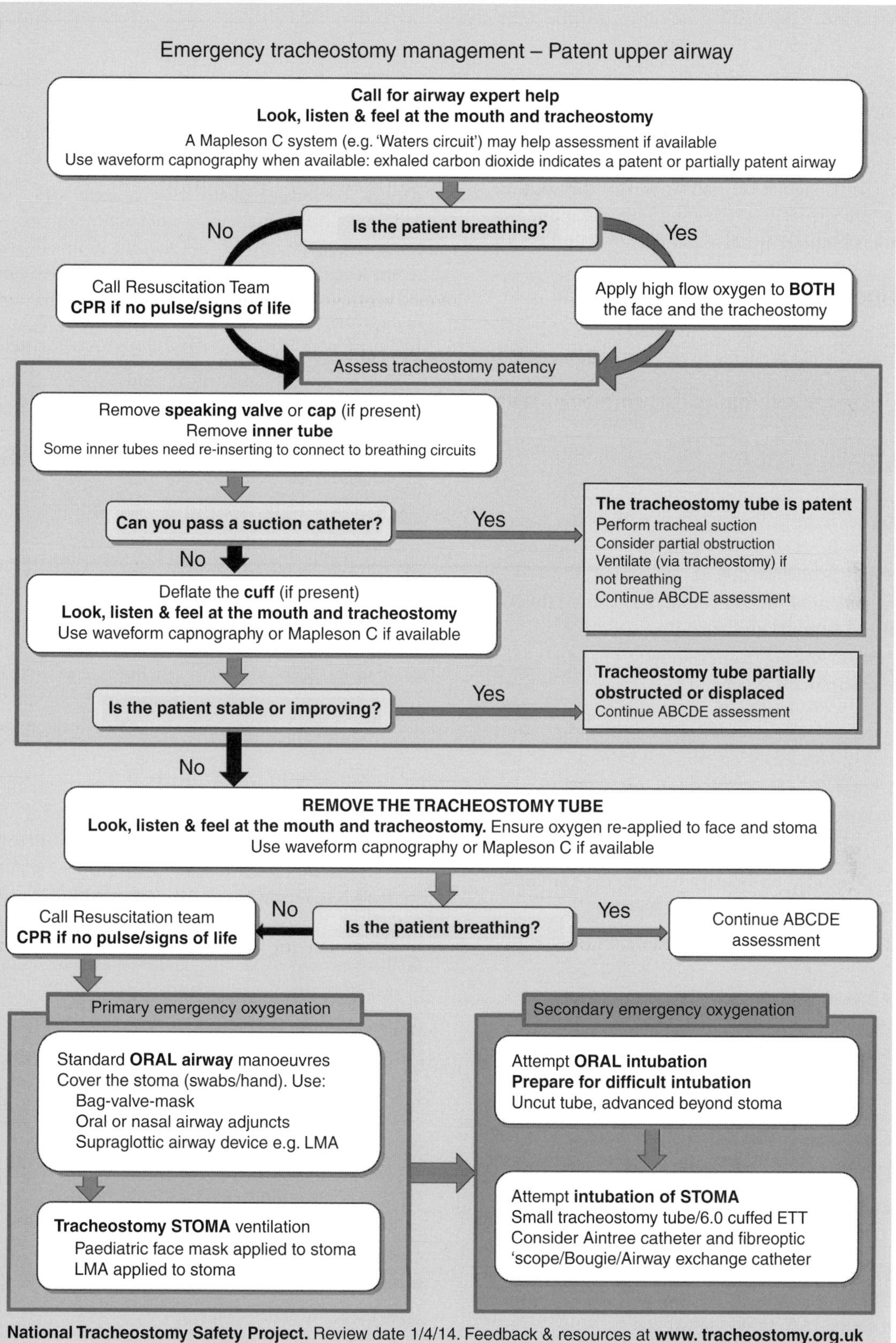

Figure 8.1 Emergency tracheostomy management. Reproduced from McGrath et al. *Anaesthesia*. 2012; 67: 1025–1041, with permission from the Association of Anaesthetists of Great Britain & Ireland/Blackwell Publishing Ltd. (A black and white version of this figure will appear in some formats. For the colour version, please refer to the plate section.)

ventilatory support via an endotracheal tube or tracheostomy tube. Extra care must be taken not to miss tube dislodgement in the setting of reduced CO_2 delivery to the lungs, i.e. in cardiac arrest, or in VA-ECMO support. Anticoagulation can increase the risk of bleeding into the airway following manipulation, and extra care is required in these patients.

Learning Points

- Equipment for emergency intubation should be immediately available in the cardiothoracic critical care unit alongside equipment for management of the difficult airway.
- Extra care is needed to avoid airway bleeding in patients receiving anticoagulation.
- Oesophageal intubation may be difficult to diagnose in the presence of low pulmonary blood flow: use direct assessment via laryngoscopy or fibreoptic bronchoscopy in case of doubt.
- Management of the difficult airway should follow local and national guidance.
- Safe airway management requires multidisciplinary input.

Further Reading

American Society of Anesthesiologists Task Force on Management of the Difficult Airway. Practice Guidelines for Management of the Difficult Airway: An Updated Report. *Anesthesiology*. 2013; 118: 1–20.

Cook TM, Woodall N, Frerk C; 4th National Audit Project of The Royal College of Anaesthetists and the Difficult Airway Society. Major complications of airway management in the United Kingdom. Report and findings March 2011. Available from: www.rcoa.ac.uk/document-store/nap4-full-report

Difficult Airway Society UK Guidelines. 2015. Available from: www.das.uk.com/guidelines/downloads.html

McGrath BA, Bates L, Atkinson D, et al. Multidisciplinary guidelines for the management of tracheostomy and laryngectomy airway emergencies. *Anaesthesia*. 2012; 67: 1025–1041.

Young D, Harrison DA, Cuthbertson BH, et al. Effect of early vs late tracheostomy placement on survival in patients receiving mechanical ventilation. The Tracman randomized trial. *Journal of the American Medical Association*. 2013; 309: 2121–2129.

MCQs

Please identify whether the below statements are true or false.

1. **Difficult intubation management in the cardiothoracic critical care unit should involve:**
   (a) At least five attempts at intubation before help is called
   (b) A logical approach guided by local and national protocols
   (c) Preparation of the patient, equipment, drugs and team if time allows
   (d) Administration of the same doses of induction agents as in an elective setting
   (e) Clear communication of team roles

2. **Regarding tracheostomy:**
   (a) A fenestrated inner tube should be used with positive pressure ventilation
   (b) Tracheostomy should be performed routinely after 4 days of endotracheal intubation
   (c) Decannulation can occur as soon as the patient is weaned from positive pressure ventilation
   (d) The tube with deflated cuff should be a tight fit in the trachea so that no air can escape around it

3. **Endotracheal intubation:**
   (a) Requires specific training under supervision by an expert in airway management
   (b) Should always be performed by an anaesthetist
   (c) Should always have waveform capnography available continuously to aid with assessment of tube position
   (d) Requires chest X-ray to exclude oesophageal intubation
   (e) Can be more difficult to perform in the critically ill patient

4. **Cardiothoracic patients may experience airway com plications due to:**
   (a) Presence of anticoagulation

(b) Low pulmonary blood flow reducing the level of expected end-tidal carbon dioxide

(c) Airway oedema secondary to critical illness

(d) Cerebrovascular accident following surgery

(e) Prolonged endotracheal intubation

5. **Predictors of difficult intubation include:**

   (a) Limited neck extension

   (b) Prominent overbite

   (c) Short legs

   (d) Marfan's syndrome

   (e) Mallampati score of I

Exercise answers are available on p.467. Alternatively, take the test online at www.cambridge.org/CardiothoracicMCQ

Chapter 9

Chest Drainage

Alia Noorani and Yasir Abu-Omar

Introduction

The pleural space is a thin, fluid filled space between the visceral and parietal pleura. In a healthy 70 kg individual, this space contains a few millilitres of serous pleural fluid, the function of which is to allow the pleurae to slide easily over the lungs during ventilation. The presence of air or fluid (pus, blood, chyle or excessive pleural fluid) impedes the normal function of the lungs, and depending on the symptoms and signs affecting the patient, will require chest drainage.

Usually, the pressure in the pleural space is less than atmospheric. This negative pressure helps maintain partial lung expansion and the magnitude of negativity changes during the respiratory cycle. In inspiration the pressure is approximately −8 cmH_2O and in expiration this falls to −4 cmH_20. A breach of the pleural cavity leads to development of a positive pressure in this space either equal to or more than atmospheric pressure, leading to a pneumothorax.

History

The earliest known reference to chest drainage dates back to the fifth century Hippocratic texts. Here conservative management of empyemas is described using plants and herbs, and open drainage for persistent infections is well documented including the surgical technique for doing this. Hippocrates gave detailed descriptions of using a scalpel to cut between the ribs, evacuating pus and leaving a hollow tube in for 2 weeks.

Since this, other physicians have described the technique including the leading French physician surgeon Guy de Chauliac in 1395. The first description of a closed chest drainage system was by Hewett in 1876.

Indications

The indications for chest drain insertion are to remove fluid, air or both from the pleural space. Table 9.1 shows the common indications for chest drainage.

Table 9.1 Common indications for chest drainage

Traumatic haemothorax
Large spontaneous or traumatic pneumothorax
Benign or malignant pleural effusion
Chylothorax
Following cardiac or thoracic surgery

Figure 9.1a shows a chest radiograph of a patient with a large pneumothorax following cardiac surgery, and Figure 9.1b shows the same patient post chest drain insertion. Figure 9.2a shows a chest radiograph of a patient with a left pleural effusion and Figure 9.2b shows the same patient post drain insertion.

Technique

The emergency insertion of a large bore chest drain for the relief of a tension pneumothorax is well described in the Advanced Trauma Life Support guidelines and there are many published step-by-step descriptions of the procedure.

The British Thoracic Society guidelines for the insertion of chest drains were originally developed in 2003 and subsequently updated in 2010. These guidelines were in effect aimed at training and guiding physicians to safely perform this procedure. Figure 9.3 shows the BTS guidelines as an algorithm.

Anatomical Landmarks

The BTS describes the triangle of safety within which chest drains should be placed (Figure 9.4). This triangle is the area bounded by the anterior border of latissimus dorsi and the lateral edge of pectoralis major with the base formed by a line superior to the horizontal line of the nipple.

The advantages of this position are to minimise potential damage to underlying nerve and vascular structures such as the long thoracic nerve and the lateral thoracic artery. Additionally, placement in this

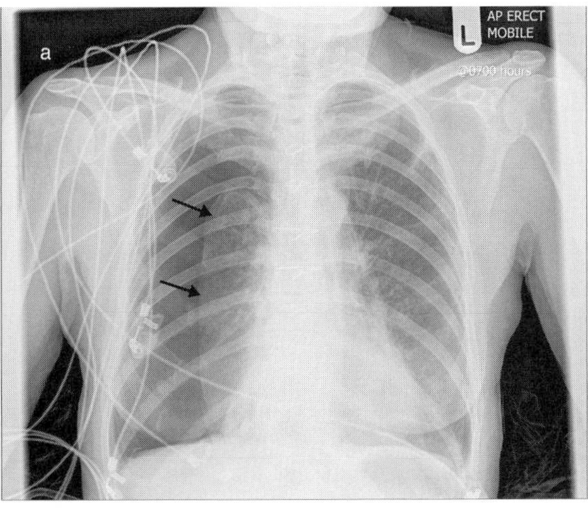

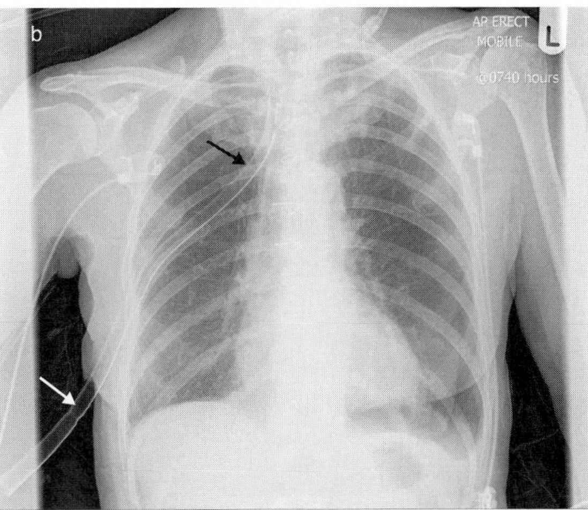

Figure 9.1 (a) Radiograph of a patient with a large right pneumothorax (black arrows). (b) The same patient with a right sided chest drain in situ (white arrow) and reinflation of the right lung.

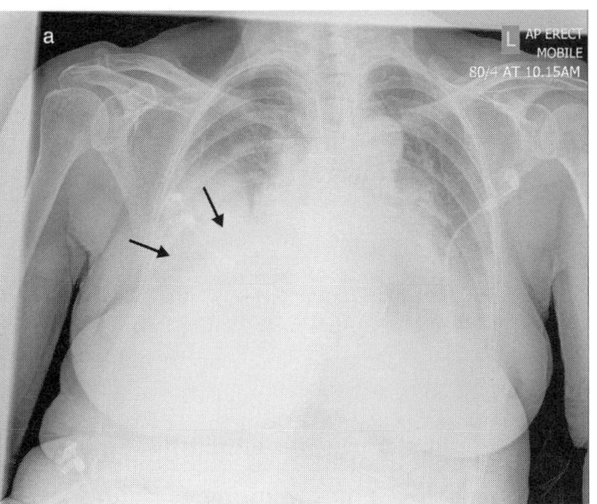

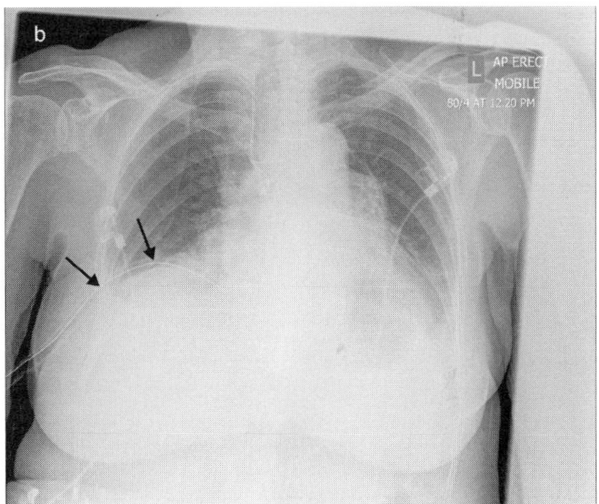

Figure 9.2 (a) Chest radiograph of a patient with a large right pleural effusion (black arrows) and (b) resolution of the effusion with the insertion of a right sided chest drain (black arrows).

area may prevent excessive breast or muscle tissue dissection, reducing the risk of scarring. The presence of a loculated effusion may require a more posterior drain placement but this should be undertaken under the supervision of a specialist or under image guidance. Posteriorly placed drains are more likely to cause discomfort.

Preinsertion Preparation

All patients requiring a chest drain should be consented for the procedure (unless unable to do so due to their clinical status) and this consent should be recorded in the clinical notes. Appropriate premedication prior to the procedure can include midazolam or an opioid. Caution with these drugs should be exercised in patients with underlying respiratory disease.

Patients with abnormal coagulation or platelet defects should have these corrected before an elective drain insertion, and for those on warfarin the INR should be allowed to reach 1.5 or below if possible.

Patient Positioning

The ideal position for drain insertion is with the patient upright or at a 45° angle, with the arm on the affected side abducted and externally rotated and

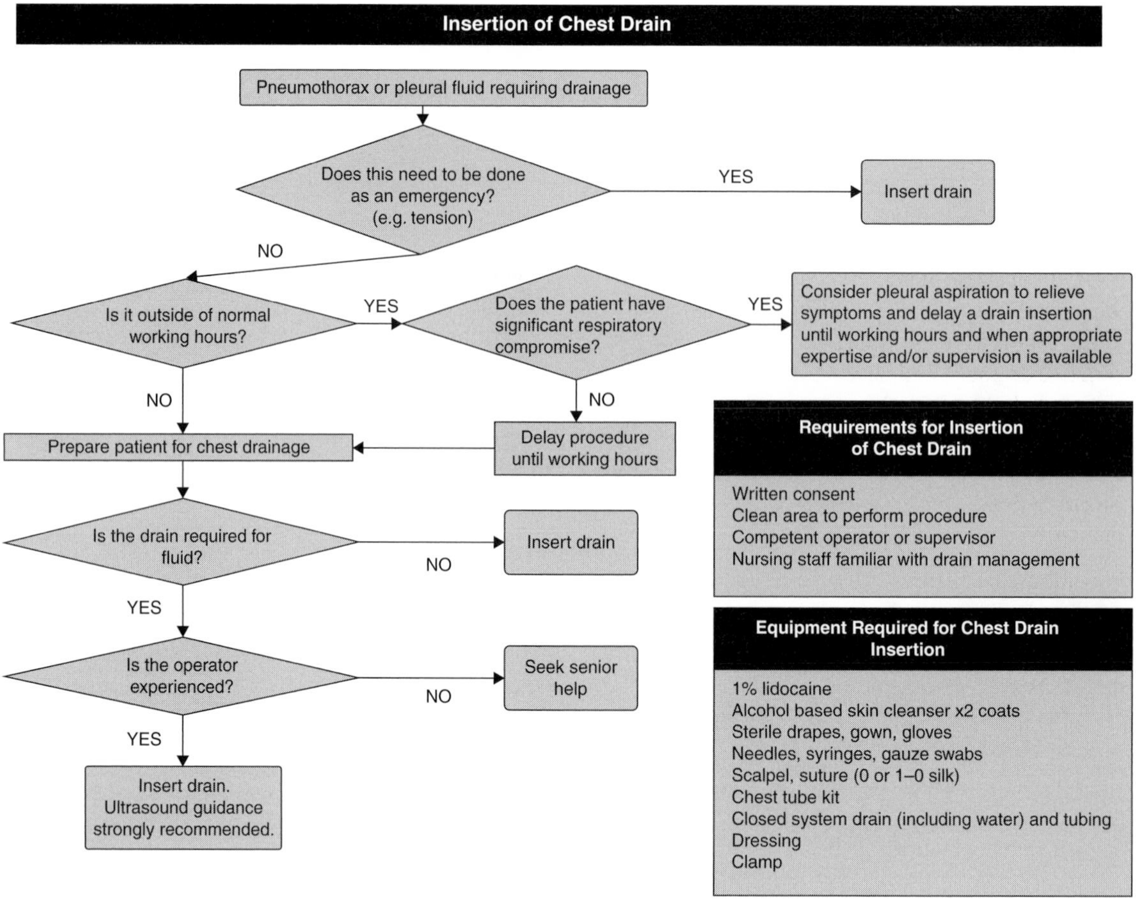

Insertion of Chest Drain

Pneumothorax or pleural fluid requiring drainage

Does this need to be done as an emergency? (e.g. tension)

YES → Insert drain

NO → Is it outside of normal working hours?

YES → Does the patient have significant respiratory compromise?

YES → Consider pleural aspiration to relieve symptoms and delay a drain insertion until working hours and when appropriate expertise and/or supervision is available

NO → Delay procedure until working hours → Prepare patient for chest drainage

NO → Prepare patient for chest drainage

Is the drain required for fluid?

NO → Insert drain

YES → Is the operator experienced?

NO → Seek senior help

YES → Insert drain. Ultrasound guidance strongly recommended.

Requirements for Insertion of Chest Drain

Written consent
Clean area to perform procedure
Competent operator or supervisor
Nursing staff familiar with drain management

Equipment Required for Chest Drain Insertion

1% lidocaine
Alcohol based skin cleanser x2 coats
Sterile drapes, gown, gloves
Needles, syringes, gauze swabs
Scalpel, suture (0 or 1–0 silk)
Chest tube kit
Closed system drain (including water) and tubing
Dressing
Clamp

Figure 9.3 British Thoracic Society algorithm for the insertion of chest drains.

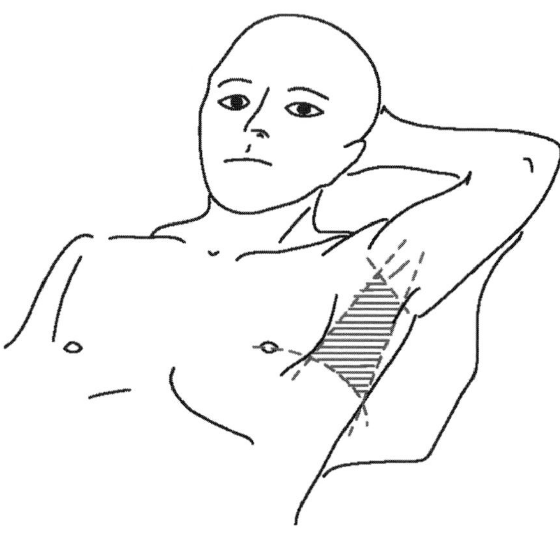

Figure 9.4 The triangle of safety. Anteriorly the lateral border of pectoralis major, laterally the anterior border of latissimus dorsi and inferiorly a line superior to the fourth nipple.

placed behind the patient's head. This exposes the axillary area.

Prior to insertion it is imperative to undertake a clinical examination to confirm the presence of pleural fluid or pneumothorax and to confirm the side of the pathology on a recent chest radiograph. The only exception is in the case of a tension pneumothorax where clinical signs alone are sufficient.

The increasing use of thoracic ultrasonography to identify the presence of an effusion is highly recommended.

Procedure

1. Once the patient is positioned appropriately, the triangle of safety is prepped with antiseptic and draped. The entire procedure must be carried out in an aseptic manner to avoid infection ascending into the thoracic cavity. The rates of empyema

following chest drain insertion after trauma are approximately 3% and lead to significant morbidity. One study has identified no infections in a group of 80 patients requiring a chest drain for trauma carried out in an aseptic manner.

2. The procedure equipment is usually available sterile and prepacked in most hospitals. Chest tubes are made of clear plastic and are available in a variety of sizes (diameters) based on the French scale (multiples of 4, e.g. 12F, 16F, 20F, up to 36F). These drains have multiple side holes to allow effective drainage and have a radio-opaque marker strip to help identification on chest radiography. Trocars are occasionally present within chest drains but the routine use of these is not recommended as they can cause undue visceral damage.

The kit should contain:

- Sterile drapes
- 1% lidocaine (in a dose of up to 2 mg/kg)
- 20 ml syringe
- Green and yellow needles (21–25 gauge)
- Sterile skin preparation solution (chlorhexidene)
- Scalpel
- Curved instrument such as a Roberts's clamp or Spencer Wells
- Chest drain (sizes vary, usually 28F and larger for effusions and smaller for pneumothorax)
- Skin suture (nylon or silk)
- Chest drain tubing
- Chest drain bottle primed with sterile water (underwater seal)
- Dressing to cover drain insertion site.

3. Next, local anaesthesia is infiltrated using a small gauge needle and by raising a dermal bleb. Lidocaine in a safe dose (up to 2 mg/kg) or an alternative local anaesthetic is used. The next step is to freely aspirate either air in the case of pneumothorax or fluid in the case of an effusion to confirm the pathology. If neither can be done, a chest drain should **not** be inserted without further image guidance. Studies have shown that image guided placement of drains has a low complication rate of pneumothorax at 3% and a successful insertion rate of over 70%.
4. Once a successful aspirate has been obtained and the local anaesthetic deemed successful, a skin incision just above and parallel to the ribs is made. This incision should be similar in size to the diameter of tube being inserted and the operator's index finger.
5. Much debate has been had about the size of the chest tubes used. General recommendations are to use a large bore tube in the setting of trauma or acute haemothorax, to facilitate drainage and monitor on-going losses (28–30F). Smaller drains are more comfortable and can be used for pneumothoraces. Blunt dissection into the pleural cavity, skirting the upper border of the ribs to avoid injury to the neurovascular bundle, should be performed, with a finger sweep manoeuvre into the pleural space, in particular with larger drains, to avoid injury to the lung parenchyma and other thoracic organs.
6. Once a chest drain is inserted into the pleural cavity it should be connected to an underwater seal and secured to the skin. A chest radiograph should be requested to assess the position.

Underwater Seals

All chest drains should be connected to a single flow drainage system which can comprise an underwater seal bottle or a flutter valve. The purpose of such a system is to maintain a negative intrapleural pressure and although there are different methods of achieving this, in a traditional underwater seal, a tube is placed at a depth of 3 cm with a side vent that allows the escape of air. Often a suction system is required to maintain a negative pressure. The newer thoracic drainage systems such as the Thopaz (Medela, IL) are compact devices that allow for patient mobility, without restriction.

Contraindications

There are no contraindications to chest drain insertion in a clinically urgent scenario. For non-urgent cases, however, if a patient is anticoagulated, the INR should be less than 1.5. Any other clotting abnormalities should also be corrected.

Nursing Care

The aftercare of chest drains is extremely important. Patients should be managed on a ward where staff are experienced in the routine care of chest drains. A daily record of the volume of drainage, the type of fluid drained and the presence or absence of an air leak and swing should be clearly documented to facilitate decision making with regards to the timing of drain removal. Additionally, drains should routinely be inspected for non-function as heralded by lack of fluctuation of fluid within the tube with respiration or coughing. Non-function may be due to kinking, debris or malposition. Tension pneumothorax is a serious complication within the context of an on-going air leak and a blocked drain. Due care with adequate fixation of the drain and subsequent patient education are important to avoid inadvertent chest drain dislodgement.

Removal of Drains

Chest drains should be removed once the clinical indication for their use has been fulfilled. For pneumothoraces this is when the lung has reinflated on the chest radiograph and when the drain has stopped bubbling. For pleural effusions this depends on the pathology that prompted drain insertion and the volume of fluid drained. An empyema will require a prolonged period of drainage compared to a postoperative drain inserted in a cardiac patient.

Chest drain removal is a two-person job whereby both professionals are trained in the procedure. One removes the drain while the patient performs a Valsalva or during expiration. The assistant then pulls the purse string present and ties it to close the insertion site.

Complications

Chest drainage is a fairly common procedure but it is not without risk. The NPSA reported over 2000 patient safety incidents relating to chest drains between January 2005 and March 2008. Of these there were 12 deaths and 15 cases of severe harm associated with chest drains between January 2005 and March 2008. The main reasons for these incidents were deemed to be:

- Inadequate level of supervision, training or operator experience,
- Incorrect site of insertion and poor patient positioning,
- Inadequate preprocedure imaging,
- Excessive insertion of the dilator when using a Seldinger technique.

Details of some complications are given below.

Drain Malposition

Malpositioning of drains is the commonest complication of chest drain insertion and understandably this is commoner in the emergency setting than the elective setting where the speed of the procedure can lead to injury. Intraparenchymal positioning of drains can occur in the presence of pleural adhesions. Chest wall placement has been reported to occur in up to 18% of cases and can be diagnosed with a lack of swinging in the drain tubing and bottle. Drains placed too far into the chest cavity can result in perforation of other intrathoracic organs such as the heart, major vessels, nerves, and oesophagus as well as the diaphragm. Abdominal placement of drains can occur when the insertion point is lower than the base of the triangle of safety. Injury to the liver, spleen, stomach and bowel have all been reported.

Nerve Injuries

Horner's syndrome has been reported due to direct pressure of the tip of the chest tube on the sympathetic chain in the medial portion of the apex of the thoracic cavity. Phrenic nerve injury can cause diaphragmatic paralysis and severe cases may require plication. Injury to the long thoracic nerve of Bell during insertion too far laterally in the triangle of safety can lead to winging of the scapula. Ulnar neuropathy due to injury of the posterior cord of the brachial plexus has also been reported.

Heart

Inadvertent injury to the heart is a potentially fatal complication of chest drain insertion. Injuries to all chambers have been reported and the continued drainage of fresh blood should raise the suspicion of this injury. Urgent surgical intervention is required.

Intercostal Vessels

Injury to the intercostal vessels can lead to significant haemorrhage. Knowledge of intercostal bundle anatomy and the technique of dissecting above a rib are essential to avoid this complication.

Re-expansion Pulmonary Oedema

This is an uncommon but potentially fatal complication following chest drain insertion for pleural effusion or pneumothorax. Mortality rates of up to 20%

have been reported. The aetiology of re-expansion pulmonary oedema is unclear and it can affect the ipsilateral, contralateral or both lungs. It is thought that increased endothelial permeability and loss of alveolar integrity are the main factors leading to exudation of proteinaceous fluid. Rapid drainage of large volumes of pleural fluid resulting in sudden re-expansion may be a contributing factor as can re-expansion of a lung which has been collapsed for several days. Clinical findings can be quite profound with the patient developing symptoms and signs within 2 hours following chest drainage and lung re-expansion. Signs include tachypnoea, tachycardia and central cyanosis. Chest radiography may show ground glass appearance. Close cardiorespiratory monitoring with symptomatic support is key to survival.

Oesophageal Perforation

This is a rare complication following chest drain insertion. The drainage of enteric contents should raise the suspicion of an injury and contrast imaging will confirm the diagnosis.

Chylothorax

Injury to the thoracic duct can lead to the development of chylothorax. Appropriate investigations include medium chain triglycerides levels, which directly enter the portal system, thereby avoiding the lymphatic system.

Infection

Ascending infection leading to empyema is a serious complication following chest drainage and can occur in up to 8% of cases. Cases of infection are higher for emergency insertions of drains than for elective procedures. Routine antibiotics are not indicated, except in trauma cases where gross contamination is expected.

Summary

Chest drain insertion is a vital part of the management of the trauma, cardiothoracic surgical and chest medical patient. It should be undertaken by experienced operators to avoid significant injury to other intrathoracic or intra-abdominal structures leading to morbidity and mortality. Routine aftercare should be undertaken by experienced staff who can monitor the functionality of the drain and observe closely for complications.

Further Reading

Adegboye VO, Falade A, Osinusi K, Obajimi MO. Reexpansion pulmonary oedema as a complication of pleural drainage. *Nigerian Postgraduate Medical Journal.* 2002; 9: 214–220.

Havelock T, Teoh R, Laws D, Gleeson F. Pleural procedures and thoracic ultrasound: British Thoracic Society Pleural Disease Guideline 2010. *Thorax.* 2010; 65(Suppl 2): 61–76.

Hewett FC. Thoracentesis: the plan of continuous aspiration. *British Medical Journal.* 1876; 1: 317.

Kesieme EB, Dongo A, Ezemba N, et al. Tube thoracostomy: complications and its management. *Pulmonary Medicine.* 2012; 256878.

Lamont T, Surkitt-Parr M, Scarpello J, et al. Insertion of chest drains: summary of a safety report from the National Patient Safety Agency. *British Medical Journal.* 2009; 339: b4923.

MCQs

1. **Indications for insertion of a chest drain include:**
   (a) Pneumothorax
   (b) Chylothorax
   (c) Empyema
   (d) Haemothorax
   (e) All of the above

2. **The boundaries of the triangle of safety are:**
   (a) Anterior border of latissimus dorsi, lateral border of pectoralis major and inferiorly a line superior to the nipple
   (b) Lateral border of serratius anterior, medial border of latissimus dorsi and superiorly the nipple
   (c) Medial border of pectoralis minor, lateral border of pectoralis major and the sixth costal interspace
   (d) None of the above

3. **The commonest complication of chest drain insertion is:**
   (a) Malposition
   (b) Bleeding
   (c) Infection
   (d) Tension pneumothorax

4. **The purpose of an underwater seal is to:**
   (a) Maintain a positive intrapleural pressure
   (b) To allow drainage of pleural contents
   (c) To prevent infection
   (d) To maintain a negative intrapleural pressure
5. **A 65 year old female had a right chest drain inserted for a large pleural effusion 2 hours ago. She drained 3 litres of serosanguinous fluid within the first 45 minutes. You are asked to see her because she is in respiratory distress with tachypnoea, tachycardia and mild cyanosis. The most likely cause for this is:**
   (a) Tension pneumothorax
   (b) Haemothorax
   (c) Re-expansion pulmonary oedema
   (d) Bronchopleural fistula
   (e) Cardiac herniation

Exercise answers are available on p.467. Alternatively, take the test online at www.cambridge.org/CardiothoracicMCQ

Chapter 10

Cardiac Pacing and Defibrillation

Sérgio Barra and Patrick Heck

Introduction

Patients admitted to a cardiothoracic critical care unit (CCU) are at increased risk for cardiac arrhythmias and severe conduction disturbances, which represent an important cause of morbidity and can be potentially life threatening. Sustained arrhythmias may occur in up to 20% of critically ill patients admitted to the CCU. Atrial fibrillation (AF) and ventricular tachycardia (VT) represent the majority of tachyarrhythmias, while conduction disturbances with severe bradycardia can account for up to 20%.

These events may represent the primary reason for admission, but are often the result of a series of insults commonly seen in the context of a CCU, such as hypoxia, myocardial ischaemia, infection, sepsis, adrenergic hyperactivity, QT interval prolongation and electrolyte imbalance. Additional causes or triggers include cardiac surgery, mechanical ventilation, mechanical irritation from central venous catheters, inotropic and vasopressor agents and drugs known to prolong the QT interval.

The presence of significant structural heart disease, chronic obstructive pulmonary disease or other significant extracardiac comorbidities, systemic inflammatory response syndrome, sepsis, high central venous pressure and low arterial oxygen tension are known predictors of a higher arrhythmic risk. However, it is often not possible to predict or prevent the occurrence of severe arrhythmias or conduction disturbances and therefore a prompt diagnosis and treatment are required.

Management includes the correction of a known trigger as well as treatment directed at the arrhythmia itself (such as antiarrhythmic drugs, pacing, cardioversion or defibrillation). The impact of a certain arrhythmia depends on the patient's underlying cardiac and respiratory function and the characteristics of the arrhythmia itself (rate, duration, irregularity), and these parameters will also influence the urgency and type of treatment required.

In addition, patients in the cardiothoracic CCU may have previously implanted cardiac electronic devices such as standard pacemakers, cardiac resynchronisation therapy (CRT) devices and implantable cardioverter-defibrillators (ICD). Although implantation, follow-up and troubleshooting of these devices should be in the domain of a trained cardiologist, it is imperative that intensive care physicians are familiar with the patients' underlying cardiac diagnoses, the reason for the device implant, the basics of the current cardiac electronic device technology and the most frequent issues relevant in the context of a cardiothoracic CCU.

The purpose of this chapter is to discuss the role of pacing and defibrillation in patients admitted to a cardiothoracic CCU and the most frequently encountered issues involving pacemakers and ICDs.

Pacing in the Cardiothoracic Critical Care Unit

The most common indication for pacing, either temporary or permanent, is bradycardia. Bradyarrhythmias are relatively common in patients admitted to the CCU following cardiac surgery. In most cases, these events are temporary and due to sick sinus syndrome, slow AF or atrioventricular (AV) block.

Causes of Bradycardia

The most common cause of bradycardia in the cardiothoracic CCU is postoperative heart block. Up to 8% of patients undergoing aortic valve replacement were shown to require permanent pacemaker implantation. Local oedema may prolong conduction times, but direct injury to the conduction system during removal of penetrating calcium or insertion of deep stiches placed during valve surgery are the main cause. Postoperative complete AV block is seen in approximately 4% of patients undergoing mitral valve replacement and ring annuloplasty, although any degree of AV block may be seen in nearly 25%. Damage to the AV nodal artery may play a role in these cases. Proximal left anterior descending artery and septal artery disease have also been shown to increase risk of postoperative AV block. Predictors of need for permanent pacemaker implantation include older age, female sex, greater preoperative end-systolic diameter and left ventricular septum hypertrophy, pre-existing conduction system disease, severe annular calcification, prolonged total perfusion time, re-do operations and history of renal dysfunction, hypertension and bicuspid aortic valve. Predictive models have been developed for the prediction of perioperative need for permanent pacemaker implantation.

When to Pace

Acutely, the decision to pace is based on the haemodynamic impact caused by the underlying bradycardia, rather than the specific rhythm disturbance per se. When pacing is required, it may be temporary or permanent. Temporary pacing options include surgically implanted epicardial pacing wires, transvenous pacing leads implanted fluoroscopically or using floatation balloons or, in emergency situations, transcutaneous pacing via external defibrillator pads. Decisions on permanent pacemaker implantation are based on whether the bradycardia is expected to resolve or not.

The American College of Cardiology/American Heart Association guidelines recommend permanent pacemaker implantation for patients with postoperative third-degree or advanced second-degree AV block *that is not expected to resolve*, although the timing for implant is left to the physician's discretion. Most authors recommend pacemaker implantation 5–7 days after the operation if conduction disturbances persist, especially in patients in whom these disturbances are unlikely to recover, namely those at advanced age, with pre-existing conduction system disease and submitted to valve surgery. Recovery is common in patients with sick sinus syndrome, but unlikely in the case of complete heart block. Predictors of long-term pacemaker dependency are complete AV block as the indication, bypass time longer than 105–120 minutes, preoperative history of syncope and body mass index ≥28.5 kg/m^2.

The cost of prolonged occupation of intensive care beds and prolonged hospital stay, as well as the increased morbidity, reduced mobilisation, comfort and safety associated with prolonged temporary pacing should be weighed against the cost and risks of unnecessary pacemaker implantation in patients who would otherwise demonstrate a full recovery.

Basic Pacemaker Functioning

A detailed review of pacemaker function is beyond the scope of this chapter, but certain considerations regarding basic pacemaker types and function are worth mentioning. In its simplest form a pacing system delivers regular electrical impulses to the heart at a programmed rate. The minimum energy required to be delivered by the pacing system in order to achieve electrical capture is called the **pacing threshold**. Most modern pacing systems are designed to also look for intrinsic electrical activity first, before pacing, in order to minimise any unnecessary pacing but also to prevent delivery of a ventricular pacing stimulus on a T wave, which can be dangerous and trigger arrhythmias. To do this the pacing system has to be able to **sense** intrinsic electrical activity.

Pacing Mode

Whether permanent implanted systems or temporary external pacing boxes, all pacing systems have different pacing modes that dictate their function. The North American and British Group (NBG) pacemaker code is a three- to five-letter code designed to describe pacemaker mode.

- The first letter designates the chamber paced: A stands for atrium, V for ventricle, D for both (dual), O if the pacemaker has been deactivated.
- The second letter designates the chamber sensed (A, V, D, O): O represents asynchronous pacing without sensing.
- The third letter describes the pacemaker's response to a sensed signal: I (inhibition) means the pacemaker discharge is inhibited by a sensed signal; T (trigger) means the pacemaker discharge is actually triggered by a sensed signal; D (dual) means both inhibition and triggering responses are available (for example, in a DDD pacemaker, an atrial sensed signal will *inhibit* atrial pacing but *trigger* ventricular pacing after a prespecified delay).

Table 10.1 Pacemaker modes of potential applicability to patients in the cardiothoracic critical care unit

MODE	Applicability
AOO and VOO	• Asynchronous pacing without any sensing • Useful during surgery or when a patient is exposed to external sources of noise (such as diathermy) • AOO should only be selected if the underlying condition is sick sinus syndrome, but with normal AV conduction
VVI	• Ventricular demand pacing • This is the most common mode used for patients with severe bradycardia • Spontaneous ventricular activity is sensed and therefore there is a low risk of R-on-T phenomenon with subsequent ventricular arrhythmias • There is also a low risk of pacemaker mediated tachycardia • The lack of AV synchrony may reduce cardiac output
DDD	• Pacing and sensing in both chambers with AV synchrony • Optimal pacing mode in patients with sick sinus syndrome or AV block • The response to DDD pacing depends on the underlying rhythm • There is a small risk of pacemaker mediated tachycardia
DDI	• Sensing occurs in both chambers, but a sensed atrial signal does not trigger ventricular pacing • Tracking of rapid atrial rates (in patients with atrial fibrillation, atrial flutter or atrial tachycardia) will not occur • Pacemaker mediated tachycardia is not possible in this mode

- Position four refers to the rate-response algorithm and is only relevant for permanent systems. Rate-response means the pacemaker will be able to increase its pacing rate in response to increasing physiological needs. This is possible due to the incorporation of either activity sensors with vibration detectors or minute-ventilation sensors.
- Position five is used to indicate whether multisite pacing is present.

A three-letter code is adequate to describe emergency temporary pacing and most forms of permanent pacing in the context of a cardiothoracic CCU. Table 10.1 gives examples of pacemaker modes, which the CCU physician should be familiar with. Although the VVI mode is potentially applicable to all cases of bradycardia, it should be kept in mind that the lack of AV synchrony may reduce cardiac output by up to 25%, which is particularly relevant in patients with structural heart disease. A DDD mode, where possible, will ensure appropriate AV synchrony.

Pacemaker Type

Permanent pacemakers can be single chamber (usually right ventricle), dual chamber (right atrium and right ventricle) or biventricular systems. The choice of system is decided based upon underlying cardiac conditions and indication for the device, and will be made by an appropriately trained cardiologist.

Biventricular pacemakers (also referred to as CRT) deserve special mention. These devices are indicated in patients who may not actually have any bradycardia, but have a LV ejection fraction ≤35%, QRS duration ≥120 ms and heart failure symptoms, especially in the presence of left bundle branch block. CRT can improve cardiac output, haemodynamics, heart failure symptoms, functional capacity and quality of life in appropriately selected patients. It is therefore reasonable to expect that a patient on the CCU who already has a CRT device in situ has advanced heart failure, and maintaining correct device function in these patients is even more critical.

Implantable Cardioverter Defibrillators

ICDs are seeing more widespread use within cardiology and are therefore likely to be seen in patients on the cardiothoracic CCU. They are implanted in patients at high risk of life-threatening ventricular arrhythmias, most commonly due to structural heart disease such as ischaemic or dilated cardiomyopathies. All ICDs have pacemaker functions in addition to their defibrillator function. Accordingly, they can be single, dual or biventricular systems.

Figure 10.1a illustrates a simple single chamber pacemaker with a solitary lead in the right ventricle. Figure 10.1b shows a more complex CRT-D device with leads in the right atrium, right ventricle and in a branch of the coronary sinus (for left ventricular pacing).

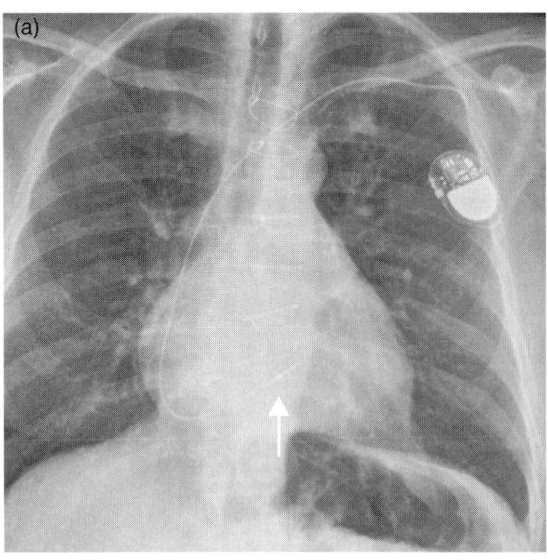

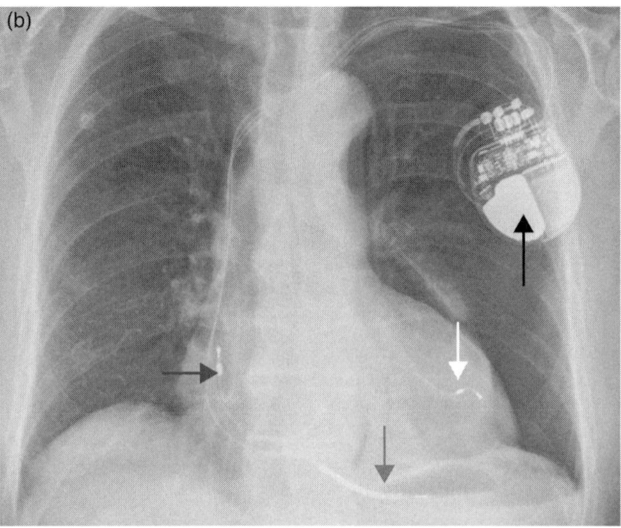

Figure 10.1 Single chamber pacemaker (a) and cardiac resynchronisation therapy defibrillator (b). (a) White arrow, right ventricular lead placed in the interventricular septum. (b) Black arrow, right atrial lead placed in the right atrial appendage; grey arrow, single-coil ICD lead placed in the right ventricular apex; white arrow, left ventricular lead placed in a branch of the coronary sinus; black arrow, high-energy device.

Pacing Related Complications

Pacing related complications can either be as a consequence of the implant procedure itself or due to abnormal or unexpected pacemaker function. Although intensive care physicians do not implant or program pacemakers, it is important to be aware of potential environmental factors that may impact on pacemaker function and possible acute complications related with the temporary or permanent pacing system implantation.

Implant Complications

With any transvenous system, permanent or temporary, the following acute implant related complications may occur: myocardial perforation with pericardial effusion and tamponade, pneumothorax, haemothorax, lead displacement or acute infection.

Other Complications

Other potential issues involving patients with pacemakers include the precautions needed when performing direct current cardioversion or defibrillation, the applicability and utility of magnet application, the possibility of electromagnetic interference and apparent or real system malfunction with failure to pace, failure to capture, failure to sense or increasing pacing threshold.

Pacemaker–Patient–Environment Interactions and Special Considerations

Certain precautions should be taken when performing specific procedures or manoeuvres in patients carrying cardiac electronic devices and this list is by no means exhaustive:

- When externally defibrillating a patient with a pacemaker the external electrodes should not be placed close to the pacemaker, the minimal effective energy should be used and the device must be checked afterwards.
- Certain situations may cause a temporary rise in pacing threshold and thereby impair device function, including electrolyte disturbance and immediately after CPR.
- Subclavian puncture should be avoided ipsilateral to implanted devices when inserting a central venous line due to the risk of lead insulation tear.
- Pulmonary artery catheters should also be avoided, if possible, in patients with recent device implantations due to the risk of lead displacement.
- Atrial pacing spikes might be misinterpreted as QRS complexes by intra-aortic balloon pumps

Table 10.2 Troubleshooting issues encountered in patients with pacemakers

	Causes	Manifestations	Troubleshooting
Failure of output	• Battery depletion • Component failure • Total lead fracture • Loose connections between generator and lead • Oversensing	Absence of pacing spikes, with or without magnet application Asystole or bradycardia, depending on the patient's underlying rhythm	• Perform chest X-ray to exclude lead fracture • Pacemaker interrogation will reveal battery voltage depletion if true output failure is due to battery end-of-life or very high or infinite impedance in the presence of lead fracture • Replace lead or generator if needed • Reduce sensitivity if oversensing is the cause of pacing inhibition
Failure to capture	• Increase in pacing threshold above programmed value • Defective pacing leads (partial fracture or insulation breach; the latter may be caused by central venous catheter placement through subclavian route) • Battery depletion • Lead displacement • Severe hyperglycaemia, hyperkalaemia, acidosis and alkalosis	Presence of pacing spikes without subsequent myocardial capture (shown by the absence of an electrogram) Higher than normal amplitude of pacing spikes if insulation failure Asystole or bradycardia, depending on the patient's underlying rhythm	• Reprogram energy output (increase voltage output or pulse duration) • Pacemaker interrogation will reveal high impedance in the presence of lead fracture or low impedance if insulation failure • Perform chest X-ray to exclude lead displacement • Replace lead if needed • Correct electrolyte and metabolic disturbances
Rapid pacing	• Oversensing of the atrial channel (due to partial lead fracture or electromagnetic interference) • Underlying atrial tachyarrhythmia with tracking of p waves to the programmed upper rate limit	Rapid ventricular paced rhythm – there is 'tracking' of the atrial sensed events	• Adjust sensitivity to prevent oversensing • Program pacemaker to VVI or DDI mode to prevent tracking of atrial tachyarrhythmia

and interfere with triggering. Using arterial waveform is an alternative.

- The use of electrocautery can cause interference with both pacing and ICD systems. In pacemakers it might result in inappropriate inhibition of pacing as the device misinterprets the electrical interference as intrinsic rhythm. In ICDs it may result in the delivery of shock therapy as the high frequency noise from electrocautery may be interpreted as a tachycardia requiring treatment.

Troubleshooting Pacing and ICD Systems

Temporary pacing, either with epicardially or transvenously placed leads, is often needed following cardiac surgery. Problems associated with temporary pacing include the displacement of the lead, myocardial perforation, which may lead to tamponade, increasing pacing threshold, lack of capture and lack of sensing. When lack of pacing or lack of capture are detected, all connections should be immediately checked, the ventricular output set to maximum and the generator programmed into asynchronous mode. Lack of capture is usually the result of lead displacement or threshold rise.

Whilst there are many similarities to the approach taken with troubleshooting a permanent pacing system, it is a more complex device and often will require the assistance of a physician familiar with pacemakers. Pacing and sensing problems can originate in the generator, the pacing leads, the lead–myocardium interface or the patient. Table 10.2 lists the most frequent troubleshooting issues encountered in patients with pacemakers, their most frequent causes and recommendations to overcome the problem. Figure 10.2 illustrates ECGs of different pacemaker malfunctions.

Most of the considerations made for pacemaker troubleshooting are equally valid in patients with ICDs. Other important occurrences in these patients include the delivery of inappropriate ICD shocks, ICD storms or

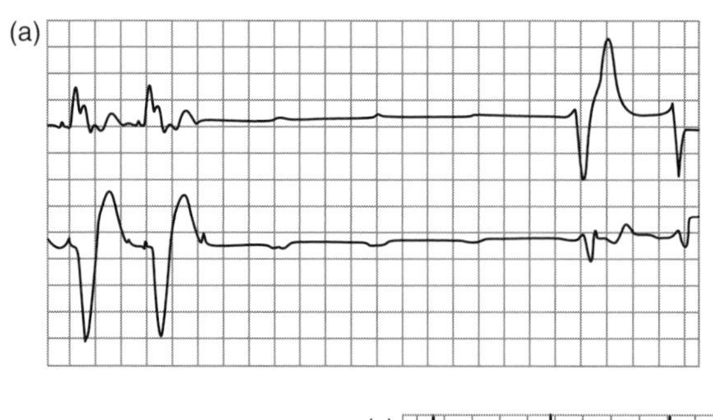

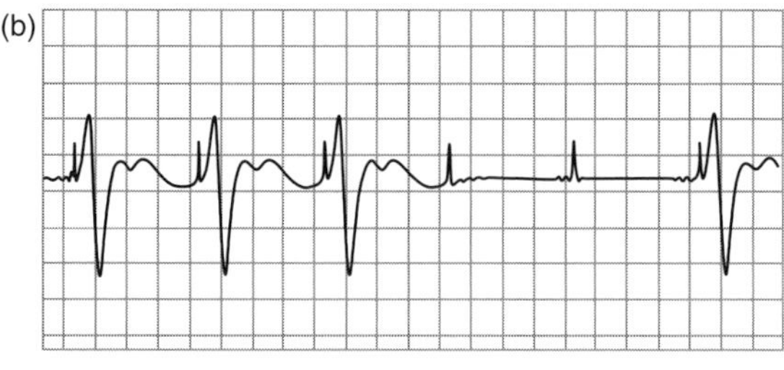

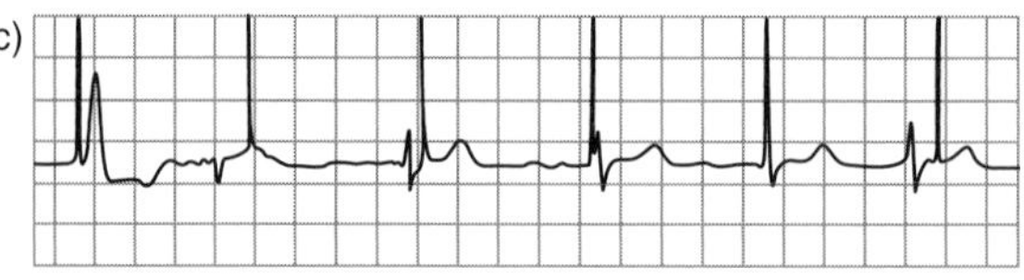

Figure 10.2 Pacemaker troubleshooting. (a) Failure to output (absence of pacing spikes causing a 3 second pause). (b) Failure to capture (4th and 5th pacing spikes are not followed by ventricular electrograms). (c) Undersensing (all but the first pacing spike are delivered inappropriately due to undersensing of electrical signals). (A black and white version of this figure will appear in some formats. For the colour version, please refer to the plate section.)

ineffective ICD therapies in patients with true life-threatening ventricular arrhythmias. As ICD systems are even more complex than pacing systems, specialist input is invariably required in troubleshooting these devices.

Pacemaker and ICD 'Magnet' Mode

Intensive care physicians should also be familiar with the typical response of pacemakers and ICDs to magnet application but this should generally only be used when appropriate reprogramming of the device to the desired function is not possible. Magnet modes can vary between manufacturers and can permanently alter device function. Some new devices allow for programming to 'off' function.

A magnet placed over a pacemaker, but not an ICD, will usually make it pace in an asynchronous mode at a fixed heart rate. This is useful to protect pacemaker dependent patients during diathermy or other sources of electromagnetic interference. However, not all pacemakers switch to a continuous asynchronous mode when a magnet is applied, as the response to magnet application may vary across models.

Magnet application over an ICD will prevent the device from sensing and delivering any therapies, which is useful in patients having inappropriate ICD shocks or ICD storms or when electrocautery is being used. However, different ICD models may respond differently, if at all, and in some cases therapies may be turned off completely until the magnet is removed and then reapplied.

Cardioversion and Defibrillation in the Cardiothoracic Intensive Care Unit

Defibrillation and cardioversion are occasionally required in the CCU. Any atrial or ventricular tachyarrhythmia causing severe haemodynamic compromise may need to be immediately dealt with using electrical cardioversion and local advanced life support guidelines should be followed. Unsynchronised high energy shocks should be used to treat ventricular fibrillation or very fast polymorphic VT, whereas synchronised shocks should be used for cardioverting AF and haemodynamically stable VT. Defibrillators delivering biphasic waveforms should be preferably used.

Electrical cardioversion is very effective in the treatment of tachyarrhythmias, but it should be borne in mind that unless the underlying cause of the arrhythmia is identified and treated, such as ischaemia or electrolyte disturbance, there is a high probability of the arrhythmia recurring.

Special Considerations for Defibrillation or Cardioversion

- Electrical cardioversion is contraindicated in patients with known digitalis toxicity, not only due to the lower efficacy in this context, but also because junctional or paroxysmal atrial tachycardia and even VF may occur within a few minutes of cardioversion.

- Ipsilateral pneumothorax can increase defibrillation threshold in patients with an ICD and may result in unsuccessful defibrillation by the device.
- Patients with atrial fibrillation lasting for longer than 24 to 48 hours and without appropriate anticoagulation are at risk of stroke following cardioversion and therefore this should not be performed without previously excluding left atrial appendage thrombus with a transoesophageal echocardiogram, unless there is significant haemodynamic compromise. Consideration of anticoagulation should be made following cardioversion even in the absence of clots, as the thromboembolic risk is higher in the postcardioversion period.
- When external cardioversion fails, potential solutions include applying additional pressure to the paddles during the shock, changing the electrodes to an anteroposterior orientation or administering intravenous antiarrhythmics such as amiodarone (for both atrial and ventricular arrhythmias) or ibutilide (for atrial fibrillation), which lower the energy required to restore sinus rhythm.

Conclusions

Cardiac arrhythmias and conduction disturbances are frequent in the context of a cardiothoracic critical care unit. Furthermore, an increasing number of patients with cardiac electronic devices are currently admitted to these units. It is imperative that the intensive care physician is aware of the basic function of pacemakers and implantable cardioverter-defibrillators, possible complications associated with the use of these devices, the most frequent troubleshooting issues and the diagnostic and therapeutic options that pacemakers and ICDs may offer to critical patients.

Learning Points

- In patients admitted to the cardiothoracic CCU and presenting with bradycardia, the decision to pace is based on the haemodynamic impact caused by the underlying bradycardia, rather than the specific rhythm disturbance per se.
- Recovery of severe conduction disturbances is common in patients with sick sinus syndrome, but unlikely in the case of complete heart block, especially in patients at advanced age, with pre-existing conduction system disease or history of syncope and submitted to valve surgery.
- With any transvenous pacing system, intensive care physicians should be aware not only of any potential periprocedural complications, but also issues such as the precautions required when performing direct current cardioversion, the utility of magnet application, electromagnetic interference and apparent or real system malfunction with failure to pace, capture or sense and increasing pacing threshold.
- Appropriate management of an electrical storm includes the correction of the underlying cause, the use of intravenous amiodarone or beta-blockers and reprogramming the ICD if the arrhythmia is well tolerated. Magnet application may be useful to prevent subsequent therapies, while deep sedation or general anaesthesia may in some cases provide complete, albeit temporary, control.
- Electrical cardioversion is very effective in the treatment of tachyarrhythmias, but unless the underlying cause of the arrhythmia is identified and treated there is a high probability of recurrence. When cardioversion fails, applying additional pressure to the paddles during the shock, changing the electrodes to an anteroposterior orientation or administering intravenous antiarrhythmics which lower the energy required to restore sinus rhythm may be useful.

Further Reading

Berdajs D, Schurr UP, Wagner A, et al. Incidence and pathophysiology of atrioventricular block following mitral valve replacement and ring annuloplasty. *European Journal of Cardiothoracic Surgery.* 2008; 34: 55–61.

Dawkins S, Hobson AR, Kalra PR, et al. Permanent pacemaker implantation after isolated aortic valve replacement: incidence, indications, and predictors. *Annals of Thoracic Surgery.* 2008; 85: 108–112.

El-Chami MF, Sawaya FJ, Kilgo P, et al. Ventricular arrhythmia after cardiac surgery: incidence, predictors, and outcomes. *Journal of the American College of Cardiology.* 2012; 60: 2664–2671.

Epstein AE, Di Marco JP, Ellenbogen KA, et al. ACC/AHA/HRS 2008 Guidelines for Device-Based Therapy of Cardiac Rhythm Abnormalities: a report of the American College of Cardiology/American Heart

Association Task Force on Practice Guidelines (Writing Committee to Revise the ACC/AHA/NASPE 2002 Guideline) *Journal of the American College of Cardiology.* 2008; 51: e1–62.

Erdogan HB, Kayalar N, Ardal H, et al. Risk factors for requirement of permanent pacemaker implantation after aortic valve replacement. *Journal of Cardiac Surgery.* 2006; 21: 211–215.

Glikson M, Dearani JA, Hyberger LK, et al. Indications, effectiveness, and long-term dependency in permanent pacing after cardiac surgery. *American Journal of Cardiology.* 1997; 80: 1309–1313.

Gordon RS, Ivanov J, Cohen G, Ralph-Edwards AL. Permanent cardiac pacing after a cardiac operation: predicting the use of permanent pacemakers. *Annals of Thoracic Surgery.* 1998; 66: 1698–1704.

Knotzer H, Mayr A, Ulmer H, Lederer W. Tachyarrhythmias in a surgical intensive care unit: a case-controlled epidemiologic study. *Intensive Care Medicine.* 2000; 26: 908–914.

Liu Q, Kong AL, Chen R, et al. Propofol and arrhythmias: two sides of the coin. *Acta Pharmacologica Sinica.* 2011; 32: 817–823.

Merin O, Ilan M, Oren A, et al. Permanent pacemaker implantation following cardiac surgery: indications and long-term follow-up. *Pacing and Clinical Electrophysiology.* 2009; 32: 7–12.

Mosseri M, Meir G, Lotan C, et al. Coronary pathology predicts conduction disturbances after coronary artery bypass grafting. *Annals of Thoracic Surgery.* 1991; 51: 248–252.

Nardi P, Pellegrino A, Scafuri A, et al. Permanent pacemaker implantation after isolated aortic valve replacement: incidence, risk factors and surgical technical aspects. *Journal of Cardiovascular Medicine (Hagerstown).* 2010; 11: 14–19.

Onalan O, Crystal A, Lashevsky I, et al. Determinants of pacemaker dependency after coronary and/or mitral or aortic valve surgery with long-term follow-up. *American Journal of Cardiology.* 2008; 101: 203–208.

Reinelt P, Karth GD, Geppert A, Heinz G. Incidence and type of cardiac arrhythmias in critically ill patients: a single center experience in a medical-cardiological ICU. *Intensive Care Medicine.* 2001; 27: 1466–1473.

Trappe H-J, Brandts B, Weismueller P. Arrhythmias in the intensive care patient. *Current Opinion in Critical Care.* 2003; 9: 345–355.

MCQs

1. **In patients admitted to the cardiothoracic CCU following cardiac surgery, which features predict the need for pacing in the event of significant bradycardia?**
   (a) Valve surgery rather than coronary revascularisation
   (b) Advanced age
   (c) History of syncope
   (d) Previous left bundle branch block
   (e) All of the above

2. **In patients admitted to the cardiothoracic CCU following cardiac surgery and with temporary pacing systems showing failure to capture, which underlying mechanisms should be considered?**
   (a) Increase of the pacing threshold above programmed value
   (b) Lead displacement
   (c) Loose connections
   (d) Hyperkalaemia, acidosis or alkalosis
   (e) All of the above

3. **In patients admitted to the cardiothoracic CCU and presenting with a fast atrial arrhythmia, which acute measure should not be taken?**
   (a) Direct current cardioversion in the case of severe haemodynamic compromise
   (b) Unsynchronised direct current cardioversion
   (c) Correction of any electrolyte disturbance
   (d) Administration of an appropriate antiarrhythmic medication, such as amiodarone, in the first hours of well-tolerated atrial fibrillation
   (e) Correction of underlying heart failure, myocardial ischaemia, bleeding or anaemia

4. **A patient is day 1 post cardiac surgery and pacing dependent with epicardial temporary pacing wires. Brief periods of asystole are seen on the monitor. Which of the following measures should not be considered?**
   (a) Retesting the pacing threshold and increasing output if required

(b) Checking the connectors of the pacing wires and pacing box

(c) Placement of transcutaneous pacing pads in case of need

(d) Increasing the sensitivity of the pacing system to detect any intrinsic rhythm

(e) Replacing the batteries in the pacing box

5. **A patient has a permanent pacemaker in situ in VVI mode and a lower heart rate limit of 60 beats per minute and is functioning normally. Which of the following statements is correct?**

(a) The atrium will be paced by the device when needed

(b) The pacemaker will provide adequate AV synchrony

(c) The pacemaker will prevent the heart from going slower than 60 beats per minute

(d) The pacemaker will be unaffected by the use of electrocautery

(e) The pacemaker will increase the patient's heart rate beyond 60 beats per minute with exercise

Exercise answers are available on p.467. Alternatively, take the test online at www.cambridge.org/CardiothoracicMCQ

Chapter 11

Arterial and Venous Catheterisation and Invasive Monitoring

Stuart A Gillon, Nicholas A Barrett and Christopher IS Meadows

Principles of Vascular Access

Vascular catheters are ubiquitous to cardiothoracic critical care. They may be defined or described on the basis of numerous factors (Table 11.1). For the purposes of this chapter, vascular access relates to catheters within the arterial or central venous system.

Insertion

Vascular catheter insertion within the critical care unit is almost universally by the Seldinger technique: a needle is inserted into the target vessel (or a tributary of the target vessel); a guide wire is passed into the vessel; one or more dilators are passed over the guide wire to create a tract through the skin and soft tissues; and the catheter is advanced over the guide wire, into the vessel.

Traditionally, the target vessel was sought using a combination of anatomical landmarks and palpation. The increasing availability of point-of-care ultrasound technology within the critical care environment has led to a gradual move towards real-time ultrasound guided vascular access. The use of ultrasound for vascular access has been demonstrated to increase success and reduce complications and is now considered a standard of care by the National Institute of Clinical Excellence.

Position may be confirmed by ensuring free aspiration of blood, by transduction of pressure (thereby confirming arterial or venous placement), by measurement of the oxygen content of aspirated blood (suggestive of arterial or venous placement) or by imaging (either X-ray or ultrasound).

Complications

The complications associated with line placement, and potential strategies to minimise risk are listed in Table 11.2.

Table 11.1 Factors defining vascular catheters

Type of vessel: arterial, venous; peripheral, central
Site of insertion: jugular, femoral, central, etc.
Duration of access: short term, medium term, long term
Pathway from skin to vessel: tunnelled, non-tunnelled
Length: short, mid, long
Additional features: number of lumens, antibiotic, antiseptic or heparin impregnated

Pressure Monitoring

Transducers

A transducer converts mechanical energy (hydrostatic pressure within the vascular system) into an electrical signal; the hydrostatic pressure within the catheter is quantified and displayed as both a value and a waveform.

A continuous column of fluid maintains contact between the transducer and the vascular system. Changes in pressure are transmitted down the column of fluid, leading to distortion of the transducer membrane. The membrane contains a strain gauge: distortion of the membrane stretches a wire, altering its resistance. The wire is integrated into a Wheatstone bridge, which allows accurate determination of changes in resistance. The change in resistance equates to change in pressure and this is displayed on the monitor.

A valve within the transducer system permits flow of 3–4 ml of saline per hour through the arterial line, to maintain line patency. Some units heparinise the saline flush on the basis that this may reduce the risk of intracatheter thrombus formation. The use of heparin, however, exposes the patient to heparin (and associated reactions) and may interfere with the accuracy of coagulation samples drawn from the line if the flush fluid is incompletely removed prior to sampling.

Table 11.2 Complications related to central venous catheter placement and strategies to reduce risk

Immediate	Damage to adjacent structure (e.g. arterial puncture, pneumothorax)	Ultrasound guidance, experienced operator (particularly in the presence of anatomical abnormalities)
	Air embolism	Head-down position in jugular and subclavian approaches
	Bleeding	Correction of coagulopathy prior to insertion
Late	Infection	Introduction of CVC insertion 'bundles', full barrier precautions during insertion, use of antibiotic impregnated catheters, use of antimicrobial impregnated patches over the insertion site, avoidance of the femoral vein as an insertion site, removal of catheters when no longer required
	Thrombosis	Avoidance of femoral insertion, use of heparin impregnated catheters, early removal

Systematic review of studies examining the efficacy of heparinised saline in this context found no convincing evidence of improved catheter patency.

Resonance and Damping

Every material has a natural frequency: the frequency at which it freely resonates. If a material is exposed to a frequency close to its natural frequency it will resonate, or oscillate, at its maximum amplitude. This physical phenomenon is of significance to pressure monitoring systems as, if the frequency of one of the components of the measured pressure wave is close to the natural frequency, the excessive oscillation generated will distort the measured pressure.

In order to avoid this phenomenon, the natural frequency of a pressure monitoring system must be several orders of magnitude greater than the component frequencies of the waveform being measured. Using longer tubing, of wider diameter and using a low density fluid within the tubing, will increase the natural frequency of a system.

Damping describes the dissipation of energy in a resonant, oscillating system. A pressure monitoring system may be over-damped by tubing, which is of excessive length, insufficient diameter, or made from highly compliant material. Additionally, kinks, clots or air bubbles within the system will contribute to damping.

The optimal system strikes a balance between resonance and damping. A system with excessive resonance will tend to over-measure peak (systolic) pressures and under-measure trough (diastolic) pressures; mean pressure should be unaffected. Such systems are described as under-damped. In contrast, a system with excessive damping and insufficient resonance (damped system) will under-measure peak and over-measure trough pressures; again mean pressure is unaffected. Whilst pressure measurement systems are produced with material and dimensions most suited to optimal damping, over-damping and under-damping may occur.

Zeroing

Accurate measurement of physiological pressure requires the transducer to be 'zeroed' to atmospheric pressure (a system pressure of zero equates to atmospheric pressure, as physiological pressures are described as relative to atmospheric pressure). Calibration involves opening the pressure system to air, and referencing this pressure to zero on the system. Transducers are prone to baseline drift and therefore this process should be undertaken several times per day.

The height of the transducer relative to the patient is also important. By convention, the transducer should be at the same height above the floor as the left atrium of the patient. A transducer placed above or below the height of the atrium will lead to under-reading and over-reading of pressure respectively.

Arterial Catheters

There are three major indications for placement of an arterial catheter.

1. Haemodynamic instability (either current or expected) in which beat to beat measurement of arterial pressure allows close monitoring of haemodynamic state and safe titration of inotropic and vasoactive drugs.
2. Need for frequent arterial blood sampling (e.g. respiratory failure or severe, persistent metabolic disturbance).
3. Non-pulsatile flow (for example in cardiac bypass or venoarterial ECMO) as there is no alternative method of measuring systemic pressures.

Arterial catheters may be inserted into:

- Peripheral arteries (e.g. most commonly radial, also ulnar, brachial, dorsalis pedis);
- Central arteries (e.g. most commonly femoral, also axillary).

The arterial pressure in peripheral arteries differs from that in central arteries.

- A decrease in arterial compliance with increasing distance from the heart leads to a higher systolic and lower diastolic pressure measurement in peripheral compared with central arteries; the mean pressure should be comparable.
- The tone of peripheral arteries will demonstrate a more significant response to temperature and vasoactive medications than central arteries; measurement of peripheral arterial pressure could therefore be a poor reflection of the central arterial pressure perfusing vital organs.
- These differences between central and peripheral pressure are more pronounced in the elderly and in those with vascular disease.

Information Derived from the Arterial Waveform

- Pulse rate
- Systolic blood pressure
- Diastolic blood pressure
- Mean blood pressure
- The shape of the arterial waveform is determined by numerous factors:
  - The stroke volume,
  - Left ventricular contractility,
  - Capacitance of the central arterial tree (the ability to distend and accommodate ejected blood),
  - Peripheral resistance (the rate at which blood dissipates from the central arteries into peripheral circulation).
- The dichrotic notch is the positive deflection in the downstroke of the arterial waveform, which represents closure of the aortic valve:
  - Typically occurs at one third into the pressure wave descent when aortic pressure (AoP) exceeds left ventricular pressure (LVP);
  - If peripheral resistance is reduced (e.g. sepsis), AoP > LVP later in the cycle and the dicrotic notch shifts down the curve.

Pulse Pressure Variation

- The intrathoracic pressure varies throughout the respiratory cycle; this alters the loading conditions of the heart and results in variation in stroke volume and pulse pressure between inspiration and expiration.
- The magnitude of this variation is greater on the steep portion of the Frank–Starling curve (where a patient is likely to increase cardiac output in response to fluid) than on the flat portion (with less likelihood of fluid responsiveness).
- Meta-analysis of studies relating to pulse pressure variation (PPV) (and the closely related stroke volume variation) suggests that variation of >13% is strongly predictive of fluid responsiveness.
- The studies relating to PPV were however largely conducted in highly controlled environments, in deeply sedated patients, with no spontaneous ventilation; analysis of the intensive care population shows that few patients are comparable to the subjects of the initial studies; the practical application of PPV in the clinical setting therefore has significant limitations.

Central Venous Catheters

A central venous catheter (CVC) is a vascular catheter with a tip sitting in the central venous system. These may be short catheters (15–20 cm) inserted into a central vein (femoral, jugular or subclavian) or longer catheters inserted into a peripheral vein and advanced to the central circulation (peripherally inserted central catheter, PICC).

Indications for CVC placement include the following.

- Administration of drugs which may only be safely delivered directly into a central vein (e.g. amiodarone, noradrenaline, concentrated potassium, cytotoxic agents, total parenteral nutrition).
- Measurement of central venous pressure (CVP) or central venous oxygen saturation ($ScvO_2$).
- To facilitate a procedure which requires access to the central venous circulation (e.g. renal replacement therapy, pulmonary artery catheter

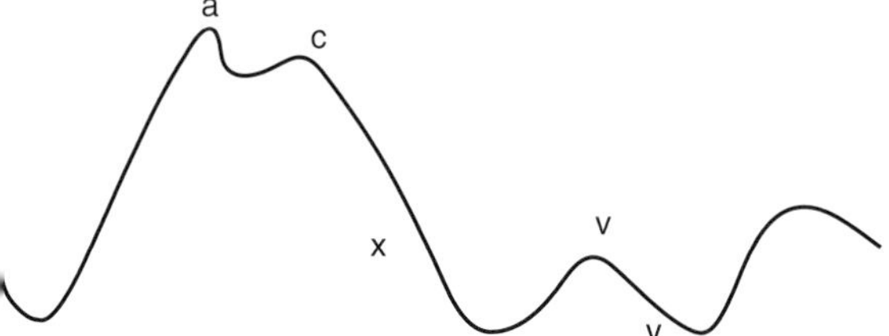

Figure 11.1 CVP trace: a atrial contraction; c closure of tricuspid valve; x atrial relaxation; v ventricular contraction; y opening of the tricuspid valve.

flotation, temporary pacing wire insertion, extracorporeal membrane oxygenation).
- If peripheral venous access proves impossible.

Central Venous Pressure Trace

The central venous pressure (CVP) trace is outlined in Figure 11.1.

Central Pressures

The CVP, when measured in the superior vena cava (SVC) equates to right atrial pressure (RAP). The significance of CVP in terms of the global haemodynamic state is complex and its role in management of the haemodynamic state is controversial.

At the end of the nineteenth century, Otto Frank and Ernest Starling described the relationship between myocardial stretch and stroke volume and demonstrated an increase in cardiac output in response to increasing preload. This so-called Frank–Starling mechanism became a cornerstone of cardiovascular physiology and remains an important concept in haemodynamic management.

Some 50 years after this original work, Arthur Guyton built upon the Frank–Starling concept. Guyton concluded, on the basis of a series of animal models, that venous return (Vr) was the key determinant of cardiac output. According to the Guyton model, Vr is determined by three factors: the *mean circulatory filling pressure* (MCFP) (generated by the elastic properties of the vasculature and the hydrostatic force exerted by volume within the vessels, the so-called stressed volume); *RAP* (against which the MCFP must drive); and the *venous resistance* (which may be altered by changes in regional blood flow to organ vascular beds). The accuracy of this complex model remains the subject of significant debate, not least because it is impossible to test in an intact human circulation. It remains therefore primarily a theoretical construct.

One key practical product of Guyton's work has however arisen: the use of the RAP (in the form of CVP) in the clinical optimisation of cardiac output. Guyton considered RAP to be an independent determinant of SV (and therefore cardiac output). He proposed RAP and SV to have a similar relationship to that between end-diastolic volume and SV reported by Starling. Given its ease of measurement, CVP was thus widely integrated into clinical practice as a measure of left ventricular preload.

The intervening six decades have witnessed significant technological advances in terms of haemodynamic monitoring. Yet the use of CVP as a marker of left ventricular preload persists. The Surviving Sepsis Campaign, for example, recommends a CVP of 8–12 mmHg as a target for volume resuscitation in the shocked septic patient.

The clinical utility of CVP in the assessment of preload is however questionable. Manipulation of preload in the shocked patient is undertaken with a view to optimising cardiac output; any assessment of preload is therefore beneficial only if it reliably identifies those patients in whom increase in preload (by fluid administration) is likely to increase cardiac output. In clinical trials, the CVP has consistently been shown to be a poor determinant of fluid responsiveness. As such, there are calls from some quarters for the CVP as a marker of preload to be abandoned.

Pulmonary Artery Catheter

History

The pulmonary artery catheter (PAC) evolved during the twentieth century as a means of measuring pressure and flow within the pulmonary vasculature. Ronald Bradley of St Thomas' Hospital, London, first described the placement of a catheter in the pulmonary circulation of humans in the 1950s. This original catheter was, however, difficult to site. Harold Swan (an alumnus of St Thomas' Medical School) and his colleague William Ganz (Cedars-Sinai Medical Center, Los Angeles) adapted Bradley's design by adding a flotation balloon, thereby enhancing ease of insertion. The names of Swan and Ganz have since become eponymous with the PAC.

Components

- A typical adult PAC is 110 cm in length and 7–8 F in diameter; distance markers are found every 10 cm to guide insertion.
- It is made of radio-opaque polyvinyl chloride.
- There are typically four lumens, the most distal is located at the tip and used for measuring pulmonary pressures; the most proximal is located around 30 cm from the tip, measures RAP and serves as the route of injection of cold saline for cardiac output measurement.
- A thermistor is located close to the tip for the purposes of cardiac output and core temperature measurement.
- A balloon, 1–1.5 ml in volume, is located close to the tip of the catheter; this is inflated for the purposes of flotation into the pulmonary artery, and measurement of the pulmonary artery wedge pressure.

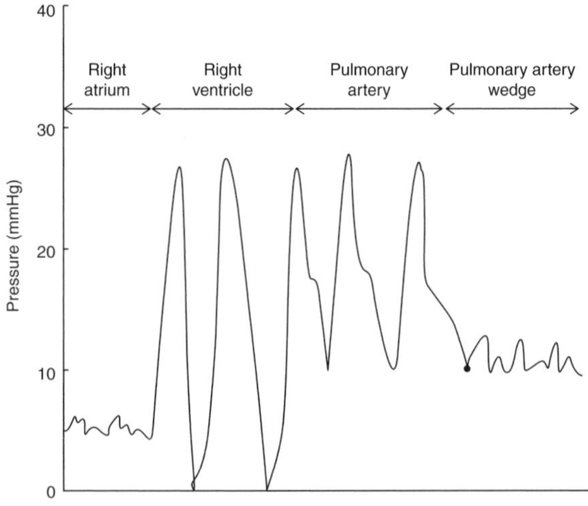

Figure 11.2 Pulmonary artery catheter waveform as it is 'floated' through the heart into pulmonary circulation.

Indications

Indications for insertion of the PAC include:

- Cardiac output monitoring;
- Measurement of right heart pressures, pulmonary artery pressure, and left atrial pressure;
- Measurement of central venous oxygen saturation ($ScvO_2$) and mixed venous oxygen saturation (SvO_2).

Insertion of the Pulmonary Artery Catheter

- The procedure is undertaken using an aseptic technique; all lumens of the catheter are flushed; the distal port is connected to a pressure transducer.
- An insertion sheath is placed using a Seldinger technique into a central vein (right internal jugular and left subclavian provide the most direct route for the flotation catheter).
- The PAC is introduced via the sheath; once the tip is sitting within the vena cava or right atrium, the balloon is inflated and the catheter advanced in a smooth motion; the passage of the catheter from atrium to ventricle to pulmonary artery may be tracked by:
  - The changing pressure waveform (Figure 11.2), the most common approach;
  - Fluoroscopy;
  - Transoesophageal echocardiography.

Pulmonary Artery Measurements

The PAC allows measurement of pressure and flow within the pulmonary vasculature. Table 11.3 outlines direct and indirect variables, which may be obtained from the PAC.

Cardiac Output Monitoring

The PAC measures cardiac output by means of thermodilution. A known volume of cold saline is rapidly injected into the proximal, RA, port. The resultant change in temperature of blood is measured by the thermistor at the tip of the PAC and a washout curve is generated. Blood flow, which equates to cardiac output, is inversely proportional to the rate of temperature change; flow is quantified by means of the Stewart–Hamilton equation:

$$CO = \frac{\dfrac{k(\text{core temperature} - \text{indicator temperature})}{\text{volume of indicator}}}{\text{Change in blood temperature}}$$

Table 11.3 Direct and indirect variables obtained from the pulmonary artery catheter

	Variable	Equation	Normal values
Direct measurements	Right atrial pressure (RAP)		2–6 mmHg
	Right ventricular pressures (RVP)		systolic 20–30 mmHg diastolic 0–5 mmHg
	Pulmonary artery pressures (PAP)		systolic 20–30 mmHg diastolic 8–12 mmHg mean 10–20 mmHg
	Pulmonary artery wedge pressure (PAWP)		4–12 mmHg
	Cardiac output (CO)		4–8 l/min
Derived variables	Cardiac index (CI)	$\frac{CO}{BSA}$	2.5–4 l/min
	Systemic vascular resistance (SVR)	$\frac{MAP - RAP}{CO}$	800–1200 dyne s/cm^5
	Pulmonary vascular resistance (PVR)	$\frac{mPAP - PAWP}{CO}$	37–250 dyne s/cm^5
	DO_2	$CO(SpO_2 \times Hb \times 1.34) + (0.003PaO_2)$	
	VO_2	$10(CaO_2 - CvO_2) \times CO$	

where k is a constant.

The traditional means of cardiac output monitoring via the PAC relies upon intermittent bolus studies and cannot therefore provide continuous cardiac output monitoring. Variants of the PAC are now available which have a heating element in the region of the proximal injection port. This element intermittently heats the passing blood, allowing regular washout curves to be created and near-continuous cardiac output to be calculated.

Evidence Basis

The PAWP may be used in a similar manner to the CVP, as a static marker of preload. However, like the CVP, the PAWP has been demonstrated to be a poor predictor of fluid responsiveness and has therefore, in many centres, been replaced by other, dynamic assessments.

The impact of PAC monitoring upon outcome has been tested in randomised control trials in the general intensive care population (PACMAN study), in patients admitted with acute respiratory distress syndrome (ARDSnet group), in high risk cardiac surgical patients and those with severe heart failure (ESCAPE study). No study demonstrated improved outcomes with the additional information provided by the PAC and there was an increased incidence of adverse, catheter related, events.

The appropriateness of the randomised control trial as a means of testing a monitoring tool is however questionable, since the utility of the PAC is dependent upon clinician ability to correctly interpret the results. Therefore, whilst there have been calls to remove the PAC from clinical practice based upon the results of the above named trials, the PAC proponents remain, particularly amongst those clinicians managing complex cardiac patients.

Transpulmonary Dilution and Pulse Contour Analysis

PiCCO

- The PiCCO system utilises a modified arterial line to provide advanced cardiovascular monitoring.
- The PiCCO arterial line is inserted in a central artery (usually femoral, alternatively axillary).
- The PiCCO connects to a transducer, providing standard arterial line information.
- A thermistor, at the tip of the PiCCO line, allows performance of transpulmonary thermodilution.
  - 15 ml of cold saline is injected into a central line placed in the internal jugular or

subclavian vein; a sensor placed in the CVC port monitors the timing of injection and the temperature of the injectate.
  - The cold injectate crosses the pulmonary circulation and enters the systemic circulation; the resultant change in blood temperature is monitored by the PiCCO thermistor; a temperature washout curve – similar to that generated by a PAC – is used to determine cardiac output.
  - PiCCO transpulmonary thermodilution also provides volumetric data.
    - **Global end diastolic volume (index) (GEDVI)** (650–1000 ml/m^2), volume of blood within the cardiac chambers at end-diastole; indicative of preload. Typically indexed to body surface area.
    - **Intrathoracic blood volume (index) (ITBVI)** (800–1000 ml/m^2), volume of blood within the chest, derived from thermodilution technique; indicative of preload.
    - **Extravascular lung water (index) (EVLWI)** (3–7 ml/m^2), volume of water lying within the lung parenchyma, a marker of pulmonary oedema.
- Following calibration using the described thermodilution technique, the PiCCO system uses mathematical analysis of the pulse waveform to provide continuous measurement of stroke volume (and therefore cardiac output).

LiDCO

- The LiDCO, like the PiCCO, utilises a transpulmonary dilutional technique to determine cardiac output. There are however a number of differences.
  - The LiDCO utilises a standard arterial line, in any artery; the LiDCO system is attached externally to the arterial line.
  - Lithium is used for the dilution technique, rather than cold saline; the dependence upon lithium makes the LiDCO unreliable in those patients on therapeutic lithium or who have recently received non-depolarising muscle relaxants (which cross react with the molecular sensor).
  - The lithium injectate does not require a CVC; a peripheral cannula will suffice.
  - LiDCO does not provide the volumetric measurements offered by the PiCCO.

Non-calibrated Systems

In addition to the PiCCO and LiDCO, several non-calibrated systems are available. Like the continuous cardiac output monitoring offered by calibrated counterparts, these non-calibrated systems utilise waveform analysis to determine stroke volume and subsequently cardiac output. They may offer stroke volume variation (as described in the arterial waveform section). The lack of calibration has called the accuracy of these systems into question and comparison to calibrated systems demonstrates a discrepancy between measured cardiac output.

Learning Points

- Vascular access is a common undertaking in critical care; the use of insertion bundles and real-time ultrasound appears to reduce the incidence of complications.
- Central venous pressure appears to be a poor predictor of fluid responsiveness in clinical practice, it may however offer information regarding the venous system not obtainable by other means.
- The pulmonary artery catheter offers a means of measuring pulmonary pressures, cardiac output and a surrogate of left atrial pressure; its use has not however been demonstrated to change patient outcomes.
- Transpulmonary thermodilution and pulse contour analysis techniques are more commonly employed means of measuring cardiac output than the pulmonary artery catheter; performance in trials is comparable to the pulmonary artery catheter.
- Dynamic markers of cardiovascular performance, such as pulse pressure analysis, may be more accurate in determining volume status than traditional static parameters; whether this accuracy is maintained in the complex critical care population is not clear.

Further Reading

Binanay C, Califf R, Hasselblad V, et al. Evaluation study of congestive heart failure and pulmonary artery catheterization effectiveness: the ESCAPE trial. *Journal of the American Medical Association.* 2005; 294: 1625–1633.

Guyton AC. Determination of cardiac output by equating venous return curves with cardiac response curves. *Physiological Reviews.* 1955: 35: 123–129.

Harvey S, Harrison DA, Singer M, et al. Assessment of the clinical effectiveness of pulmonary artery catheters in management of patients in intensive care (PAC-Man): a randomised controlled trial. *Lancet.* 2005; 366: 472–477.

Marik PE, Cavallazzi R. Does the central venous pressure predict fluid responsiveness? An updated meta-analysis and a plea for some common sense. *Critical Care Medicine.* 2013; 41: 1774–1781.

Marik PE, Lemson J. Fluid responsiveness: an evolution of our understanding. *British Journal of Anaesthesia.* 2014; 112: 617–620.

McGee DC, Gould MK. Preventing complications of central venous catheterization. *New England Journal of Medicine.* 2003; 348: 1123–1133.

Pronovost P, Needham D, Berenholtz S, et al. An intervention to decrease catheter-related bloodstream infections in the ICU. *New England Journal of Medicine.* 2006; 355: 2725–2732.

Sakka S, Kozieras J, Thuemer O, van Hout N. Measurement of cardiac output: a comparison between transpulmonary thermodilution and uncalibrated pulse contour analysis. *British Journal of Anaesthesia.* 2007; 99: 337–342.

Sandham JD, Hull RD, Brant RF, et al. A randomized, controlled trial of the use of pulmonary-artery catheters in high-risk surgical patients. *New England Journal of Medicine.* 2003; 348: 5–14.

Wheeler A, Bernard G, Thompson B, et al. Pulmonary-artery versus central venous catheter to guide treatment of acute lung injury. *New England Journal of Medicine.* 2006; 354: 2213–2224.

MCQs

1. **What degree of pulse pressure variation is suggestive of fluid responsiveness?**
   (a) >5%
   (b) <5%
   (c) >13%
   (d) <13%
   (e) >100%
2. **Which of the following parameters is *derived* from pulmonary artery catheter measurements?**
   (a) Cardiac output
   (b) Systolic pulmonary artery pressure
   (c) Pulmonary artery wedge pressure
   (d) Pulmonary vascular resistance
   (e) Right atrial pressure
3. **Which of the following is NOT associated with decreased incidence of central line associated infection?**
   (a) Full barrier precautions at time of insertion
   (b) Early removal of central line
   (c) Insertion into the femoral vein
   (d) Antimicrobial impregnated patch over insertion site
   (e) Introduction of an insertion 'bundle' into the department
4. **At which point in the cardiac cycle does the dichrotic notch occur?**
   (a) End systole
   (b) Mid systole
   (c) End diastole
   (d) Mid diastole
   (e) None of the above
5. **Which of the following pulmonary artery catheter measurements is most in keeping with a patient with cardiogenic shock secondary to an anterior myocardial infarction?**
   (a) Cardiac index 1.6 l/min/m^2; pulmonary artery wedge pressure 22 mmHg; mean pulmonary artery pressure 27 mmHg; central venous oxygen saturation 44%
   (b) Cardiac index 1.6 l/min/m^2; pulmonary artery wedge pressure 4 mmHg; mean pulmonary artery pressure 10 mmHg; central venous oxygen saturation 44%

(c) Cardiac index 4.6 l/min/m^2; pulmonary artery wedge pressure 8 mmHg; mean pulmonary artery pressure 12 mmHg; central venous oxygen saturation 84%

(d) Cardiac index 2.6 l/min/m^2; pulmonary artery wedge pressure 9 mmHg; mean pulmonary artery pressure 14 mmHg; central venous oxygen saturation 64%

(e) Cardiac index 2.2 l/min/m^2; pulmonary artery wedge pressure 12 mmHg; mean pulmonary artery pressure 36 mmHg; central venous oxygen saturation 64%

Exercise answers are available on p.467. Alternatively, take the test online at www.cambridge.org/CardiothoracicMCQ

Chapter 12

Antibiotics in the Cardiothoracic Intensive Care Unit

Oana Cole and Olly Allen

The modern era of antibiotics starts with the discovery of penicillin by Alexander Fleming in 1928. Since then, antibiotics have transformed the face of modern medicine and enabled major advances in the treatment of patients. So much so that antibiotics could partially be credited for the staggering increase in the general population's life expectancy from around 60 years old in the UK in the 1920s, according to the Office for National Statistics, to 81 years old in 2015.

Critical care is a young specialty whose evolution has largely been shaped by the evolution of antimicrobial therapy. It can be argued that the only treatment we can offer our patients is antimicrobials, the rest – vasoactive medications, mechanical ventilation, diuretics and so on – are merely supportive measures.

The aim of this chapter is to present the aspects of antimicrobial therapy most pertaining to a cardiothoracic critical care context. Data are presented as valid in 2016. We do not assume to give an exhaustive representation of the myriad of issues faced by the modern intensivist, but to offer a brief update of the most important issues we are currently confronting.

'Appropriate' Antibiotic Therapy

There is no universal recipe for which antibiotics should be used first in a critically ill patient. As shown in Figure 12.1, the choice is individualised for the patient, unit, hospital and geographical area. Most clinicians, when faced with a patient with a severe infection or septic shock, would choose to start with a broad spectrum antibiotic or combination and narrow down as pathogens and their susceptibilities are identified.

The comparative effects of appropriate and inappropriate antibiotic therapy are well illustrated in a recent retrospective study by Neinaber et al. conducted over 6 years in a single institution in the USA. In this study, the risk of nosocomial infections, the median length of stay and the hospital mortality were significantly higher in the inappropriate antibiotic group.

An example of an algorithm for presumptive antibiotic therapy for pneumonia in a critically ill patient is presented in Figure 12.2.

Critically ill patients have multiple risk factors for serious and life-threatening infections. Exposure to antibiotics and other treatments which eradicate and modify the commensal flora, compromised host defences due to nutritional deficiencies, critical illness, compromised integument (intravascular devices, percutaneous interventions and devices) and disruption of cellular and humoral immunity as in the transplant patients lead to a high susceptibility to sepsis. In the context of severe infections, Table 12.1 highlights the most prevalent microorganisms in Western world critical care patients.

Antibiotic Administration in the Critically Ill Patient

In the last few years there has been a focus on the most appropriate way of administering and dosing antibiotics in intensive care. This has been triggered by a better understanding of the critical illness pathophysiology, as well as the emergence of new technologies that alter the pharmacodynamics and pharmacokinetics of drugs in this patient population (Figure 12.3).

Time dependent antimicrobials ($fT_{>MIC}$) include beta-lactams, glycopeptides, macrolides and linezolid. Their concentrations have to be well above the minimum inhibitory concentration (MIC) for the pathogen for at least 40% of the interval between doses in order to achieve their therapeutic targets. There is a growing body of research concerning the administration of beta-lactams as a continuous or prolonged infusion so that the optimum concentration is achieved for sustained periods of time.

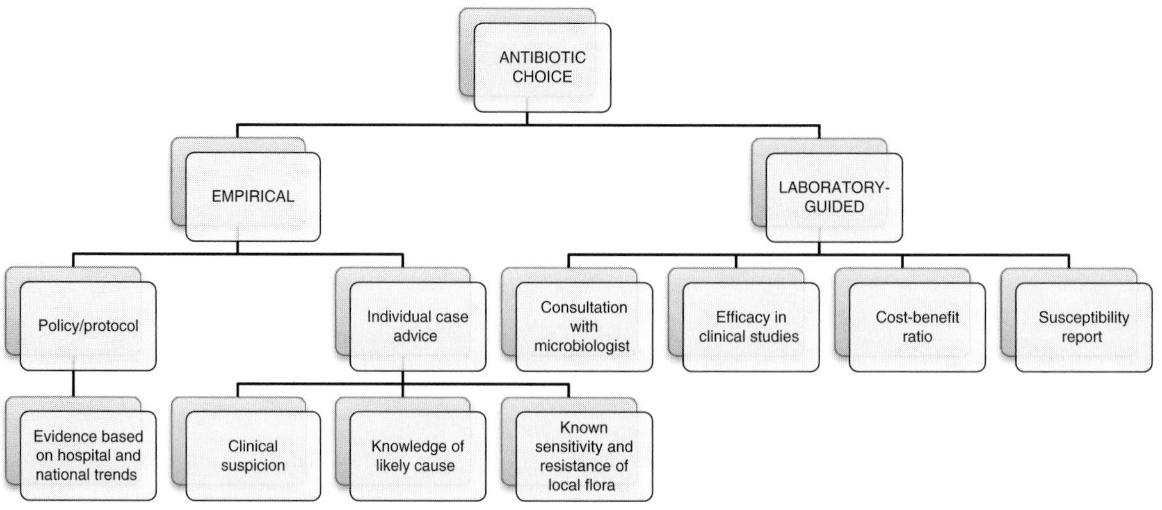

Figure 12.1 Flow chart for choice of antibiotic.

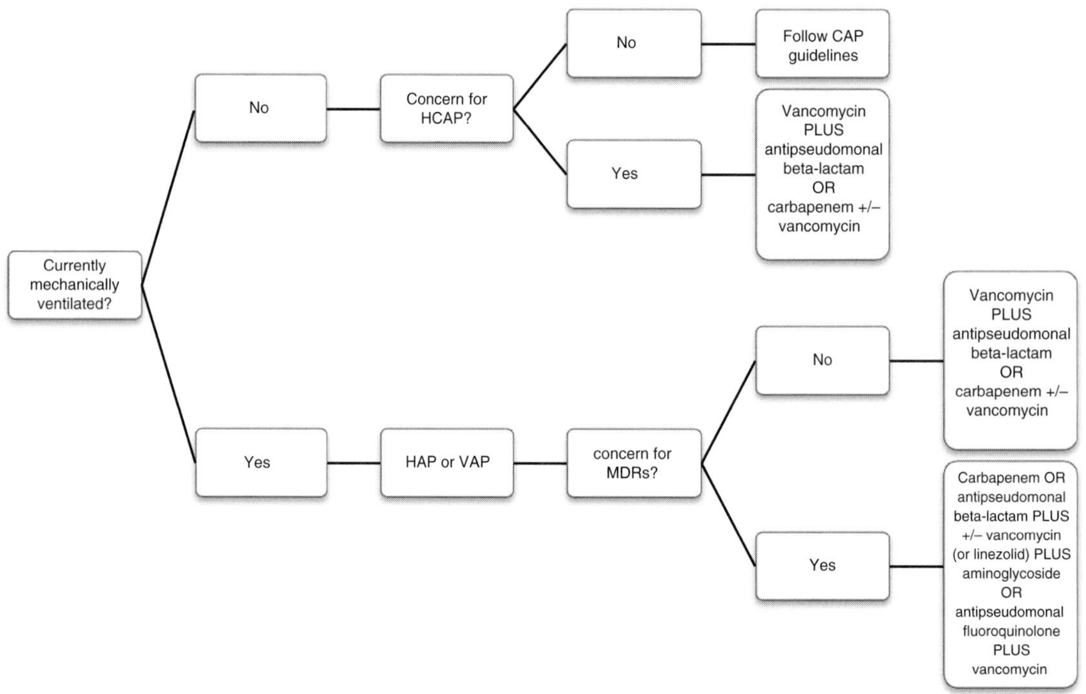

Figure 12.2 Presumptive antibiotic therapy for pneumonia in the ICU. HCAP Health Care Associated Pneumonia; HAP hospital acquired pneumonia.

Concentration dependent antimicrobials (fCmax/MIC) include aminoglycosides, fluoroquinolones, metronidazole, echinocandins, polyenes and daptomycin. These antibiotics need to be administered in doses which achieve target concentrations well above 8–9 times MIC of the pathogen.

The antibiotic concentrations in the target tissues are influenced by the pharmacokinetic changes in the critically ill patient.

1. Volume of distribution, Vd – increased for hydrophilic drugs due to increased total body water; unchanged for lipophilic drugs.

Table 12.1 Most prevalent organisms in Western world critical care patients

Diagnosis	Potential pathogens	Initial therapy	Alternative therapy
Catheter-related blood stream infections	*S. aureus*, coagulase-negative staphylococci, Gram-negative rods *Candida* spp.	Flucloxacillin Vancomycin Tazocin Fluconazole	Vancomycin Linezolid Ciprofloxacin Echinocandins
Infectious endocarditis	Streptococci, *S. aureus*, Enterococci	Amoxicillin Flucloxacillin Vancomycin ± gentamicin ± rifampicin	Flucloxacillin – MSSA Vancomycin – MRSA Gentamicin if *Enterococci* Rifampicin if prosthetic valve
Pneumonia, including VAP	Gram-negative rods, *Haemophilus*, *S. pneumoniae*	Piperacillin-tazobactam	Carbapenems Ciprofloxacin Penicillins
Sepsis/bacteraemia	*S. aureus*, Gram-negative rods *Candida* spp. *Aspergillus*	Piperacillin-tazobactam Flucoxacillin Vancomycin Fluconazole Voriconazole Echinocandins	Fluoroquinolone Vancomycin Echinocandins Amphotericin B

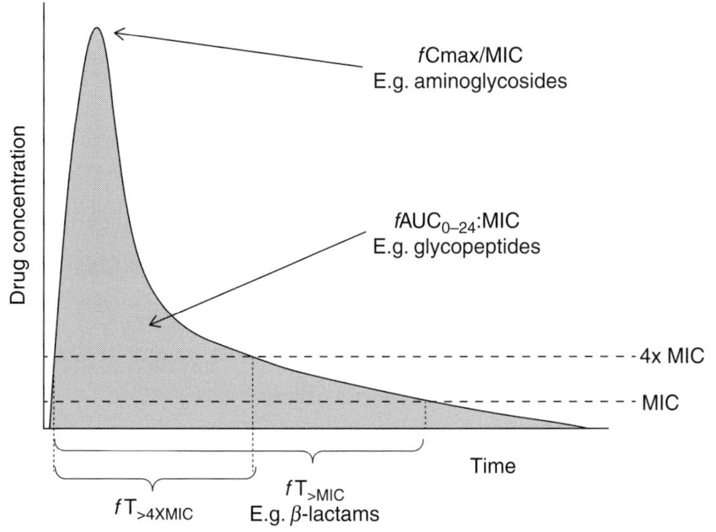

Figure 12.3 The kill characteristics of antibiotics. Modified from Tsai et al. (2015).

2. Clearance and elimination – may change according to the renal and hepatic blood flows and function; severely deranged in septic shock; drug clearance and elimination also dependent on whether renal replacement therapy is instituted.
3. Decreased albumin levels – the volume of distribution and clearance of protein-bound drugs increase, decreasing their efficacy.
4. End-organ dysfunction – cardiac dysfunction in the context of septic shock increases the elimination half-time and the risk of toxicity and drug accumulation.
5. Tissue penetration – can be variable due to microcirculatory dysfunction.

Special Case – Antibiotics and Extracorporeal Circuits

The pharmacokinetics of antibiotics in patients on extracorporeal circuits is a growing area of research. The volume and distribution and clearance of drugs

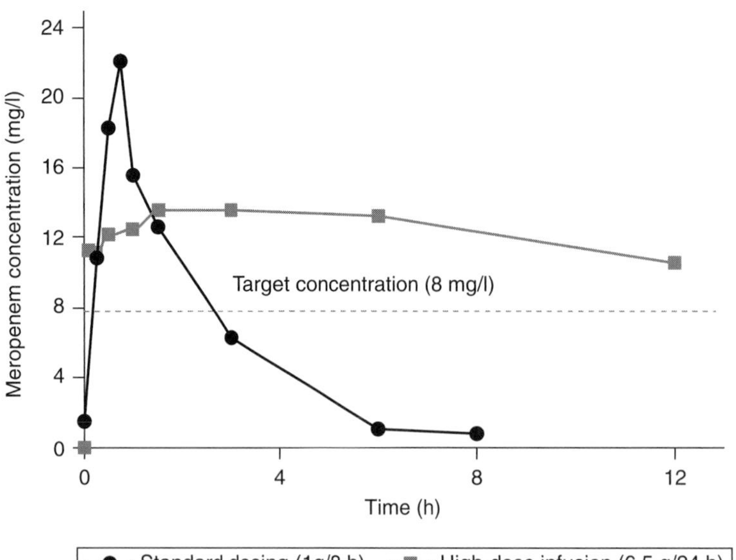

Figure 12.4 Meropenem concentration during ECMO run with two different dosing regimens.

is altered and these are compounded by the added potential for sequestration in the circuit. The importance of understanding the pharmacology and changing the doses and intervals of administration of antimicrobials is colossal, since subtherapeutic doses are associated with worse outcomes.

An example is provided in Figure 12.4, which shows the effect of two dosing regimens of meropenem, as described by Shekar et al. (2013).

Unfortunately, data are very limited to be able to generalise these results for all antimicrobials. What is certain, though, so far, is that 'one size does not fit all' when it comes to drug dosing in patients on extracorporeal circuits. If feasible, drug levels should be monitored in this category of patients in order to establish the appropriate therapeutic regime.

Endocarditis and Intracardiac Device Infection

Infective endocarditis (IE) is a deadly disease. Despite major improvements in diagnosis and treatment, IE remains associated with high morbidity and mortality. IE patients admitted to critical care are among the sickest the intensivist will have to deal with.

The following categories of patients have the highest risk to acquire IE, as well as a poorer prognosis of the disease:

1. Patients with a prosthetic valve or with prosthetic material used for valve repair; this category includes transcatheter implanted valves and homografts.
2. Patients with previous IE; they also have a higher risk of infectious complications than patients with a first episode of IE.
3. Patients with untreated cyanotic congenital heart disease (CHD) or with prosthetic baffles or conduits as part of palliative management; the European Society of Cardiology (ESC) guidelines 2015 recommend that patients with definitive repair of CHD with prosthetic material should only receive antibiotic prophylaxis for the first 6 months, while endothelialisation of the prosthetic material occurs.

Diagnosis of infective endocarditis is based on the modified Duke criteria and the ESC 2015 guidelines, as shown in Table 12.2.

Successful treatment of IE involves primarily pathogen eradication. Surgical treatment and the treatment of complications are beyond the scope of this chapter. With respect to antimicrobials in IE, there are currently the following recommendations, according to the British Society of Antimicrobial Chemotherapy, 2012 guidelines.

1. Initial empirical treatment of native valve endocarditis (NVE) depends on the clinical presentation.
   (i) NVE indolent presentation: amoxicillin + gentamicin.

Table 12.2 Diagnosis of infective endocarditis

Definite IE	
Pathological criteria	• Positive blood cultures for IE • Microorganisms identified on histological analysis of vegetation or embolic material • Vegetation or embolic material identified by histology
Clinical criteria	• 2 major criteria • 1 major criterion and 3 minor criteria • 5 minor criteria
Possible IE	
• 1 major criterion and 1 minor criterion • 3 minor criteria	
Unlikely/rejected IE	
• Firm alternative diagnosis • Resolution of symptoms with antibiotic treatment ≤4 days • No histological evidence of IE	

Major and minor criteria of IE (ESC, 2015)

Major criteria
Blood cultures positive Typical IE microorganisms from 2 separate cultures *Viridans streptococci*, *Streptococcus gallolyticus* (*Streptococcus bovis*), HACEK group, *Staphylococcus aureus*; or Community acquired enterococci in the absence of a primary focus; or Microorganisms consistent with IE from persistently positive blood cultures: ≥2 positive blood culture drawn >12 hours apart; or All 3 or a majority of ≥4 separate blood cultures (with first and last sample drawn >1 hour apart); or Single positive blood culture for *Coxiella burnetii* or phase I IgG antibody titre >1:800
Imaging positive for IE Echocardiogram positive for IE Vegetation Abscess, pseudoaneurysm or intracardiac fistula Valvular perforation or aneurysm New partial dehiscence of prosthetic valve Abnormal activity around the site of prosthetic valvular implantation detected by radiolabelled WBC SPECT/CT Definite paravalvular lesions by cardiac CT
Minor criteria
Predisposition – heart condition or intravenous drug administration Temperature >38 °C Vascular phenomena: major arterial emboli, septic pulmonary infarcts, intracranial haemorrhage, conjunctival haemorrhages and Janeway's lesions Immunological phenomena – glomerulonephritis, Osler's nodes, Roth's spots, and rheumatoid factor Microbiological evidence – positive blood culture but does not meet the major criteria above or serological evidence of active infection with a microorganism consistent with IE

(ii) NVE severe sepsis: vancomycin + gentamicin.
(iii) NVE severe sepsis + risk of MDR: vancomycin + meropenem.

2. Prosthetic valve endocarditis (PVE): vancomycin + gentamicin + rifampicin; this applies to all PVE irrespective of time.
3. Antibiotic treatment of IE due to oral streptococci and *Streptococcus bovis* group depends on minimum inhibitory concentration, MIC (usual course is 4 weeks for NVE and 6 weeks for PVE).
   (i) Penicillin-susceptible strains, non-penicillin allergic patients:

      (a) Benzylpenicillin, or
      (b) Amoxicillin, or
      (c) Ceftriaxone.
   (ii) Penicillin-susceptible strains, penicillin-allergic patients: Vancomycin BD.
   (iii) Strains relatively resistant to penicillin (higher MIC required), non-penicillin allergic patients:
      (a) Benzylpenicillin, double the dose for penicillin-susceptible strains and gentamicin, or
      (b) Amoxicillin, double the dose for penicillin-susceptible strains and gentamicin, or
      (c) Ceftriaxone and gentamicin.
   (iv) Strains relatively resistant to penicillin (higher MIC required), penicillin-allergic patients: Vancomycin and gentamicin.
4. Antibiotic treatment of IE due to *Staphylococcus* spp., for NVE:
   (i) Methicillin-susceptible *Staphylococcus* spp., non-penicillin-allergic patients: Flucloxacillin.
   (ii) Methicillin-susceptible *Staphylococcus aureus*, alternative strategy: Vancomycin or daptomycin.
   (iii) Penicillin-allergic patients or methicillin-resistant *Staphylococcus* spp.:
      (a) Vancomycin for 4–6 weeks, intravenous administration,
      (b) Daptomycin for 4–6 weeks, intravenous administration.
5. Antibiotic treatment of IE due to *Enterococcus* spp.:
   (i) Beta-lactam and gentamicin-susceptible strains:
      (a) Amoxicillin and gentamicin for 4 weeks for NVE or 6 weeks for PVE,
      (b) Ampicillin with ceftriaxone for 4 weeks for NVE or 6 weeks for PVE, for *E. faecalis*,
      (c) Vancomycin and gentamicin for 6 weeks if penicillin allergy known or suspected.
   (ii) Gentamicin-resistant species – replace gentamicin with streptomycin, if susceptible to the latter.
   (iii) Multiresistance to beta-lactams, aminoglycosides and vancomycin:
      (a) Daptomycin and ampicillin,
      (b) Linezolid,
      (c) Vancomycin, if beta-lactam resistance but vancomycin susceptibility detected.

We must stress that these are only guidelines, and that individual hospitals in different regions may have different antibiotic policies, depending on the local ecology.

Catheter Related Bloodstream Infections

The definition of catheter related bloodstream infections, also known as central line associated bloodstream infections (CLABSI), is bacteraemia or fungaemia in a patient with an intravascular catheter, sepsis and at least one positive blood culture taken from a peripheral vein, in the absence of another apparent source except for the catheter. In addition, there should be evidence that the catheter was infected based on quantitative or semi-quantitative methods. Another diagnostic method for CLABSI is differential time to positivity – blood cultures taken from the central line presumed to be infected may turn positive at least 2 hours before blood cultures taken simultaneously from a peripheral vein. This is due to the almost three-fold increase in the micro-organism load of an infected catheter compared to blood.

Prevention of CLABSI relies on several measures, as follows:

1. Choice of insertion site – femoral lines should be a last resort; they should be changed as soon as possible, within a maximum time frame of 48 hours.
2. Insertion techniques – experienced personnel, avoidance of haematoma formation around the insertion site.
3. Adoption of a care bundle; the Matching Michigan campaign has shown that CLABSI decreased by more than 60% over 2 years in ICUs in England after introduction of a care bundle.
4. Antibiotic-coated central venous catheters have been proposed and adopted with success across intensive care units worldwide. The catheters are impregnated with minocycline-rifampicin and are effective in inhibiting the development of

Table 12.3 Systemic treatment of CLABSI – a possible guide

Pathogen	First line antibiotic	Alternative treatment
Coagulase-negative staphylococci		
Methicillin-sensitive	Flucloxacillin *mecA* gene negative	Vancomycin
Methicillin-resistant	Vancomycin	Daptomycin or linezolid
S. aureus		
MSSA	Flucloxacillin	Vancomycin
MRSA	Vancomycin	Daptomycin or linezolid
Enterobacteriaceae		
ESBL –ve	Piperacillin/tazobactam	Ciprofloxacin or aztreonam
ESBL +ve	Carbapenem	Ciprofloxacin
Pseudomonas	Carbapenem or piperacillin-tazobactam	Ciprofloxacin or aztreonam May consider the addition of an aminoglycoside
Candida spp.	Echinocandins or fluconazole	Amphotericin
Candida glabrata	Echinocandins or fluconazole at higher doses if susceptible strains	Amphotericin

Table 12.4 Retrospective analysis of all VAD patients from the Mayo Clinic between 2005 and 2011

Infection type	Cases per 100 patient-years of LVAD support (95% CI)
All	32.8 (26.7–39.9)
Endocarditis	1.6 (0.5–3.8)
Pump and/or cannula infection	4.9 (2.7–8.0)
Bloodstream infection	
VAD related	7.5 (4.7–11.2)
Non-VAD related	6.8 (4.2–10.4)
CLABSI related	3.3 (1.6–6)
CLABSI associated	1.6 (0.5–3.8)
Pocket infection	2.3 (0.9–4.7)
Driveline infection	15 (10.9–20)
Permanent pacemaker/CRT-D infection	1.6 (0.5–3.8)
Mediastinitis, VAD related	2 (0.7–4.2)

biofilm of both Gram-negative and Gram-positive bacteria, with the exception of *P. aeruginosa* and *Candida* spp.

Table 12.3 shows possible systemic treatment for CLABSI.

Mechanical Circulatory Support Device (MCSD) Infections

Infections in MCSD patients are difficult to treat and have been associated with poor prognosis and poor quality of life. Ventricular assist devices differ from other cardiac devices by the fact that they have a percutaneous drive-line, which has been termed the 'Achilles' heel' of these devices. The most recent INTERMACS report (March 2016) has shown that major infections in MCSD are the third highest cause of death with an overall death toll of 9% (June 2006 to March 2016), surpassed only by neurological dysfunction and multiorgan failure.

The results of a retrospective analysis of all VAD patients from the Mayo Clinic between 2005 and 2011 are shown in Table 12.4.

The salient points of international standards for the management of MCSD infections as valid in June 2016 are presented below.

1. Bacterial infections:
   (a) Gram-positive cocci are the most prevalent pathogens, followed by Gram-negative rods.
   (b) Nosocomial pathogens – *Pseudomonas, Serratia* and *Enterobacter* – account for the second most common cause after *Staphylococcus* spp.
   (c) The duration of antimicrobial treatment is not clearly established; most centres recommend courses of at least 2 weeks for superficial driveline infections and at least 4 weeks for deep-seated infections.
   (d) Due to the wide variety of possible scenarios, there are currently no international guidelines on the treatment of bacterial infections associated with MCSD. The antibiotic agents should be administered after consultation with the local microbiology department, infectious diseases specialist and the transplant or heart failure specialist teams.
2. Fungal infections:
   (a) The prevalence of fungal infections has increased over the years.
   (b) Most fungal infections are caused by *Candida* spp., with a few other case reports of *Aspergillus* spp. and other yeasts.
   (c) No evidence has demonstrated that the routine use of antifungal prophylaxis decreases the rate of fungal infections in MCSD patients; however, preimplantation prophylaxis should be considered in high-risk patients.
   (d) *Candida* spp. pump or cannula infection should be treated with 8–12 weeks of amphotericin, echinocandin intravenously or high dose fluconazole if susceptible *Candida* strains.
   (e) Deep-seated pocket or driveline infection should be treated with 8–12 weeks of echinocandin or amphotericin intravenously followed by prolonged suppressive oral therapy.
   (f) Superficial driveline infections should be treated with 2 weeks of azole therapy.

Antifungals in the ICU

Fungal infections are associated with high morbidity and mortality in the critically ill patient and lead to very high healthcare costs. The prevalence of fungal infections in intensive care is increasing due to the increasing complexity of medical and surgical ICU patients, the presence of medium- and long-term devices, such as ECMO and VAD cannulae, and the use of broad spectrum antibiotics.

Although all species of yeasts can be encountered, *Candida* and *Aspergillus* spp. are by far the most prevalent in cardiothoracic ICU patients, so we will refer to treatment for these two pathogens in the discussion below.

1. *Candida* spp:
   (a) The 2012 European guidelines recommend that fungicidal agents – echinocandins or lipid-based polyenes – be used for the initial treatment of invasive *Candida* infection; once the species of *Candida* and the sensitivities are identified, treatment can be de-escalated to azoles for susceptible strains.
   (b) Polyenes are preferred to other classes for the treatment of deep-seated infections, such as mediastinitis or endocarditis.
2. *Aspergillus:*
   (a) Caspofungin is the only echinocandin approved for the treatment of invasive aspergillosis; however, it is an inferior choice to voriconazole and amphotericin.
   (b) Voriconazole is recommended as first line agent for aspergillosis; notably, it interacts with tacrolimus and cyclosporine by interfering with the hepatic metabolism pathways; the therapeutic levels of the immunosuppressants should be monitored and higher doses may be required.
   (c) Lipid-based polyenes (amphotericin B) are recommended as second line therapy for aspergillosis, where voriconazole is contraindicated.

Antibiotic Resistance and the Development of New Agents

The last decade has seen worrying levels of increased antimicrobial resistance, prompting the Centre for Disease Control in the USA and similar organisations worldwide to declare the current situation an emergency. The Review of Antimicrobial Resistance has recently published a report outlining the problem and proposing several strategies of tackling the issue of the increase in antimicrobial resistance.

Table 12.5 Microorganisms showing resistance

Urgent threats	*C. difficile* Carbapenem-resistant Enterobacteriaceae (CRE)
Serious threats	Multidrug-resistant *Acinetobacter* spp. Fluconazole-resistant *Candida* spp. Extended spectrum beta-lactamase-producing Enterobacteriaceae (ESBL) Multidrug-resistant *Pseudomonas* Carbapenemase-producing *Pseudomonas* Methicillin-resistant *S. aureus* (MRSA)
Concerning threats	Vancomycin-resistant *S. aureus* (VRSA)

Which are the microorganisms causing these issues and where are they most likely to be encountered?

The Centre for Disease Control has published a list of the current microorganism resistance threats. We present the ones most likely to be encountered in a cardiothoracic critical care unit in Table 12.5.

There have been volumes written on how to best tackle the emergence of these infections in the ICU. The key message from organisations all over the world is to implement antibiotic stewardship programmes and improve the education of the 'jobbing' intensivists in the pharmacology of antimicrobials.

Antimicrobial stewardship is a bundle of interventions designed to optimise and measure the appropriate use of antimicrobials based on pharmacodynamics and pharmacokinetic data available, local ecology and patient and unit characteristics. A well-run stewardship programme is a two-stage process.

Stage 1:

(a) Identification of patients with infection;
(b) Empirical antibiotics according to local policy and microbiological advice;
(c) Optimised dosing according to pharmacokinetics(PK)/pharmacodynamics(PD).

Stage 2:

(a) Review within 72 hours with laboratory results and clinical progress;
(b) Switch to narrow spectrum antibiotics (if broad spectrum antibiotics started initially);
(c) Stop antibiotics if the pathology is unlikely to be infection.

In Spain, a country with a high prevalence of multidrug resistant organisms (MDR), a recently implemented 'zero resistance' programme recommends that antimicrobials against MDR should only be administered in patients with septic shock and a high risk of MDR based on risk factors or knowledge of local ecology.

The following are risk factors for carriage of MDR.

1. Hospital admission for more than 5 days in the last 3 months.
2. Institutionalised patients (prison, healthcare, social centre).
3. Known previous colonisation or infection with MDR.
4. Antibiotic course of at least a week in the previous month, especially with one or more of the following:
   (a) Third or fourth generation cephalosporins;
   (b) Fluoroquinolones;
   (c) Carbapenems.
5. End-stage renal disease or renal-replacement therapy.
6. Comorbid conditions associated with colonisation or infection with MDR, such as:
   (a) Cystic fibrosis;
   (b) Bronchiectasis;
   (c) Chronic skin ulcers.

Even though these risk factors were highlighted in the context of the Spanish healthcare system, they are internationally recognisable as the situations which should alert most clinicians to the possibility of the patient being colonised by or having an infection with a MDR pathogen.

The arsenal available to combat these infections is, as explained earlier, getting more and more limited. Commonly used antibiotics to treat potential MDRs are complemented by some new preparations and combinations. Table 12.6 lists some of the most commonly available.

Learning Points

- The most common approach to empirical antibiotic treatment in severe infections in the critically ill is to 'start broad and narrow down'.
- Consider the most likely source of sepsis when deciding which antibiotics to start.

Table 12.6 Most commonly available new preparations against MDRs

Antibiotic	Active against	No activity	Remarks
Colistin (polymyxin E)	*Acinetobacter* spp. *P. aeruginosa* Enterobacteriaceae Most other Gram-negative aerobic bacilli	*Serratia* spp. *Providencia* spp. *Burkholderia cepacia* Gram-positive and Gram-negative aerobic cocci Gram-positive aerobic bacilli Anaerobes	• Emergent strains of colistin-resistant KPC • Serious nephrotoxicity and neurotoxicity
Tigecycline	MRSA VRE Carbapenemase-producing Enterobacteriaceae Several ESBL strains	*P. aeruginosa* *Proteus* spp. *Providencia* spp.	Can be used for deep-seated infections, note poor lung penetration of this antibiotic
Carbapenems	Most Enterobacteriaceae MSSA *P. aeruginosa* ESBL Anaerobes	Strains of Gram-positive cocci with reduced penicillin sensitivity	Emerging strains of carbapenemase-producing microorganisms (KPO)
Glycopeptides (vancomycin, teicoplanin)	Gram-positive cocci *Clostridium difficile*	Gram-negative bacteria	
Daptomycin	MDR Gram-positive cocci, especially MRSA and VRSA VRE MSSA right-sided endocarditis	Gram-negative bacteria	Inactivated by alveolar surfactant – ineffective in pneumonias
Linezolid	MRSA VRSA VRE Penicillin-resistant *S. pneumoniae*	Gram-negative bacteria	• Reversible thrombocytopenia • Interacts with SSRIs – serotonin syndrome
Fosfomycin	*S. aureus*, including MRSA *Enterococcus* spp. including VRE ESBL-producing *K. pneumoniae* and *E. coli*	Some *Pseudomonas* and *E. coli* strains	High potential for development of resistance under prolonged therapy
Ceftolozane/tazobactam	Indications: • Complicated UTI • Complicated intra-abdominal infections • Complicated ventilator associated pneumonia		
Tedizolid	MRSA VRSA VRE	Gram-negative bacteria	• Fewer side effects than linezolid • More bactericidal activity than linezolid
Avibactam	ESBL Carbapenemase-producing *K. pneumoniae*		
Plazomicin	Metallo-beta-lactamase-producing strains MRSA		Phase 3 clinical trials
Echinocandins	Fluconazole-resistant *Candida* spp. *Aspergillus*		

- The rate of discovery of new antibiotics is lower than the rate of development of multidrug resistant strains in pathogens.
- In the current context of drug resistant pathogens, antibiotic stewardship is a must.
- In certain cases, be mindful of the pharmacokinetic and pharmacodynamics changes which occur due to critical illness pathophysiology.

Further Reading

Bion J, Richardson A, Hibbert P, et al. 'Matching Michigan': a 2-year stepped interventional programme to minimise central venous catheter–blood stream infections in intensive care units in England. *British Medical Journal Quality and Safety*. 2013; 22: 110–123. doi:10.1136/bmjqs-2012-001325

Coley CJ II, Miller MA. *Ventilator-Associated Pneumonia in Healthcare Associated Infections*. Oxford: American Infectious Disease Library OUP, 2013.

De Pascale G, Tumabarello M. Fungal infections in ICU: advances in treatment and diagnosis. *Current Opinion in Critical Care*. 2015; 21: 421–429.

Husain S, Sole A, Alexander BA, et al. The 2015 International Society for Heart and Lung Transplantation Guidelines for the management of fungal infections in mechanical circulatory support and cardiothoracic organ transplant recipients: Executive summary. *Journal of Heart and Lung Transplantation*. 2016; 35: 261–282.

Neinaber JJ, Kusne S, Riaz T, et al. Clinical manifestations and management of left ventricular assist device-associated infections. *Clinical Infectious Diseases*. 2013; 57: 1438–1448.

Shekar K, Roberts JA, Ghassabian S, et al. Altered antibiotic pharmacokinetics during extracorporeal membrane oxygenation: cause for concern? *Journal of Antimicrobial Chemotherapy*. 2013; 68: 726–727.

Tsai D, Lipman J, Roberts JA. Pharmacokinetic/pharmacodynamics considerations for the optimisation of antimicrobial delivery in the critically ill. *Current Opinion in Critical Care*. 2015; 21: 412–420.

MCQs

1. **A 19 year old girl is admitted to the ICU following double lung transplant for cystic fibrosis. She was known to be previously colonised with multidrug resistant *Pseudomonas*. After initial satisfactory progress, the patient develops severe pneumonia on day 3 postoperatively. Talking to the anaesthetist for the case, it was a difficult intubation with a small double lumen tube and incomplete tracheobronchial toilet may have been performed. Suspecting that this is possible contamination with the patient's previous flora, choose which antibiotic you would consider starting.**
   (a) Tigecycline
   (b) Linezolid
   (c) Piperacillin-tazobactam ± gentamicin
   (d) Vancomycin with ciprofloxacin
   (e) Colistin

2. **A 57 year old male presents to the A&E department of a peripheral hospital with a history of 3 weeks of fever, chills and malaise. In the last few hours, though, he is increasingly dyspnoeic and has started to cough pink, frothy sputum. His medical history is unremarkable apart from an aortic valve replacement for a stenotic bicuspid aortic valve 3 years previously. The cardiology registrar does a 'quick TTE' and, despite the poor windows, detects free aortic regurgitation and a rocking valve. What would you do next?**
   (a) Send the patient urgently to the regional cardiac surgical centre and give a dose of intravenous flucloxacillin and gentamicin, with instructions to be continued for 6 weeks or until microbiological advice
   (b) Keep the patient in overnight, start a vasoconstrictor to help increase the perfusion pressure to the brain and start piperacillin/tazobactam and gentamicin intravenously
   (c) Send the patient urgently to the regional cardiac surgical centre and give a dose of intravenous vancomycin with gentamicin and rifampicin, with instructions to be continued for 6 weeks or until microbiological advice
   (d) Intubate the patient prior to transfer and give fluids to compensate for increased capillary permeability with sepsis; start a course of rifampicin
   (e) Keep the patient in overnight, start a diuretic, give fluid boluses and a vasoconstrictor to maintain MAP > 65 mmHg; start vancomycin with ciprofloxacin and fluconazole

3. **An acceptable initial choice of antibiotics for presumed ventilator associated pneumonia in a non-penicillin-allergic patient who is otherwise progressing well would be:**
   (a) Meropenem
   (b) Piperacillin/tazobactam

(c) Nebulised colistin

(d) Metronidazole and piperacillin/tazobactam

(e) Levofloxacin

4. **A 36 year old woman with a LVAD for postpartum cardiomyopathy is referred to the parent cardiac centre with fever and chills. The device has been alarming increased power for the last 24 hours. She has a history of frequent driveline infections with MSSA and *C. albicans*. What is the choice of antibiotics if we presume that LVAD infection is a possible diagnosis?**

(a) Echinocandin for 8–12 weeks and vancomycin and gentamicin for at least 6 weeks

(b) Rifampicin for 6 weeks and fluconazole for 6–8 weeks

(c) Flucloxacillin, rifampicin and gentamicin and an echinocandin for 6 weeks

(d) Amphotericin for 12 weeks, metronidazole and ceftriaxone for 6 weeks

(e) Linezolid and amphotericin for 12 weeks

5. **The risk of CLABSI is highest with:**

(a) Line insertion in an emergency

(b) Line insertion in a septic patient

(c) Line insertion at a prior infected line site

(d) Multiple line insertions in the same vein

(e) Long-term catheter insertion in the radiology department

Exercise answers are available on p.467. Alternatively, take the test online at www.cambridge.org/CardiothoracicMCQ

Chapter 13

Blood Products and Transfusion

Martin Besser

Introduction

Along with cardiothoracic operating departments, cardiothoracic intensive care units are some of the greatest consumers of blood products in the world; so for example UK cardiac surgical centres use approximately 10% of the national supply. Furthermore, use of blood products is currently on the increase due to a combination of factors, including advancing patient age, increasing burden of comorbidities, expanding use of antiplatelet therapy and greater surgical complexity. Importantly, transfusion of blood products is associated with increased morbidity and mortality thus it is imperative to employ strategies such as patient blood management (PBM) to avoid unnecessary transfusion and conserve precious resources.

Blood Products

More than 2 million donations are made each year in the UK to National Health Service Blood and Transfusion (NHSBT). From these donations, approximately 2,000,000 units of red cells, 300,000 units of platelets, 350,000 units of FFP and 126,000 units of cryoprecipitate are prepared. The current commonly prescribed blood products in the UK are listed in Table 13.1.

Blood components are not blood group specific due to pooling of donors in the production process. This means equilibration of interindividual variation from donor to donor and the dilution of hazardous antibodies such as antineutrophil antibodies. It is important to note that some products have traces of heparin and may be potentially contraindicated in heparin induced thrombocytopenia. Red cells are considered suitable in the UK for transfusion for up to 35 days post donation and are stored at 4 °C ±2 °C, FFP and cryoprecipitate are usable for up to 2 years and are stored at −30 °C. Platelets have a shelf life of 7 days if stored at room temperature with agitation.

To reduce the risk of transmission of infection, all donors complete a health questionnaire prior to donation to identify those that may be unsuitable. Any donations taken are then tested for a range of infections including HIV 1 and 2, syphilis, HTLV1 and 2, hepatitis B and hepatitis C. As of April 2016, NHSBT also commenced screening for hepatitis E negative blood for transfusion to some patients who are immunosuppressed due to haematological malignancy or who are scheduled for or have undergone solid organ or bone marrow transplantation. Several initiatives are also in place to reduce the risk of transmission of Variant Creutzfeldt-Jakob disease including leukodepletion (1999) and the use of non-UK methylene blue treated plasma components or commercial solvent/detergent fresh frozen plasma (SD FFP) treated pooled plasma for patients born after 1995.

Red Blood Cells

It has been shown that isovolaemic haemodilution of normal volunteers and non-anaemic patients is tolerated to a haemoglobin of 50 g/l. Studies that have assessed patients who refuse blood found that the degree of preoperative anaemia affected the risk of death but did not have an effect on mortality. Hebert showed in a randomised controlled trial (TRICC) that a restrictive (70 g/l) transfusion strategy was superior to a liberal (90 g/l) one in ICU patients. However, some doubt has been cast on this in the setting of cardiothoracic surgery after a recent study reported improved outcomes with a liberal strategy. In the TITRe2 trial, patients undergoing elective cardiac surgery were randomised between 90 g/l and 75 g/l as the transfusion threshold. Ischaemic cerebral events, myocardial infarction, infection or acute renal failure within 3 months of surgery were non-significantly different. This leads to transfusion rates of 92.7% versus 53.4%. Strikingly, the mortality was different, 2.6% versus 4.2%, in the two groups with a hazard ratio

Table 13.1 Comparison of blood products and components currently in use in the UK

		Commercial product	Protein	Platelet	Fibrinogen	II	V	VII	VIII	vWF	IX	X
Blood components	Packed red cells		Haemoglobin <40 g/l	trace	trace	trace	trace	trace	trace	trace	trace	trace
	Platelets			>240 × 10^9/l	trace	trace	trace	trace	trace	trace	trace	trace
	FFP		>50 g/l	nil	0.9 g/l	variable	variable	variable	>70 U	variable	variable	variable
	Cryoprecipitate			nil	>0.7 g/pool	variable	variable	variable	350 U/pool	variable	variable	variable
	Methylene blue FFP		>50 g/l	nil	0.7 g/l	variable	variable	variable	50 U	variable	variable	variable
	Methylene blue cryo			nil	0.7 g/pool (80% of untreated)	variable	variable	variable	350 U/pool (80% of untreated)	variable	variable	variable
Blood products	Fibrinogen concentrate	Riastap®	Albumin	nil	20 g/l							
	Prothrombin complex	Beriplex®	6–14 g/l	nil	NA	20–60**	NA	10–25**	NA	NA	20–31***	22–60***
		Octaplex®	1.3–4.1 g/l	nil	NA	20–76***	NA	18–48**	NA	NA	50***	36–60***
	SD FFP		45–70 g/l	nil	NA	NA	31	NA	28	NA	NA	NA

* Assumed to be 100% activity but donors will vary 70–100%.
** Prior to freezing.
*** Per ml reconstituted.
Beriplex® and Riastap® are trademarks of CSL Behring.
Octaplex® is a ® trademark of Octapharma.

of 1.67 (1.00–2.67) ($p = 0.045$) favouring the higher threshold.

Accepted side effects of transfusion are infection, immune reactions, volume overload, immune suppression, and red cell and HLA allo-immunisation. General recommendations agree that a Hb of <70 g/l is an indication for transfusion; however when the Hb is >70 g/l the circumstances of the patient need to be taken into account and the risk/balance of transfusion assessed. In patients with a Hb of 80–100 g/l, the transfusion decision should be individualised and generally a transfusion is not indicated with a Hb of >100 g/l. However, these recommendations do not include patients with coronary artery disease.

Platelets

We usually apply the threshold of platelets <100 × 10^9/l in the immediate postoperative setting. Controversies exist for patients with concomitant antiplatelet therapy. Patients exposed to antiplatelet therapy take several days to recover normal platelet function: clopidogrel (7 days), aspirin (7 days), ticagrelor (5 days) and prasugrel (7 days). Cangrelor is an interesting alternative ADP-inhibitor that allows rapid platelet function recovery within a few hours of stopping administration. Despite the recent development of near patient platelet function testing, the problem remains that the platelet function testing becomes abnormal with reducing platelet count (around 75 × 10^9/l for the Multiplate). Moreover, the treatment of confirmed or assumed platelet dysfunction is platelet transfusion. The British Commission for Standards in Haematology have published guidance for platelet transfusion. The evidence for the use of platelet transfusion is marred by the impact of ongoing antiplatelet therapy on both the patient's own and transfused platelets. The general advice is to discontinue antiplatelet therapy where possible, taking into account the time required to normalise platelet function. Platelet transfusion in patients requiring antiplatelet therapy may increase the risk of atherosclerotic complications while not positively affecting platelet function.

During the intensive care stay there is controversy about the optimal platelet count for preventing bleeding with a number of invasive procedures. The

XI	XII	XIII	Protein C	Protein S	Antithrombin	Heparin	Red cell stroma	Blood group specific	White cell contaminant	Clinically important subtypes	Donor exposure	Pathogen inactivation or reduction
trace	trace	trace	trace	trace	trace	No	Yes	Yes	<5106/unit	washed, CMV, negative, irradiated	1	Leukodepletion (UK)
trace	trace	trace	trace	trace	trace	No	trace	Yes	<5106/unit**	pool, single donor apheresis, HLA matched	1 to 6	Leukodepletion (UK)
variable	variable	variable *	variable *	variable *	variable *	No	trace**	Yes	<5106/unit**		1	Leukodepletion (UK)
variable	variable	variable	variable	variable	variable	No	trace**	Yes	<5106/unit**		5	Leukodepletion (UK)
variable	variable	variable	variable	variable	variable	No	trace**	Yes	<5106/unit**		1	Methylene blue
variable	variable	variable	variable	variable	variable	No	trace**	Yes	<5106/unit**			Methylene blue
						No	nil	No	No		>20,000	Pasteurisation
NA		NA	15–45	12–38	Yes	Yes	nil	No	No		>20,000	Filtration, pasteurisation
NA			26–62**	24–64**	NA	Yes	nil	No	No		>20,000	Filtration, pasteurisation
NA		NA	NA	50	NA	No	nil	Yes	No		>20,000	Solvent detergent

insertion or removal of epidural catheters is considered safe with platelet counts >(80–100) × 10^9/l. The majority of procedures, such as line insertions or chest drain removals, are safe with platelet counts over 50 × 10^9/l provided concomitant anticoagulation has been corrected or stopped. Our practice, with the exception of epidurals and lumbar punctures, is to transfuse platelets for counts $<50 \times 10^9$/l prior to intervention and to not transfuse platelets for counts of >80 × 10^9/l. Between 50 and 80 × 10^9/l we will reserve a unit of platelets for 8 hours for the patient in case of excessive bleeding or if the clinician requests these.

In patients on ECMO the agreed platelet threshold is currently debated. We accept 100 × 10^9/l in a bleeding patient but have had individual patients where we tried to achieve higher platelet counts due to concomitant intracranial bleeding with a continued need for heparin anticoagulation. Others advocate thresholds as low as 20 × 10^9/l. The coagulation system in adults and children is fundamentally different and therefore it is not likely that the same threshold can be applied for both groups of patients.

In individual patients who develop thrombocytopenia while on ECMO, a number of possible causes such as drugs, mechanical factors or immune mechanisms have to be considered. Where there is an associated bleeding pattern this is important and the need for ongoing anticoagulation needs to be reviewed. Where reduced anticoagulation therapy can be compensated with measures such as increasing the flow of the ECMO circuit, this is likely to be more effective than a small increment in platelet count. Any transfused platelets will be subjected to the same causes of thrombocytopenia as the patient, and particularly in moderate thrombocytopenia are unlikely to have a prolonged effect.

We assume that a unit of platelets will contain a minimum of 250 × 10^9/l per adult therapeutic dose. In a healthy adult we assume a daily platelet production of 10 × 10^9/l. A platelet transfusion is clinically most effective in a patient with thrombocytopenia. The platelet recovery following a fixed dose infusion of platelets is highly variable and is dependent on the original reason for thrombocytopenia in the patient. It is bound to be optimal in a patient with lack of production but far less satisfactory in a patient with platelet destruction. There are a number of specific cardiothoracic interventions that will reduce the platelet recovery in a given patient such as extracorporeal membrane oxygenation (ECMO) and intra-aortic balloon pump (IABP).

Human platelet concentrates express very few AB antigens and are suspended in less than 50 ml of plasma. For this reason ABO groups can be overridden in case of an emergency. Platelets do however express HLA class I antigens, which can lead to antibody formation causing platelet refractoriness (defined as repeated platelet increments of $<5 \times 10^9/l$). Red cells are more potent HLA type sensitisers than platelet transfusions and multiparous women are particularly at risk. The UK national blood service is able to provide HLA class I typing and antibody screening with a view to providing HLA selected/matched platelets. These products are considerably more expensive than standard platelets but may lead to better increment and thus overall reduction in platelet usage. All HLA matched platelets must be irradiated.

Cryoprecipitate and Fibrinogen Concentrate

Fibrinogen is a critical haemostatic factor for the development of effective local clotting in all surgical patients, and in particular for the management of perioperative bleeding in cardiac surgical patients. Normal fibrinogen levels are 200–400 mg/dl in the non-parturient, but may be >400 mg/dl during the third trimester of pregnancy. The optimal transfusion threshold for fibrinogen replacement is unknown. There is no RCT evidence for the transfusion threshold of 1 g/dl but it has been accepted in clinical practice. More recently, higher thresholds for fibrinogen replacement have been advocated with thresholds of up to 2 g/dl. The massive transfusion guidelines published by the BCSH advise use of a cut-off of 1.5 g/dl as the threshold, as do the NICE transfusion guidelines of November 2015.

An adult dose of cryoprecipitate (10 units or 2 pools) is equivalent to 2–4 g of fibrinogen concentrate. Based on the relative content of fibrinogen per ml, fibrinogen concentrate should be superior to cryoprecipitate in restoring low fibrinogen levels. However, cryoprecipitate also contains factors such as vWF and factor XIII which may be of therapeutic benefit. Importantly, a therapeutic dose of 4 g of fibrinogen is four times as expensive as cryoprecipitate.

Ranucci et al. recently reported a prospective, randomised, blind study of 116 patients undergoing high risk cardiac surgery with an expected cardiopulmonary bypass duration of >90 minutes. Patients received fibrinogen concentrates after protamine administration and prothrombin complex concentrates (PCCs) if bleeding persisted. Patients receiving fibrinogen had a significantly lower rate of any allogeneic blood product transfusions, including PRBCs and FFP. Postoperative bleeding was also reduced in the fibrinogen treated patients (median, 300 ml; interquartile range, 200 to 400 ml) compared with the control patients (median, 355 ml; interquartile range, 250 to 600 ml). However, the recently published REPLACE-trial comparing the early aggressive use of fibrinogen concentrate in patients undergoing aortic surgery with placebo, on the background of a defined transfusion algorithm with platelets and FFP, did not demonstrate clinical benefit.

Fresh Frozen Plasma and Prothrombin Complex Concentrate

Fresh frozen plasma may increase clotting factor activity by up to 30% with administration of 15 ml/kg. The absolute increment depends on the baseline factor activity in 40 ml/kg of patient plasma and may be considerably smaller if the clotting factor levels are nearly normal. There may be considerable variation in the concentration of individual factors such as factor XI or IX between donors. In some congenital coagulation factor deficiencies, it may therefore be advisable to use pooled products to minimise these effects between donors.

Prothrombin complex is a pooled plasma product that contains factors II, VII, IX and X as well as Protein C and S. It is licensed for use in acquired deficiency of the vitamin K dependent clotting factors. The most recent guidelines (2015) on the treatment of massive haemorrhage explicitly advise against the use of prothrombin complex in massive transfusion outside studies. The main advantage of using PCC over FFP is the reduced volume and easier administration. An FFP equivalent dose is 15 U/kg, and there are published dosing recommendations for warfarin reversal based on baseline INR with up to 50 U/kg. The available PCCs also contain traces of heparin so are contraindicated for the reversal of warfarin in patients with HIT.

Recombinant Activated Factor VIIa

Recombinant FVIIa is used off-label as a prohaemostatic agent for life threatening hemorrhage. Its mechanism of action is thought to be related to binding with tissue factor (TF) expressed at the site of vascular injury to locally produce thrombin and amplify haemostatic activation. Controlled clinical trials report the incidence of thrombotic complications among patients who received rFVIIa to be relatively low and similar to that among patients who received placebo. In the most recent cardiac surgical study, patients bleeding postoperatively >200 ml/hour were randomised to placebo, 40 μg/kg rFVIIa or 80 μg/kg rFVIIa. Primary endpoints were the number of patients suffering critical serious adverse events. Secondary endpoints included rates of reoperation, blood loss and transfusions. Although more adverse events occurred in the rFVIIa groups, they did not reach statistical significance. However, after randomisation, significantly fewer patients in the rFVIIa group underwent a reoperation because of bleeding or needed allogeneic transfusions.

Bleeding and Coagulopathy

About 50% of cardiac surgical patients receive red cells, 30% of which also receive blood product combinations including platelets or plasma. Established risk factors for transfusion include preoperative anaemia, low body mass index, complexity and urgency of surgery.

The cell based model of haemostasis is complex and not easily reproducible in vitro (Figure 13.1). Haemostasis is initiated following tethering of platelets to a site of vascular injury through vWF and GPIb/V/IX. The platelet membrane undergoes activation and mediators are released. Traces of tissue factor stabilise the factor VIIa, which in turn activates traces of IXa, Xa and thrombin. This sets off an autofeedback mechanism that propagates self-activation and results in fibrin polymerisation, followed by thrombin inactivation.

The effects of CPB on haemostasis are also complex and multifactorial. During surgery the majority of the surgical field is bypassed by the circulating blood; the patient's blood is haemodiluted with crystalloid and albumin. Hypothermia in combination with partial activation of the clotting cascade prolongs the clotting reaction further. Primary haemostasis is impaired by platelet consumption and degranulation. Platelets may also have been exposed to antiplatelet agents in the immediate preoperative phase, which will have reduced platelet activation further. High doses of unfractionated heparin inhibit the majority of the serin proteases in an antithrombin dependent manner. If administered in high doses, the half-life of heparin is prolonged, ranging between 30 and 90 minutes. Elimination is via renal and hepatic mechanisms in addition to poorly delineated pathways involving the macrophages and endothelial cells. Sequestration sites can be a source of heparin rebound, which is sometimes observed in patients who have received exceedingly high doses of heparin during CPB for up to 12 hours. Tissue debris is aspirated by cardiotomy suckers from the surgical field and mixed with the other blood and recirculated, adding a source of extrinsic clotting factor activation.

Diagnostic Testing

The majority of cardiac patients have postoperative thrombocytopenia and the clotting factors, if measured, can be as low as 25–50% of baseline immediately after separating from CPB. A gradual recovery occurs over the next 2–4 days. No single laboratory test has been shown to be predictive of postoperative clinical bleeding and unselected correction of platelet count or fibrinogen has had only disappointing results.

Preoperative Screening

It is currently accepted practice to screen aPTT and PT preoperatively along with full blood count (FBC). The reason for screening PT and aPTT is an anachronism dating back to when warfarin and unfractionated heparin were the main anticoagulants in use. The FBC is more important than ever in that it allows screening for preoperative anaemia or thrombocytopenia, which may be amenable to preoperative intervention. Generally we accept platelet counts $>90 \times 10^9/l$, aPTT <38 s and PT <18 s, assuming the patient is not on anticoagulants. A bleeding score is more useful to identify patients with a potential undiagnosed bleeding disorder.

Blood Tests Used To Assess and Direct Treatment of Post CPB Coagulopathy

The majority of centres now use a combination of laboratory and point-of-care assays in combination with clinical assessment to guide transfusion of products according to predefined algorithms (see Figure 13.2); for further details see Chapter 36.

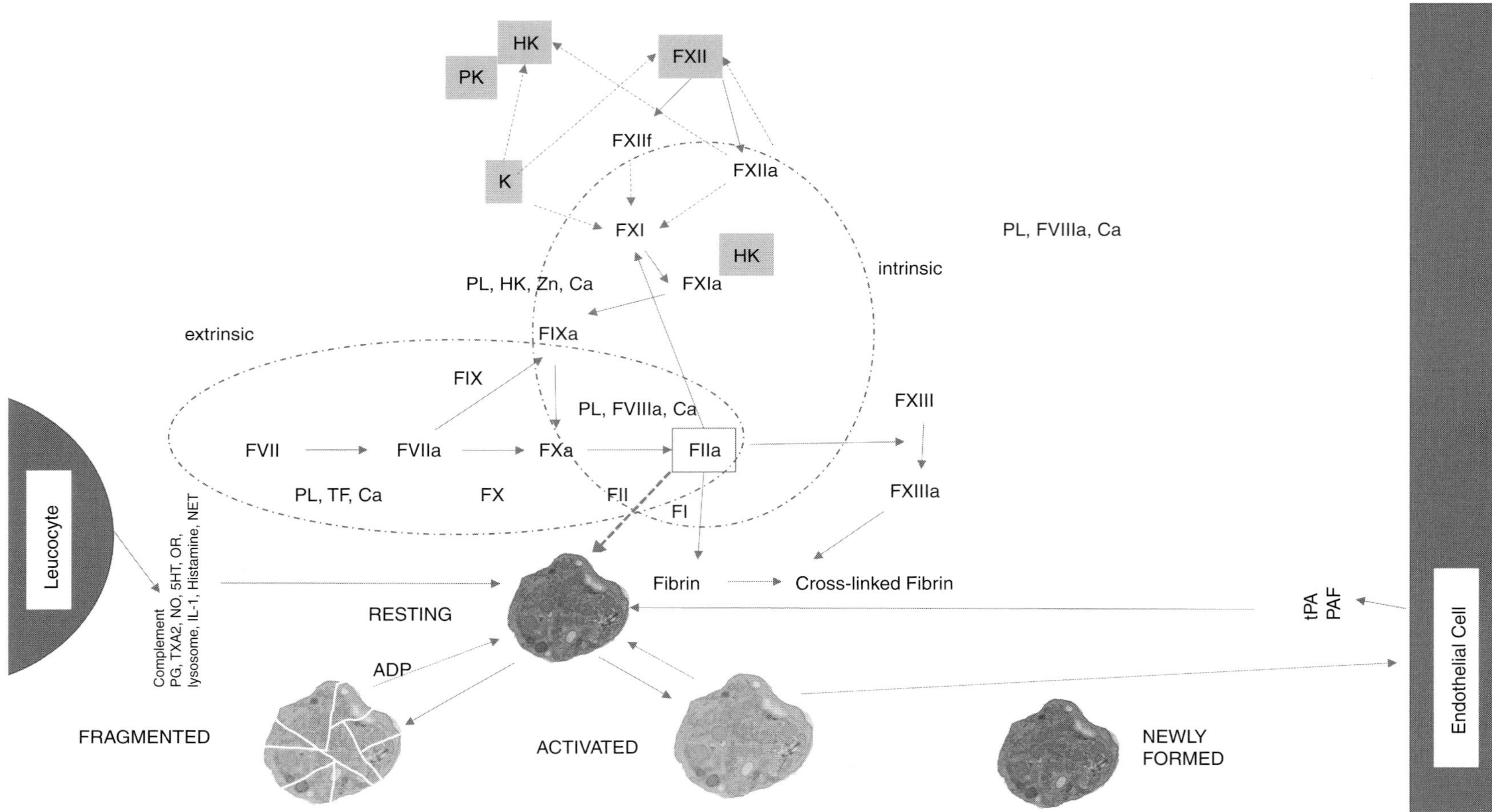

Figure 13.1 Cell based model of haemostasis. Contact activation occurs with activation of the four contact factors: K, PK, HK and XII. This leads to activation of the intrinsic pathway and activated complement. Both the activation of the complement pathways and the formation of thrombin activate platelets and lead to platelet aggregation and fragmentation. Platelet activation, in turn, activates endothelial cells and causes release of tPA platelet activation.

K kallikrein, PK prekallikrein, HK high-molecular-kininogen, F factor, a activated form, f fragmented form, PG prostaglandin, NO nitrous oxide, TXA2 thromboxane A2, OR oxygen radicals, 5HT serotonin, IL1 interleukin 1, PAF platelet activating factor, tPA tissue plasminogen activator. (A black and white version of this figure will appear in some formats. For the colour version, please refer to the plate section.)

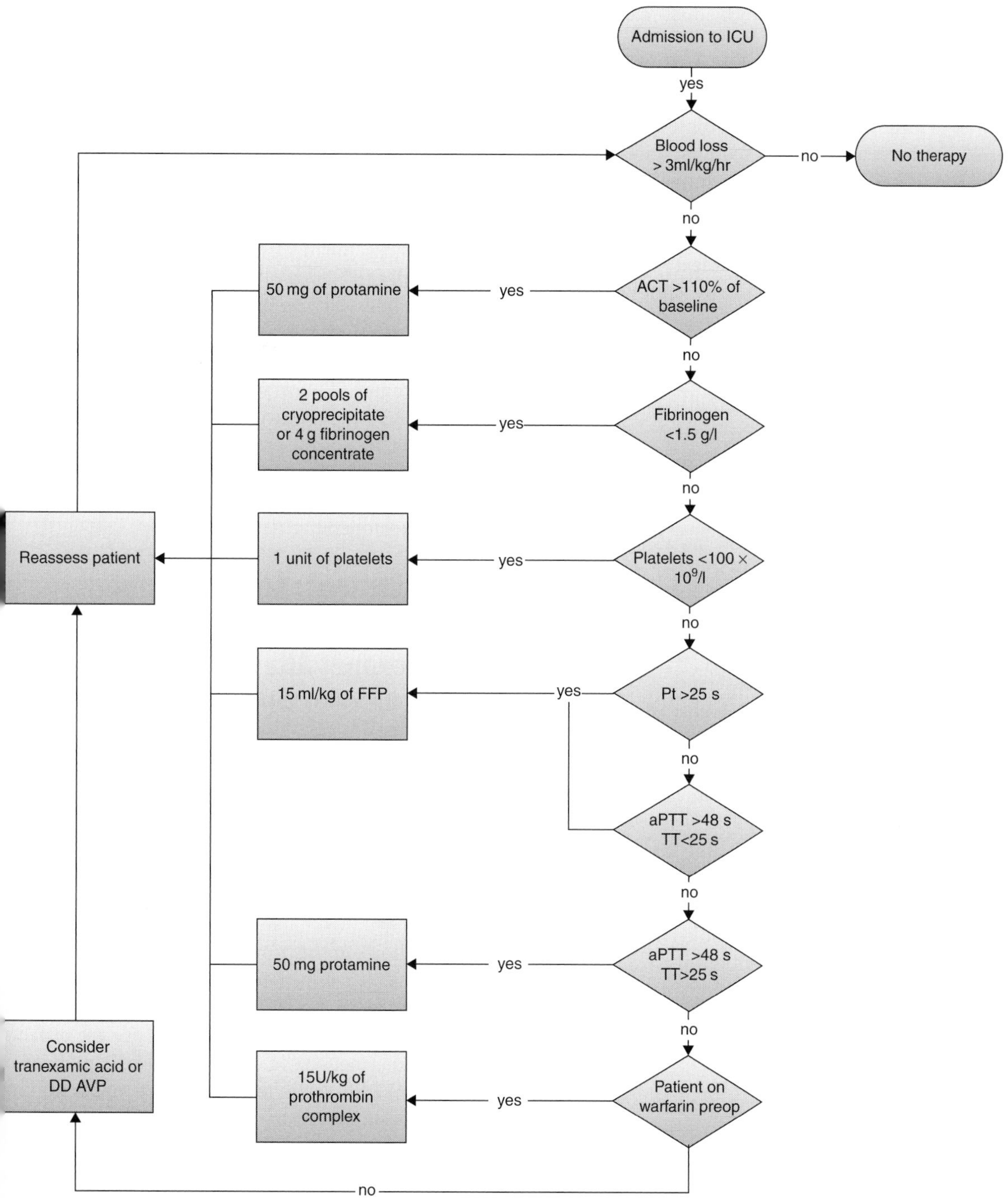

Figure 13.2 Part of the rationale for use of blood products is the use of preagreed transfusion algorithms to restore near normal haemostasis.

Laboratory Based Tests

The conventional laboratory tests in use are the PT/INR, aPTT, Clauss fibrinogen and thrombin time. Others include anti-Xa level. FBC is also essential. Generally it is assumed that thrombocytopenia will respond clinically to platelet transfusions up to 100 $\times 10^9$/l. PT >20 s and aPTT >48 s correct with FFP. These screening tests tend to become prolonged when the levels of some individual factors have decreased to 40% or less.

The main drawback of using laboratory based assays is the slower turnaround time, which may be as long as 40 minutes. Furthermore, these assays are sensitive to high heparin levels. Thrombin time allows the detection of heparin and interpretation of prolonged clotting tests in complex patients. It is more sensitive to heparin than aPTT, and a TT value >25 s suggests heparin contamination. In the context of recently discontinued warfarin therapy, mildly prolonged aPTT and PT may hint at potentially correctable deficits in a patient with protracted bleeding. Dabigatran or argatroban may similarly potentially produce falsely low fibrinogen results.

Point-of-Care (POC) Testing

POC testing is firmly establishing itself in the setting of cardiothoracic surgery. The benefit of these tests is the rapid turnaround and the ability to detect hypofibrinogenaemia at the POC. The drawback is the relative insensitivity to some of the more subtle imbalances of coagulation such as warfarin or heparin therapy for which laboratory based assays have been validated and have a long track record.

The two dominant technologies are thromboelastography (TEG) and rotational thromboelastometry (ROTEM). A third, the Sonoclot, was evaluated by NICE in 2014 but was not deemed suitable to be used outside a clinical trial. All the viscoelastic assays benefit from a number of activator kits which usually include a PTT like reagent with kaolin or celite, a tissue factor based activator (EXTEM or fastTEG), a fibrinogen activator (functional fibrinogen, or FIBTEM) and a heparinase containing Celite or kaolin assay. Manufacturers are developing a cartridge based solution that allows the simultaneous assessment of several of the assays at once in varying combinations to improve reliability.

The TEG is able to assess platelet function in addition to the above tests by making the reaction dependent on ADP platelet activation or arachidonic acid based activation. Another potentially useful test is the Multiplate platelet function assay. This utilises electric impedance to detect platelet function/aggregation in whole blood. Results are available in under 10 minutes but one of the problems with the test is the interference from low platelet counts, which may be a secondary reason for a lack of detectable platelet function perioperatively.

Blood Conservation

PBM is an international initiative based on the Australian experience of using a multimodal approach to optimise red cell mass, minimise blood loss and harness the physiological tolerance of anaemia, so as to reduce the need for transfusion, improve patient outcomes and ensure that blood products are available for those patients that absolutely require transfusion. The UK Department of Health has published guidelines which can be downloaded freely and encompass a range of interventions beginning with rapid diagnosis of preoperative anaemia and correction of reversible causes when possible prior to surgery, the use of cell salvage and adjuncts such as fibrin glue, along with targeted reversal of anticoagulants and algorithms to correct coagulopathy, so as to minimise perioperative blood loss, and use of a restrictive policy of diagnostic testing to reduce the impact of repeated blood sampling on postoperative haemoglobin.

Future Outlook: Anticoagulant Reversal with Beriplex, Idaricuzimab and Adexanet Alfa

Four new oral anticoagulants have come on the market over the past 5 years. While the adoption was slow initially, now patients present for urgent or elective surgery while on these drugs. There are set recommendations by the manufacturers with regard to pausing treatment prior to surgery based on renal function and risk of surgery. Tranexamic acid and correcting other correctable factors like thrombocytopenia may also help.

Prothrombin complex has become the reversal agent of choice of the novel anticoagulants with doses of 25–50 IU/kg (albeit not licensed). This has now been superseded for dabigatran by idaricuzimab, a monoclonal antibody for dabigatran. We are expecting that adexanet alfa (a dummy factor Xa molecule) will receive a license in the near future for Xa inhibitors for specific reversal.

Learning Points

- Blood products and components vary in their indications, and internationally and randomised control trials to determine their optimal use are lacking.
- Recombinant products are only available for a minority of indications such as congenital factor VIII deficiency.

- Recombinant factor VIIa was inferior to best conventional management in cardiothoracic surgery.
- Point-of-care testing has advantages over laboratory testing of turnaround time and global nature. Laboratory assays by comparison have a defined advantage in their reproducibility and use in transfusion algorithms.
- Prothrombin complex has become the unlicensed reversal agent of choice for direct oral anticoagulants (DOACs). Specific reversal agents will probably be available in the near future.

Further Reading

http://www.b-s-h.org.uk/guidelines/guidelines/use-of-platelet-transfusions/

www.nice.org.uk/guidance/ng24

http://transfusion.com.au/transfusion_practice/blood_conservation

Weiskopf RB, Viele MK, Feiner J, et al. Human cardiovascular and metabolic response to acute, severe isovolemic anemia. *Journal of the American Medical Association*. 1998; 279(3): 217–221.

MCQs

Which of the following statements is true?

1. **UK Plasma:**
   (a) Is being used to manufacture plasma derived single factor concentrates where so far there is no recombinant option
   (b) Is no longer used
   (c) Is used in patients born after 1.1.1996 only if treated with methylene blue
   (d) Is now only used for FFP, cryoprecipitate and platelets
   (e) Is pooled before use
2. **Point-of-care testing:**
   (a) Has been endorsed by NICE after cardiothoracic surgery
   (b) Is advocated for warfarin reversal
   (c) Leads to more restrictive cryoprecipitate or fibrinogen use
   (d) Increases the use of FFP
   (e) Should not be performed intraoperatively
3. **Laboratory based testing:**
   (a) The thrombin time is sensitive to heparin overhang
   (b) The anti-Xa levels may be falsely low in HIT
   (c) Clauss fibrinogen is unaffected by thombin inhibitors such as dabigatran
   (d) There is no role for the aPTT and PT in postoperative quantification of coagulopathy
   (e) DOAC should be reversed with activated prothrombin concentrate
4. **Blood products:**
   (a) Red cells can be stored for up to 2 years
   (b) FAC sorted platelets can be ordered by the NHSBT
   (c) Platelets express class I HLA antigens
   (d) Red cell transfused patients will not develop HLA class I antibodies
   (e) Platelet increments should be performed 7 days after administration
5. **Transfusion associated risks:**
   (a) Greatest risk to the patient is viral transmission
   (b) Patients who refuse blood on grounds of lack of safety of the blood supply should be offered concomitant antiretrovirals
   (c) Patients who refuse blood should be offered autologous predeposit of blood
   (d) Prothrombin complex is a recombinant product
   (e) A liberal transfusion threshold >90 g/l was superior to 75 g/l in the T2 study

Exercise answers are available on p.468. Alternatively, take the test online at www.cambridge.org/CardiothoracicMCQ

Chapter 14

Fluid Administration

Vasileios Zochios and Kamen Valchanov

Introduction

Intravenous fluid administration is performed in critically ill patients to maintain fluid volume homeostasis and to achieve many other goals. Intensivists and perioperative physicians who care for the cardiothoracic critically ill patient must appreciate that fluids are 'drugs' and therefore it is necesssary to understand their physiology and pharmacology. Appropriate fluid resuscitation is often the first intervention for the haemodynamically unstable patient. There is ongoing debate regarding whether the fluid chosen for these patients should be a crystalloid solution (i.e. isotonic saline, Ringer's lactate) or a colloid containing solution (i.e. albumin solution, hyperoncotic starch). Large international surveys have shown that choice of fluid is mostly a matter of institutional preference rather than due to specific procedural/patient related factors.

Pathophysiology

There are several determinants in assessing the need for intravascular volume replacement in the context of cardiac surgery: (i) blood loss, (ii) increasing vascular capacitance as often occurs with patient rewarming, (iii) third space fluid losses secondary to cardiopulmonary bypass (CPB) induced systemic inflammation, and (iv) increased cardiac preload requirements in the setting of transient cardiac ischaemia – reperfusion injury, myocardial stunning and reduced ventricular compliance.

Total body water for the average 70 kg adult male is about 45 l of which 30 l (65%) is intracellular and 15 l (35%) is extracellular fluid. The extracellular space can be subdivided into interstitial space (10l) and intravascular space (5 l). All three compartments also contain electrolytes, including ions and larger molecules. The cellular membranes maintain potential differences via a complex differential concentration between intracellular (potassium) and extracellular (sodium) ions. In addition, proteins and large molecules maintain the colloid distributions between intracellular, interstitial and intravascular spaces.

The fate of any intravenous fluid given into the vascular compartment depends on many factors including the electrolyte and colloid (if any) compositions, the patient's intravascular volume status, the total volume of fluid administered, and the integrity of endothelial glycocalyx. The endothelial glycocalyx modulates vascular permeability and inflammation and according to the Starling model it is a key determinant of fluid disposition. The primary forces defining transcapillary fluid movement and the counterbalancing process of fluid movement into the vascular space in a normal and damaged vasculature are shown in Figure 14.1. It has been shown that CPB is associated with loss of glycocalyx integrity and microvascular dysfunction. Interestingly, significant shedding of the glycocalyx also occurs during off-CPB procedures. In critical illness, including post-CPB postoperative states, endothelial glycocalyx denudation causes high transcapillary movement of fluid leading to tissue oedema and inadequate intravascular volume expansion after intravenous fluids are administered.

Fluids in the Cardiothoracic ICU

Colloids Versus Crystalloids

There is a lack of prospective data with special regard to 'ideal' fluid in the cardiac surgical patient population. Colloid fluids would be expected to produce a much larger volume expanding effect. Usual teaching suggests that the colloid to crystalloid volume expansion efficacy is 1:3 (300% greater efficacy for colloids), whereas the colloid to crystalloid ratio for volume expansion in adequately powered and well-designed

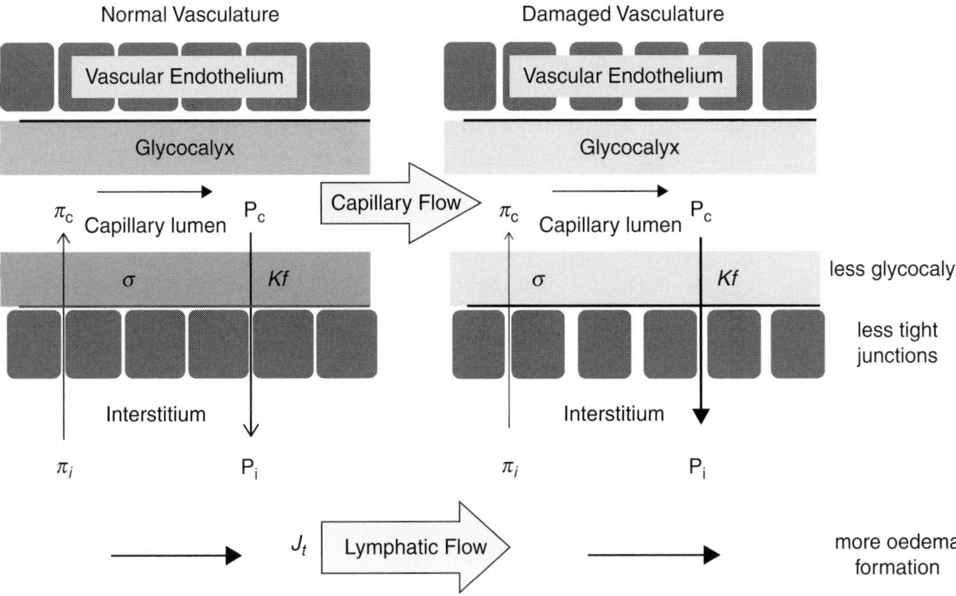

Figure 14.1 The opposing forces defining the steady state net flow of fluid from the capillary into the interstitial space are defined by the hydrostatic pressure differences between the capillary lumen pressure (P_c) and interstitial pressure (P_i) as opposed by the filtration coefficient (*Kf*) which itself is a function of the vascular endothelial cell integrity and the intraluminal glycocalyx. This net efflux of fluid out of the capillary into the interstitium is blunted by an opposing oncotic pressure gradient moving fluid in the opposite direction because capillary oncotic pressure (π_c) is greater than interstitial oncotic pressure (π_i). And like hydrostatic pressure dependent flow, oncotic dependent flow is blunted by the reflection coefficient (σ), which like K_f is a function of the glycocalyx and vascular endothelial integrity. Under normal conditions (left side), both K_f and σ are high, minimising fluid flux resulting in a slight loss of plasma into the interstitium which is removed by lymphatic flow. However, if the vascular endothelium and glycocalyx are damaged (right side), oncotic pressure gradients play a minimal role because a large amount of protein-rich plasma translocates into the interstitial space, minimising the oncotic pressure gradient, whereas the constant P_c promotes massive fluid loss and interstitial oedema.

Adapted from Lira and Pinsky (2014), permission to reproduce granted under SpringerOpen general terms.

randomised controlled trials (RCTs) was 1:1.2–1:1.4 (approximately 30% greater efficacy for colloids). The contents of solutes in colloid and crystalloid solutions are presented in Tables 14.1 and 14.2.

It would stand to reason that early during elective cardiac surgery colloid fluids may have a better volume expansion effect than crystalloids as capillary pressures are likely to be normal and loading with crystalloids would produce a dilutional effect on plasma oncotic pressure leading to tissue oedema and a reduced volume expansion effect.

Crystalloids are preferred over colloid containing solutions for the management of patients with severe hypovolaemia not due to bleeding. Saline solutions seem to be as effective as other crystalloid solutions and colloid containing solutions, and are much less expensive. It is recommended that hyperoncotic starch solutions are avoided as they increase the risk of acute kidney injury, need for renal replacement therapy (RRT) and mortality. They may also lead to hypernatraemia, hyperchloraemia and acidosis. There was a black box warning from FDA for heat starch.

In a 9 year multicentre open label trial (CRISTAL), 2857 patients with hypovolaemic shock, due to any cause, were randomly assigned to fluid resuscitation with colloid or crystalloid. There was no difference in 28 day mortality or need for RRT between the two arms. Patients treated with colloids had more mechanical ventilation free days (13.5 versus 14.6 days) and vasopressor therapy (15.2 versus 16.2 days), as well as a lower 90 day mortality (31% versus 34%). However, the open label design and heterogeneity of fluids that were compared between the groups limit confidence in the apparent benefit of colloid solutions in this population.

Albumin

In theory, albumin has two possible advantages over crystalloid solutions: (i) more rapid plasma volume expansion, since the colloid solution remains intravascularly (in contrast to saline, three quarters of which

Table 14.1 Composition of currently available crystalloid solutions

Fluid/solute	Na^+ mEq/l	K^+ mEq/l	Cl^- mEq/l	Ca^{2+} mEq/l	Mg^{2+} mEq/l	Osmolarity mOsm/l	Lactate mEq/l	Gluconate mEq/l	Acetate mEq/l	Glucose g/l
Plasma	142	4	103	5	3	290	2	—	—	1
NaCl 0.9% Dextrose 5%	154	—	154	—	—	230	—	—	—	50
NaCl 0.45% Dextrose 5%	77	—	77	—	—	203	—	—	—	50
NaCl 0.9%	154	—	154	—	—	308	—	—	—	—
Lactated Ringer's	130	4	109	3	—	273	28	—	—	—
Dextrose 5%	—	—	—	—	—	252	—	—	—	50
Plasmalyte 148	140	5	98	—	3	294	—	23	27	—
Normasol	140	5	98	—	3	294	—	23	27	—

Table 14.2 Composition of currently available colloid solutions

Fluid/solute	Osmolarity mOsm/l	pH	Na^+ mEq/l	K^+ mEq/l	Ca^{2+} mEq/l	Cl^- mEq/l
Gelofusine	274	7.4	154	<0.4	<0.4	125
Hetastarch	308	4.0–5.5	154	—	—	154
Haemaccel	301	7.4	145	5	6.25	145
Pentastarch	326	5.0	154	—	—	154
Albumin 4.5%		7.4	<160	<2	—	136

enters the interstitium) and (ii) lesser risk of pulmonary oedema, since dilutional hypoalbuminaemia will not occur. Well-designed RCTs and meta-analyses have failed to demonstrate benefits from the use of albumin. However, in some cardiothoracic intensive care units albumin remains the colloid of choice for patients undergoing lung transplantation and pulmonary endarterectomy when volume expansion is needed in the immediate postoperative period, in an attempt to reduce the risk of early reperfusion lung injury.

Hydroxyethyl Starch (HES)

Use of hyperoncotic starch solutions has been associated with increased incidence of acute kidney injury (AKI) and high mortality in some studies. In a RCT, 7000 patients were randomised to receive 6% HES or normal saline for all fluid resuscitation until ICU discharge. There was an increased incidence of AKI requiring RRT in the HES group compared with the saline group (5% versus 5.8%). Two meta-analyses, one of which excluded seven trials that were retracted due to scientific misconduct of one investigator, found that compared to conventional fluid resuscitation regimens, HES was associated with increased risk of mortality and need for RRT. HES associated AKI appears to be related to pinocytosis of metabolites into renal proximal tubular cells after glomerular filtration. HES has also been associated with increased risk of bleeding, which is probably due to impaired fibrin polymerisation and decreased factor VIII, vWF and XIII levels and not associated with haemodilution. Given the fact that the cardiac surgical patient population is at risk of AKI and coagulopathy anyway, the use of HES in the setting of cardiac surgery is not recommended.

Crystalloids

One of the most commonly used crystalloid solutions is 0.9% sodium chloride or 'normal' saline, which is anything but 'normal' or 'physiological' as it is slightly hypertonic and contains equal amounts of sodium and chloride making it hypernatraemic and very hyperchloraemic relative to plasma. Administration of high volume 'normal' saline will result in hypernatraemia, hyperchloraemic acidaemia leading to renal vasoconstriction and reduction in renal blood flow. This has led to suggestions that physiologically buffered fluids with a chemical composition that approximates extracellular fluid (e.g. Ringer's lactate solution, Hartman's solution, Plasma-lyte 148, Accusol) are used instead of 'isotonic' saline for large volume resuscitation. A recent RCT which enrolled healthy volunteers, and large observational series, have demonstrated that adverse effects associated with saline use were not evident when physiologically buffered fluids were used.

Hypertonic Solutions

Hypertonic solutions typically used in cardiac surgery include 2–7% saline. They have been used in an attempt to minimise volume overload and produce cellular dehydration in the context of cerebral oedema. The majority of the trials of hypertonic solutions have been in patients with traumatic brain injury. The results cannot be extrapolated for the general cardiac surgical population. However, cardiac surgical patients with cerebral oedema may benefit from hypertonic saline solutions on an individual basis. Studies examining use of hypertonic solutions did not examine their effect on renal function and reported a high incidence of hypernatraemia.

Fluid Balance Management

Positive fluid balance has been associated with worse outcomes in some but not all critically ill patient populations. A recent observational study that included a large cohort of medical, surgical and cardiothoracic ICU patients showed that positive fluid balance at the time of ICU discharge was associated with increased risk of death, after adjusting for markers of illness severity and chronic medical conditions, particularly in patients with underlying heart or kidney disease.

A secondary analysis of the FACTT trial demonstrated that patients with ARDS who developed AKI had a higher mortality (independent of a conservative or liberal fluid administration strategy). This study demonstrated some evidence of causality, as diuretic use was associated with a protective effect, potentially due to its effect on fluid balance. When the diuretic effect was adjusted for fluid balance, the protective effect was attenuated, thus potentially suggesting that the modulation of fluid balance promoted the benefit.

Intravenous fluid administration is a common intervention used for both the prevention and treatment of AKI. The pathogenesis of AKI in cardiac surgical patients is multifactorial, not only due to perturbed haemodynamics but also the result of direct cellular injury as well as indirect injury from inflammation and microcirculatory changes. AKI with oliguria as well as fluid resuscitation often results in accumulation of excess total body fluid. This fluid accumulates in all tissues of the body, and through the interstitial space, as well as remaining within the vascular space, resulting in increased venous pressure. The presence of oliguria is associated with a poor prognosis; however, it remains unclear whether this is due to severity of injury or due to fluid overload. Most studies to date have been conducted in the general ICU population. Similar findings have been reproduced in the cardiac surgery population, as early administration of fluid can lead to AKI. In a prospective observational cohort of 100 patients undergoing cardiac surgery, those patients in the quartile receiving the highest volume of fluid suffered the highest degree of AKI. This study was limited by the small number of patients included.

It has been demonstrated that positive fluid balance in the first 3 postoperative days is associated with primary graft dysfunction after lung transplantation. Patients undergoing pulmonary endarterectomy constitute a unique patient population at risk of development of ARDS due to high permeability lung injury. Therefore restrictive fluid management strategies and adequate diuresis in the first 48 hours (aiming for 2 l negative fluid balance) is of paramount importance. Negative fluid balance should also be maintained during the first week after lung resection surgery. Fluids should be limited because lung resection decreases the pulmonary vascular bed and overhydration will result in impaired gas exchange, need for prolonged mechanical ventilation, prolonged length of stay and high mortality.

Fluid Responsiveness

In the cardiothoracic intensive care populations, reduced cardiac output is treated by correcting the main determinants: heart rate, myocardial contractility, afterload and preload. When preload is reduced and fluid replacement is needed then the strategy is usually to administer the minimum fluid required to achieve optimising of cardiac output for the particular moment of time. Overenthusiastic fluid administration in the cardiac surgical population can lead to increased preload (which is more difficult to treat), overstretching of myocardial fibres, pulmonary oedema and generalised oedema. However, on occasions fluid administration in cardiothoracic critically ill patients is required. In general this is guided by imaging of the heart and IVC or cardiac output monitors. Sometimes, a more pragmatic way of monitoring fluid administration can be measuring fluid responsiveness.

The definition of fluid responsiveness varies according to the clinical or research setting. A recently proposed definition is 'an increase in a physiologic parameter, preferably cardiac output, within 15 minutes superseding twice the error of the measuring technique after a 15-minute administration of 6 ml kg^{-1} of crystalloids'. In the critical care setting, only 50% of haemodynamically unstable patients are 'fluid-responders' when the fluid bolus is given on 'clinical grounds'. This emphasises that fluid loading is not always the correct therapy for a clinically hypoperfused patient and that 'non-responders' are exposed to the risks of volume overload, systemic and pulmonary oedema and tissue hypoxia. In other words, fluid responsiveness is a measure of 'preload dependence' or 'preload reserve' but not all 'fluid-responders' necessarily need volume loading.

Examples of clinical measures include static and dynamic parameters. The static parameters (such as central venous pressure) are described as having little value; however, the dynamic parameters (stroke volume variation and pulse pressure variation, as measured using a number of monitors) are shown to be good physiological determinants of fluid responsiveness. Passive leg raise is an increasingly popular fluid responsiveness assessment tool. In patients receiving mechanical circulatory support (extracorporeal life support, ventricular assist devices, intra-aortic balloon pump), transthoracic and transoesophageal echocardiography are invaluable diagnostic tools that can be utilised to assess fluid responsiveness and intravascular volume status.

Learning Points

- Fluids are drugs.
- The integrity of the endothelial glycocalyx appears to have a major role in fluid exchange and distribution.
- Starch solutions should be avoided during and after cardiothoracic surgery.
- Physiologically buffered fluids have some advantages including maintenance of renal perfusion and avoidance of acid-base imbalance.
- Bedside assessment of fluid responsiveness should always precede fluid loading.

Further Reading

Annane D, Siami S, Jaber S, et al. Effects of fluid resuscitation with colloids vs crystalloids on mortality in critically ill patients presenting with hypovolemic shock: the CRISTAL randomized trial. *Journal of the American Medical Association*. 2013; 310: 1809.

Banks DA, Pretorius GV, Kerr KM, et al. Pulmonary endarterectomy: part I. Pathophysiology, clinical manifestations, and diagnostic evaluation of chronic thromboembolic pulmonary hypertension. *Seminars in Cardiothoracic and Vascular Anesthesia*. 2014; 18: 319–330.

Bouchard J, Soroko SB, Chertow GM, et al. Fluid accumulation, survival and recovery of kidney function in critically ill patients with acute kidney injury. *Kidney International*. 2009; 6: 422–427.

Bruegger D, Rehm M, Abicht J, et al. Shedding of the endothelial glycocalyx during cardiac surgery: on-pump versus off-pump coronary artery bypass graft surgery. *Journal of Thoracic and Cardiovascular Surgery*. 2009; 138: 1445–1447.

Cherpanath TG, Aarts LP, Groeneveld JA, et al. Defining fluid responsiveness: a guide to patient-tailored volume titration. *Journal of Cardiothoracic and Vascular Anesthesia*. 2014; 28: 745–754.

Chowdhury AH, Cox EF, Francis ST, et al. A randomized, controlled, double-blind crossover study on the effects of 2-L infusions of 0.9% saline and Plasma-lyte® 148 on renal blood flow velocity and renal cortical tissue perfusion in healthy volunteers. *Annals of Surgery*. 2012; 256: 18–24.

Finfer S, Bellomo R, Boyce N, et al. A comparison of albumin and saline for fluid resuscitation in the intensive care unit. *New England Journal of Medicine*. 2004; 350: 2247–2256.

Fulop T, Pathak MB, Schmidt DW, et al. Volume-related weight gain and subsequent mortality in acute renal failure patients treated with continuous renal replacement therapy. *ASAIO Journal*. 2010; 56: 333–337.

Gheorghe C, Dadu R, Blot C, et al. Hyperchloremic metabolic acidosis following resuscitation of shock. *Chest*. 2010; 138: 1521.

Hahn RG. Volume kinetics for infusion fluids. Anesthesiology. 2010; 113: 470–481.

Lee J, de Louw E, Niemi M, et al. Association between fluid balance and survival in critically ill patients. *Journal of Internal Medicine*. 2015; 277: 468–477.

Lira A, Pinsky MR. Choices in fluid type and volume during resuscitation: impact on patient outcomes. *Annals of Intensive Care*. 2014; 4: 38.

Marik PE, Baram M, Vahid B. Does central venous pressure predict fluid responsiveness? A systematic review of the literature and the tale of seven mares. *Chest*. 2008; 134: 172–178.

Michard F, Teboul JL. Predicting fluid responsiveness in ICU patients: a critical analysis of the evidence. *Chest*. 2002; 121: 2000–2008.

Morgan TJ. The meaning of acid-base abnormalities in the intensive care unit: part III – effects of fluid administration. *Critical Care*. 2005; 9: 204.

Myburgh JA. Fluid resuscitation in acute medicine: what is the current situation? *Journal of Internal Medicine*. 2015; 277: 58–68.

Myburgh J, Cooper D, Finfer S, et al. Saline or albumin for fluid resuscitation in patients with traumatic brain injury. *New England Journal of Medicine*. 2007; 357: 874–884.

Myburgh JA, Finfer S, Bellomo R, et al. Hydroxyethyl starch or saline for fluid resuscitation in intensive care. *New England Journal of Medicine*. 2012; 367: 1901–1911.

O'Dell E, Tibby SM, Durward A, Murdoch IA. Hyperchloremia is the dominant cause of metabolic acidosis in the postresuscitation phase of pediatric meningococcal sepsis. *Critical Care Medicine*. 2007; 35: 2390.

Perel P, Roberts I. Colloids versus crystalloids for fluid resuscitation in critically ill patients. *Cochrane Database of Systematic Reviews*. 2012; 2012(6): CD000567.

Perner A, Haase N, Guttormsen AB, et al. Hydroxyethyl starch 130/0.42 versus Ringer's acetate in severe sepsis. *New England Journal of Medicine*. 2012; 367: 124.

Raghunathan K, McGee WT, Higgins T. Importance of intravenous fluid dose and composition in surgical ICU patients. *Current Opinion in Critical Care*. 2012; 18: 350–357.

Shaw A, Raghunathan K. Fluid management in cardiac surgery: colloid or crystalloid? *Anesthesiology Clinics*. 2013; 31: 269–280.

Tollofsrud S, Noddeland H. Hypertonic saline and dextran after coronary artery surgery mobilises fluid excess and improves cardiorespiratory functions. *Acta Anaesthesiologica Scandinavica*. 1998; 42: 154–161.

Woodcock TE, Woodcock TM. Revised Starling equation and the glycocalyx model of transvascular fluid exchange: an improved paradigm for prescribing intravenous fluid therapy. *British Journal of Anaesthesia*. 2012; 108: 384–394.

MCQs

1. **The main determinant of fluid disposition after cardiopulmonary bypass is:**
   (a) Total volume of fluid given
   (b) Electrolyte composition
   (c) Endothelial glycocalyx integrity
   (d) The patient's intravascular fluid status
   (e) Serum albumin level

2. **Fluid responsiveness in the postoperative cardiac surgical patient is assessed by:**
   (a) Increase in central venous pressure
   (b) Increase in stroke volume
   (c) Increase in mean arterial pressure
   (d) Decrease in lactate levels
   (e) Increase in urine output

3. **Fluid overload in the cardiothoracic critically ill:**
   (a) Is associated with poor clinical outcomes
   (b) Is associated with acute kidney injury
   (c) Is associated with postoperative acute respiratory distress syndrome (ARDS)
   (d) Is associated with prolonged mechanical ventilation
   (e) Is associated with late graft dysfunction in lung transplant recipients

4. **Regarding physiologically balanced solutions:**
   (a) They can cause hyperchloraemic metabolic acidosis
   (b) Their use is associated with maintenance of renal blood flow
   (c) Administration of physiological solutions is an acid-base intervention
   (d) They are preferred to colloids in cardiac surgical patients
   (e) Their use is contraindicated in hypoalbuminaemic patients

5. **Regarding colloids in the cardiothoracic ICU:**
   (a) Their use has been associated with impairment of the blood-brain barrier
   (b) Starch solutions can cause acute kidney injury and should be avoided
   (c) Albumin has a role in hypoalbuminaemic patients with clinical tissue oedema
   (d) They are the fluid of choice to assess fluid responsiveness
   (e) The incidence of anaphylaxis relating to use of gelatin solutions is 0.04%

Exercise answers are available on p.468. Alternatively, take the test online at www.cambridge.org/CardiothoracicMCQ

Chapter 15

Inotropes and Vasopressors

Gabriel Kleinman, Shahzad Shaefi and Charles Shayan

Introduction

Ahlquist's discovery in animal models of two distinct types of adrenergic receptors in 1948 set the foundation for the modern day critical care use of inotropic drugs. He named these receptors in relation to their activity as activators (alpha) or blockers (beta). His original work has been expanded exponentially by discovery of subtypes of the originally identified receptors as well as many other discrete types of vasoactive receptors. Though it was uniquely postulated that these vasoactive receptors respond only to sympathin (epinephrine), we now know that these G protein coupled receptors (GPCRs) are regulated by a variety of agonists and antagonists and play a key role in prevalence of sympathetic nervous system activity. In the cardiac ICU, these vasoactive receptors are stimulated with various natural and synthetic molecules, resulting in augmented cardiac output (CO), chronotropy and mean arterial pressure (MAP), and in some cases enhanced lusiotropy in the postsurgical cardiac setting. Norepinephrine, epinephrine, dopamine, dopexamine, dobutamine, milrinone, enoximone, levosimendan and phenylephrine are the most commonly encountered vasoactive agents in the intensive care unit. We will review the current evidence for the use of inotropic agents in the perioperative care of cardiac patients.

Alpha-1 Receptors

Furthering Ahlquist's work, Piascik elucidated the mechanism of action of GPCRs. Upon agonist binding to the alpha-1 receptor (A1r), Gq protein stimulates the phospholipase C (PLC) system, which in its turn activates the 1,2-diacylglycerol (DAG) protein kinase C (PKC) pathway through hydrolysis. The consequence of this enzymatic process is an increased release of calcium from the sarcoplasmic reticulum (SR) and increased protein phosphorylation (Figure 15.1). The end result is vascular smooth muscle constriction. This leads to globally increased systemic vascular resistance (SVR). In the perioperative setting, A1r agonists are used to counter the decreased SVR seen with a variety of physiological and pathophysiological processes. The A1r does not undergo sensitisation, or internalisation, though at maximal supratherapeutic agonist doses, it could produce organ ischaemia or substantially increase SVR, which can be widely distributed in epicardial, renal, splanchnic, cerebral and pulmonary vascular beds.

Beta Receptors

B receptors (Br) are subtyped into B1, B2 and B3 variants and regulate inotropy and chronotropy as well as smooth muscle relaxation in various vascular beds. Their distribution is not uniform. Although B1r and B2r are both present in myocardium, thoracic aorta and carotid artery, and epigastric and pulmonary artery, B1 is the predominant receptor subtype in the myocardium. B1 agonism exerts its effect through the Gs GPCR pathway. This interaction in cardiac cells leads to calcium induced calcium release from the myocardial sarcoplasmic reticulum, thereby allowing increased actin-myosin cross linkages and an enhanced chronotropic and inotropic state.

In contrast to the action of beta agonists on cardiac cells, in smooth muscle, B2r stimulation leads to increased activity of cAMP dependent protein kinase, increased phosphorylation and activation of phospholamban, increased cellular calcium reuptake through the ryanodine receptors and, ultimately, vasodilation.

Dobutamine

Dobutamine is a synthetic Br (B1, B2) agonist, which entered clinical use in 1978 as a promising replacement for dopamine in the treatment of acute

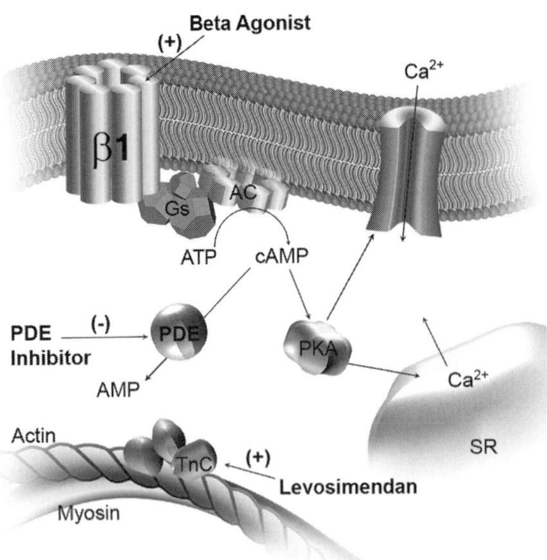

Figure 15.1 β1 receptor: AC adenylyl cyclase, cAMP cyclic adenosine monophosphate, PDE phosphodiesterase, PKA phosphokinase A, SR sarcoplasmic reticulum, TnC troponin C. Please refer to the text for detailed explanation.

decompensated heart failure. It has a 3:1 B1:B2 agonist activity and a trivial alpha-1 effect. Dobutamine is used in clinical practice for the treatment of acute decompensated heart failure in a dose dependent fashion, usually starting with an infusion of 2–3 μg/kg/min and rapidly uptitrated to a therapeutic dose of 7.5–15 μg/kg/min. It increases CO, stroke volume and coronary perfusion with minimal pulmonary vascular effect. Furthermore it has moderate chronotropy as it improves the atrioventricular (AV) conduction. Tachycardia has been reported to be more significant compared to use of milrinone, hence overall oxygen (O_2) consumption may be increased with its use. Dobutamine has a mean plasma half-life of 2–3 minutes titratable, though after a 72 hour infusion, many patients become resistant to dobutamine, due to tachyphylaxis, with resultant rebound hypertension on discontinuation probably due to beta receptor downregulation and internalisation. Dobutamine has been shown to increase myocardial oxygen consumption, as well as malignant ventricular arrhythmias, at any dose. Even though dobutamine improves cardiac output, it has not been shown to optimise regional O_2 delivery to ischaemic vascular beds that need O_2 the most. A recent randomised controlled trial comparing norepinephrine-dobutamine to epinephrine in patients with acute non-ischaemic cardiogenic shock requiring inotropic support found no difference in overall metabolic and objective parameters (O_2 delivery and renal perfusion) between the two groups. Thus, in patients with non-ischaemic HF requiring inotropic support, dobutamine may be the better agent compared to epinephrine given the tendency of epinephrine to aggravate lactic acidosis and, conversely, its lower effectiveness in an acidotic milieu. Though dobutamine infusions are frequently used as pharmacological therapy for bridge to cardiac transplantation or for long-term management of heart failure in patients not eligible for transplant, eosinophilic hypersensitivity reactions have been reported. The relationship between dobutamine and eosinophilia appears to be related to dose of dobutamine and duration of treatment, eventually resulting in eosinophilic myocarditis with unfortunate further decompensation of the patient's underlying cardiac disease. It is well documented that chronic infusions of dobutamine are associated with higher risk for mortality.

Norepinephrine (NE)

The primary endogenous neurotransmitter in humans, norepinephrine, has a more profound effect at A1r than at B1r and B2r at clinically relevant doses. Extensive research has been done focusing on the effects of NE in the setting of sepsis, and in clinical practice it has a profound vasoconstrictive effect with less heart rate variability when compared to dopamine and epinephrine. This finding, along with the decreased mortality associated with NE as compared to other vasoactive medications, makes it the gold standard choice in the setting of septic shock. In the cardiac ICU it is used to increase systolic and diastolic pressures and therefore coronary perfusion pressure, in a variety of vasoplegic states, thus giving it a favourable cardiac profile compared to dopamine and phenylephrine. It appears that the overall effect of NE on CO is determined through the interplay of systemic vascular resistance, heart rate and stroke volume variation (SVV). Patients with a SVV greater than 8.4% are likely to increase their CO in response to NE, while those with a SVV less than 8.4% are likely to decrease their cardiac output in the same setting. Prolonged infusions of NE may have direct toxic effects on cardiac myocytes, though this has only been demonstrated in animal models.

Epinephrine (Epi)

Epinephrine has a dose dependent affinity for A1r, B1r and B2r. At low doses, it acts primarily on B1r, increasing chronotropy, inotropy and lusitropy. As the dose is increased, a profound A1r effect is noted. Epi acts to increase coronary blood flow at low doses by increasing the relative time the myocardium is in diastole. At higher doses, it acts by increasing diastolic and therefore coronary perfusion pressure. Epi also acts to increase blood flow to the pulmonary vasculature through alpha-1 mediated pulmonary vasoconstriction, and dilates bronchioles through B2 mediated smooth muscle dilation. Levy et al. compared Epi to combination norepinephrine-dobutamine in cardiogenic shock patients without acute coronary syndrome and found that although Epi is as effective as norepinephrine-dobutamine at achieving haemodynamic goals, it was also associated with increased rates of lactic acidosis, tachycardia, arrhythmias and worsened perfusion to gastric mucosa. Furthermore, use of Epi in treatment of myocardial depression and low cardiac output syndrome may be associated with more adverse effects on the end-organ function such as kidneys in the postoperative period.

Isoproterenol

Isoproterenol is a purely synthetic B1 and B2 receptor agonist at clinical doses. While the B1 effects in cardiac cells lead to increased inotropic and chronotropic states, the increased cAMP in smooth muscles of the respiratory bronchioles and vasculature leads to bronchodilation with an increase in lung compliance and decrease in SVR respectively. Isoproterenol is used in the EP laboratory to induce AV nodal re-entrant tachycardias, as well as to initiate Wolff–Parkinson–White (WPW) syndrome re-entry and to chemically pace patients in third degree heart block, a property that is very useful in heart transplants particularly at the time of separation from CPB. Experimentally, isoproterenol is used to induce acute myocardial infarctions and HF due to the myocardial ischaemia it induces during long infusions.

Dopamine

Dopamine is the immediate in vivo precursor to norepinephrine. The actions of dopamine are mediated by five distinct GPCRs (D1–D5). These receptors are found in various densities on the surface of cells in the nervous system, pulmonary artery, splanchnic circulation and renal tubules. Dopamine-1 receptors (DA1) are found in the proximal convoluted tubules, ascending loop of Henle and collecting ducts. DA2 receptors are mainly located in the renal vascular endothelium. These receptors couple to Gs which peripherally increases cAMP, causing vasodilation. At low dose infusions up to 3 μg/kg/min, dopamine stimulates DA1 predominantly and results in vasodilation by increasing the intracellular cAMP (and therefore lowering calcium influx) at the level of vascular endothelium in renal, mesenteric beds. In the kidneys, dopamine inhibits the NaCl cotransporter at the distal convoluted tubule causing diuresis. Despite improving renal blood flow, dopamine has not been shown to improve glomerular filtration rate. At the level of myocardium DA1–DA4 receptors are found mainly in atria. At escalating doses (3–10 μg/kg/min) dopamine binds to these receptors as well as B1r and causes both chronotropy and inotropy, although it is not quite clear whether these effects are indirect (via presynaptic NE release) or by direct B1r stimulation. At doses higher than 10 μg/kg/min, dopamine binds to A1r causing peripheral vasoconstriction. A trial comparing dopamine to NE in patients with diagnosis of shock found that among the subset of patients with cardiogenic shock, the rate of death was significantly higher in the group treated with dopamine than in the group treated with NE.

Milrinone

While most of the vasoactive medications used in the cardiac ICU directly exert their effects on GPCRs, milrinone, a bipyridine PDE-3 inhibitor, utilises a novel mechanism, and is therefore not subject to receptor phosphorylation, internalisation of deactivation, and thus does not demonstrate the need for therapeutic dose escalation due to tachyphylaxis. Milrinone exerts its inotropic effect by inhibiting the conversion of cAMP to AMP, which causes smooth muscle relaxation in peripheral vasodilation, while in cardiac cells increased cAMP causes increased lusitropy and inotropy (Figure 15.2). Due to its lack of receptor internalisation and downregulation, like direct B2r, milrinone can be used in a beta receptor depleted state, such as stage D heart failure awaiting heart transplant. Milrinone has been shown to improve diastolic dysfunction and increases flow in coronary artery bypass grafts after cardiopulmonary bypass, however this effect is not demonstrable if milrinone is given prior to initiation of cardiopulmonary bypass. On the other hand if milrinone is administered in inhaled fashion prior to initiation of CPB it is beneficial in the first 24 hours postoperatively in cardiac patients with

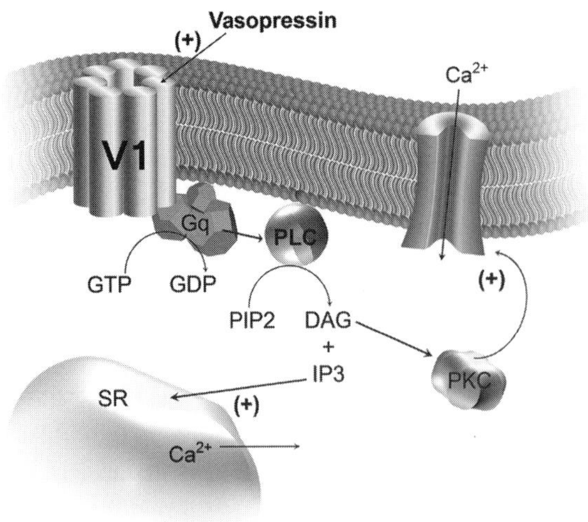

Figure 15.2 V1 receptor: DAG diacylglycerol, GDP guanosine diphosphate, IP3 inositol triphosphate 3, PIP2 phosphatidylinositol 4,5-biphosphate, PKC phosphokinase C, PLC phospholipase C. Please refer to the text for detailed explanation.

pulmonary hypertension. The clinical effect of long-term administration of milrinone in ambulatory patients was evaluated by Packer who found an excessive mortality rate in the milrinone treated group. Milrinone home infusion may be an alternative in stage 1B patients awaiting OHT, although the presence of ICD is advisable given the possibility of ventricular tachycardia. Milrinone may also be combined with beta-blockers in stage D heart failure, although large scale studies still need to be designed to evaluate outcomes in these patients. A 2012 meta-analysis of milrinone treatment in adult cardiac surgery suggests that milrinone is associated with a significantly increased risk of dying when compared with other drugs (mainly levosimendan). Even though OPTIME-CHF investigation showed that milrinone infusion in CHF exacerbation does not improve the mortality, it demonstrated that it may have a positive impact on renal functions when secondary outcomes were analysed. However, the full extent of this effect would have to be evaluated further.

Dopexamine

Dopexamine is a dopamine analogue that has activity at DA1, DA2, B1r and B2r. It has more significant B2r activity than B1r and hence, along with DA receptors, activation leads to cerebral, coronary and renal vasodilation and increased perfusion. Despite its particular vasodilatory property, in certain vascular beds it is considered an inotrope. Animal studies initially demonstrated that dopexamine may have immunomodulatory effect (B2 interaction), notably decreased lactataemia and cytokine release in animal models of endotoxaemia. This effect has not been duplicated in clinical observations. Dopexamine was compared to dobutamine in a randomised double blind, crossover fashion, in a paediatric population undergoing cardiac surgery for non-complex congenital correction, for separation from CPB and mitigating myocardial stunning. Both agents had a similar increase in CI. Obviously patients treated with dopexamine had lower systemic vascular resistance (SVR).

Calcium Sensitisers

In normal cardiac cells, tropomyosin and troponin C (TnC) inhibit the binding of thick to thin filaments. TnC, in the presence of calcium released from the sarcoplasmic reticulum, causes a conformational change in the troponin-tropomyosin complex, allowing extensive thick and thin filament interaction and thereby myocardial contraction (Figure 15.2). Once calcium diffuses off its binding site on TnC, tropomyosin again returns to its resting position, blocking the thick and thin filament contractile apparatus. Under typical physiological conditions, a large cardiac contractile reserve exists. Experimental and in vivo models have demonstrated that increasing calcium concentration in the sarcoplasmic reticulum leads to increased binding of TnC and, therefore, increased heart rate and inotropic state. It was this contractile reserve that led to the development of calcium sensitising agents that either increase the affinity of TnC for calcium or act directly on the thick and thin filaments to allow interaction with little endogenous calcium required. Two drugs that act to increase the affinity of TnC for calcium are currently available outside the USA, pimobendan and levosimendan.

Pimobendan is an oral agent that exerts its inotropic effect through calcium sensitising as well c-AMP dependent pathway. It has only been studied in the EPOCH study in a randomised double blind fashion, which demonstrated a non-statistically significant decrease in sudden cardiac death, hospitalisation for HF, and death from HF in the pimobendan treatment group. This study also found significantly decreased adverse cardiac events in the treatment group.

Levosimendan, which has a similar mechanism of action to pimobendan, has been shown not only to improve inotropy as well as lusitropy, but also to cause vasodilation by activating ATP dependent K channels on the smooth muscles. Levosimendan has been demonstrated to increase SV and CI by 28% and 39% respectively, while marginally increasing heart rate and meanwhile decreasing the left and right filling pressures and systemic arterial pressures when compared to placebo in a double blind RCT. The LIDO trial, which compared levosimendan to dobutamine, demonstrated that levosimendan exerted superior haemodynamic effects and in secondary and post hoc analyses was associated with a lower risk of death after 31 and 180 days. In addition, the second Randomized Multicenter Evaluation of Intravenous Levosimendan Efficacy (REVIVE II) study showed that patients with ADHF who received levosimendan in addition to standard therapy were more likely to show clinical improvement and less likely to deteriorate than patients on standard therapy alone. However, there was no significant change in 90 day mortality and there were more adverse side effects (tachyarrhythmia and hypotension) in the levosimendan group. As the previous studies had only compared levosimendan to placebo, the SURVIVE trial compared levosimendan to dobutamine in a double blind RCT in patients requiring inotropic support for ADHF and found that despite an initial reduction in plasma B-type natriuretic peptide level in patients in the levosimendan group compared with patients in the dobutamine group, levosimendan did not significantly reduce all-cause mortality at 180 days or affect any secondary clinical outcomes. Like milrinone, levosimendan used in combination with a beta adrenergic antagonist may have beneficial effects in patients with cardiogenic shock who exhibit tachycardia in response to inotropic agents.

Vasopressin

Pathophysiology of vasoplegia post cardiac surgery involves generation of interleukins, decreased endogenous vasopressin and increased production of NO by endothelial cells. Vasopressin is a peptide synthesised by the paraventricular and supraoptic nuclei of the posterior hypothalamus and is released in the capillary bed of the posterior pituitary gland where there is no blood-brain barrier. Its release is potently regulated by plasma osmolality and haemodynamic parameters such as decreased blood pressure producing hormones that are essential for osmotic as well as cardiovascular homeostasis. Vasopressin receptors are GPCRs, and there are three subtypes of these receptors: V1 is found in vascular smooth muscles; liver, platelets and most peripheral tissues; V2 is only found in renal collecting ducts; and V3 is limited to the anterior pituitary. Stimulation of the V1 receptor leads to vasoconstriction through a mechanism similar to that of alpha-1 receptor agonists, Gq activation of PLC leading to calcium release from intracellular stores (Figure 15.2). This vasoconstriction is apparent when there is a severe dysregulation of sympathetic, renin-angiotensin systems. Interestingly, vasopressin has a vasodilatory effect in the cerebral, pulmonary and coronary vascular bed at low doses while increasing the vascular tone in splanchnic, skeletal and cutaneous circulations. Recent studies have shown that a deficiency in vasopressin exists in some shock states, and numerous case studies and small trials show vasopressin increases arterial pressure in septic shock. The largest randomised prospective controlled study was published in 2003 by Dunser and colleagues. In this study, 48 patients with catecholamine-resistant vasodilatory shock were prospectively randomised to receive a combined infusion of vasopressin and norepinephrine or norepinephrine alone to maintain a MAP above 70 mmHg. The vasopressin group showed a significant increase in MAP, cardiac index, systemic vascular resistance index, and left ventricular stroke work index as well as reduced norepinephrine requirements and heart rates. Compared with the norepinephrine group, there was better preservation of gut mucosal blood flow and a significantly lower incidence of tachyarrhythmias. In survivors of cardiac arrest, vasopressin levels have also been demonstrated to be higher than in those cardiac arrest patients who do not survive, a finding which led to the inclusion of vasopressin in the ACLS algorithm.

Phenylephrine

The principal alpha agonist used in clinical practice is phenylephrine, which is a direct-acting synthetically derived alpha-1 agonist. It exerts no beta effects due to its lack of a hydroxyl group at position 4 on its benzene ring and it causes its vasoconstrictive effects through inhibition of cAMP production. In the perioperative period, it is used to rapidly increase the mean arterial pressure and maintain forward flow in patients with systolic outflow tract obstruction and single ventricle physiology. The rapid increase in

MAP caused by phenylephrine can lead to a carotid baroreceptor-mediated bradycardia. At clinically relevant doses, phenylephrine reduces CO and increases myocardial work, and oxygen requirements. Though not definitive, this may be associated with myocardial injury and significantly decreased coronary perfusion. In addition to its usefulness as both a bolus and infusion perioperative medication, phenylephrine has also been described in case reports to correct smooth muscle vascular tone in patients who coingest both PDE-5 inhibitors and nitrates.

Methylene Blue

Methylene blue, which is normally used as a cell dye and as a treatment for cyanide poisoning, when given as an intravenous bolus or infusion, binds to and inhibits guanylate cyclase, scavenges nitric oxide and inhibits synthesis of nitric oxide via iNOS. All three of these actions lead to decreased systemic levels of cGMP and NO, which act to synergistically minimise the overall response to endogenous vasodilators. Methylene blue has been used successfully for the treatment of vasoplegic syndrome, for which fluid resuscitation and conventional vasopressors are ineffective, as well as vasopressor resistant septic shock. Two studies have specifically looked at the role of methylene blue in cardiac surgery patients at highest risk for developing vasoplegic syndromes (preoperative ACE inhibitors, calcium channel blockers). When administered in the preoperative period, the treated patients had greater haemodynamic stability, less vasopressor requirements, less fluid administration, fewer blood transfusions, and decreased intensive care unit and overall hospital stays. None of the patients who received methylene blue developed vasoplegic syndrome, while 26% of the placebo patients did go on to develop some degree of vasoplegic syndrome. The same haemodynamic stability and decreased ICU and hospital stay held true for patients that were given methylene blue after the development of vasoplegic syndrome. Though a rapid and effective treatment for vasoplegic syndrome, methylene blue is not a completely benign drug. Severe renal impairment is an absolute contraindication, as it is excreted predominantly by the kidney. Relative contraindications include G6PD deficiency and other oxidiser initiated haemolytic anaemias. Methylene blue also inhibits MAO and must be used cautiously in patients on SSRIs, who are at a higher risk for serotonin syndrome.

Further Reading

Alhashemi JA. Treatment of cardiogenic shock with levosimendan in combination with β-adrenergic antagonists. *British Journal of Anaesthesia*. 2005; 95: 648–650. doi: 10.1093/bja/aei225

Bellomo R, Chapman M, Finfer S, Hickling K, Myburgh J. Low-dose dopamine in patients with early renal dysfunction: a placebo-controlled randomised trial. Australian and New Zealand Intensive Care Society (ANZICS) Clinical Trials Group. *Lancet*. 2000; 356: 2139–2143.

De Backer D, Biston P, Devriendt J, et al. Comparison of dopamine and norepinephrine in the treatment of shock. *New England Journal of Medicine*. 2010; 362: 779–789.

Klein L, Massie BM, Leimberger JD, et al. Admission or changes in renal function during hospitalization for worsening heart failure predict postdischarge survival: results from the Outcomes of a Prospective Trial of Intravenous Milrinone for Exacerbations of Chronic Heart Failure (OPTIME-CHF). *Circulation: Heart Failure*. 2008; 1: 25–33.

Laflamme M, Perrault LP, Carrier M, et al. Preliminary experience with combined inhaled milrinone and prostacyclin in cardiac surgical patients with pulmonary hypertension. *Journal of Cardiothoracic and Vascular Anesthesia*. 2015; 29: 38–45.

Levy B, Perez P, Perny J, Thivilier C, Gerard A. Comparison of norepinephrine-dobutamine to epinephrine for hemodynamics, lactate metabolism, and organ function variables in cardiogenic shock. A prospective, randomized pilot study. *Critical Care Medicine*. 2011; 39: 450–455.

Majure DT, Greco T, Greco M, et al. Meta-analysis of randomized trials of effect of milrinone on mortality in cardiac surgery: an update. *Journal of Cardiothoracic and Vascular Anesthesia*. 2013; 27: 220–229.

Mebazaa A, Nieminen MS, Packer M, et al. Levosimendan vs dobutamine for patients with acute decompensated heart failure: the SURVIVE Randomized Trial. *Journal of the American Medical Association*. 2007; 297: 1883–1891.

Movsesian M, Stehlik J, Vandeput F, Bristow MR. Phosphodiesterase inhibition in heart failure. *Heart Failure Reviews*. 2009; 14: 255–263.

Nathan Coxford R, Lang E, Dowling S. Dopamine versus norepinephrine in the treatment of shock. *Canadian Journal of Emergency Medicine*. 2011; 13: 395–397.

Ozal E, Kuralay E, Yildirim V, et al. Preoperative methylene blue administration in patients at high risk for vasoplegic syndrome during cardiac surgery. *Annals of Thoracic Surgery*. 2005; 79: 1615–1619.

MCQs

1. A 45 year old male is presenting to CTICU for postoperative management after a heart transplant. His past medical history is significant for arrhythmogenic right ventricular hypertrophy. His immediate postoperative vitals include a BP = 100/70, HR = 65.
   What inotropic agent would be MOST appropriate to start at this point?
   (a) Dopamine
   (b) Milrinone
   (c) Dobutamine
   (d) Norepinephrine
   (e) No need for inotropic agent
2. A 65 year patient with longstanding history of CAD is presenting to CTICU for further postoperative management. His preoperative systolic and diastolic functions are severely reduced.
   What would be the LEAST appropriate inotropic agent in this patient?
   (a) Dopamine
   (b) Milrinone
   (c) Dobutamine
   (d) Epinephrine
   (e) Levisomendan
3. A 75 year old patient with longstanding history of non-ischaemic cardiomyopathy and chronic heart failure (CHF), necessitating multiple hospitalisations and volume overload management in the past, is readmitted for acute exacerbation of his CHF.
   What is the MOST desirable inotropic agent to use in this patient?
   (a) Milrinone
   (b) Dobutamine
   (c) Epinephrine
   (d) Dopamine
   (e) Centre dependent
4. A 55 year old patient s/p MVR/TVR/AVR is presenting to CTICU. On admission the patient is on infusion of high dose milrinone, dobutamine and dopamine. Patient BP = 80/40, HR = 100, CI = 2.1.
   What agent would be the MOST useful to infuse at this time?
   (a) Phenylephrine
   (b) Norepinephrine
   (c) Epinephrine
   (d) Vasopressin
5. A 66 year old African American male is presenting s/p heart transplant (complicated intraoperative course), with profound thrombocytopenia and high pyrexia. His past medical history is significant for anxiety, severe depression and opioid abuse.
   Administration of all the following agents may contribute to his symptomology EXCEPT:
   (a) Odansetron
   (b) Fluoxetine
   (c) Trazadone
   (d) Methylene blue
   (e) Methadone

Exercise answers are available on p.468. Alternatively, take the test online at www.cambridge.org/CardiothoracicMCQ

Chapter 16

Sedation and Analgesia

Lachlan Miles and Barbora Parizkova

Introduction

Analgesia and sedation are ubiquitous in the management of the intubated ICU patient, and attitudes towards them have undergone a paradigm shift in recent years. Where once the ICU was viewed as an extension of the operating room environment, the 'anaesthetic triad' of deep sedation, potent analgesia and neuromuscular blockade is now rarely indicated beyond the doors of theatre.

The problems of **delirium**, **agitation** and **pain** are intrinsically connected. It is perhaps best to conceptualise this 'ICU triad' as a three-legged stool – if any 'leg' is neglected, the stool cannot function as intended.

Infusion Pharmacokinetics

The administration of sedative and analgesic medications in the ICU is frequently via intravenous infusion.

When administering any drug via continuous intravenous infusion, a steady state concentration will eventually be achieved, as determined by the dose rate and the clearance of the drug.

The time taken for an infusion to reach this steady state is determined by the half-life of the drug (the time taken for the plasma concentration of the drug to decrease by 50%). It takes 3–5 half-lives for a drug to reach steady state.

For agents with a prolonged half-life, an increase in the infusion rate is an inefficient means of achieving desired depth of sedation within a short timeframe. Increasing the infusion rate to a level such that the target concentration is achieved quickly will result in a relative overdose if the infusion is allowed to continue at that rate (Figure 16.1).

To achieve the target concentration of a drug whilst maintaining a continuous infusion at a safe dose rate, a loading dose is used.

If the loading dose is sufficient to achieve the target concentration for a given infusion rate, then the target concentration will be immediately achieved and maintained by the infusion without needing to wait the requisite 3–5 half-lives. If the loading dose yields a drug concentration more or less than the target concentration, it will still take 3–5 half-lives for steady state to be reached, but the starting concentration will be closer to the steady state concentration than if the loading dose had not been given (Figure 16.2).

Sedation

Oversedation is an important cause of morbidity in the ICU. The initiation of a sedative or analgesic agent should not be based on anticipated distress but rather on that which is perceived by the clinical team at the bedside.

In the postcardiac surgery setting, sedation may be misused to mask a variety of problems without considering the underlying issue (particularly pain). With a few exceptions (status epilepticus, raised intracranial pressure and severe respiratory failure), it is recognised that maintaining light levels of sedation leads to improved clinical outcomes (i.e. shorter duration of mechanical ventilation, decreased length of ICU stay). Whilst lighter levels of sedation lead to a more pronounced physiological stress response, this has not been linked to an increased incidence of myocardial ischaemia.

Consequently, it is vital to identify the underlying cause of any distress, rather than resorting to sedation in the first instance. Anxiety, pain, delirium and residual neuromuscular paralysis are amongst the most common causes in the intensive care setting. A common underlying cause of anxiety amongst this population is patient-ventilator dys-synchrony, and the adjustment of ventilator settings (despite acceptable blood gas values) may negate the need for sedation.

Non-pharmacological strategies are equally important. Whilst attention must be paid to addressing the

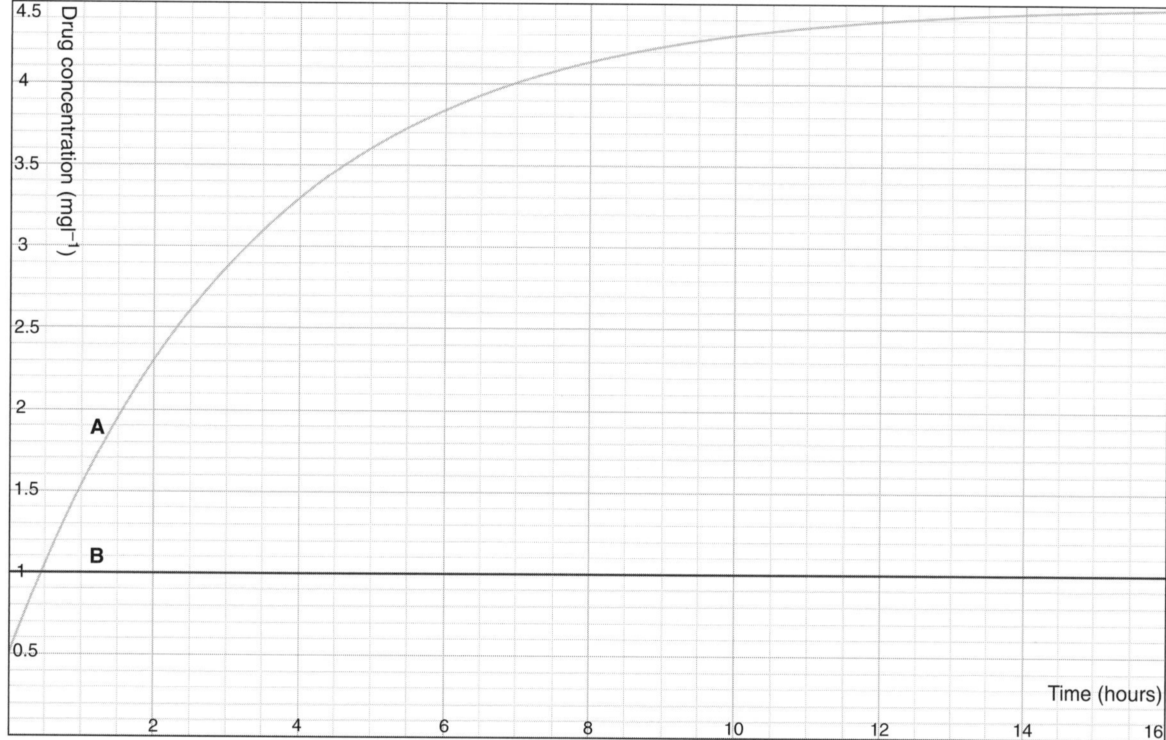

Figure 16.1 The effects of increasing the rate of infusion to achieve a rapid clinical effect with a hypothetical drug with a half-life of approximately 4 hours. An increase in the infusion rate (from a steady state of 0.5 mg l^{-1}) is performed. The desired clinical effect is achieved relatively rapidly, within 15 minutes (at a blood concentration of 1 mg l^{-1}). However, due to the prolonged half-life of the drug, the blood concentration steadily rises over the next 16 hours, a situation which, if left unchecked, will result in a steady state blood concentration nine-fold that of the original level, with potentially deleterious effects.

cause of agitation and distress, frequent reassurance and communication is equally important. Regular family visits, preservation of regular sleep-wake cycles and cognitive-behavioural therapies (music therapy, relaxation therapy) where available should also be incorporated into patient care.

Monitoring Sedation

A variety of different structured, subjective sedation assessment scores have been proposed. Of these, the **Richmond Agitation-Sedation Scale (RASS)** (Table 16.1) and the **Sedation-Agitation Scale (SAS)** (Table 16.2) are the most psychometrically reliable (particularly in terms of inter-rater variability) in measuring the quality and depth of sedation in adult ICU patients. In direct comparisons, neither of these measures is clearly superior.

A variety of different devices have been evaluated for the objective measurement of cerebral function in the sedated ICU patient. These include:

- Bispectral index (BIS);
- State entropy (SE);
- Auditory evoked potentials (AEP);
- Narcotrend index (NI);
- Patient state index (PSI).

Whilst these have some use in patients who cannot be clinically assessed (i.e. patients receiving neuromuscular blockade), or in whom monitoring of EEG is particularly important (i.e. non-convulsive status epilepticus), it is generally recognised that they are inferior to subjective scoring systems in the non-paralysed, non-comatose patient.

Planning Sedation

As previously mentioned, lighter levels of sedation lead to improved patient outcomes when combined with effective analgesia. This has led to the advent of **protocolised sedative-analgesic strategies**, whereby the bedside clinician titrates sedation to a set of predefined goals, guided by routine, structured, subjective

Table 16.1 The Richmond Agitation-Sedation Scale (RASS)

Score	Classification	Description
4	Combative	Overly combative or violent; immediate danger to staff
3	Very agitated	Pulls on or removes tube(s) or catheter(s) or has aggressive behaviour towards staff
2	Agitated	Frequent non-purposeful movement or patient-ventilator dys-synchrony
1	Restless	Anxious or apprehensive but movements not aggressive or vigorous
0	Alert and calm	
−1	Drowsy	Not fully alert but has sustained (more than 10 seconds) awakening with eye contact to voice
−2	Light sedation	Briefly (less than 10 seconds) awakens with eye contact to voice
−3	Moderate sedation	Any movement (but no eye contact) to voice
−4	Deep sedation	No response to voice, but movement to physical stimulation
−5	Unarousable	No response to voice or physical stimulation

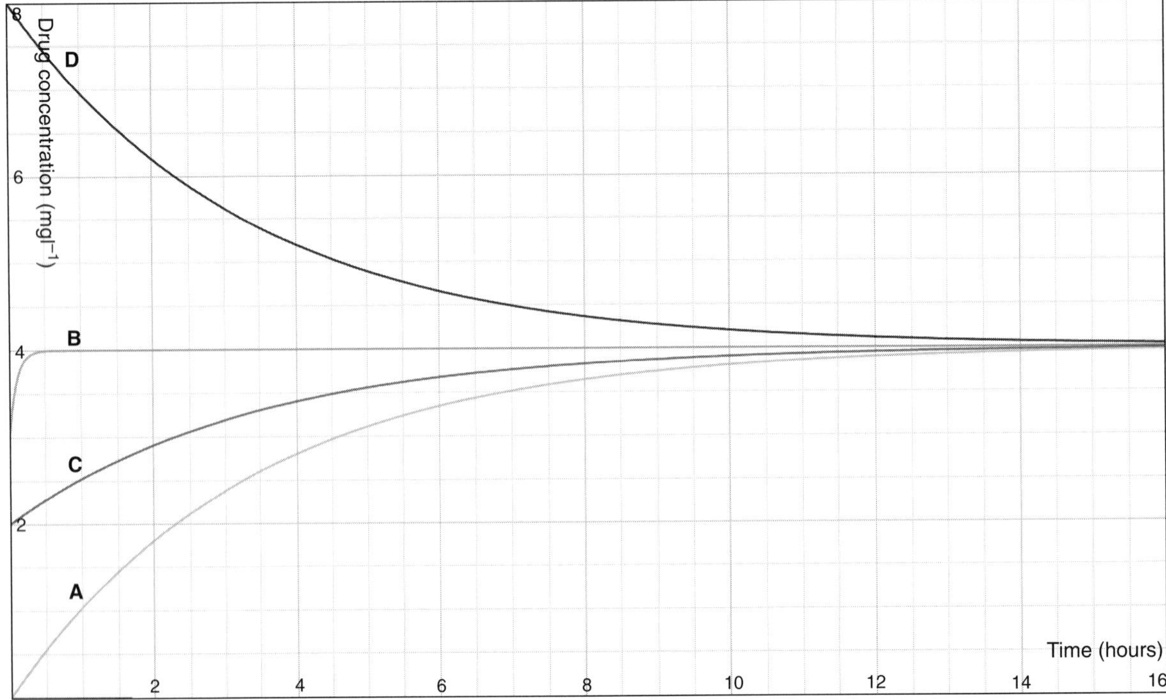

Figure 16.2 This graph demonstrates the effects of a loading dose for a hypothetical drug with a half-life of approximately 4 hours. Curve A demonstrates the effect of no loading dose, and the target steady state of 4 mg l^{-1} is reached after 4 half-lives. Curve B shows the effect of a perfectly calculated loading dose – the target steady state is reached immediately, and maintained by the infusion. Curve C shows the effect of a partial loading dose. The starting concentration is higher, but it still takes 4 half-lives until steady state is reached. Finally, curve D shows the effect of an excessive load. The starting concentration is extremely high, and takes 4 half-lives to fall to the target steady state concentration. Drug concentration in mg l^{-1}. (A black and white version of this figure will appear in some formats. For the colour version, please refer to the plate section.)

assessments. The ability to undertake such intensive monitoring is dependent on bedside staffing and training, but it is effective in orientating practice towards sedation minimisation.

Another strategy is the use of **daily sedation interruption (DSI)**. This involves ceasing sedation for a period to allow comprehensive, formal assessment of underlying neurological function. The use of this technique in isolation has met with controversy in the literature. If a unit is already practising sedation minimisation and/or protocolised sedation, the use of DSI offers little benefit.

Table 16.2 The Sedation-Agitation Scale

Score	Classification	Description
7	Dangerous agitation	Pulls at endotracheal tube, tries to remove catheter, climbs over bed rail, strikes at staff, thrashes side to side
6	Very agitated	Does not calm despite frequent verbal reminding of limits, requires physical restraints, bites endotracheal tube
5	Agitated	Frequent non-purposeful movement or patient-ventilator dys-synchrony
4	Calm and cooperative	Is calm, awakens easily, follows commands
3	Sedated	Is difficult to arouse, awakens to verbal stimuli or gentle shaking but drifts off again, follows simple commands
2	Very sedated	Arouses to physical stimuli but does not communicate or follow commands, may move spontaneously
1	Unarousable	Has minimal or no response to noxious stimuli, does not communicate or follow commands

Despite years of use, the common agents used for sedation (propofol and benzodiazepines) in the ICU have only recently been assessed by large, randomised controlled trials, many of which have significant limitations. This renewed interest came about as a result of the introduction of dexmedetomidine. Sodium thiopentone and the other barbiturates are rarely used outside of neurosurgical intensive care. They will not be discussed in this chapter.

In general, the choice of sedative agent is driven by:

1. The specific clinical circumstances and sedation goals for the individual patient including haemodynamic compromise and end-organ impairment;
2. The pharmacokinetic profile of the agent, including half-life, context sensitive half-time, metabolism and active metabolites, clearance and side-effects; and
3. Pharmacoeconomic factors and overall cost.

Benzodiazepines

These agents act at the α/γ subunit of the $GABA_A$ receptor to produce sedative effects, mostly by enhancing neurotransmitter binding. They exhibit anxiolytic and skeletal muscle relaxant properties, although their sedative-hypnotic effects are not as pronounced as those of some other classes of agent. Cheap and readily available, there is some evidence that protracted use can lead to prolongation of mechanical ventilation and length of ICU stay, resulting in diminished popularity especially when sedation is required for more than 96 hours. They all demonstrate a similar side effect profile, with respiratory depression and systemic hypotension being the major manifestations. These are often seen when benzodiazepines are used in combination with other sedating agents. All benzodiazepines undergo extensive hepatic metabolism by cytochrome P450 enzymes, particularly CYP3A4 and CPY2C19. This leads to prolonged action in low cardiac output states due to diminished hepatic extraction.

Midazolam

Midazolam is possibly the most popular of the benzodiazepines, with a relatively short median half-life of 6.6 hours. It rapidly equilibrates across the blood-brain barrier, with duration of action of approximately 30 minutes after a bolus dose. Accumulation in the setting of prolonged infusion is a common problem, especially in the elderly or in renal and hepatic failure. Metabolised by CYP3A4 to the equipotent active metabolite α-hydroxy-midazolam, it competes with other drugs (particularly fentanyl) for elimination.

Diazepam

No longer used as an infusion in the ICU setting as it binds to PVC, diazepam has an elimination half-time roughly ~20-fold that of midazolam (20–50 hours), leading to gross prolongation of effect relative to other sedatives. This issue is further compounded by its multiple active metabolites, including desmethyldiazepam, N-methyloxazepam and oxazepam. It cannot be removed by dialysis and is extremely irritant when extravasated.

Lorazepam

More potent than midazolam or diazepam, lorazepam is less lipid soluble, with a slower onset of effect following a bolus dose. Uncommonly used in the ICU setting relative to midazolam, the major advantage of lorazepam is the lack of active metabolites, theoretically leading to more rapid offset when the drug is ceased, although the elimination half-life is still 8–15 hours. The clinical effects and duration of action are still prolonged by hepatic dysfunction. Parenteral formulations of lorazepam contain propylene glycol, which has toxic effects. Thought initially to only occur with very high doses, it has been seen with cumulative doses as low as 1 mg kg^{-1} day^{-1}, manifesting as renal dysfunction and metabolic acidosis. Both of these occur frequently in the postcardiac surgical patient, and hence propylene glycol toxicity may be overlooked as a cause.

Propofol

Propofol is an intravenous sedative that has a number of useful properties for use in the ICU. It demonstrates sedative, hypnotic, anxiolytic, amnestic and anticonvulsant effects, but is not an analgesic. Whilst acting as a $GABA_A$ agonist, it also acts at a number of other receptors in the CNS, such as glycine, nicotinic and muscarinic cholinergic receptors.

As a sedative, propofol is characterised by a relatively rapid offset of action. This is due to its high lipid solubility and redistribution away from the site of action, but also its unusual hepatic and extra-hepatic clearance. This results in a short context sensitive halftime (despite a prolonged duration of infusion), allows for rapid changes in sedation depth and facilitates daily sedation interruptions.

Despite its many positive qualities, the use of propofol is not without risk, particularly in the postcardiac surgery patient. Similar to other sedative agents, it causes dose dependent respiratory depression, and hypotension due to systemic vasodilation. These changes are more pronounced in the patient with pre-existing circulatory instability.

The propofol infusion syndrome (PRIS) is caused by the inherent mitochondrial toxicity of the drug, and resembles the mitochondrial myopathies. The underlying pathophysiology is impaired entry of long-chain fatty acids, disruption of fatty acid oxidation and failure of the respiratory chain. Manifestation is uncommon, but presents with an unexplained metabolic acidosis, hypertriglyceridaemia, arrhythmia and escalating vasopressor and inotrope requirements. The risk of PRIS is increased by high infusion rates (>70 μg kg^{-1} min^{-1}) over prolonged periods, but it has been reported with low dose infusion. The incidence of PRIS has been estimated to be as high as 1%. The syndrome is difficult to diagnose as these patients frequently have multiple aetiologies for clinical instability. Management involves early recognition and cessation of the infusion, followed by supportive care. This may not be sufficient to arrest its progress, and consequently, PRIS has a mortality of 33% in some series.

α_2-Adrenoceptor Agonists

Frequently used as second line agents, the α_2-agonists act on spinal and supraspinal α_2-adrenoceptors to accelerate the reuptake of adrenaline and noradrenaline into the presynaptic nerve terminal, thus mitigating their excitatory effects. This produces a different quality of sedation to the more traditional agents, typified by a more arousable state, with less respiratory depression, as well as demonstrating analgesic (and hence opioid-sparing) effects. These agents are rapidly finding a role in the management of the ICU patient with delirium, both intubated and extubated. However, despite the absence of respiratory depression, these agents have been known to cause loss of oropharyngeal tone at higher doses, and hence close monitoring of patients receiving them is still required to detect airway obstruction. In keeping with their site of action, the α_2-agonists have cardiovascular side effects, particularly hypotension and bradycardia. As a result, α_2-agonists are relatively contraindicated in patients with haemodynamic instability or rate dependent cardiac output.

Clonidine

Despite its relatively unfavourable pharmacokinetics (with an elimination half-life of 8 hours), clonidine can be administered as an intravenous infusion for sedation in the ICU. The drug has an α_2:α_1 selectivity ratio of 200:1, and is classified as a partial agonist by some as increasing doses lead to inevitable α_1-adrenoceptor stimulation. Because of the relatively low α-adrenoreceptor selectivity, a rise in blood pressure due to α_1 stimulation following a bolus dose is not uncommon, followed by a more sustained fall in blood pressure and heart rate. Rebound hypertension can be seen following sudden cessation of high dose infusion (>1.2 g day^{-1}).

Dexmedetomidine

The D-stereoisomer of medetomidine, this agent is a relatively recent addition to the ICU sedation armamentarium, and is frequently used for the management of severe delirium. The drug has an α_2:α_1 selectivity ratio of 1600:1, and is classified as a full agonist. Onset of action is within 15 minutes after starting an infusion, with peak sedation reached at 60 minutes. This may be hastened with the use of a loading dose, albeit at a greater risk of haemodynamic instability. The drug is rapidly redistributed and broken down by the liver to inactive metabolites, with an elimination time of 2–3 hours; however hepatic dysfunction can prolong this. Some studies suggest dexmedetomidine offers decreased time to extubation and decreased incidence of delirium relative to midazolam.

The uptake of dexmedetomidine has been slow relative to other agents. This is largely because of cost, although the aforementioned benefits offered relative to benzodiazepines may represent a cost saving when the drug is used routinely.

Analgesia

The recognition that agitation and pain are separate entities in ICU patients has been incorporated into recent clinical guidelines. This is an important distinction, as the intubated, sedated ICU patient may still have some awareness and recollection of their experience, but no way of communicating unpleasant sensations to clinical staff. Most patients will experience pain as part of their ICU stay, whether this is due to tracheal intubation, the postoperative state or pre-existing conditions. This can have both short-term and long-term consequences.

In the short term, pain results in an acute stress response, with increases in circulating catecholamines, increasing cardiac afterload, heart rate and contractility, all of which increase myocardial oxygen consumption. Tissue perfusion may be impaired due to peripheral vasoconstriction. The release of other stress hormones such as glucocorticoids results in a hypermetabolic response, with increased rates of lipolysis and glycolysis being compounded by insulin resistance and hyperglycaemia, with resultant impaired wound healing. The presence of a catabolic state increases the risk of disuse myopathy, and, in theory, impairs weaning from mechanical ventilation, and increases the risk of lower respiratory tract infection and deep venous thrombosis.

In the long term, the experience of pain, and an inability to communicate this, is a common source of psychological sequelae, even after physical recovery is complete. Those patients who have poorly controlled pain during their ICU stay have a higher incidence of post-traumatic stress disorder, chronic pain and an overall poorer quality of life.

Monitoring Analgesia

There has not been the same focus on analgesia monitoring scales for the ICU patient as there has been on sedation scales in the literature. In many centres, crude measures such as vital signs are still in use as the primary means of assessing pain. Whilst such tools may be occasionally of use in the more robust patient, the postcardiac surgical state is frequently typified by haemodynamic disturbance, meaning that the characteristic nociceptive response of hypertension and tachycardia may not be present despite the patient experiencing pain.

Monitoring scales for analgesia do exist, and the realisation that pain and agitation are potentially separate entities implies that clinical staff should employ separate rating scales and pharmacological strategies in their management. In observational studies, the **behavioural pain scale (BPS)** (Table 16.3) and **critical care pain observation tool (CPOT)** (Table 16.4) score consistently well on psychometric evaluation. They can be implemented quickly and have been shown to improve patient outcome when used routinely.

Planning Analgesia

A complete overview of all the factors in planning an effective analgesic strategy for a critically ill postoperative patient is beyond the scope of this chapter. However, some general principles are worthy of discussion when planning an analgesic regimen, and have been highlighted in recent consensus guidelines.

1. A therapeutic plan and goal of analgesia should be established and communicated to care givers.
2. Assessment of pain and response to therapy should be performed regularly.
3. The level of pain reported by the patient is the standard for assessment but subjective observation and physiological indicators may be used when the patient cannot communicate.

Table 16.3 Behavioural pain scale, scores in the range 4–12

Item	Description	Score
Facial expression	Relaxed	1
	Partially tightened (i.e. brow lowering)	2
	Fully tightened (i.e. eyelid closing)	3
	Grimacing	4
Upper limb movements	No movement	1
	Partially bent	2
	Fully bent with finger flexion	3
	Permanently retracted	4
Compliance with mechanical ventilation	Tolerating movement	1
	Coughing but tolerating ventilation for most of the time	2
	Fighting ventilator	3
	Unable to control ventilation	4

4. Sedation of critically ill patients should only be commenced after providing adequate analgesia and treating reversible physiological causes.

Needless to say, the involvement of a specialist acute pain service for those patients with complex or difficult to treat pain is invaluable (see Figure 16.3).

Opioid Analgesia

Currently, opioids are recommended as the first line agents in the management of non-neuropathic pain in the critically ill. This is largely because of their relative efficacy and predictable side effect profile. The analgesic effects of opioids are achieved through the μ_1-receptor, which is found at a variety of spinal and supraspinal locations. Indeed, pure μ_1-receptor stimulation provides excellent pain relief. However, there is more than one type of opioid receptor, and stimulation of the μ_1-receptor and these additional sites leads to the characteristic acute side effects of respiratory depression, sedation, reduced gut motility and bradycardia, and the longer term issues of tolerance, dependence and opioid induced hyperalgesia. Consequently, opioids should always be prescribed with caution, and the use of non-opioid analgesia considered in all cases. All opioids exhibit similar analgesic efficacy and are associated with similar outcomes (duration of intubation, length of stay) when titrated to similar endpoints.

Morphine

Based around three benzene rings, and hence classified as a phenanthrene (along with codeine and oxycodone), morphine has formed the mainstay of opioid therapy for decades. It has relatively low lipid solubility, and hence the onset of effect following a bolus dose is between 15 and 30 minutes with peak effect at 45–90 minutes. The drug is metabolised via hepatic conjugation into morphine-3-glucuronide (a metabolite with known neurotoxic side effects), morphine-6-glucuronide (an active metabolite considerably more potent than morphine) and normorphine. These metabolites are then excreted unchanged in the urine, and dose reduction is required in patients with renal and hepatic dysfunction.

Oxycodone

Another phenanthrene similar to morphine, oxycodone is rarely used in the ICU setting due to the expense of the parenteral formulation. However, it undergoes hepatic conjugation to inactive or weakly active metabolites, noroxycodone and oxymorphone, meaning that accumulation in renal failure is not as pronounced.

Fentanyl

Fentanyl is a potent phenylpiperadine, or synthetic opioid. It has onset of action within 3 minutes due to lipid solubility 700–800 fold, and potency 100 fold compared with morphine. Consequently, bolus doses, if not administered with caution, have a greater potential to cause sedation and respiratory depression.

In bolus doses, the duration of action (20 minutes) is limited by redistribution away from the effect site

Table 16.4 Critical care pain observation tool (CPOT), scores in the range 0–8

Indicator	Description	Score	
Facial expression	No muscular tension observed	Relaxed, neutral	0
	Presence of frowning, brow lowering, orbit tightening and levator contraction	Tense	1
	All of the above plus eyelids tightly closed	Grimacing	2
Body movements	Does not move at all	Absence of movement	0
	Slow, cautious movements, touching or rubbing the pain site, seeking attention through movements	Protection	1
	Pulling tube, attempting to sit up, moving limbs, thrashing, not following commands, striking at staff, trying to climb out of bed	Restlessness	2
Muscle tension	No resistance to passive movements	Relaxed	0
	Resistance to passive movements	Tense, rigid	1
	Strong resistance to passive movements, inability to complete them	Very tense or rigid	2
Compliance with the ventilator (if intubated)	Alarms not activated, easy ventilation	Tolerating ventilator or movement	0
	Alarms stop spontaneously	Coughing but tolerating	1
	Asynchrony; blocking ventilation, alarms frequently activated	Fighting ventilator	2
OR			
Vocalisation (extubated patients)	Talking in normal tone or no sound	Talking in normal tone or no sound	0
	Sighing, moaning	Sighing, moaning	1
	Crying out, sobbing	Crying out, sobbing	2

However, with a prolonged infusion, these peripheral sites (particularly adipose tissue) may become saturated, leading to a depot of drug and a marked increase in half-life once these compartments equilibrate with the plasma. Fentanyl is often recommended in the setting of renal impairment due to the relative lack of active metabolites. The accumulation of norfentanyl has, however, been reported, and is a potential cause of toxic delirium.

Remifentanil

Remifentanil has been used in anaesthetic practice for a number of years. An extremely potent opioid, remifentanil has a unique metabolic pathway, being rapidly metabolised by plasma esterases. This limits the redistribution of the drug to peripheral compartments and keeps the half-life of the drug at 4–5 minutes, regardless of the duration of the infusion. Consequently, it is ideal for those patients in whom rapid weaning of sedation to assess neurological status is desirable, or in those patients at high risk of excessive opioid accumulation. However, possibly due to its potency, remifentanil carries a high risk of opioid induced hyperalgesia, and many studies have suggested a higher incidence of chronic pain after using remifentanil in the operative setting, including in cardiac surgery. This risk may also translate to the ICU.

Non-opioid Analgesia

Whilst current guidelines recommend opioids as first line therapy for the management of nociceptive pain in the ICU, multiple other classes of analgesic agents exist. These drugs are useful, for two reasons:

1. Minimisation of opioid dose, and hence opioid related side effects; and
2. Management of pain that is not responsive to opioids.

It is assumed that the mechanism of action and side effect profile of commonly used drugs such as paracetamol and the non-steroidal anti-inflammatories are

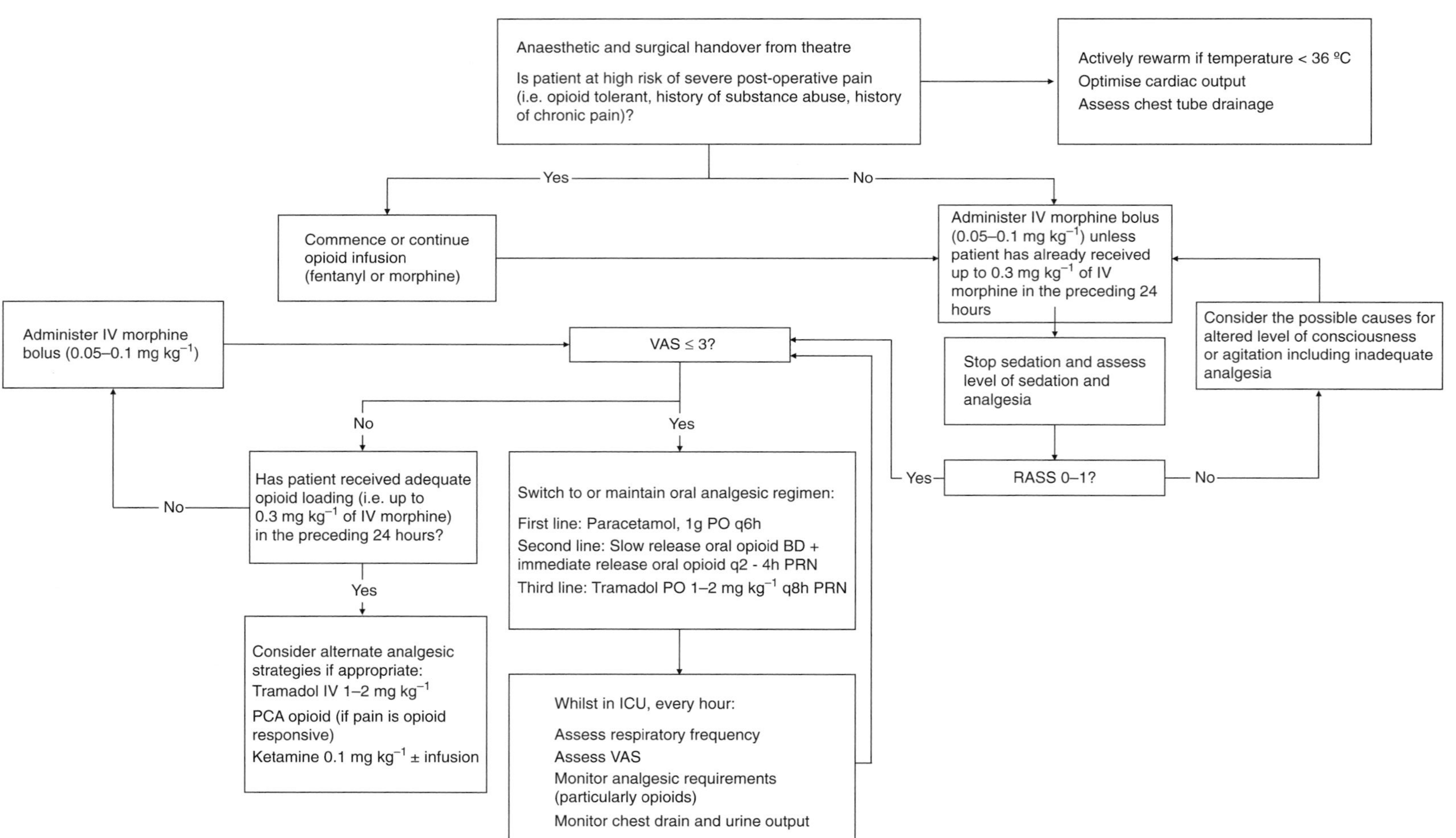

Figure 16.3 This algorithm presumes that the patient returns to the ICU on some form of sedation (i.e. propofol, 1–2 mg kg^{-1} hour−1, and has received some form of opioid loading in the operating theatre (i.e. morphine bolus, morphine infusion, etc.), and that the patient is receiving regular paracetamol (1 g NG or intravenous q6h). Unless stated otherwise, all medications should be dosed according to ideal body weight. It is valid only for management of pain in the ICU.

well understood, and hence they will not be discussed here. However, there are other classes of drug that are less commonly used that should be examined.

Ketamine

A phencyclidine derivative, ketamine acts via blockade of the N-acetyl-D-aspartate (NMDA) receptor. It effectively has two roles:

1. Prevention and management of pain due to 'central sensitisation', particularly neuropathic pain, severe 'acute' pain and opioid resistant pain; and
2. Reducing the overall dose of opioid required in a given pain situation.

At relatively low doses of 0.1–0.2 mg kg^{-1} $hour^{-1}$, ketamine acts primarily as an analgesic. Bolus doses of 0.1–0.25 mg kg^{-1} can be used as a loading dose or as rescue therapy. Beyond this infusion rate, adverse effects begin to emerge with relatively little incremental analgesic benefit. Vivid dreams and hallucinations are often limiting factors in its use. These effects are entirely dose dependent, and a cessation of the infusion will reliably eliminate neurocognitive phenomena within the drug half-life of 1–2 hours. The drug is metabolised to norketamine, an active metabolite that is renally excreted.

At high bolus doses (1–2 mg kg^{-1}), ketamine can be used to induce anaesthesia. It is often popular in trauma situations as it affords a degree of haemodynamic stability relative to other agents by increasing the peripheral effects of circulating catecholamines. However, in a state of maximal sympathetic tone, ketamine cannot increase these effects further, and may act as a negative inotrope. Ketamine also preserves respiratory drive, although the airway may be compromised by increased muscle tone and hypersalivation.

Tramadol

A cyclohexanol derivative, tramadol has a triphasic mechanism of action. Given intravenously, tramadol inhibits the reuptake of noradrenaline and serotonin (5-HT), enhancing the action of the descending noxious inhibitory control system. In addition, one of its metabolites (M_1 or O-desmethyltramadol) is a weak opioid agonist. This opioid effect is enhanced with oral administration due to hepatic first-pass metabolism.

Intravenously, tramadol is administered as a bolus dose of 1–2 mg kg^{-1} (based on ideal body weight) every 6 hours. A loading dose of 3 mg kg^{-1} is occasionally used in anaesthetic practice, although the use of such a dose in the awake patient increases the risk of side effects. Rapid administration causes nausea and vomiting, and hence slow administration over 20 minutes is recommended.

In equianalgesic doses, tramadol is far less likely to cause respiratory depression than morphine. Respiratory depression has only been observed in patients with severe renal impairment. Tramadol also has a reputation for provoking seizures. However, when given within the recommended dose limits, tramadol does not increase seizures relative to other analgesic agents.

Due to the enhancement of 5-HT release and inhibition of reuptake, tramadol is a theoretical cause of serotonergic syndrome. In practice, this is rare. Caution should be exercised when prescribing tramadol in the elderly, in patients with renal impairment, and with concurrent high doses of serotonergic medications, particularly selective serotonin reuptake inhibitors, noradrenaline-serotonin reuptake inhibitors and monoamine oxidase inhibitors. Note that drugs that block the effect of serotonin (particularly the 5-HT_3 receptor blockers such as ondansetron) will diminish the analgesic efficacy of tramadol.

Regional Analgesia

First described in 1984, high thoracic epidural analgesia (HTEA) in cardiac surgery has found sporadic acceptance. Proponents argue that the diminished catecholamine release and central neuraxial blockade attenuates the sympathetic response to the surgical insult, leading to a diminished inflammatory response, superior analgesia and earlier postoperative extubation. It is also argued that the postulated risk of epidural haematoma with cardiopulmonary bypass has not eventuated, provided the epidural is placed sufficiently in advance of systemic heparinisation. Depending on the preference of surgeon and anaesthetist, patients having cardiac surgery may occasionally arrive in the intensive care unit with an epidural catheter in situ, delivering a mixture of local anaesthetic and opioid according to local preference. Serious complications of epidural analgesia, such as epidural haematoma or abscess, will often manifest with lower limb neurological signs. Hence, sedation should be titrated to allow continuous assessment of lower limb motor function as the consequences of late detection of such a complication are catastrophic.

A well-functioning, high thoracic epidural will inevitably cause a degree of sympathetic blockade, which may manifest as hypotension. This can normally be managed with judicious intravascular volume replacement; however, particularly in patients unable to tolerate further fluid therapy, vasopressors may be required. Clinicians may be tempted to stop the epidural as part of managing hypotension. It is worth noting that the prolonged half-life of the local anaesthetic agents commonly used in epidural analgesia (ropivacaine, bupivacaine and levo-bupivacaine) means that the benefit of such an action will not be reaped for some hours, and that it is often best to initiate a more definitive plan from the outset whilst continuing the epidural.

Regional analgesia is practised commonly in thoracic surgery, where a continuous infusion of local anaesthetic provides excellent analgesia of the surgical site, and minimises the use of oral or intravenous opioid, with the associated risk of respiratory depression. For unilateral thoracic surgery where the pleura has not been breached adjacent to the vertebral column, many authors advocate a paravertebral block, arguing that the quality of analgesia provided is just as good, with a lower incidence of common side effects such as hypotension, urinary retention, nausea and vomiting.

Neuromuscular Blockade

In the new era of 'daily sedation interruptions' and 'sedation minimisation', the indications for neuromuscular blockade (beyond short-term paralysis for invasive procedures such as intubation, bronchoscopy, etc.) in the ICU are limited. Effectively, they can be summarised into three categories:

1. Facilitation of invasive modes of ventilation, when they are not tolerated by an adequately sedated patient.
2. Open chest: surgical bleeding or indwelling vascular cannulae may necessitate the patient's chest being left open for a short time and the patient being kept completely still.
3. Raised intracranial pressure or status epilepticus.

The association with prolonged weakness has been the biggest factor in the decline in popularity of neuromuscular blockade. This phenomenon may be more common when aminoglycoside antibiotics or corticosteroids are administered concurrently, because of their interaction at the neuromuscular junction. Spontaneous muscle breakdown during total muscle inactivity has also been postulated.

In practice, neuromuscular blockade can be a useful, albeit last line, clinical tool. This is especially true in the presence of significant, persistent hypoxia. Neuromuscular blockade in this scenario reduces VO_2, and hence reduces tissue perfusion requirements in skeletal muscle. Patient synchronisation with the ventilator is also improved.

The choice of drug for neuromuscular blockade is often clinician dependent; however, the benzylisoquinoliums (atracurium and cisatracurium) are often preferred as they undergo organ independent metabolism. Rather than undergoing hepatic modification, these drugs are hydrolysed by plasma esterases, or undergo Hoffman elimination. This is a pH and temperature dependent process that is prolonged by hypothermia and acidosis. The breakdown products of this process (in particular laudanosine) can be neurotoxic, but at doses well in excess of those encountered clinically.

Further Reading

Barr J, Fraser GL, Puntillo K, et al. Clinical practice guidelines for the management of pain, agitation and delirium in adult patients in the intensive care unit. *Critical Care Medicine*. 2013; 41: 264–306.

Macintyre PE, Scott DA, Schug SA, et al. (Eds). Acute pain management in intensive care. *Acute Pain Management: Scientific Evidence*, 3rd Edition. Melbourne: Australian and New Zealand College of Anaesthetists and Faculty of Pain Medicine, 2010, Section 9.8, pp. 286–289.

Reade MC, Finfer S. Sedation and delirium in the intensive care unit. *New England Journal of Medicine*. 2014; 370: 444–454.

Shehabi Y, Bellomo R, Mehta S, et al. Intensive care sedation: the past, present and future. *Critical Care*. 2013; 17: 322–329.

MCQs

1. **Which of the following represents the 'ICU triad' of sedatoanalgesia?**
   (a) Pain, neuromuscular blockade, sedation
   (b) Analgesia, sedation, delirium
   (c) Delirium, agitation, pain
   (d) Agitation, sedation, pain
   (e) Analgesia, neuromuscular blockade, sedation

2. **Which of the following determines the time taken for an intravenous infusion of a drug to reach steady state?**
   (a) Half-life
   (b) Clearance
   (c) Dose rate
   (d) Lipid solubility
   (e) Molecular weight

3. **Which of the following statements is NOT true? In general, lighter levels of sedation lead to:**
   (a) Shorter duration of mechanical ventilation
   (b) Decreased ICU length of stay
   (c) Increased patient-ventilator dys-synchrony
   (d) Diminished haemodynamic perturbation
   (e) Decreased myocardial oxygen demand

4. **Which of the following is the superior modality for the monitoring of sedation in the standard cardiothoracic ICU patient?**
   (a) Bispectral index
   (b) Auditory evoked potentials
   (c) Multichannel electroencephalography
   (d) Richmond agitation-sedation scale
   (e) Glasgow coma score

5. **Poorly controlled postoperative pain in the ICU setting leads to an increased long-term incidence of which of the following:**
   (a) Major depressive disorder
   (b) Post-traumatic stress disorder
   (c) Complex regional pain syndrome
   (d) Drug induced psychosis
   (e) Improved quality of life

Exercise answers are available on p.468. Alternatively, take the test online at www.cambridge.org/CardiothoracicMCQ

Chapter 17

Mechanical Ventilation

Anja Schneider and Erik Ortmann

Introduction

Most patients admitted to the cardiothoracic critical care unit will require a form of mechanical ventilation at some point during their journey. However, the spectrum of indications is wide and ranges from patients on a 'fast-track' concept, who are only being ventilated for a very short period of time directly after surgery, to very complex patients with severe cardiovascular and respiratory failure due to their underlying disease or the impact of major cardiothoracic surgery. Therefore a sound knowledge of the various techniques of invasive and non-invasive mechanical ventilatory support is essential to develop the appropriate strategy for the individual patient and their current clinical state.

Technical Aspects

The basic principle of modern intensive care ventilators is a positive pressure gradient, which creates gas flow into the lungs during inspiration. Expiration is usually passive due to fall of the pressure gradient to an expiratory level (PEEP). The gas flow is delivered either invasively through an endotracheal tube or a tracheostomy cannula, or non-invasively via a tight fitting facemask or similar device.

Traditionally ventilation modes have been described as either volume or pressure controlled. Modern ventilators however provide a variety of different sophisticated modes, some of which combine characteristics of both, and are controlled by the so-called 'phase variables' *triggering*, *limiting* and *cycling*.

Triggering Phase

The *triggering variable* sets the start of inspiratory gas flow and can be time, pressure, flow or volume. Thus the trigger can be controlled by the ventilator, the patient, or a combination of both. When time is the trigger variable, the breath is considered mandatory.

Limiting Phase

The *limiting variable* defines the length or size of inspiratory gas flow. It can also be set to a certain pressure, volume, flow or time. The type of waveform produced for pressure, flow and volume defines a breath delivery. Depending on the chosen limiting variable the ventilation pattern may be one of the three following types:

Volume controlled: A constant volume and constant flow waveform; the pressure waveform will vary depending on lung characteristics.

Pressure controlled: The pressure waveform has a preselected specific pattern but volume and flow will vary depending on lung characteristics.

Time controlled: Pressure, volume and flow waveforms all vary depending on lung characteristics.

Cycling Phase

The *cycling variable* starts the expiration phase by ending inspiratory gas flow. This may also be pressure, volume, flow or time. For example the ventilator may cycle to the expiratory phase after a certain time (i.e. preset frequency for mandatory ventilation), when the pressure reaches a certain set maximum during inspiration, or cycle to the expiratory phase when flow falls to a set level (commonly 5 l/min) or percentage (commonly 25%) of peak flow (patient trigger).

By combining various settings to the different phase variables, modern ventilators can create a large number of ventilation patterns, which can be further individualised to specific clinical situations. These are all based on three types of breath:

A *mandatory breath* is one in which the ventilator does all the work of breathing and controls the transition between phases of the breath.

An *assisted breath* is one where the patient begins or 'triggers' inspiration but the ventilator controls the inspiratory phase and the cycling of inspiration to expiration.

A *spontaneous breath* is one in which the patient controls the transition between all breathing phases.

Ventilation Modes

Nomenclature of modes of ventilation has become confusingly complex, with different names being used for similar modes by different manufacturers. We want to review the most common terms and explain the technical principles of the different ventilator modes.

In principle, there are two different techniques of ventilation: the mandatory technique and the spontaneous technique. In mandatory modes, ventilation is fully or partially controlled by the respirator. Spontaneous modes allow either independent breathing of the patient or respirator assisted spontaneous breathing.

Three main subgroups can be classified:

Mandatory ventilation	– volume controlled modes
	– pressure controlled modes
Spontaneous ventilation	– spontaneous/assisted modes.

However, this classification is not static and an overlap with spontaneous/assisted ventilator modes is possible, as the elaborated mandatory techniques can provide assisted or augmented ventilation as well. This is an important option, especially during weaning from mechanical ventilation. Even though modern ventilators have factory presets, to assist application under common conditions, a profound understanding of the control variables is necessary to adjust mechanical ventilation to individual patient needs.

Variables of Mechanical Ventilation

Inspiration

The inspiration phase is preceded by a *triggering phase* during which the ventilator is 'waiting' for a signal to start the inspiration. There are two trigger options:

Patient triggered: Via flow or pressure trigger, the ventilator identifies the inspiration effort of the patient after which a mandatory breath is delivered. An adjustable trigger threshold guarantees individual patient sensitivity. If no patient effort is detected during a set time window, a mandatory inspiration can be triggered (time trigger) to guarantee a certain ventilation frequency.

Respirator triggered: A mandatory breath is triggered by set parameters such as inspiratory time, frequency and I:E (inspiration:expiration) ratio. The timing is obligatory and the patient has no influence.

Expiration

The variable that ends inspiratory gas flow can be either flow or time:

Flow cycled: Dependent on the inspiratory flow of the patient, the expiratory period is triggered as soon as the inspiratory flow has reached a selected part of the maximum inspiratory flow.

Time cycled: Inspiratory time is defined and expiration begins as soon as a set inspiratory time is terminated.

Principles of Mechanical Ventilation

Volume Control Ventilation

The parameter remaining constant during this ventilation technique is the tidal volume, which is delivered by a constant inspiratory flow. The frequency of the mandatory breaths and the tidal volume can be adjusted, producing a certain minute volume. Inspiratory pressure is dependent on patient conditions (for example lung mechanics). As patient physiologies vary, it is important to adjust pressure limits when using volume control ventilation.

Special Feature PRVC and Autoflow®

Closed loop/servo control modes utilise feedback monitoring systems within the ventilator to assess breath delivery, compare and contrast the actual breath delivered with the set target parameters, and then adjust flow and pressure to match these set parameters more closely. The pressure regulated volume controlled ventilation (PRVC) combines a constant tidal volume with the minimum necessary airway pressure. The inspiratory pressure level is adapted to lung condition with every mandatory breath. Autoflow® provides additionally the possibility of patient triggering during the whole breathing cycle.

Pressure Control Ventilation

Two parameters are remaining constant during pressure control ventilation: the lower pressure level (i.e. PEEP) and the upper pressure level (i.e. inspiratory pressure). Tidal volume results from patient conditions, i.e. inspiratory effort, as well as lung mechanics and especially from the difference between the two pressure levels. The inspiration time determines the inspiration period and the upper pressure level is constant during the whole inspiration time whereas the decelerating gas flow and tidal volumes are dependent variables

PEEP (Positive End Expiratory Pressure)

A positive airway pressure level during the expiration period can be achieved by either flow resistance or threshold resistance. *Flow resistors* work as an expiratory retard device. Pressure across the resistor is regulated by flow. *Threshold resistors* allow continuity of expiratory flow until pressure within the breathing cycle has reached PEEP level (according to threshold value). If possible, ventilators with threshold resistance technique should be preferred as they reduce resistance during the expiration period and decrease the risk of barotrauma.

Intrinsic PEEP (or auto-PEEP) is defined as the fixed recoil pressure of the respiratory system at end-expiration. It is caused by airway obstruction, or incomplete exhalation, which generates flow resistance.

The application of PEEP may improve ventilation conditions of the patient and optimise oxygenation and decarboxylation in different ways, including:

- increase of the functional residual capacity (FRC) with improvement of the alveolar oxygen reservoir,
- recruitment of collapsed alveoli, which improves lung compliance and reduces pulmonary shunting,
- redistribution of lung oedema from the alveoli to the interstitium.

However, application of PEEP might also increase dead space, increase the risk of barotrauma and potentially reduce cardiac output. These factors have to be taken into account when finding the 'optimum PEEP' for an individual patient.

Which Mode for Which Patient?

There is a spectrum of indications for mechanical ventilation in patients admitted to cardiothoracic critical care. Therefore different ventilation strategies and ventilation modes need to be applied according to the indication but also according to the clinical phase.

Most patients after cardiac surgery are admitted to the ICU sedated and mechanically ventilated to allow an initial stabilisation phase. Once the patient's clinical situation is deemed stable with regard to cardiovascular and respiratory stability, bleeding and coagulopathy, a structured process of weaning from mechanical ventilation should be started as early as possible in order to keep the ventilation phase as short as possible. As soon as sedation reduction has begun, there should be a protocol based repetitive spontaneous breathing trial, to evaluate muscle weakness and breathing control of the patient. In general, after routine surgery, breathing control and adequate muscle strength return quickly.

However, a proportion of patients experience a complex ICU journey with prolonged phases of mechanical ventilation, and require differentiated strategies. If sedation can be decreased, breathing control returns potentially unstable. Breathing muscles may be weak due to critical illness myopathy and neuropathy. Thus, mixed ventilation modes are required, which enable the patient to trigger a mandatory breath or in the next step to take spontaneous breaths. Breathing effort is shared between equipment and patient. By the time breathing control improves, but muscle weakness is still present, a supported spontaneous breathing mode might be adequate. After a long phase of critical illness with ventilator support, a phase of non-invasive ventilation (NIV) might be required to stabilise the patient's spontaneous breathing and prevent further respiratory failure needing invasive mechanical ventilation.

Ventilation Modes

CMV (Continuous Mandatory Ventilation)

This ventilation mode is ventilator triggered and time cycled. Volume (VC-CMV) or pressure control (PC-CMV) mode is possible. There is no ability to sense patient respiratory effort. This ventilation mode guarantees maximum security for controlled ventilation of a patient, for example directly after admission or for transport, but requires the patient to be sufficiently sedated.

AC (Assist/Assist-Control Ventilation)

This ventilation mode allows the patient triggering of a mandatory breath due to sensing mechanisms for patient respiratory effort. Thus, it is a time cycled respirator or patient triggered mode. Volume (VC-AC) or pressure control (PC-AC) is possible. In the case of absence of a patient trigger, a mandatory breath will be automatically applied after end of expiration. Dependent on patient breathing, this respirator mode performs an assist mode or assist-control mode.

SIMV (Synchronised Intermittent Mandatory Ventilation)

This ventilation mode is ventilator or patient controlled and time cycled. The mandatory breaths are synchronised with the patient's inspiration effort. The defined SIMV rate determines the SIMV cycle. If the triggering effort occurs in a defined time slot, a mandatory breath is applied. This adjustment avoids alteration of the frequency of the mandatory breaths. Volume (VC-SIMV) or pressure control (PC-SIMV) mode is possible.

MMV (Mandatory Minute Ventilation)

This ventilation mode is ventilator or patient controlled and time cycled. The patient always obtains defined minute ventilation. Any successful patient breath is counted towards this target. Volume (VC-MMV) or pressure control (PC-MMV, volume guarantee enabled) mode is possible.

APRV (Airway Pressure Release Ventilation)

This is a pressure controlled (PC-APRV), ventilator triggered and time cycled ventilator mode. The patient can breathe spontaneously at inspiration pressure level. Active expiration is induced with short pressure reduction (to the low pressure level), to enable optimised CO_2 elimination. The change between the two pressure levels is machine triggered and time cycled.

BIPAP (Biphasic or Bilevel Positive Airway Pressure)

This ventilation mode is ventilator or patient controlled and time cycled. It is a pressure control mode (PC-BIPAP), which allows the patient to breathe between two set pressure levels, i.e. PEEP and inspiratory pressure. The number of mandatory breaths is defined. A spontaneous breathing attempt is enabled during the whole breathing cycle synchronised to inspiration and expiration. If the mandatory breath is reduced due to synchronisation with expiration, the next mandatory breath is prolonged. Synchronisation with inspiration shortens the expiration period.

During spontaneous breathing at PEEP level a pressure support can be applied. In the case of absence of a patient trigger during the inspiration trigger period, a mandatory breath will be delivered.

This is one of the most common ventilator modes in modern ICU treatment. Tidal volume, and in consequence minute volume, change based on lung resistance and compliance (i.e. patient conditions) and have to be carefully monitored.

PSV (Pressure Support Ventilation)

This ventilation mode is patient or ventilator triggered and flow cycled with a backup frequency preset. It is a pressure control mode (PC-PSV). The patient breathes spontaneously at PEEP level and every inspiration attempt can be pressure supported. Patient conditions define time, duration and frequency of the mandatory breath. In the case of absence of patient triggering, mandatory breaths at inspiratory pressure level will be delivered.

CPAP (Continuous Positive Airway Pressure/Pressure Support)

This ventilation mode requires spontaneous breathing (SPN-CPAP). It is patient triggered and flow cycled. Compared to atmospheric conditions, this ventilation mode enables an increased, continuous pressure level during the entire breathing cycle. Every inspiration effort triggers a flow cycled mandatory breath. Pressure support or variable pressure support (SPN-CPAP/PS) and volume support (SPN-CPAP/VS) can be added dependent on patient conditions (i.e. weakness of respiratory muscles). Backup time cycled frequencies of mandatory breaths can be adjusted (i.e. apnoea ventilation).

Special Ventilation Modalities

IRV (Inversed Ratio Ventilation)

The inspiration to expiration ratio (I:E) is physiologically about 1:2. Inversed ratio ventilation means prolongation of the inspiration period to up to four times the expiration period and is therefore not a defined mode of ventilation. The mean airway pressure of the breathing cycle is increased to support the re-expansion of the collapsed, non-compliant lung in patients with acute lung injury. A combination with increased PEEP can also be reasonable for patients with acute compromised lung, high FiO_2 requirements and restricted decarboxylation, for example after cardiac surgery, with a history of COPD or pneumonia. Please note that besides improving the residual capacity, oxygenation and/or decarboxylation, there is an increased risk of barotrauma with IRV.

HFV (High Frequency Ventilation)

This ventilation mode uses much higher respiratory rates and therefore much lower tidal volumes than conventional mechanical ventilation. There are five different types:

- HFPPV high frequency positive pressure ventilation
- HFJV high frequency jet ventilation
- HFOV high frequency oscillatory ventilation
- HFFI high frequency flow interruption
- HFPV high frequency percussive ventilation.

As examples, three more commonly used types of high frequency ventilation will be explained.

- HFPPV: use of conventional volume or pressure limited ventilation, low compliance and respiratory rates of 60–100/minute with tidal volumes of 100 to 400 ml (danger of inadequate tidal volume and air trapping).
- HFJV: pulses of high pressure gas flow (tidal volume up to 150 ml) are delivered with a respiratory rate of 100–600/minute over a specialised endotracheal tube or an attachable catheter, which creates an open system for continuous expiration.
- HFOV: during the entire respiratory cycle a special pump mechanism generates an oscillating pressure (500 to 3000 cycles/minute). This leads to positive pressure during the inspiration period and negative pressure during the expiration phase, which in contrast to the above modes creates active expiration. Mean airway pressure and FiO_2 determine oxygenation, whereas decarboxylation is influenced by the oscillatory amplitude.

The mechanisms of ventilation and oxygenation in these ventilation modes are not fully understood and are beyond the scope of this chapter. Alveoli located close to the airways are ventilated by convection, for more distant alveoli gas mixing mechanisms such as gas streaming, 'Pendelluft', and helical diffusion seem to play a major role. The use of HFV is reserved for special indications, such as short intrapulmonary interventions and newborn RDS syndrome.

NAVA® (Neurally Adjusted Ventilatory Assist)

One of the problems in weaning from mechanical ventilation can be a lack of synchronisation between the patient's increasing spontaneous efforts and the mechanical assistance of the ventilator, especially in the case of severe critical illness myopathy and neuropathy. One attempt to improve this synchronisation is to move from the common flow or pressure trigger indicating patient effort and move to the neural level by capturing the electrical activity of the diaphragm. In theory this should allow the patient's attempt to breathe to be sensed, even if there is not sufficient movement of the diaphragm. Therefore neural activity and mechanical ventilation can be synchronised to start an assisted breath earlier and better match the patient's spontaneous activity. Only a few ventilator types offer this feature. A special nasogastric sensor tube has to be placed and synchronised with the ventilator sensing, which requires a certain routine.

Differential Lung Ventilation

Differential or single lung ventilation is a frequently used anaesthesia technique in thoracic surgery, with increasing indication in cardiac surgery. An example is minimally invasive mitral valve surgery, which is undertaken using this technique in some centres. Commonly used devices are double lumen endotracheal tubes and bronchial blockers.

To date in the ICU setting, differential ventilation has rarely been applied.

Differential ventilation can be divided into anatomical and physiological lung separation. Its ICU indications can be summarised in the treatment of severe unilateral lung disease (after trauma) or lung disease with an asymmetrical distribution (pneumonia, unilateral oedema), aspiration and bronchopleural fistula. Differential lung ventilation offers the opportunity to use different levels of PEEP, inspiratory pressure and volumes. Optimised inspiration to expiration ratio, and even different gas mixtures to the two lungs can be provided.

Non-invasive Ventilation (NIV)

This ventilation mode offers mechanical ventilation support without any artificial endotracheal airway (i.e. endotracheal tube, tracheostomy). A variety of masks and even helmets are available.

Spontaneous breathing and the patient's ability to protect the airway are mandatory. Most commonly used is the CPAP ventilation mode, with or without pressure support. Indications are acute respiratory failure due to decompensated heart failure with pulmonary oedema, exacerbated COPD and obstructive sleep apnoea.

High flow nasal oxygen therapy is worth mentioning. This technique delivers heated and humidified oxygen with a continuous flow over a specialised nasal cannula. Advantages are the creation of a constant positive airway pressure, a reduction of oxygen dilution and a minimised dead space.

Physiology of Mechanical Ventilation

Cardiovascular System and Circulation

The technique of positive pressure ventilation, today quite obligatory combined with PEEP, may create adverse side effects in the cardiovascular system. Positive pressure ventilation, as well as PEEP, lead to an increased intrathoracic pressure and a continuously changing lung volume, both affecting the cardiovascular system.

Cardiac output depends on four variables: preload, afterload, contractility and heart rate. Generally, the increased intrathoracic pressure, and especially PEEP, lead to a decrease in cardiac output (CO). This causes reduced venous return and therefore a reduction of right ventricular (RV) preload as well as an increase in RV afterload due to increased pulmonary vascular resistance especially at higher levels of PEEP (>10–15 cmH_2O). The effects on RV preload are more pronounced in the presence of hypovolaemia and autonomic neuropathy. Variation of the systolic arterial blood pressure between the inspiratory and expiratory periods of positive pressure ventilation, usually referred to as 'pulse pressure variation', can even be used to predict the patient's fluid responsiveness.

The reduced cardiac output of the right ventricle leads to a decrease in left ventricular (LV) preload. Even though LV contractility remains unaffected, the LV compliance and filling might be affected by increased intrathoracic pressure due to direct effects and ventricular interdependence. However, patients with LV failure still benefit from positive pressure ventilation and PEEP (see NIV-CPAP therapy) as it may reduce work of breathing and pulmonary oedema.

Renal and splanchnic blood flow might be affected by positive pressure ventilation and intracranial pressure may rise due to reduced venous drainage.

Dependent on patient conditions and ventilation-perfusion ratio, PEEP reduces intrapulmonary shunt but potentially increases alveolar dead space. Thus an adequate modification and regular evaluation of PEEP level is important.

Effects on the Respiratory System

Mechanical ventilation can have detrimental effects on the lung itself, especially if it is needed for prolonged periods or if an 'invasive' ventilation strategy with high peak airway pressures, high tidal volumes and high FiO_2 is used. Even though mechanical ventilation probably is not the sole cause of respiratory complications in a complex intensive care setting, two conditions have been described in that context: *ventilator associated pneumonia* (VAP) and *ventilator associated lung injury* (VALI). Lung infections developing after more than 48 hours of mechanical ventilation are usually referred to as VAP and have a significant impact on outcome.

The exact mechanisms leading to ventilator associated lung injury (VALI) are still unclear. VALI is mostly associated with a pre-existing pulmonary disease. Important effects are alveolar overexpansion due to high tidal volume (*volutrauma*), and *barotrauma* because of high airway pressures and prolonged alveolar atelectasis (atelectrauma). Inflammation of the alveolar tissue and the potential toxicity of high FiO_2 levels may play a role as well (*biotrauma*).

Several strategies for *protective ventilation* have been established to prevent VAP (ventilator care bundle) and VALI:

- low tidal volume (maximum 5–7 ml/kg);
- adequate PEEP level and limitation of peak inspiratory pressure, pressure support ventilation;
- IRV (for example protocol based in case of increasing FiO_2 and hypercapnia);

- permissive hypercapnia;
- disinfectant oral care (avoidance of mucosal drying, secretion retention);
- airway humidification;
- elevated head;
- cuff pressure monitoring, subglottic suction;
- minimal sedation strategy;
- early protocol driven weaning from ventilation.

Effects on Other Physiological Systems

Gut distension and dysmotility are common during invasive ventilation. Both bleeding and ischaemia of the GI tract due to injury of the mucosal wall can occur. Protocolised feeding tube management in combination with stepwise enteral food intake and assessment of gastric motility should be applied.

The prolonged requirement of sedation to facilitate a complex ventilator strategy can also have adverse effects including the risk of delirium.

The majority of patients requiring invasive ventilator therapy for more than 2 weeks develop serious critical illness neuropathy and myopathy. Protocol based sedation breaks, standardised weaning strategies and a periodically conducted delirium screen can help to reduce patient ventilator time.

Further Reading

Anantham D, Jagadesan R, Tiew PE. Clinical review: independent lung ventilation in critical care. *Critical Care*. 2005; 9: 594–600.

Gattinoni L, Protti A, Caironi P, Carlesso E. Ventilator-induced lung injury: the anatomical and physiological framework. *Critical Care Medicine*. 2010; 38: S539–S548.

Skjeflo GW, Dybwik K. A new method of securing the airway for differential lung ventilation in intensive care. *Acta Anaesthesiologica Scandinavica*. 2014; 58: 463–467.

Yamakawa K, Nakamori Y, Fujimi S, et al. A novel technique of differential lung ventilation in the critical care setting. *BMC Research Notes*. 2011; 4: 134.

MCQs

1. **Which phase variables in a modern ventilator define a pressure controlled ventilation?**
   (a) Trigger phase
   (b) Limiting phase
   (c) Cycling and limiting phase
   (d) Trigger and limiting phase
   (e) Cycling phase
2. **Pressure regulated volume controlled ventilation (PRVC) provides the following feature(s):**
   (a) Constant volume with peak and plateau pressure levels
   (b) Constant pressure with variable tidal volume
   (c) Pressure controlled ventilation
   (d) Set tidal volumes with minimum necessary pressure
   (e) Tidal volume adjusted to a minimum airway pressure
3. **Positive end expiratory pressure (PEEP) does NOT have the following effects:**
   (a) Recruitment of collapsed alveoli
   (b) Increase of the functional residual capacity (FRC)
   (c) Improvement in lung compliance
   (d) Reduction in cardiac preload, especially in hypovolaemic patients
   (e) Reduction of peak airway pressure
4. **The following ventilator mode is NOT appropriate for a patient admitted to the ICU after uncomplicated aortic valve replacement:**
   (a) BiPAP
   (b) HFJV
   (c) CPAP/PS
   (d) SIMV
   (e) VC-CMV
5. **Protective ventilation does NOT include the following strategy:**
   (a) Adequate PEEP level
   (b) Airway humidification
   (c) Low tidal volume (10–12 ml/kg)
   (d) Elevated bed-head
   (e) Early protocol driven weaning from ventilation

Exercise answers are available on p.468. Alternatively, take the test online at www.cambridge.org/CardiothoracicMCQ

Chapter 18

Renal Replacement Therapy

Jonah Powell-Tuck, Matt Varrier and Marlies Ostermann

Introduction

Acute kidney injury (AKI) is a common complication of cardiovascular surgery affecting >20% of patients. The aetiology is complex and includes ischaemia-reperfusion injury, pro-inflammatory processes following prolonged cardiopulmonary bypass, haemodynamic instability, haemolysis, nephrotoxins and radiocontrast dye. It commonly develops on the background of pre-existing comorbidities such as vascular disease, older age and chronic kidney disease (CKD). Following cardiac surgery, patients are particularly vulnerable to the consequences of AKI, especially electrolyte derangement, metabolic acidosis and fluid accumulation. Between 1 and 5% of patients require renal replacement therapy (RRT). Several risk prediction models for RRT have been developed.

The main indications for starting RRT are:

- removal of excess fluid;
- correction of electrolyte abnormalities (most importantly hyperkalaemia);
- removal of metabolic byproducts (e.g. urea, ammonia, sulphates);
- correction of metabolic acidosis;
- removal of toxins, including drugs;
- removal of inflammatory mediators.

RRT is considered a supportive therapy during a period where metabolic and fluid demands exceed native kidney function. It can also help to limit non-renal organ dysfunction that may be exacerbated by the consequences o f AKI. Although it achieves solute clearance, acid-base homeostasis and fluid removal, it does not fully replace all kidney functions, such as reabsorption of amino acids, activation of vitamin D and erythropoietin production.

Types of Renal Replacement Therapy

There are several techniques of administering RRT, which can be classified according to the technique used (modalities) and the duration of therapy (modes).

Modalities

Renal replacement therapy can be administered either by utilising an extracorporeal circuit containing an artificial membrane (haemodialysis or haemofiltration) or by utilising the abdominal cavity and the patient's own peritoneal membrane (peritoneal dialysis).

- Haemodialysis (HD) refers to the removal of solute and water across a semipermeable membrane by means of diffusion across a concentration gradient. Blood is pumped through a filter whilst electrolyte containing dialysate fluid flows in the reverse direction on the opposite (non-blood) side of the filter membrane (see Figure 18.1).
- Haemofiltration (HF) relies on the principle of convection. A pressure gradient is applied across a semipermeable membrane resulting in removal of solute and water. A balanced replacement fluid is added pre-filter and/or post-filter to maintain electrolyte concentrations and fluid balance (see Figure 18.2). It should be remembered that the addition of pre-filter replacement fluid reduces the delivered RRT dose.
- Haemodiafiltration (HDF) incorporates the removal of solute and water across a semipermeable membrane by means of the application of both a concentration gradient and a transmembrane pressure (see Figure 18.3).
- Peritoneal dialysis (PD) uses the patient's peritoneum as a membrane. Dialysate fluid is instilled into the abdominal cavity and drained out several hours later. Fluids, electrolytes

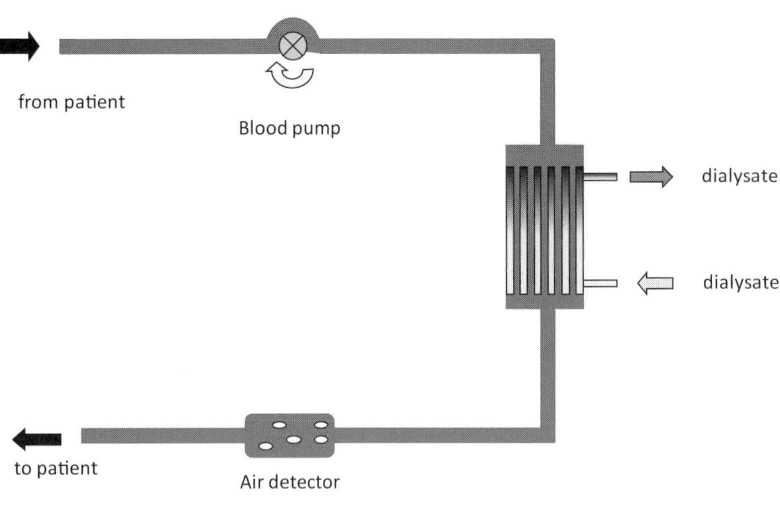

Figure 18.1 Haemodialysis. (A black and white version of this figure will appear in some formats. For the colour version, please refer to the plate section.)

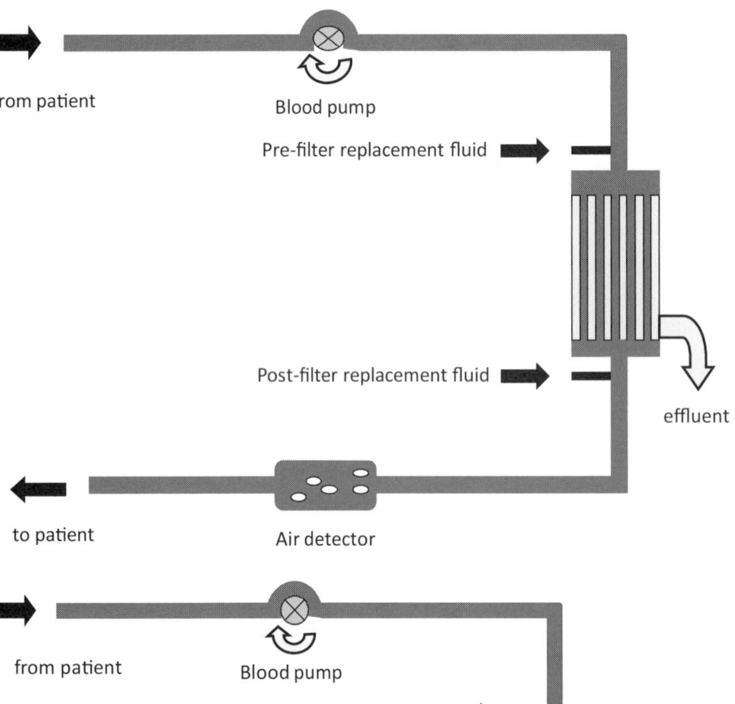

Figure 18.2 Haemofiltration. (A black and white version of this figure will appear in some formats. For the colour version, please refer to the plate section.)

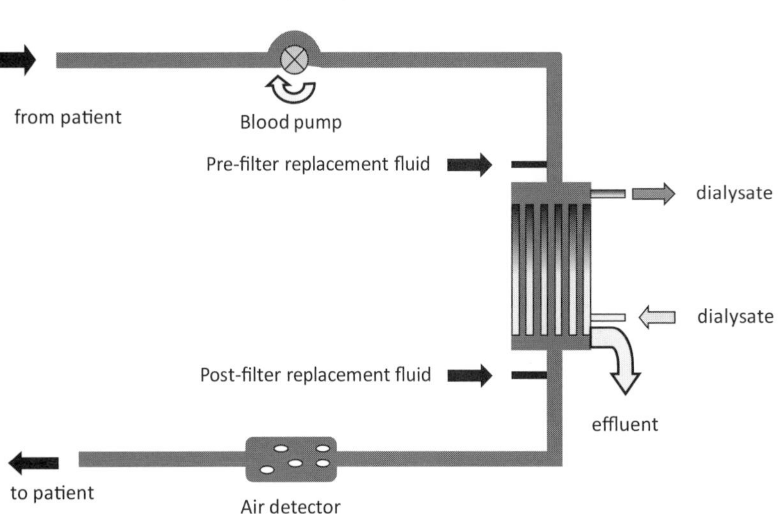

Figure 18.3 Haemodiafiltration. (A black and white version of this figure will appear in some formats. For the colour version, please refer to the plate section.)

Table 18.1 Advantages of intermittent and continuous RRT

Continuous RRT	Intermittent RRT
Continuous removal of toxins and electrolytes	Rapid clearance of toxins and electrolytes
Slower removal of excess fluid (i.e. better haemodynamic tolerability)	More time for diagnostic and therapeutic procedures
Less fluid and metabolic fluctuations	More time for physiotherapy/rehabilitation
	Reduced exposure to anticoagulation
	Lower financial costs

Abbreviations: RRT renal replacement therapy.

and small molecules are exchanged across the peritoneal membrane by diffusion.

HD, HF and HDF should be viewed as equivalent therapies for AKI after cardiac surgery. Middle molecular weight molecules may be removed more effectively by convection than by diffusion but there is no evidence to suggest that this leads to clinically important differences in outcome.

PD has theoretical advantages in that haemodynamic disturbance is rare and anticoagulation is not necessary. However, the efficiency and control of fluid and solute balance is inferior to HD, HF and HDF. In chronic PD patients, PD has a role for maintenance RRT during the recovery period post surgery.

Modes

RRT can be provided intermittently (≈4 hours daily or alternate days) or continuously (24 hours/day). During continuous renal replacement therapy (CRRT), solute clearance and fluid removal occur over a longer time resulting in less fluctuation in the concentrations of osmotically active molecules, such as urea and ammonia. Intermittent RRT (IRRT) is more effective at clearing small solutes and fluid rapidly.

CRRT is recommended for patients who are haemodynamically unstable and/or do not tolerate rapid fluid removal. It is also superior to intermittent RRT in patients with cerebral injury or cerebral oedema who may not tolerate fluctuations in osmotically active molecules. However, the potential advantages of CRRT are offset by the need for immobilisation, longer exposure to anticoagulation and increased health care costs (Table 18.1). Intermittent RRT has a role in situations where patients are haemodynamically more stable and where the focus of care has shifted to rehabilitation.

Haemodialysis is usually IRRT but can be provided as CRRT. Haemofiltration is usually CRRT, and haemodiafiltration can be performed as CRRT or IRRT.

Hybrid therapies such as slow low efficiency dialysis (SLED) or prolonged intermittent renal replacement therapy (PIRRT) are variations of RRT, which are usually provided daily for 6–12 hours. They offer the advantages of both intermittent and continuous RRT and are often employed during the transition period from CRRT to IRRT.

Indications and Timing

In patients with life threatening complications of AKI such as severe hyperkalaemia, marked metabolic acidosis or fluid overload, the decision to urgently start RRT is generally unequivocal (Table 18.2).

In the absence of overt or impending life threatening complications, the optimal threshold for starting RRT after cardiac surgery remains uncertain. Important considerations include the severity of illness, non-renal organ dysfunction, degree of fluid overload, severity of metabolic acidosis, clinical reserve to tolerate fluid overload and metabolic disturbances, anticipated fluid administration and likelihood of spontaneous recovery of renal function.

Potential advantages of earlier RRT initiation may be offset by the risks of catheter insertion, bleeding, treatment related haemodynamic instability, infectious complications and unwanted losses of nutrients and drugs (Table 18.3). In contrast, delays in initiating RRT may put patients at risk of serious fluid overload and other life threatening complications.

A recent meta-analysis of two randomised controlled trials (RCTs) and nine retrospective cohort studies which included a total of 841 patients following cardiac surgery concluded that the early initiation of RRT was associated with a lower 28-day mortality and shorter stay in ICU. However, there was marked heterogeneity between the studies including the definitions of 'early' and 'late' initiation.

Table 18.2 Summary of absolute and relative indications for starting RRT in critically ill patients with AKI

Absolute indications	• Refractory hyperkalaemia ($K^+ > 6.5$ mmol/l or rapidly rising) • Refractory metabolic acidosis (pH ≤ 7.2) • Refractory pulmonary oedema due to fluid overload • Uraemic pericarditis • Uraemic encephalopathy • Overdose/toxicity from a dialysable drug/toxin
Relative indications (in the absence of life threatening complications of AKI)	• Progressive fluid accumulation • Non-renal organ dysfunction worsened by the effects of AKI • Need for large volume fluid administration • Limited physiological reserve to tolerate the consequences of AKI • Progressive AKI with little chance of immediate recovery of renal function • Concomitant accumulation of poisons or drugs which can be removed by RRT

Abbreviations: AKI acute kidney injury; RRT renal replacement therapy.

Table 18.3 Benefits and drawbacks of early RRT

Benefits	Drawbacks
Avoidance and/or early control of fluid accumulation and overload	Risk of complications associated with dialysis catheter insertion
Avoidance and/or earlier control of complications of uraemia	Risk of complications from anticoagulation
Avoidance and/or earlier control of electrolyte/metabolic derangement	Risk of haemodynamic instability
Avoidance and/or earlier control of acid-base derangement	Clearance of micronutrients and trace elements
Avoidance of unnecessary diuretic exposure	Excess clearance of dialysable medications (i.e. antimicrobials, antiepileptics)
Clearance of inflammatory mediators	Workload for providers
	Immobilisation
	Healthcare costs

Abbreviations: AKI acute kidney injury; RRT renal replacement therapy.

Clinical practice is often variable. Ideally, the decision to start RRT should be individualised and based on the dynamic context and trajectory of the patient, illness severity, non-renal organ dysfunction, along with physiological and laboratory data, rather than relying on absolute laboratory values. Figure 18.4 shows an algorithm which incorporates these principles.

Dose of RRT

The dose of RRT is a measure of the quantity of a solute that is removed from the patient during extracorporeal treatment. In patients on intermittent haemodialysis, dose of treatment is expressed as urea reduction ratio (URR) or Kt/V (K is dialyser clearance of urea, t is dialysis time and V is the volume of distribution of urea). Both parameters have important limitations in critically ill patients with AKI where neither urea generation rate nor volume of distribution can be clearly defined. In patients receiving CRRT, the dose may be estimated considering the effluent flow rate indexed by the patient's body weight. It is usually described as ml/kg/hour.

Based on two large RCTs, the current recommendation is to deliver a target dose of 20–25 ml/kg/hour. However, unintended interruptions in treatment often occur which will reduce the effective dose. Therefore, doses higher than 20–25 ml/kg/hour may have to be prescribed but there is no role for high volume RRT.

Although the dose of RRT classically refers to solute clearance, ultrafiltration rate and target fluid balance should also be considered as important components of the prescription. Cardiac surgery results in an inflammatory state and capillary leak, which may result in fluid accumulation. Progressive tissue and pulmonary oedema can be attenuated by

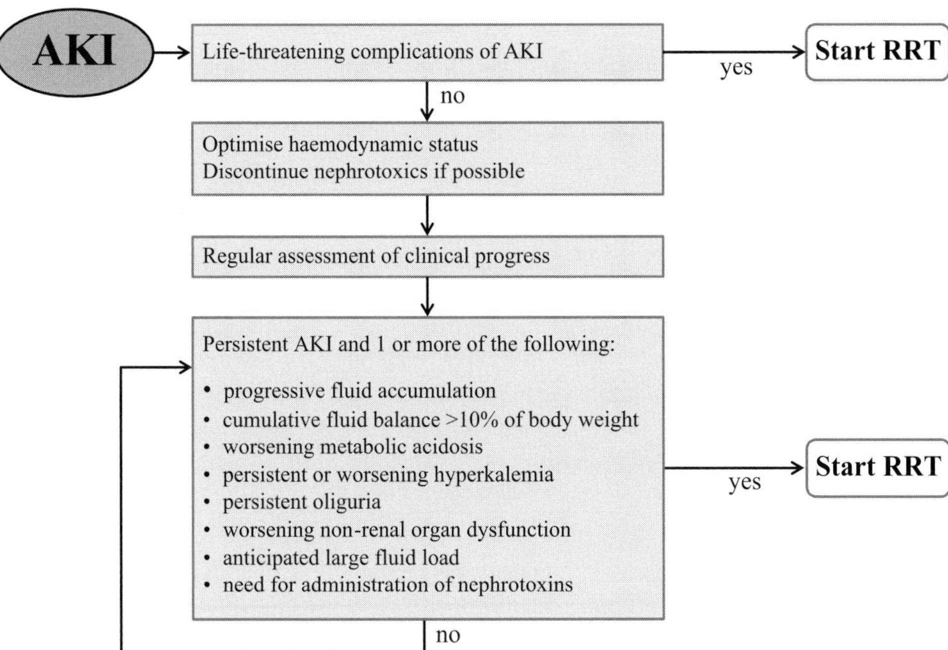

Figure 18.4 Algorithm for deciding whether to begin RRT.

close attention to fluid balance and judicious use of ultrafiltration.

Anticoagulation

In patients with AKI requiring RRT, contact of blood with the extracorporeal circuit results in activation of the coagulation cascade. Additionally, the haematocrit within the filter increases as a result of fluid removal, which adds to the risk of the filter clotting. Premature clotting of the circuit reduces effective clearance, leads to blood loss and increases the workload and financial costs. The goal of anticoagulation is to maintain filter patency, and thus avoid these complications.

The most commonly used anticoagulation strategies include unfractionated heparin delivered systemically or via the circuit, low molecular weight heparin (LMWH), systemic epoprostenol, regional anticoagulation with citrate and non-pharmacological measures. Other options are thrombin inhibitors such as argatroban, factor Xa inhibitors such as danaparoid or fondaparinux, or serine proteinase inhibitors, for example nafamostat mesylate. The choice should be individualised and based on characteristics of the patient, potential risks and benefits of the anticoagulant, availability and local expertise (Table 18.4).

Heparin is still the most commonly used anticoagulant worldwide; however, the use of citrate for regional anticoagulation is becoming increasingly popular. Citrate acts by chelating calcium, thereby inhibiting the clotting cascade at several levels. Citrate is infused into the circuit prior to the filter to achieve an ionised calcium concentration [Ca_i] of <0.35 mmol/l in blood passing through the filter. Calcium replacement occurs after the filter to correct the calcium deficit in the blood returning to the patient. As a result, the extracorporeal circuit is fully anticoagulated whilst the patient is not. Thus better circuit patency is achieved with fewer bleeding complications. Additionally, citrate serves as a source for the generation of bicarbonate.

Several RCTs and meta-analyses have demonstrated improved safety, less bleeding complications and better circuit patency with citrate anticoagulation when compared to heparin. It is particularly useful in patients with a high bleeding risk, including patients in the immediate postoperative period.

Non-pharmacological strategies of prolonging circuit patency include using higher pump speeds, pre-diluting blood with replacement fluid prior to the filter or flushing the filter at regular intervals with saline.

Table 18.4 Characteristics of commonly used anticoagulants

Characteristics	Unfractionated heparin	Low molecular weight heparin	Epoprostenol	Citrate
Action	Inactivation of thrombin and other proteases involved in the clotting cascade	Inactivation of thrombin and other proteases involved in the clotting cascade	Inhibition of platelet function	Chelation of calcium
Extent of anticoagulation	Systemic	Systemic	Systemic	Regional
Most common side effects	Bleeding HIT	Bleeding HIT	Vasodilation	Citrate accumulation metabolic alkalosis Hypo-/hypercalcaemia
Absolute/relative contraindications	Bleeding HIT	Bleeding HIT	Severe haemodynamic instability due to vasodilation	Severe liver failure Severe intracellular hypoxia

Abbreviations: RRT renal replacement therapy; HIT heparin induced thrombocytopenia.

Official recommendations by the Kidney Disease: Improving Global Outcomes (KDIGO) expert group include the following. For patients not already receiving effective systemic anticoagulation:

(i) use either unfractionated or low molecular weight heparin for anticoagulation in patients receiving intermittent RRT;

(ii) use regional citrate anticoagulation for patients treated with CRRT provided they have no contraindications to citrate;

(iii) use either unfractionated or low molecular weight heparin for patients with contraindications to citrate receiving CRRT.

Monitoring

The indication and prescription of RRT needs to be reviewed and adjusted on a daily basis, as the condition of the patient and treatment goals may change. This review should include an assessment of the overall aims of RRT, the delivered dose, target fluid balance and filter patency. Particular attention also needs to be given to the patient's drug chart and nutritional requirements since RRT affects the clearance of certain medications and is associated with losses of nutrients and trace elements.

Discontinuation of RRT

RRT should be discontinued when it is no longer required, either because the patient's native kidney function has recovered sufficiently to meet the metabolic and fluid demands, or because the goals of care have changed. The process of stopping RRT may consist of simple discontinuation of RRT, or may include a change in the modality, frequency, or duration of RRT. For example, switching from CRRT to IRRT or decreasing the frequency of IRRT from daily to alternate days are two methods of testing underlying kidney function.

Urine output appears to be the best predictor of successful discontinuation. A large prospective observational study showed that in 529 patients who survived the initial period of CRRT, 313 were successfully removed from RRT, whereas 216 patients needed to restart RRT within 7 days of discontinuation. Multivariate logistic regression analysis showed that patients who achieved a urine output of greater than 400 ml/24 hours without diuretic use had an 81% chance of successful discontinuation of RRT. Patients receiving diuretics with a urine output of 2330 ml/24 hours had an 87.9% chance of remaining off RRT.

Outcome

The initiation of RRT represents an escalation in both the complexity and costs of care. It is well established that the development of AKI is an independent risk factor for in-hospital mortality and this holds true post cardiac surgery. Patients with severe AKI receiving RRT are at increased risk of major morbidity, including non-recovery of kidney function, rapid progression to end-stage renal disease (ESRD) and long-term dialysis dependence, and premature mortality even with recovery of renal function. The risk of ESRD is particularly high in patients with pre-existing CKD.

Although it is widely recognised that AKI survivors represent a high risk group, the optimal strategy for long-term management has yet to be established.

Learning Points

- Patients undergoing cardiac surgery are at high risk of AKI including the need for renal replacement therapy.
- The indication for renal replacement therapy should be individualised based on the patient's severity and trajectory of illness, degree of fluid accumulation, metabolic control and severity of non-renal organ dysfunction.
- Haemodialysis, haemofiltration and haemodiafiltration are all acceptable techniques post cardiac surgery; continuous renal replacement therapy is preferred in the setting of haemodynamic instability.
- The target dose of RRT should be 20–35 ml/kg/hour although this should be adjusted to account for interruptions to treatment.
- Several techniques to avoid filter clotting are available. Regional citrate anticoagulation offers the best risk-benefit ratio in patients at high risk of bleeding.

Further Reading

Bai M, Zhou M, He L, et al. Citrate versus heparin anticoagulation for continuous renal replacement therapy: an updated meta-analysis of RCTs. *Intensive Care Medicine*. 2015; 41: 2098–2110.

Bastin AJ, Ostermann M, Slack AJ et al. Acute kidney injury after cardiac surgery according to Risk/Injury/Failure/Loss/End-stage, Acute Kidney Injury Network, and Kidney Disease: Improving Global Outcomes classifications. *Journal of Critical Care*. 2013; 28: 389–396.

Bellomo R, Kellum JA, Ronco C. Acute kidney injury. *Lancet*. 2012; 380: 756–766.

Chertow GM, Lazarus JM, Christiansen CL, et al. Preoperative renal risk stratification. *Circulation*. 1997; 95: 878–984.

Fortescue EB, Bates DW, Chertow GM. Predicting acute renal failure after coronary bypass surgery: cross-validation of two risk-stratification algorithms. *Kidney International*. 2000; 57: 2594–2602.

Goldstein SL, Jaber BL, Faubel S, Chawla LS. AKI transition of care: a potential opportunity to detect and prevent CKD. *Clinical Journal of the American Society of Nephrology*. 2013; 8: 476–483.

Hobson CE, Yavas S, Segal MS, et al. Acute kidney injury is associated with increased long-term mortality after cardiothoracic surgery. *Circulation*. 2009; 119: 2444–2453.

Mehta RH, Grab JD, O'Brien SM, et al. Bedside tool for predicting the risk of postoperative dialysis in patients undergoing cardiac surgery. *Circulation*. 2006; 114: 2208–2216.

Morabito S, Pistolesi V, Tritapepe L, et al. Regional citrate anticoagulation in cardiac surgery patients at high risk of bleeding: a continuous veno-venous hemofiltration protocol with a low concentration citrate solution. *Critical Care*. 2012; 16: R111.

Wald R, Quinn RR, Luo J, et al. Chronic dialysis and death among survivors of acute kidney injury requiring dialysis. *Journal of the American Medical Association*. 2009; 302: 1179–1185.

Wijeysundera DN, Karkouti K, Dupuis JY, et al. Derivation and validation of a simplified predictive index for renal replacement therapy after cardiac surgery. *Journal of the American Medical Association*. 2007; 297: 1801–1809.

Zarbock A, Kellum JA, Schmidt C, et al. Effect of early vs delayed initiation of renal replacement therapy on mortality in critically ill patients with acute kidney injury: the ELAIN randomized clinical trial. *Journal of the American Medical Association*. 2016; 315: 2190–2199.

Zhang Z, Hongying N. Efficacy and safety of regional citrate anticoagulation in critically ill patients undergoing continuous renal replacement therapy. *Intensive Care Medicine*. 2012; 38: 20–28.

Zou H, Hong Q, Gaosi X. Early versus late initiation of renal replacement therapy impacts mortality in patients with acute kidney injury post cardiac surgery: a meta-analysis. *Critical Care*. 2017; 21: 150.

MCQs

1. **Which of the following is not an indication for renal replacement therapy?**

   (a) Pulmonary oedema

   (b) Metabolic acidosis

   (c) Uraemic pericarditis

   (d) Respiratory acidosis

   (e) Hyperkalaemia

2. **Which of the following is an advantage of continuous RRT over intermittent RRT?**
   (a) Faster clearance of toxins
   (b) Improved haemodynamic stability
   (c) Reduced exposure to anticoagulation
   (d) Improved rehabilitation
   (e) Faster fluid removal

3. **Regarding RRT, which of the following statements is false?**
   (a) Haemodialysis relies on the principle of convection
   (b) Haemofiltration removes middle weight molecules more effectively than haemodialysis
   (c) In haemodiafiltration, diffusion occurs across the filter membrane
   (d) Pre-diluting circuit blood can prolong filter lifespan
   (e) Spontaneous urine output of >400 ml/24 hours has been associated with successful cessation of RRT

4. **Which of the following statements regarding anticoagulation for RRT is correct?**
   (a) Citrate inhibits platelet activation
   (b) Epoprostenol causes vasoconstriction
   (c) Citrate is recommended as the anticoagulant of first choice
   (d) Heparin has a better safety profile than citrate
   (e) Citrate dose is not titrated against anti-Xa levels

5. **Which statement regarding RRT dose is incorrect?**
   (a) Following cardiac surgery, higher RRT doses are associated with decreased 30-day mortality
   (b) In CRRT, dose is estimated as the effluent rate divided by patient's weight per hour
   (c) Dose refers to the amount of solute removed from the patient
   (d) In intermittent RRT, dose is referred to as urea reduction ratio
   (e) Interruptions to dialysis will reduce the effective delivered dose

Exercise answers are available on p.468. Alternatively, take the test online at www.cambridge.org/CardiothoracicMCQ

Chapter 19

Nutritional Support for Cardiac Surgery and Intensive Care

Peter Faber

As most patients after routine cardiac surgery quickly resume baseline nutritional intake, specific dietetic assessment and support is rarely required. However, patients with pre-existing malnutrition, especially underweight, and those requiring prolonged intensive care due to perioperative complications are at risk of further nutritional derangement and early interventions to optimise nutritional requirements are recommended.

Nutritional Assessment

At hospital admission patients should be assessed for baseline nutritional status. In the simplest and most useful form this includes:

Body weight, height and body mass index (BMI, kg/m^2); with normal weight defined as a BMI between 18.5–24.9 kg/m^2;

Physical examination with an emphasis on muscle mass and mobility to assess strength and coordination;

The presence of oedema, body temperature and oral health.

For example, elderly patients with poor muscle strength and oral health will be at increased risk of not being able to independently feed themselves during the recovery period. These patients and the critically ill intensive care (ICU) patients are likely to require either supplementary or full nutritional support.

To further identify patients at risk of malnourishment, screening questionnaires such as the Subjective Global Assessment (SGA), Nutritional Risk Screening (NRS 2002), the Malnutrition Universal Screening Tool (MUST) and the NUTRIC Score should be used.

Unless patients have specific metabolic diseases, biochemical indicators of nutritional status (e.g. plasma transferrin and 3-methylhistidine concentration) rarely offer additional information to a thorough clinical examination and assessment as outlined above.

If additional assessment is required, measurements of body composition can be applied to measure body fat content, lean body mass, bone mass and water content. Although some of these techniques, for example skin fold thickness to measure body fat and bioimpedance to measure water, fat and lean tissue, are simple to perform at initial hospital admission, most methodologies have not been validated for consecutive measurements in ICU patients. Hence, wrongly applying such techniques may at best obtain misleading results. Table 19.1 gives normal values for BMI and percentage body fat.

More accurate methods of estimating body composition increase the complexity and may not be useful in clinical practice. Table 19.2 briefly summarises the principles behind some methods of estimating body composition.

Normal Nutritional Requirements

Energy Balance

To achieve energy balance (energy intake – energy expenditure = energy balance), in a normal healthy individual an average daily energy intake is required of approximately 2500 kcal for men and 2000 kcal for women. It follows that if an individual remains in energy balance, body weight is stable.

Energy Intake

The total chemical energy of food (determined by bomb direct calorimetry) is not available to the human body. The energy available to the human body is termed the metabolisable energy. The difference in availability of energy is due to not all food being absorbed from the gastrointestinal tract, the energy

Table 19.1 Body fat and body mass index

	Body fat (%)		BMI (kg/m^2)	
	Males	Females	Normal	18.5–24.9
Normal	12–20	20–30	Overweight	25–29.9
Borderline	21–25	31–33	Obese	30–39.9
Obese	>25	>33	Severely obese	>40

Table 19.2 Principles of body composition measurements

Method	Principle
Imaging techniques (CT, MRI, DEXA scanning)	Soft tissue distribution and bone mass can be measured
Density (body plethysmography, under water weighing)	Water or air displacement to calculate total body volume and density. From the density, body composition can be determined. Water has high density, fat has low density
Bioelectrical impedance (BIA)	Electrical resistance varies across the body compartments. Water is a good conductor, fat less so. Impedance varies with body composition
Stable isotope dilution techniques	Tracer isotopes are distributed to specific body compartments. Body compartment sizes are calculated from volumes and concentrations

Table 19.3 Metabolisable energy and recommended daily intake of macronutrients

	Metabolisable energy (kcal/g)	Recommended daily energy intake, and percentage of total energy intake
Carbohydrate	4	No more than 50% (of which free sugars no more than 5%)
Protein	4	0.8 g/kg/day (approximately 15%)
Fat	9	No more than 35% (of which saturated no more than 11%)

costs of metabolism per se, incomplete oxidation of protein and energy losses through faeces and urine. Total energy intake is mainly distributed between the three macronutrients – carbohydrate, fat and protein. Excess energy intake compared with energy expenditure is stored as deposits of glycogen, fat and protein. Fat is the preferential and most efficient way of storing excess energy, as fat tissue has a high energy density with low cell turnover. This compares favourably with carbohydrates, as intracellular glycogen is obligatory stored with water and protein stores have high energy costs due to active metabolism and cell turnover. The body has no alcohol storage capacity and thus alcohol at 7 kcal/g must be preferentially metabolised before the three main macronutrients.

Table 19.3 demonstrates the metabolisable energy of the three macronutrients and the recommended daily energy intake.

Total energy intake is measured by recording the amount and composition of food consumed. Published tables provide the energy content of food items and, correctly reported and collated, total energy intake can easily be determined.

Energy Expenditure

Energy expenditure is more difficult to measure compared with energy intake. The gold standard for measuring energy expenditure, and hence to enable individually tailored energy intake, is indirect calorimetry.

Indirect calorimetry is most often applied to measure resting metabolic rate (RMR), which is the minimum energy required by the body at rest in order to fuel essential bodily processes and keep organs and tissues in working order. It is a standardised measurement performed on an awake, supine resting person in a temperature neutral environment after overnight fasting (8–10 hours).

From measurements of oxygen consumption (VO_2), carbon dioxide production (VCO_2) and additional nitrogen excretion it is possible to accurately calculate total energy expenditure as well as macronutrient oxidation (protein, fat, carbohydrates) in health and disease. The most widely used formulae to calculate energy expenditure from indirect calorimetry in humans are those of Elia and Weir:

$$RMR\ (kcal/min) = [15.818\ VO_2\ (l/min) + 5.176\ VCO_2\ (l/min)]/4.18.$$

If nitrogen excretion is measured, accuracy is improved by applying

$$RMR\ (kcal/min) = [16.489\ VO_2\ (l/min) + 4.628\ VCO_2\ (l/min) - 9.079\ N\ (g)]/4.18.$$

An assessment of substrate being metabolised can be obtained from measurement of the respiratory quotient (RQ), which is the volumetric relationship between carbon dioxide production and oxygen consumption, VCO_2/VO_2. An RQ approximating 1 indicates carbohydrate oxidation and an RQ approximating 0.7 indicates fat oxidation.

Predictive equations, based on age and anthropometry, which negate the requirements for equipment to accurately measure RMR, have been developed.

In health, the Mifflin–St Jeor equation is accurate 75% of the time when compared with individually measured indirect calorimetry:

$$RMR\ (kcal/day) = 10 \times weight\ (kg) + 6.25 \times height\ (cm) - 5 \times age\ (years) + 5\ (males),$$

$$RMR\ (kcal/day) = 10 \times weight\ (kg) + 6.25 \times height\ (cm) - 5 \times age\ (years) - 161\ (females).$$

In disease, the modified Penn State equation can be used to account for the metabolic effects of body temperature and minute ventilation:

$$RMR\ (kcal/day) = Mifflin \times 0.96 + Tmax \times 167 + VE \times 31 - 6212\ (males),$$

$$RMR\ (kcal/day) = Mifflin \times 0.74 + Tmax \times 85 + VE \times 64 - 3085\ (females).$$

Here Mifflin is the RMR as estimated by the Mifflin–St Jeor equation, Tmax is maximum body temperature (°C) in the previous 24 hours and VE is the minute ventilation in litres/minute.

Nutritional Requirements in Disease

Apart from a few exceptions (e.g. cachexia in severe mitral stenosis, poor outcome at extremes of BMI for lung transplant patients), cardiac patients do not differ from other patients undergoing major surgery and admission to the ICU. Sepsis, stroke, renal failure, long-term ventilation and bowel ischaemia are feared perioperative complications across a range of surgical specialities as well as for cardiac surgery. These are all complications that have a direct impact on the management of nutritional rehabilitation.

Compared with healthy individuals, the critically ill exhibit an increased turnover and mobilisation of stored fuel reserves, especially protein. Due to hormonal changes and inflammatory response in the ill patient, this happens even when energy balance has been achieved and thus the resting metabolic rate in what appears to be sedentary ill patients can be increased by an average of approximately 25% compared with healthy individuals. In patients with severe burns, RMR can be double baseline value.

The increase in metabolism caused by the inflammatory response to surgery and trauma is independent of the injury type when controlled for the effect of fever. Fever compounds the increase in metabolism and protein catabolism observed after major surgery, trauma and sepsis. The resting metabolic rate in these patients can increase up to 1.5 times compared with healthy individuals. In febrile patients, the metabolic rate increases by approximately 10% per degree increase in body temperature and in the most severely ill patients energy requirements can reach 40–50 kcal/kg/day against a normal figure of approximately 25 kcal/kg/day. During the acute febrile phase of infection there is additional salt and water retention, exacerbating oedema, renal and ventilatory complications. Thus, although serial measurement of body weight is recommended to monitor energy balance and changes in body weight, in clinical practice it is very difficult to accurately weigh intensive care patients, and with the often concurrent large disturbances in fluid balance, this is of little added value for assessing nutritional status per se.

The increased concentrations of cortisol and catecholamines, and the reduced effect of insulin, compound the often significant protein catabolism observed during a sustained inflammatory response. Urinary nitrogen losses (gram protein oxidised = 6.25 × gram nitrogen excreted) can be measured to assess the protein wastage, which in the severely ill patient can reach more than 200 g/day. The amino acids released from skeletal muscle are used for gluconeogenesis and protein synthesis, i.e. in disease there is an energy increase requiring acceleration of protein turnover and enhanced lipolysis.

Indirect calorimetry remains the most accurate method for measuring patients' energy requirements. In the absence of this, predictive equations (based on the patient's hospital admission body weight) with additions for disease pathology will in most cases provide adequate nutritional support. In clinical practice, however, a value of 25–30 kcal/kg/day is often used as the initial energy requirement for most critically ill patients

Macronutrients

Protein

Compared with the dietary reference intake (DRI) of 0.8 g protein/kg/day in healthy individuals, studies have all demonstrated increased requirement of protein in critically ill patients. The consensus is to provide 1.2–1.5 g protein/kg/day with a total energy intake from protein approximating 15–20%. If protein is metabolised for gluconeogenesis there is a reduction in skeletal muscle mass as well as structural proteins, resulting in impaired wound healing and immune response. In patients with renal failure and increased gastrointestinal losses, protein intake should be re-evaluated and increased. However, in azotaemia and ureamia, an excess protein intake can worsen encephalopathy in confused patients and patients with intracranial pathology. Hence, judiciously assessed protein intake is important for the patients' recovery and although rarely done in clinical practice, the measurement of nitrogen balance will improve individually determined protein requirements.

Carbohydrate

The recommended daily intake of carbohydrates (glucose, oligosaccharides and polysaccharides) is between 2–6 g/kg/day. The optimal amount should be additionally guided by the requirement of protein sparing and the patient's ability to metabolise the carbohydrates. This is done concurrently with insulin administration under the guidance of blood glucose (8–10 mmol/l) and plasma lactate concentrations. The total daily energy intake from carbohydrates should be between 30–70%.

Fat

Generally fat can safely provide 15–35% of the total energy intake. If administered as a lipid emulsion this equates to approximately 0.5–1.5 g/kg/day with a maximum of 2 g/kg/day. If administered as an intravenous lipid emulsion, patients are at risk of metabolic complications if administered at rates exceeding 0.11 g/kg/hour. Excessive amount of lipid administration results in fat overfeeding syndrome, signs of which include hypertriglyceridaemia, respiratory distress, abnormal liver function and coagulopathies. The calorie content of 10% propofol lipid emulsion is 1.1 cal/ml and should be included in calculations of total calorie and fat intake.

Timing and Route of Administration

Enteral Nutrition

If the patient is not able to resume full oral intake within 24–48 hours, it is recommended to insert a nasogastric feeding tube to commence full or supplementary feeding. Cardiothoracic patients should as a group tolerate enteral feeding and in general there are only very few evidence based contraindications (Table 19.4). It is a common misperception that patients in inotrope requiring shock should not receive enteral feeding.

Enteral nutrition has been demonstrated to be not only simpler than parenteral nutrition, but also superior in terms of nutritional adequacy, metabolic complications and preservation of gastrointestinal integrity. This results in a decreased rate of infection, hospital length of stay and organ failure. There is no firm evidence suggesting the nasogastric feeding tube is best placed prepyloric or postpyloric. However, if there are continued large gastric aspirates it may be worth repositioning the feeding tube postpyloric before commencing parenteral nutrition.

Although simple in principle, it is often difficult to achieve the nutritional requirements by enteral delivery of nutrition and it has been found that only about 50% of patients achieve the prescribed nutritional intake. Contributing conditions are gastroparesis and

Table 19.4 Contraindications to enteral feeding

Intestinal obstruction or ileus
Intractable vomiting/diarrhoea
Severe gastrointestinal bleeding
Intestinal ischaemia
Severe pancreatitis
Abdominal compartment syndrome
Gastrointestinal fistula

ntestinal hypomotility observed in up to 50% of critically ill patients. This is compounded by for example opiates and catecholamines.

Impaired gastrointestinal motility is manifest by abdominal distension and continued gastric residual volumes of the delivered nutrition. If impairment of gastrointestinal motility prevents adequate calorie intake, supplemental or full parenteral nutrition should be considered. A 4–6 hourly gastric residual volume of between 3–500 ml can be considered as a tolerance indicator to enteral nutrition.

Feeding should be administered continuously and commenced at 20 ml/hour to assess tolerance, and increased in accordance with nutritional requirements and measured gastric aspirates. Therefore some patients may initially not achieve their nutritional goals. Often gastrointestinal motility can be facilitated by the administration of prokinetic agents, for example lactulose, erythromycin, metoclopramide and domperidone. Laxatives can be prescribed if there has been absence of stools for 3 or more consecutive days.

Composition of Enteral Feeds

Most commercially supplied enteral feeds contain 1–1.25 kcal/ml. Low volume feeds with the highest energy density are used for example for patients with renal impairment. Depending on manufacturer, the energy from protein, fat and carbohydrate is approximately 15–25%, 25–35% and 40–60%, respectively.

For a standard nutrition formula of 1.2 kcal/ml, a 75 kg patient would require approximately 80–100 ml/hour to cover energy and macronutrient requirements.

Nasogastric feeds are enriched in electrolytes, essential fatty acids, vitamins and micronutrients. In addition to nutrition, fluid requirements should be supplemented by appropriate intravenous or nasogastric fluids, the volume of which should be guided by hydration status, renal function and electrolyte balance. Daily fluid requirements are approximately 30–35 ml/kg/24 hours in non-febrile patients. Adult electrolyte, vitamin and micronutrient requirements are shown in Table 19.5.

Figure 19.1 suggests an algorithm for the initiation of enteral feeding.

Aspirate nasogastric tube before commencing. If no aspirate, check that tube is correctly placed by chest radiography and/or air insufflation.

Table 19.5 Proposed enteral reference daily intakes (RDI) of electrolytes, micronutrients and vitamins

Nutrient	RDI
Sodium	60–100 mmol/day or 1 mmol/kg
Potassium	50–100 mmol/day or 1 mmol/kg
Magnesium	12–14 mmol/day
Phosphate	25 mmol/day
Calcium	20 mmol/day
Zinc	60–190 μmol/day
Iron	180–270 μmol/day
Copper	16–32 μmol/day
Vitamin B12	2–6 μg
Vitamin B6	1.5–2 μg
Folate	180–400 μg
Thiamin	1.2–1.5 mg
Vitamin C	60 mg
Vitamin A	850–1000 mg

If aspirate >250 ml, await nasogastric feeding for 4 hours and aspirate again. Commence feeding when aspirates <250 ml. Routinely prescribe lactulose 15 ml TDS.

If gastric aspirates 250–500 ml, consider administration of:
Metoclopramide 10 mg intravenously TDS
Erythromycin 200 mg intravenously TDS
Domperidone 30–40 mg via nasogastric tube.

If within 3–5 days the patient does not receive >50% required energy intake, supplementary parenteral nutrition should be commenced.

Parenteral Nutrition

For patients in whom enteral nutrition delivers inadequate calories, supplementary or full parenteral nutrition should be commenced. Parenteral nutrition is hypertonic and needs to be administered via dedicated central venous access with formulations supplied by the hospital pharmacy after dietetic advice and guidance. In well-nourished patients it is not necessary to start parenteral nutrition until after 3–5 days of failure of attempted enteral feeding.

Parenteral nutrition is based upon essential and non-essential L-amino acids as a source of nitrogen, glucose for carbohydrates and fatty acids as fat. Parenteral formulations are relatively high in fat content, alleviating the risk of hyperglycaemia and hepatic steatosis associated with too high an energy

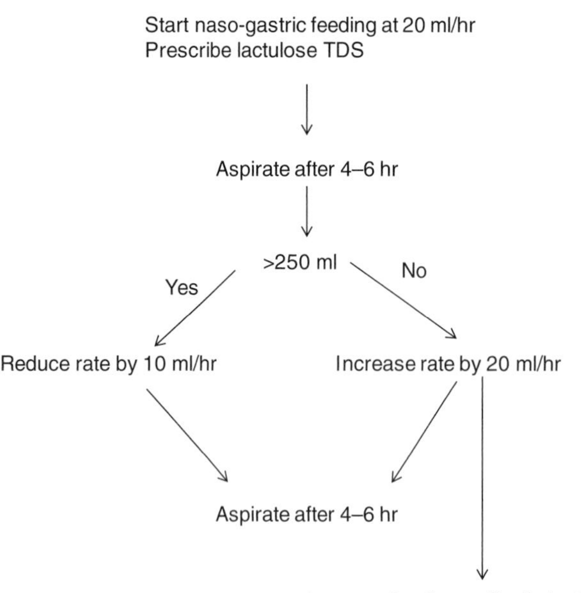

Figure 19.1 Initiation of enteral feeding.

equivalent from glucose. Fat can be administered at a rate of up to 1.2 g/kg/day. Vitamins, trace elements and phosphate are supplemented in appropriate amounts.

In clinical practice, there is often a high threshold for commencing parenteral nutrition due to the recognised complications of hyperglycaemia, infection, abnormal liver function tests and cholestasis. However, by observing judicious antibacterial care, supplemental insulin administration and frequent review of nutritional requirements, these complications should not prevent the patients from receiving adequate nutrition. It is worth remembering that enteral and parenteral nutrition can often be satisfactorily combined, with an overall reduction in complications associated with either technique.

Nutrition Adjusted to Renal Failure

Acute kidney injury after cardiac surgery has been reported to occur in up to 25–30% of patients and a significant proportion of these patients will require renal replacement therapy while admitted to the ICU. Renal impairment and failure is a common complication that directly affects the nutritional management of ICU patients. The metabolism of all three macronutrients is altered, with a decrease in insulin clearance and glucagon. Changes in the activity of lipid clearance during acute kidney injury result in an increased plasma concentration of triglycerides and there is accentuated protein catabolism and acidosis. Renal production and synthesis of hormones and amino acids will be impaired during kidney injury and renal replacement therapy. Micronutrients and water soluble vitamins are often depleted and should be substituted accordingly. The disturbances in fluid balance will add to the complications of clinically assessing nutritional status. Bed bound patients receiving renal replacement therapy will experience an accelerated loss of muscle protein in addition to the clearance of smaller peptides and amino acids by the haemofiltering membranes. Thus, protein administration should be increased to the order of 1.5–1.8 g/kg/day. Glutamine becomes conditionally essential and should be substituted judiciously as should zinc, phosphorus, selenium and thiamine together with the water soluble vitamins.

Further Reading

Bost RBC, Tjan DHT, van Zanten ARH. Timing of (supplemental) parenteral nutrition in critically ill patients: a systematic review. *Annals of Intensive Care*. 2014; 4: 31–44.

Desai SV, McClave SA, Rice TW. Nutrition in the ICU. *Chest*. 2014; 145: 1148–1157.

Faber P, Siervo M (Eds). *Nutrition in Critical Care*. Cambridge: Cambridge University Press, 2014.

Hooper MH, Marik PE. Controversies and misconceptions in intensive care nutrition. *Clinics in Chest Medicine*. 2015; 36: 409–418.

Ridley E, Gantner D, Pellegrino V. Nutrition therapy in critically ill patients – a review of current evidence for clinicians. *Clinical Nutrition*. 2015; 34: 565–571.

MCQs

True or False

1. **Assessment of nutritional status in patients should routinely comprise:**

   (a) Body weight, height and food questionnaires for total calorie intake

   (b) Biochemical markers transferrin and 3-methylhistidine

   (c) Quick and easy measurements of body composition, for example bioimpedance and skin-fold thickness

2. **When discussing energy balance:**

   (a) Energy intake is easily and simply measured by recording food intake into a diary

   (b) When in energy balance, people losing weight have a high metabolism and people gaining weight have a slow metabolism

   (c) Basic metabolic rate increases with age

3. **In disease the critically ill patient:**

   (a) Shuts down the metabolism of amino acids to preserve protein

   (b) Anti-inflammatory medication will restore a normal metabolism

   (c) Grams protein oxidised can be calculated from multiplying urinary nitrogen excretion

4. **In disease the recommended macronutrient intake of protein, carbohydrate and fat is:**

   (a) Protein intake should be approximately 0.8 g/kg/day providing 15–20% of energy intake

   (b) Carbohydrate intake should be less than approximately 1 g/kg/day

   (c) Fat intake should be approximately 0.5–1.5 g/kg/day

5. **When discussing enteral and parenteral nutrition:**

   (a) Feeding should be commenced after 24–48 hours if oral intake has not been resumed

   (b) Postpyloric placement of the feeding tube is preferable to gastric placement

   (c) The absence or presence of stool guides the initiation of nasogastric feeding

Exercise answers are available on p.468. Alternatively, take the test online at www.cambridge.org/CardiothoracicMCQ

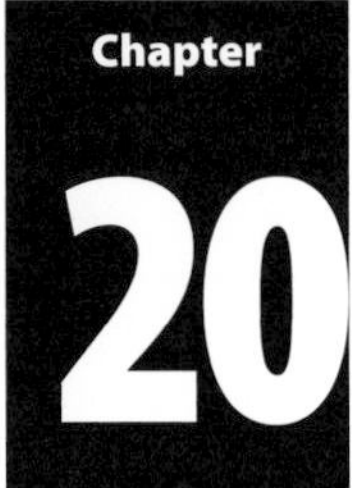

Physiotherapy and Rehabilitation

Adam Baddeley and Allaina Eden

Introduction

Physiotherapy over the last decade has evolved considerably in the areas of critical care, cardiac and thoracic surgery. This chapter will review the changes in these areas supported by research, in particular, postoperative critical care based rehabilitation, respiratory physiotherapy and physiotherapy practice in relation to cardiothoracic surgery.

Rehabilitation

Effect of Bed Rest

At some stage during the majority of critical care admissions, many patients will require sedation to maintain physiological stability during an acute period of illness and will be unable to mobilise out of bed. In addition to sedation and immobility, the use of neuromuscular blockades and the presence of sepsis lead to intensive care acquired weakness and a reduction in functional ability.

Physical and non-physical changes present in critical care patients. Below are a number of negative changes associated with sedation and bed rest, however, this is not an exhaustive list.

Neuromusculoskeletal

- Muscle atrophy
- Reduced joint range of movement
- Neuromuscular changes, i.e. the electromechanical relationship between the nerve and muscle

Respiratory

- Reduced respiratory muscle strength
- Reduced cough strength
- Reduced gas exchange
- Reduced ventilation and increased atelectasis

Cardiovascular

- Increased risk of thrombosis
- Increased heart rate
- Reduced blood volume
- Orthostatic hypotension
- Reduced stroke volume

Psychological

- Altered mental health (e.g. anxiety, depression, PTSD)
- Cognitive issues
- Delirium

Other

- Pressure sores/tissue viability
- Malnutrition
- Reduced bone density

Aims of Rehabilitation

Early rehabilitation is essential to limit the impact of changes associated with prolonged critical care stay and should be started as soon as appropriate. Providing treatment to improve the patient's overall physical ability is not just the role of the physiotherapist, but requires effective multidisciplinary team (MDT) working, involving medical and nursing staff, other therapists, the patient's family, friends and the patient. The setting of goals should be discussed and agreed with the whole team, including the patient. Those involved in rehabilitation can support the patient to achieve their goals by providing a stimulating environment that encourages independence and maintains focus and orientation for the patient.

The physiotherapist's role is to coordinate the rehabilitation pathway to enable the patient to achieve their goals, and to act as a lead in the provision of physical rehabilitative treatment. However, other members of the MDT are crucial in the delivery of rehabilitation, for example, regular functional activities such as brushing hair, cleaning teeth, assisting with eating, performance of prescribed exercise programmes and practising of bed mobility for personal care. Additional benefits of rehabilitation include a reduction in delirium, reduced time weaning from mechanical ventilation, reduced length of stay in critical care and overall hospital admission, reduction in long-term disability and a faster return to normal functional ability.

Early Rehabilitation

A large number of research studies on rehabilitation in critical care focus on 'early' rehabilitation. Many studies involve services that require referral for physical therapeutic intervention, therefore the intervention group receives expedited referrals for rehabilitation. The UK model of healthcare provides the opportunity for early rehabilitation as physiotherapists assess respiratory and physical needs at the first assessment. The research on early rehabilitation supports and recommends that rehabilitation should commence as soon as it is safe to do so. This may be passive treatment during times of sedation, or becoming more active and participative from the commencement of sedation breaks.

Physiotherapy can be provided for patients on mechanical lung ventilation. This can be in the form of stationary bicycles especially adapted to lie on the bed to early ambulation using a portable ventilator, and can also be applied to patients on ECMO.

The NICE guidance for 'Rehabilitation after Critical Illness' advises that a short clinical assessment is required to identify patients at risk of physical or non-physical morbidity whilst in critical care. Patients deemed 'at risk' should receive comprehensive clinical assessments throughout their hospital admission and multitherapeutic input.

In collaboration with the patient, rehabilitation should start as early as possible, based on agreed physical and non-physical rehabilitation goals. These goals should be short, medium and long term. Review of the assessment should be performed before discharge from critical care, during ward base care, before discharge from hospital and 2–3 months after critical care discharge. In addition to supportive rehabilitative in-patient care and community care, follow-up clinics provide an environment to identify on-going physical and non-physical issues that require referral to other healthcare providers. The provision of critical care diaries to patients and their families at follow-up clinics supports patients with memory loss and adjusting to their period of critical illness.

Adjuncts and Treatment

A standard pattern of exercise progression can be seen in Figure 20.1.

Some patients require no additional therapeutic intervention other than exercise and movement facilitation. However, patients who have received high levels of sedation, paralysing agents and steroids often develop intensive care acquired weakness characterised by very poor global muscle power. These patients require increased input to progress. Physiotherapists have a repertoire of equipment that can be used within the critical care environment to aid physical recovery and functional ability. Manual handling equipment

Sedated	Non-sedated Poor strength	Alert Increasing strength
• Passive range of movement bed exercises • Bed bike • Neuromuscular electrical stimulation	• Bed or chair based, passive and active assisted exercise programme • Hoisting/pat sliding to chair • Sitting on edge of bed • Core stability strengthening • Limb strengthening • Sit to stand practice • Bed or chair cycling • Tilt table	• Active and resistive/weighted exercise programme • Standing practice • Stepping practice • Standing transfer bed to chair • Marching on spot • Walking • Bed/chair cycling or upright cycle

Figure 20.1 Pattern of exercise progression.

such as handling belts, frames, turn aids, standing hoist, tilt table and parallel bars could be used to aid the physical facilitation of patients. However, caution should be applied in view of recent surgical wounds, i.e. sternotomy and thoracotomy, as it is advised that patients should not weight bear through their upper limbs during the acute postoperative stage, and thoracic belts used with some manual handling equipment may be uncomfortable on wounds and drain sites. Pedals that can be used in bed or the chair in passive, active assisted or resistive mode have been shown to increase quadriceps strength and functional ability at hospital discharge.

There is emerging evidence that transcutaneous neuromuscular electrical stimulation may be beneficial in preserving muscle strength, specifically in patients who are critically unwell for longer periods, and therefore more likely to develop intensive care acquired weakness. The use of interactive video games within critical care can be used to improve muscle strength, balance, coordination and cognitive state.

Practicalities and Safety

To be able to conduct rehabilitation in critical care safely, a number of factors must be considered:

- Assessment of patient's psychological state, ability to follow commands and risk/benefit analysis if patient is or becomes delirious during treatment.
- Does the patient require glasses or hearing aids to be able to participate adequately during the session?
- Is the patient receiving or has recently discontinued an infusion of inotropes; is the cardiovascular system stable?
- What indwelling cannula, attachments and monitoring does the patient require? What are the risks if these are disconnected/dislodged during treatment?
- What is the patient's weaning plan? Do they need more ventilator support during rehabilitation and therefore a plan for treatment before reduction of support is commenced?
- If the patient is physically able, it is possible to progress rehabilitation to walking whilst on the ventilator (this can be achieved with a tracheostomy or endotracheal tube in situ, if the patient is tube tolerant).
- If the patient is moving outside of the critical care environment, i.e. to a gym, for rehabilitation, ensure there are hospital guidelines to ensure this is undertaken safely.
- The key to a successful rehabilitation session is the correct staff numbers and skill mix. It is common to require at least two members of physiotherapy staff (at least one registered physiotherapist) and the nurse. Additional support from healthcare support workers may be required if moving attachments or a wheelchair is needed.

Obtaining enough staff to provide rehabilitation throughout the day can be difficult. The use of physiotherapy assistant practitioners to provide some aspects of treatment is a growing practice within critical care and ward environments.

Outcome Measures

To assess a patient's progression throughout their critical care admission, the regular use of outcome measures is strongly recommended. Outcome measures can be used to assess level of impairment, physical functional status, mental functional status and neuropsychological functioning. The use of outcome measures should improve MDT communication, provide increased direction for treatment planning and help motivate patients. Physiotherapists mainly use measures to evaluate physical changes. There are a multitude of outcome measures available, however, many do not have adequate sensitivity to detect small physical changes found within debilitated critical care patients.

A basic test is the Medical Research Council scale of muscle strength. This is a validated and reliable scoring system from 0 (no movement) to 5 (normal power). However, this test is not linked to functional ability, and therefore its application for a patient's physical capability is limited.

There are many outcome measures such as Katz's Index of Independence in Activities of Daily Living, the Barthel Index, the Rivermead Motor Index and Functional Independence Measure and Functional Assessment Measure (known as FIM and FAM) which rank the patient's ability on functional tasks. However, these tools lack sufficient sensitivity to recognise small changes in critical care patients' ability.

Recently developed critical care outcome measures are Physical Functional Intensive Care test (PFIT) and the Chelsea Critical Care Physical Assessment tool (CPAx). PFIT assesses endurance, strength, cardiovascular capacity and functional level. The assessment components are: level of assistance required for sit to stand, steps per minute whilst marching on the spot, muscle strength of shoulder flexion and knee extension. This tool has proven reliability, validity and responsiveness. Patients need to be awake and cooperative to complete the PFIT, which is not representative of many critical care patients. The volitional aspects of testing will be dependent on patient effort, which may be poorly performed in critical care.

CPAx is a critical care specific tool that is sensitive enough to recognise small changes in ability in patients. It covers 10 dimensions involving respiratory function, bed and transfer ability and grip strength. These are graded 0–5 depending on the level of assistance required. It is validated for the general adult critical care population, but not for specialist conditions.

Barriers to Rehabilitation

Despite overwhelming positive evidence in support of rehabilitation in critical care, treatment is delayed or limited. The Intensive Care Society recommends rehabilitation assessment within 24 hours and 45 minutes of rehabilitation per day, 5 days per week by each therapy. In practice, it is difficult to achieve this for various reasons:

- Staff availability within physiotherapy and nursing;
- Respiratory treatments take priority;
- Rehabilitation is often time consuming and requires higher staff numbers to complete, and therefore is not undertaken in times of reduced staffing;
- Critical care patients are often too fatigued or are having other procedures throughout the day, which means they are unable to participate in more than one session per day.

However, rehabilitation should take place at times that are best for the patient. Patients also tend to have low motivation to participate in treatment, as there is little short-term gain, and it is sometimes difficult to appreciate how the current treatment leads to discharge.

To overcome barriers, good communication and the setting of daily plans will aid a united approach to rehabilitation. Providing clear explanation of roles, treatment options, anticipated progression and plans will clarify expectations and improve compliance with patients, their families and staff. Having a clear, documented plan for weaning, treatment and rest times ensures patients receive optimal care and achieve their goals in a timely manner.

Respiratory Physiotherapy

Complications of Cardiac and Thoracic Surgery

One of the common barriers to recovery following cardiothoracic surgery is postoperative pulmonary complications (PPCs) which are defined as 'an identifiable disease or dysfunction that is clinically relevant and adversely affects the clinical course'. For patients this can lead to an increased length of stay, increased morbidity and mortality. The primary role of the physiotherapist is to aid in preventing PPCs and to provide effective treatment to enable a quicker resolution when they occur.

Examples of common respiratory complications are:

- Atelectasis or lobar collapse;
- Sputum retention;
- Poor cough function due to pain or altered respiratory mechanics;
- Pneumonia;
- Respiratory failure.

Respiratory Physiotherapy – What can it Treat?

- Reduced lung volumes
- Sputum retention
- Increased work of breathing (WOB)
- Hypoxia

Respiratory Physiotherapy Techniques

Mobilisation

Mobilisation is an important treatment for all post-surgical patients and should be performed as early as possible, ideally the first morning after surgery or even on the day of surgery. In the early stages, mobilisation may entail sitting out of bed and/or marching on the spot, with this being progressed to ambulating as soon as is safe for the patient. However, static cycling is equally as effective. The aim of mobilisation is to increase the tidal volume and minute volume, therefore aiding expansion of atelectatic regions of lung. By improving lung volumes and therefore increasing airflow, secretions are mobilised enabling the patient to expectorate more easily. Patients should mobilise at a pace that equates to 3–4 on the Borg scale, or 11–14 on the modified Borg scale and on an appropriate level of supplementary oxygen if required. Patients being ventilated, on inotropes, on extracorporeal membrane oxygenation (ECMO) or ventricular assist devices (VAD) are not contraindicated to mobilising. Each patient should be assessed individually for their clinical need and safety.

Positioning

Positioning is often used in conjunction with other treatments to help maximise their effectiveness, for example side lying whilst ventilator hyperinflation is performed. It is also an important aspect of patient care in preventing PPCs by positioning patients optimally in bed or out of bed so as to reduce the time spent in recumbent postures such as supine and slumped sitting where lung volumes (in particular functional residual capacity) are naturally reduced.

An important aspect of positioning is to optimise the patient's ventilation/perfusion (V/Q) matching to improve oxygenation and ventilation. V/Q matching varies depending on whether the patient is ventilated or breathing spontaneously; this should be considered when positioning the patient. Ventilated patients will always have an element of V/Q mismatch due to the mechanics of positive pressure ventilation with the lung tissue and the effects of gravity on the pulmonary vasculature. In extreme cases of V/Q mismatch causing severe hypoxia, prone positioning has proven to be beneficial, but is a complicated procedure that requires an MDT approach.

Positioning can also be used to reduce WOB; for example, forward lean sitting or high side lying. These positions can be used with breathing control techniques for optimal effect.

Postural drainage uses gravity in specific positions to accurately drain certain lobes and segments of the lungs. These positions can be modified if the patient is unable to tolerate them, for example head-down tilt.

Thoracic Expansion Exercises (TEEs)/Deep Breathing Exercises (DBexs)

As with other techniques, TEEs should be used when indicated, therefore they should not be used routinely with post cardiac and thoracic surgery patients or as a substitution for patients who can mobilise. TEEs should be used with patients who are unable to mobilise, for example a bed bound patient. TEEs should be performed in the most effective position for improving lung volumes. The aim of TEEs is to improve lung volumes and mobilise secretions by increasing tidal volume and using collateral ventilation channels such as the pores of Kohn, communications of Lambert and pathways of Martin.

Active Cycle of Breathing Technique (ACBT)

ACBT is a breathing technique using alternating breathing techniques in a cyclical pattern including deep breaths, inspiratory holds, end-inspiratory sniffs, breathing control, forced expiration technique (FET) and cough. An example of ACBT can be seen in Figure 20.2. To prevent fatigue a period of breathing control is used to allow the patient to recover before starting another cycle.

ACBT can be used in conjunction with postural drainage to optimise sputum clearance and also with the ventilator or IPPV to augment the tidal volume further.

FET can also be varied depending on the position of the sputum. Low lung volume FET assists with distal airway sputum whereas high volume FET assists with proximal airway sputum.

ACBT can also be used in conjunction with airway clearance adjuncts such as Acapella, Flutter and OPEP. This provides additional mechanical assistance by using a combination of expiratory airflow oscillations and resistance to provide splinting for airways, in particular for patients with chronic sputum producing diseases such as bronchiectasis.

Incentive Spirometry (IS)

Incentive spirometry is the use of a mechanical device to aid augmentation of tidal volume by providing visual feedback as a motivator. Within the cardiac and thoracic surgical population, studies have shown no benefit to the use of IS when compared with early mobilisation in preventing PPCs; however, they may have a role in high risk surgical patients.

Manual Techniques – Percussion, Vibrations and Shaking

Manual techniques are rarely used in the cardiothoracic surgical patient population due to the incisions and potential for causing additional pain and impeding wound healing. When other airway clearance techniques have not been successful, manual techniques

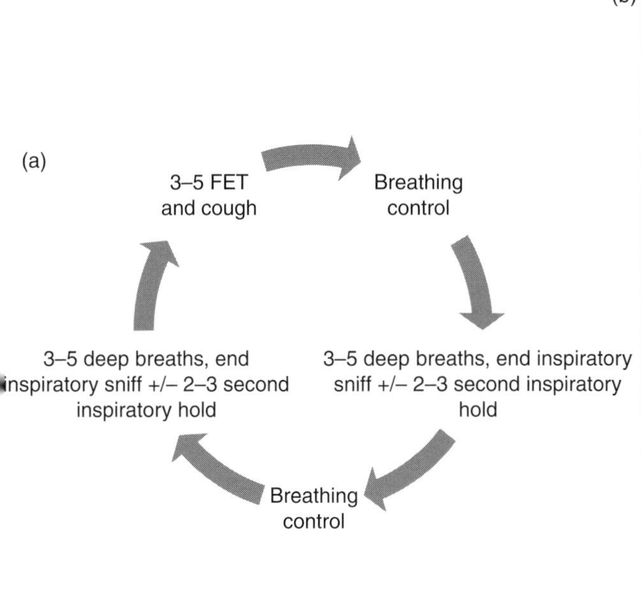

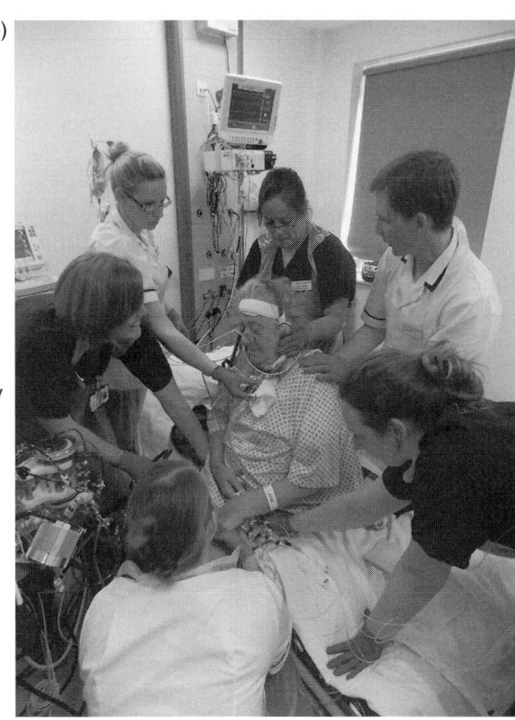

Figure 20.2 Example of ACBT. (a) Cycle of breathing exercises. (b) Sitting on the edge of the bed rehabilitation with a patient on ECMO. (A black and white version of this figure (b) will appear in some formats. For the colour version, please refer to the plate section.)

may be useful, with modification of hand position and force used dependent on wound location.

Intermittent Positive Pressure Ventilation (IPPV)

Also called the 'Bird', IPPV is a technique for delivering positive pressure during the inspiratory phase via a mouthpiece or facemask to the spontaneously ventilating patient. A PEEP valve can be applied to the exhalation port to provide airway splinting if required. An Acapella may be placed on the expiratory port to provide airway splinting and expiratory oscillation. Oxygen or medical air can be delivered via IPPV so that it may be used with patients who are CO_2 retainers. The use of IPPV requires the patient to be able to follow commands and be compliant with treatment in order to synchronise with the device. IPPV augments the patient's tidal volume to aid alveolar recruitment and sputum clearance through collateral ventilation channels. It can also improve the patient's cough through increased tidal volume. IPPV can be used in conjunction with ACBT.

Typical settings are a low trigger pressure to enable inspiratory effort without increasing WOB and an inspiratory effort of 10–15 cmH_2O, titrating these pressures up to the required level, normally 20–25 cmH_2O. Slow inspiratory flows provide optimal rise time for deep breathing; however faster flows may be required for patients who are short of breath with a high respiration rate.

Manual Hyperinflation (MHI)

MHI is a technique used with patients who have an artificial airway to augment their tidal volume up to 100% of their resting tidal volume, aiming for peak inspiratory airway pressures of between 20–35 cmH_2O so that the technique is effective (alveolar opening pressures >20 cmH_2O) and avoiding barotrauma (<40 cmH_2O). A manometer should always be used when performing MHI in combination with a rebreathe circuit using 10–15 l of oxygen. The patient should be optimally positioned for the area of lung that is to be treated, taking into consideration that air takes the path of least resistance and as this technique delivers positive pressure the uppermost lung in side lying would be preferentially ventilated. This technique should not be used with patients requiring a high positive end expiratory pressure (PEEP) (>10 cmH_2O), high FiO_2, nitric oxide, high ventilator pressures or poor lung compliance, as disconnection from the ventilator would cause a loss of pressure, lung decruitment and potential sudden hypoxaemia, for example in a patient with acute respiratory distress syndrome (ARDS).

MHI can be done with a varying technique depending on the aim of the treatment. A combination of slow inspirations with inspiratory pauses and quick releases of the bag are utilised to improve lung recruitment and sputum clearance.

Ventilator Hyperinflation (VHI)

Studies have shown that MHI and VHI are comparable as treatment techniques with the added safety benefit of VHI.

VHI works through the same mechanisms as MHI but using adjustment of settings on the ventilator avoids disconnection, therefore VHI can be used in patients with high PEEP requirements. The tidal volume and pressure limits are the same as MHI but with the added benefit of being able to assess lung compliance before and after treatment, and monitor tidal volume changes so that effectiveness of treatment and response to the technique can be measured. Inspiratory pauses are also achievable on most ventilators. The concentration of oxygen can be maintained at current settings with VHI, whereas with MHI the flow rate of oxygen and therefore concentration must be increased to allow the bag to inflate. Depending on mode of ventilation, tidal volume, inspiratory pressure, set respiratory rate and alarm limits may be adjusted to achieve increased lung volumes. Guidelines and competency assessment are required to ensure safety and standard of practice.

Manual Insufflation Exsufflation (I:E Sufflation), for example Cough Assist

In the author's opinion, the use of I:E sufflation has become more common within the critical care setting as the patient population often has problems with a weakened cough through various mechanisms such as pain, anxiety/reduced confidence, altered chest wall mechanics, phrenic or laryngeal nerve damage and intensive care acquired weakness. Manual I:E can be used on patients with either an artificial airway or spontaneously breathing, through a catheter mount or facemask respectively. Oxygen can be entrained into the circuit as required to prevent hypoxaemia during treatment. Prior to treatment the patient should be positioned optimally. The settings can be titrated as required for patient comfort and treatment optimisation. An example of settings would be an insufflation of 20–25 cmH_2O and an exsufflation of −30 to −40 cmH_2O. Devices can be set to run in manual and automated setting modes dependent on the treatment requirements.

The mechanism of action for I:E sufflation is through provision of an augmented tidal volume on inspiration and utilisation of collateral ventilation to reverse atelectasis. The sudden swing of pressure into exsufflation causes shearing forces, which loosens sputum from the airway walls. The rapid exsufflation with negative pressure aids the movement of sputum more proximally so that it can be either coughed up or suctioned out. It can be used in conjunction with the patient's own cough effort or on its own if a cough is absent.

CPAP/NIV/HFNO

Other modes of respiratory support may be instigated by a physiotherapist to support the patient in respiratory failure. CPAP and HFNO are used for type 1 respiratory failure and NIV for type 2 respiratory failure.

Suction – Endotracheal, Tracheostomy, Nasopharyngeal, Oral

Suction can be carried out via various artificial airways to aid sputum clearance when a patient is unable to do so themselves. A thorough assessment is required before suctioning a patient. Indications for suction include retained secretions secondary to:

- Sedation and paralysing agents;
- The presence of an artificial airway;
- Ineffective cough secondary to drowsiness;
- Pain;
- Ineffective cough secondary to global weakness.

The suction technique is the same for each method with the only variance being the depth the suction catheter is inserted to. The patient should receive pre-oxygenation and postoxygenation to prevent hypoxaemia. The suction catheter selected should not have an external diameter greater than one-half of the internal diameter of the airway. A pressure of −10 to −20 kPa is recommended with the application of continuous pressure rather than intermittent pressure, and no rotation of the catheter during withdrawal as this has no extra benefit for sputum removal and can lead to increased mucosal damage. A suction time of no longer than 10–15 seconds is advised as longer is associated with increased risk of mucosal damage and hypoxaemia.

Respiratory Muscle Training

Respiratory muscle training is not commonly used in critical care, however there is emerging evidence within this population that it increases inspiratory muscle strength as assessed by maximal inspiratory pressure measurements, and may contribute towards expediting the weaning process.

Considerations for Specific Patient Groups in Critical Care

Cardiac

- Haemodynamic instability can limit the use of some physiotherapy techniques.
- Adequate analgesia is important for preventing PPCs and for enabling patients to be involved with their therapy.
- Some routine cardiac surgical patients may not require physiotherapy in critical care if they are discharged within <24 hours.

Thoracic

- Enhanced recovery programmes (ERP) are used with this patient group and should be followed as soon as possible even in critical care.
- Positive pressure treatment techniques need to be carefully reasoned due to anastomosis problems.
- Adequate analgesia is important for preventing PPCs and for enabling patients to be involved with their therapy.

ECMO

- Physiotherapists provide treatment for patients on venovenous (VV) and venoarterial (VA) ECMO.
- Respiratory physiotherapy techniques can be limited in these patient groups due to cannulation sites, widespread ARDS and consolidation, and low tidal volumes despite high ventilation pressures.
- ECMO patients tend to have the same physical decline as other critical care patients due to sedation and bed rest. Therefore early rehabilitation is also essential for this group, with the additional challenge of ECMO cannulation, circuit and limited ventilator reserve.
- Each ECMO centre has their own protocol with this specialist cohort of patients.

Learning Points

- It is important to consider all of the physiological systems affected and the psychological impact of being in critical care when rehabilitating critically unwell patients.
- Rehabilitation within critical care should be commenced as soon as it is clinically safe to do so to minimise the effects of bed rest.
- Rehabilitation is safe to perform on patients in critical care, and each patient should be assessed individually for their rehabilitation needs.
- Respiratory physiotherapy is effective at treating diagnosed postoperative pulmonary complications in the cardiac and thoracic surgical populations.
- The use of prophylactic respiratory physiotherapy is not recommended or supported by evidence to prevent postoperative pulmonary complications in routine, low risk surgical patients.

Further Reading

Berney S, Denehy L. A comparison of the effects of manual and ventilator hyperinflation on static lung compliance and sputum production in intubated and ventilated intensive care patients. *Physiotherapy Research International*. 2002; 7: 100–108.

Brasher PA, McClelland KH, Denehy L, Story I. Does removal of deep breathing exercises from a physiotherapy program including pre-operative education and early mobilisation after cardiac surgery alter patient outcomes? *Australian Journal of Physiotherapy*. 2003; 49: 165–173.

Gosselink E, Bott J, Johnson M, et al. Physiotherapy for adult patients with critical illness: recommendations of the European Respiratory Society and European Society of Intensive Care Medicine Task Force on Physiotherapy for critically ill patients. *Intensive Care Medicine*. 2008; 34: 1188–1199.

Gosselink R, Schrever K, Cops P, et al. Incentive spirometry does not enhance recovery after thoracic surgery. *Critical Care Medicine*. 2000; 28: 679–683.

Hirschhorn AD, Richards DA, Mungovan SF, et al. Does the mode of exercise influence recovery of functional capacity in the early postoperative period after coronary artery bypass graft surgery? A randomized controlled trial. *Interactive Cardiovascular and Thoracic Surgery*. 2012; 15: 995–1003.

NICE. *Rehabilitation after Critical Illness*. London: NICE, 2009. Report No.: CG83.

Schweickert W, Pohlman M, Pohlman A, et al. Early physical and occupational therapy in mechanically ventilated, critically ill patients: a randomised controlled trial. *Lancet*. 2009; 373: 1874–1882.

Stiller K. Safety issues that should be considered when mobilizing critically ill patients. *Critical Care Clinics*. 2007; 23: 35–53.

Warner D. Preventing postoperative pulmonary complications. *Anesthesiology*. 2000; 92: 1467–1472.

Zeppos L, Patman S, Berney S, et al. Physiotherapy intervention in intensive care is safe: an observational study. *Australian Journal of Physiotherapy*. 2007; 53: 279–283.

MCQs

1. **What pathologies can respiratory physiotherapy treat?**
   (a) Reduced lung volumes
   (b) Sputum retention
   (c) Increased work of breathing
   (d) Reduced PaO_2
   (e) All of the above
2. **Which respiratory physiotherapy technique has no evidence to support its use in routine cardiac and thoracic surgical patients?**
   (a) Mobilising
   (b) Active cycle of breathing techniques
   (c) Incentive spirometry
   (d) Manual hyperinflation
   (e) Ventilator hyperinflation
3. **Which of these complications can occur due to bed rest within the critical care unit (choose all that apply)?**
   (a) Muscle atrophy
   (b) Reduced joint range of movement
   (c) Reduced respiratory muscle strength
   (d) Reduced cough strength
   (e) All of the above
4. **At what stage should rehabilitation commence in a critical care patient?**
   (a) Once the patient is no longer sedated
   (b) Once cardiovascularly stable
   (c) As early as is safe to do so
   (d) Once agreed by the MDT
   (e) Once the patient is off the ventilator
5. **For how long should a patient receive rehabilitation from each therapy for the 5 days a week stipulated by the NICE guidance?**
   (a) 15 minutes
   (b) 25 minutes
   (c) 30 minutes
   (d) 45 minutes
   (e) 60 minutes

Exercise answers are available on p.468. Alternatively, take the test online at www.cambridge.org/CardiothoracicMCQ

Chapter 21

Percutaneous Mechanical Circulatory Support

Evgeny Pavlushkov and Marius Berman

Short-term mechanical circulatory support (MCS) devices are used to maintain haemodynamic stability in cardiogenic shock and provide reliable oxygenation in acute cardiovascular and/or respiratory failure. Percutaneous MCS is used as a temporary measure (bridge) to recovery of definitive management. These devices may be used in the following clinical situations:

- high-risk coronary or valve interventions (complex coronary anatomy, impaired LV function);
- cardiogenic shock complicating myocardial infarction;
- acute decompensated heart failure;
- bridge to heart transplantation;
- bridge to recovery after allograft rejection;
- postcardiotomy cardiogenic shock;
- acute cardiac, lung allograft failure;
- circulatory support before and after durable LVAD implantation;
- bridge to recovery after lung transplantation for pulmonary hypertension.

The main objectives of temporary circulatory support are to provide systemic perfusion and secondly unload the heart to maximise chances of its recovery.

Several types of percutaneous MCS options are available for advanced heart/lung failure: intra-aortic balloon pump (IABP), extracorporeal membrane oxygenation, Impella axial flow pump and TandemHeart centrifugal pump.

IABP

IABP is the most commonly used device for mechanical circulatory support. It consists of two parts: the intra-aortic balloon itself (IAB), a double lumen catheter 7–8 French size; and a console containing the controller, pump and helium cylinder. The outer lumen of the balloon is a gas containing chamber and the inner lumen is open to the aorta and is used for direct arterial pressure monitoring. Helium is less soluble than some other gases (CO_2) and it is also less dense, which reduces travel time along the circuit and allows quick inflation and deflation of the balloon. IABP is usually positioned in the descending thoracic aorta through one of the femoral arteries using the Seldinger technique.

The balloon inflates during diastole and displaces the blood in the aorta, increasing diastolic and mean pressure and thus augmenting coronary perfusion. During systole, the balloon deflates, producing some vacuum effect and therefore reducing the afterload for the left ventricle (LV) and systolic pressure. This results in improved emptying of the heart, and therefore reduction of the wall stress of the heart. Other important haemodynamic effects of IABP include: reduction of the heart rate (by 20%), decrease in the pulmonary capillary wedge pressure (by 20%) and rise in cardiac output (by 0.5 l/min or by 20%). The magnitude of the effects can vary and depends on many factors: the volume of the IABP (bigger balloons, 50 cm^3, displace more volume, hence are more effective), its optimal position (the tip of the IAB should be located 2 cm caudally to the origin of the left subclavian artery which is easily confirmed by chest X-ray as 2 cm above the tracheal bifurcation, or by TOE), optimal timing of the inflation/deflation cycle, heart rate and aortic compliance.

The maximum haemodynamic effect from IABP counterpulsation is achieved when it is set to inflate just after the aortic valve closure (dichrotic notch on the arterial trace) and deflate just before aortic valve opening (upstroke part on the arterial waveform of the next cardiac cycle). Early/late inflation as well as early/late deflation could lead to suboptimal diastolic augmentation and reduced haemodynamic benefits of the IABP (Figure 21.1).

Timing of IABP is important as too early or too late inflation or deflation can in fact worsen cardiac

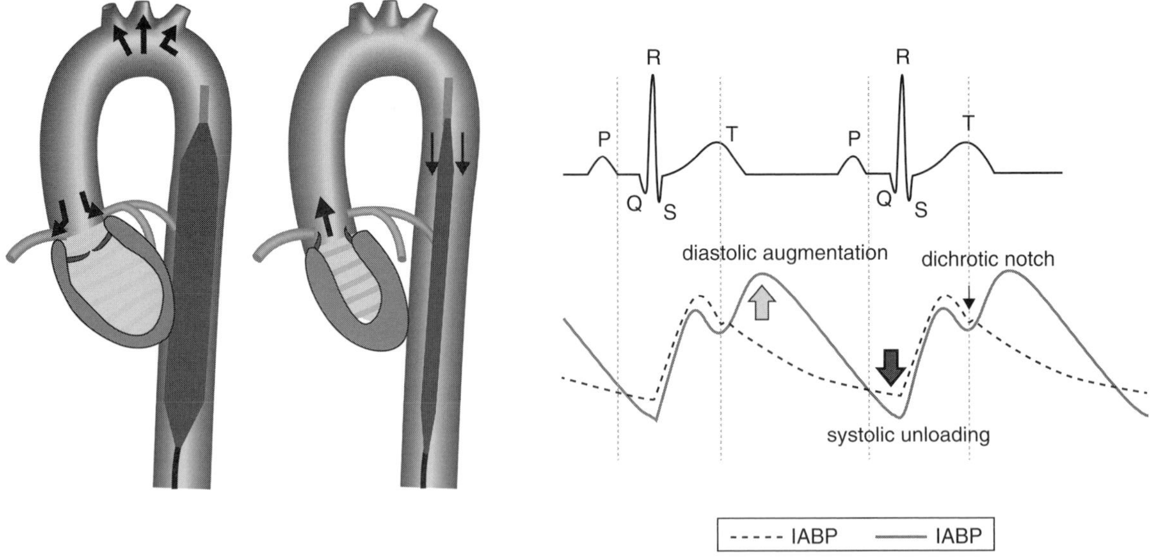

Figure 21.1 Aortic pressure waveform with IABP off and on. Inflation of the balloon corresponds to the augmented diastolic pressure. Note the decrease of systolic pressure in assisted beat.

output and increase preload. Figure 21.2 illustrates some problems with timing of IABP.

Alternative Routes for IABP Insertion

Transfemoral percutaneous method of insertion is a first choice option for IAB insertion. However, it can be technically challenging or impossible in patients with significant peripheral vascular disease or previous vascular operations on the iliofemoral segment or just small calibre arteries. Subclavian, axillary, brachial arteries have been reported to be used to access the thoracic aorta for IAB placement in different clinical settings. Direct access to the thoracic aorta can also be used as the entry site for the IABP. This technique requires an open chest and is therefore used intraoperatively during cardiac operations (Figure 21.3).

Duration and Weaning from the IABP

There is little evidence to guide the optimal duration and weaning strategy for IABP. Duration is mainly determined by patient need, institutional preferences and individual clinical circumstances of the patients. Given the invasive nature of the device, the IABP should be removed as soon as the haemodynamic situation improves to the degree when the IABP is no longer required or a more definitive treatment option becomes available. The weaning of the IABP can be achieved either by gradual (over hours) decrease of the ratio of augmented to non-augmented beats (from 1:1 to 1:2, 1:3 and so on), or by degree of inflation of the balloon, or a combination of both. According to a recent survey, 57% of centres preferred to wean by reducing the ratio.

Complications of IABP use include vascular laceration or dissection, limb ischaemia, haemorrhage, balloon rupture, cholesterol embolisation, cerebrovascular events, haemolysis, thrombocytopenia, infection and peripheral neuropathy. The incidence of major complications should not exceed 2.6% and IABP related mortality is only 0.5%.

Anticoagulation has traditionally been used with IABP to reduce thrombosis and embolisation. However, existing data suggest that omitting heparin is safe in the context of IABP counterpulsation and allows avoidance of bleeding related complications.

Common indications for IABP use have been refractory hypotension or haemodynamic instability of cardiac origin, mechanical complications of MI (MR, VSD), postcardiotomy shock, as a bridge to cardiac surgery/transplantation or as an adjunct in high-risk coronary interventions. However, the data from large randomised trials and meta-analysis (IABP-SHOCK II) downgraded the impact of IABP in patients with acute MI complicated by cardiogenic shock undergoing revascularisation as it did not reduce mortality. The routine use of IABP is no longer

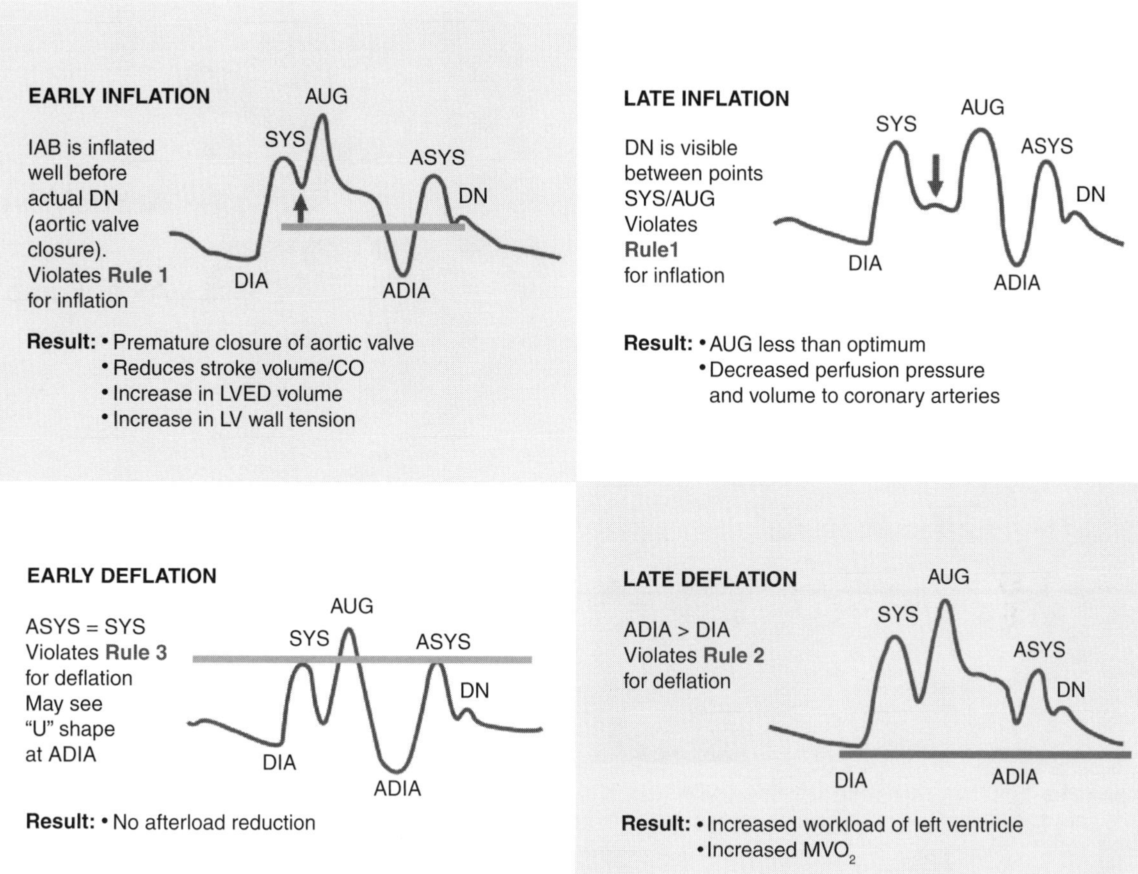

Figure 21.2 Timing problems with IABP. (A black and white version of this figure will appear in some formats. For the colour version, please refer to the plate section.)

recommended by the European Society of Cardiology (ESC) for this indication.

Impella (LV to Aorta)

The Impella (Abiomed, USA) is a temporary ventricular assist device designed for percutaneous insertion through the femoral artery, which is advanced along the aorta, across the aortic valve into the left ventricle (Figure 21.4). It employs the principle of the Archimedes screw: blood enters the inflow at the tip of the catheter and is transported to the ascending aorta, generating non-pulsatile axial flow. Four versions of the pump are currently available: Impella 2.5 (flow up to 2.5 l/min), Impella CP (3.0–4.0 l/min), Impella 5.0 (up to 5 l/min) and Impella RP (designed for right ventricular (RV) support, this drains the blood from the inferior vena cava and expels it to the pulmonary artery, providing flow above 4 l/min). Most of these modifications can be inserted using a standard Seldinger technique. Impella 5.0, although providing higher flows, requires surgical cut-down to the artery due to its bigger size, making it less convenient for insertion in an emergency setting.

Working in series with the LV (or RV in the case of Impella RP) the device unloads the ventricle, reduces wall stress and oxygen demand, reduces ventricular stroke work, and increases mean arterial pressure and cardiac output. Impella 2.5 is approved for use for up to 5 hours in the USA and up to 6 days in Europe. Impella RP can provide temporary support for up to 14 days. The safety and feasibility of Impella pumps as well as their positive impact on haemodynamics were demonstrated in trials involving different patient

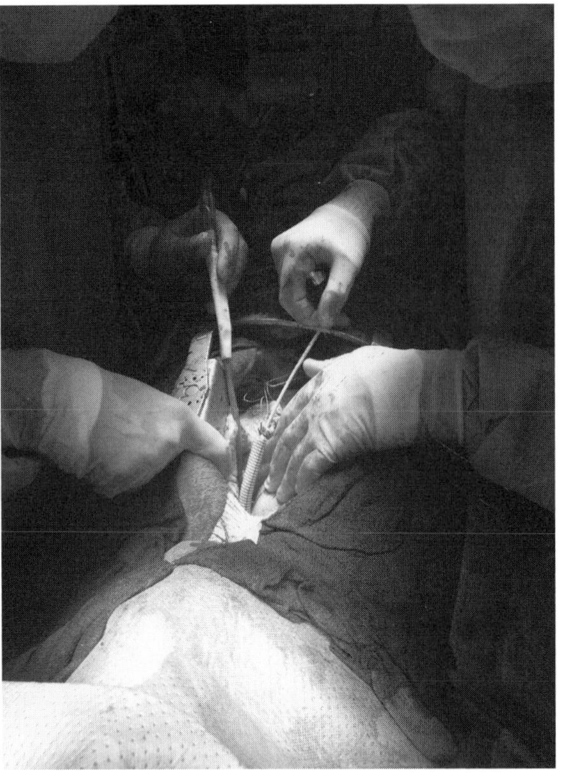

Figure 21.3 Transthoracic approach to IABP insertion. (A black and white version of this figure will appear in some formats. For the colour version, please refer to the plate section.)

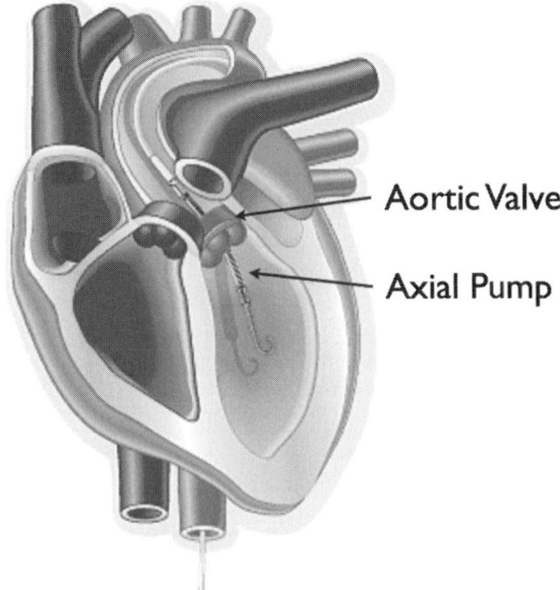

Figure 21.4 Diagram demonstrating the Impella LP2.5 axial flow left ventricular assist device sitting across the aortic valve. Reprinted with permission from Abiomed (Aachen, Germany), the manufacturer of this device. (A black and white version of this figure will appear in some formats. For the colour version, please refer to the plate section.)

populations: acute myocardial infarction complicated by cardiogenic shock (ISAR-Shock), high-risk PCI (PROTECT II) and postcardiotomy cardiogenic shock (RECOVER-I). However, the impact of these devices on mortality has yet to be established in larger randomised trials.

TandemHeart (LA to Aorta)

TandemHeart (CardiacAssist, USA) is a percutaneously inserted device, which uses an extracorporeal centrifugal pump to transfer blood from the left atrium to the aorta via the femoral artery in non-pulsatile fashion (Figure 21.5). In contrast to Impella, TandemHeart requires two cannulas: the inflow cannula inserted via the femoral vein and positioned into the left atrium through the interatrial septum, and the second cannula in the femoral artery. This configuration bypasses the left ventricle, offloads it and reduces LV workload. The circuit can be reconfigured to support the right ventricle. For this purpose, the inflow cannula is positioned into the right atrium and blood is returned to the pulmonary artery. TandemHeart can generate flow of up to 5 l/min (with 19F arterial cannula). It is approved for circulatory support for up to 6 hours in the USA and up to 30 days in Europe. Preserved RV function is essential for optimal performance of TandemHeart as well as for Impella since both devices depend on LV preload.

Similar to Impella, clinical data available suggest that TandemHeart increases blood pressure and cardiac index, decreases pulmonary capillary pressure and improves perfusion of end organs; however, evidence of influence on mortality is lacking at present.

Comparison of Percutaneous MCS Devices

Each percutaneous device for short-term mechanical circulatory support has unique characteristics and haemodynamic profile. The choice of the particular device should be guided by specific cardiovascular

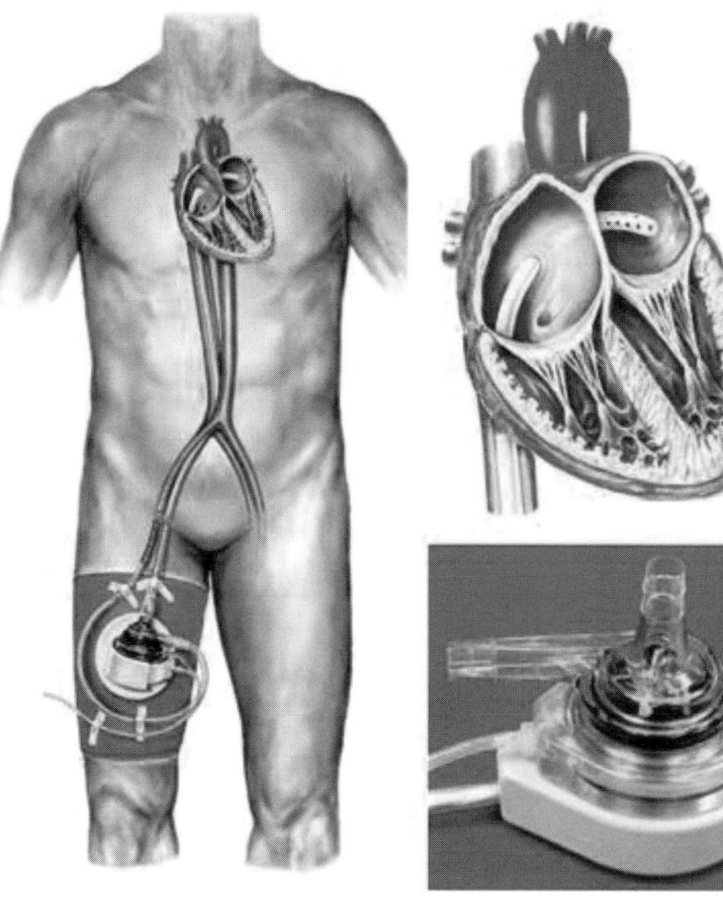

Figure 21.5 TandemHeart consists of a 21F inflow cannula in the left atrium after femoral venous access and transseptal puncture and a 15F to 17F arterial cannula in the iliac artery. Reproduced with permission from Naidu (2011). (A black and white version of this figure will appear in some formats. For the colour version, please refer to the plate section.)

goals and clinical context of the individual patient (Table 21.1).

Most of the current knowledge and guidelines for percutaneous mechanical circulatory support are based on observational data, expert opinion, retrospective studies and consensus agreement. More prospective randomised studies are needed to establish evidence-based background for this fast evolving field of cardiothoracic medicine.

Learning Points

- There are two main objectives of temporary circulatory support: (1) to provide perfusion for end organs and (2) to unload the heart to maximise chances of its recovery or bridge for further therapy.
- Each percutaneous device for short-term mechanical circulatory support has unique characteristics and haemodynamic profile.
- The choice of the particular device should be guided by specific cardiovascular and respiratory goals, and clinical context of an individual patient as well as expertise available.

Further Reading

Bignami E, Tritapepe L, Pasin L, et al. A survey on the use of intra-aortic balloon pump in cardiac surgery. *Annals of Cardiac Anaesthesia*. 2012; 15: 274–277.

Cheng JM, den Uil CA, Hoeks SE, et al. Percutaneous left ventricular assist devices vs. intra-aortic balloon pump counterpulsation for treatment of cardiogenic shock: a meta-analysis of controlled trials. *European Heart Journal*. 2009; 30: 2102–2108.

Ferguson JJ, Cohen M, Freedman RJ, et al. The current practice of intra-aortic balloon counterpulsation: results from the Benchmark Registry. *Journal of the American College of Cardiology*. 2001; 38: 1456–1462.

Table 21.1 Comparison of percutaneous MCS devices

	IABP	ECMO	TandemHeart	Impella 2.5	Impela 5.0	Impella RP
Pump mechanism	**Pneumatic**	**Centrifugal**	**Centrifugal**	**Axial flow**	**Axial flow**	**Axial flow**
Cannula size	7–9F	18–21F inflow, 15–22F outflow	21F inflow, 15–17F outflow	13F	22F	22F
Insertion technique	Descending aorta via femoral artery, Seldinger technique	Inflow cannula into RA via femoral vein, outflow cannula into descending aorta via femoral artery	21F inflow cannula into LA via femoral vein and transseptal puncture and 15–17F outflow cannula into femoral artery	12F catheter placed retrogradely across aortic valve via femoral artery	21F catheter placed retrogradely across aortic valve via surgical cutdown of femoral artery	Via the femoral vein, into the right atrium, across the tricuspid and pulmonic valves, and into the pulmonary artery
Haemodynamic support	0.5 l/min	>4.5 l/min	4 l/min	2.5 l/min	5.0 l/min	>4 l/min
Implantation time	+	++	++++	++	++++	++
Risk of limb ischaemia	+	+++	+++	++	++	+
Anticoagulation	+	+++	+++	+	+	+
Haemolysis	+	++	++	++	++	++
Management complexity	+	+++	++++	++	++	++

Modified from Ouweneel and Henriques (2012).

Kogan A, Preisman S, Sternik L, et al. Heparin-free management of intra-aortic balloon pump after cardiac surgery. *Journal of Cardiac Surgery*. 2012; 27: 434–437.

Naido SS. Contemporary reviews in cardiovascular medicine, novel percutaneous cardiac assist devices: the science of and indications for hemodynamic support. *Circulation*. 2011; 123: 533–543.

Ouweneel DM, Henriques JPS. Percutaneous cardiac support devices for cardiogenic shock: current indications and recommendations. *Heart*. 2012; 98: 1246–1254.

Pucher PH, Cummings IG, Shipolini AR, McCormack DJ. Is heparin needed for patients with an intra-aortic balloon pump? *Interactive Cardiovascular and Thoracic Surgery*. 2012; 15: 136–139.

Rihal CS, Naidu SS, Givertz MM, et al. SCAI/ACC/HFSA/STS Clinical Expert Consensus Statement on the use of percutaneous mechanical circulatory support devices in cardiovascular care. *Journal of the American College of Cardiology*. 2015; 65: e7–26.

Scheidt S, Wilner G, Mueller H, et al. Intra-aortic balloon counterpulsation in cardiogenic shock. Report of a co-operative clinical trial. *New England Journal of Medicine*. 1973; 288: 979–984.

Thiele H, Sick P, Boudriot E, et al. Randomized comparison of intra-aortic balloon support with a percutaneous left ventricular assist device in patients with revascularized acute myocardial infarction complicated by cardiogenic shock. *European Heart Journal*. 2005; 26: 1276–1283.

Thiele H, Zeymer U, Neumann F-J, et al. Intra-aortic balloon counterpulsation in acute myocardial infarction complicated by cardiogenic shock (IABP-SHOCK II): final 12 month results of a randomised, open-label trial. *Lancet*. 2013; 382: 1638–1645.

Unverzagt S, Buerke M, de Waha A, et al. Intra-aortic balloon pump counterpulsation (IABP) for myocardial infarction complicated by cardiogenic shock. *Cochrane Database of Systematic Reviews*. 2015; 3: CD007398.

Windecker S, Kolh P, Alfonso F, et al. 2014 ESC/EACTS guidelines on myocardial revascularization. *Revista Española de Cardiología (English Edition)*. 2015; 68: 144.

MCQs

1. **What are the advantages of using helium in IABP?**
   (a) High solubility
   (b) Availability
   (c) Low density
   (d) High biocompatibility
   (e) Lack of thrombogenicity

2. **What is the optimal position of the IAB tip on chest X-ray?**
   (a) 2 cm below bifurcation of the carina
   (b) 1 cm cranial to the origin of the left subclavian artery
   (c) Highest point of the aortic arch
   (d) 2 cm cephalad to bifurcation of the trachea
   (e) At the level of angle of Louis

3. **Which of the following is a haemodynamic effect of IABP?**
   (a) Decrease systolic BP
   (b) Has no effect on mean BP
   (c) Decrease diastolic BP
   (d) Has no effect on heart rate
   (e) Increase pulmonary capillary wedge pressure

4. **The least common complication of IABP is:**
   (a) Peripheral neuropathy
   (b) Bleeding
   (c) Limb ischaemia
   (d) Infection
   (e) Thrombocytopenia

5. **All statements regarding TandemHeart are true except one:**
   (a) Requires interatrial septum puncture
   (b) Reduces pulmonary capillary wedge pressure
   (c) Improves organ perfusion
   (d) Was demonstrated to reduce mortality
   (e) Is licensed for use for up to 30 days in Europe

Exercise answers are available on p.468. Alternatively, take the test online at www.cambridge.org/CardiothoracicMCQ

Chapter 22

Ventricular Assist Devices (VAD)

Harikrishna M Doshi and Steven SL Tsui

Introduction

The UK National Heart Failure Audit 2013–2014 estimated that there are 2 million people in the UK suffering from heart failure, a figure that is likely to rise due to improved survival following heart attack and more effective treatment. Heart transplant has remained a therapeutic cornerstone for patients with end stage heart failure when optimum medical therapy has failed. It offers an excellent short and long term outcome with median survival of 11 years. Major limitation in expansion of heart transplantation is the limited availability of donor organs. According to the 2015 Annual Report on Cardiothoracic Transplantation in the UK, only 30% of non-urgent heart patients were transplanted within 6 months of their listing, during which time 9% died awaiting a transplant.

Exciting new developments are being trialled to increase the donor pool, for example transplanting heart from donation after circulatory death. However, donor heart numbers will never satisfy the rapidly expanding cohort of patients who require cardiac replacement therapy. Many such patients are over 75 years of age and with comorbidities which make them unsuitable for heart transplant. Besides, many patients on the list deteriorate and cannot survive the wait for a transplant without other intervention. In 1978, Dr Denton Cooley reported the first successful bridging to transplant using mechanical heart support, and since then rapid strides have been made in the field of mechanical circulatory support devices (MCSD).

Ventricular assist devices (VAD) are mechanical blood pumps that work in parallel or in series with the native ventricle(s). Most commonly, a left ventricular assist device (LVAD) draws oxygenated blood from the left atrium or ventricle and returns it to the aorta; a right ventricular assist device (RVAD) draws venous blood from the right atrium or ventricle and returns it to the pulmonary artery. VADs provide life support for patients with failing ventricle(s) by maintaining perfusion to vital organs. The basic components of a VAD system are as follows.

1. Inflow cannula – for draining blood from the patient to the blood pump.
2. Blood pump – usually consists of a motor and an impeller for driving the blood.
3. Outflow cannula – returns blood from the pump to the patient.
4. Driveline – a composite cable for the transfer of electrical signal and power between the blood pump and the console.
5. Controller – controls blood pump operation and displays pump performance parameters.
6. Rechargeable battery pack – to power the motor of the blood pump.

Temporary MCSD

Indications

For patients who require mechanical circulatory support (MCS) over days to weeks, temporary devices may be used as a bridge to recovery, bridge to transplant or bridge to a longer term device, i.e. bridge to bridge. Temporary MCS (Table 22.1) may be indicated in patients with decompensated heart failure, acute cardiogenic shock or arrested patients with uncertain neurology, to assess recovery of end organ function before deciding on the next step (bridge to decision). They may also be considered for patients with severe symptomatic acute heart failure where myocardial recovery is anticipated, for example fulminant myocarditis. Occasionally it may be indicated in post-cardiotomy cardiogenic shock where weaning from cardiopulmonary bypass fails. The aim is to provide short term support while other medical problems such

Table 22.1 Indications of temporary MCSD

- Cardiogenic shock due to acute myocardial infarction
- Postcardiotomy shock
- High risk percutaneous coronary intervention, ventricular tachycardia ablation
- Acute rejection post cardiac transplant with haemodynamic compromise
- Bridge to LVAD or transplant
- Right ventricular failure

as infection, renal failure and neurological assessment can be dealt with and prognosis of the patient can be better defined.

Types of Temporary Mechanical Circulatory Support

1. Extracorporeal life support (ECLS) or cardiac ECMO (see Chapter 23):
   (a) Peripheral cannulation;
   (b) Central cannulation.
2. Percutaneous devices:
   (a) Intra-aortic balloon pump (IABP) (see Chapter 21);
   (b) Impella devices: 2.5, CP, 5.0, LD (Abiomed Inc., MA, USA), transaortic intraventricular pump;
   (c) TandemHeart System (CardiacAssist, Inc., PA, USA), transvenous transseptal left atrium to arterial pump.
3. Non-percutaneous devices: for example CentriMag centrifugal pump (Thoratec Corporation, CA, USA).

   Characteristics of Impella devices are given in Table 22.2, and contraindications to temporary MCSD are listed in Table 22.3.

Non-percutaneous Devices: CentriMag

The CentriMag (Thoratec Corporation, CA, USA) system is an extracorporeal circulatory support device. It has a disposable polycarbonate pump (Figure 22.1) mounted on a reusable motor. The magnetically levitated pump impeller provides a friction-free blood path which minimises blood trauma and haemolysis. It is approved for use for up to 30 days and has been widely adopted with reasonable success. This device can produce flows of up to 9.9 l min^{-1} in vitro and uses a priming volume of 31 ml. The CentriMag system can be used to provide left or right ventricular support and it can also be used in an ECMO circuit. The CentriMag system is most commonly implanted through a sternotomy incision in the operating room. Anchoring of the percutaneous vascular cannulae as they traverse the anterior abdominal wall allows the patient limited mobilisation and rehabilitation. Bedside pump changes can be performed in awake patients every 30 days, allowing patients to be supported for months on the CentriMag system.

Implantable or Durable VAD

Implantable VAD are designed to provide durable circulatory support for patients with advanced heart faiure. Patients can be supported with these devices for months or years. The main advantage of durable VAD is to allow implanted patients to return to the community and lead an active life. Currently, LVAD is the most common type of durable MCSD implanted.

Types of Long Term VAD

- First generation LVADs such as the Thoratec HeartMate XVE, PVAD and IVAD were pulsatile devices. They consisted of a pump housing with a diaphragm and unidirectional valves to pump blood in a pulsatile manner, typically ejecting 80 to 100 times per minute. In 2001, results of the REMATCH study showed that patients with end stage heart failure not eligible for transplantation who were implanted with the HeartMate VE had a significant survival advantage at 1 year compared with patients who were managed with optimal medical therapy. However, first generation LVAD were bulky, less durable and had high complication rates including bleeding, infection, stroke, device malfunction and development of right heart failure. Over the last 10 years, outcomes with continuous flow devices have been shown to be far superior to outcomes with pulsatile devices. As a result, first generation LVADs have become obsolete.
- Second generation VAD are axial flow pumps with a single moving impeller mounted on mechanical bearings spinning at high speed. They are smaller in size and more durable than their predecessors. These devices are silent in operation and provide continuous blood flow with reduced

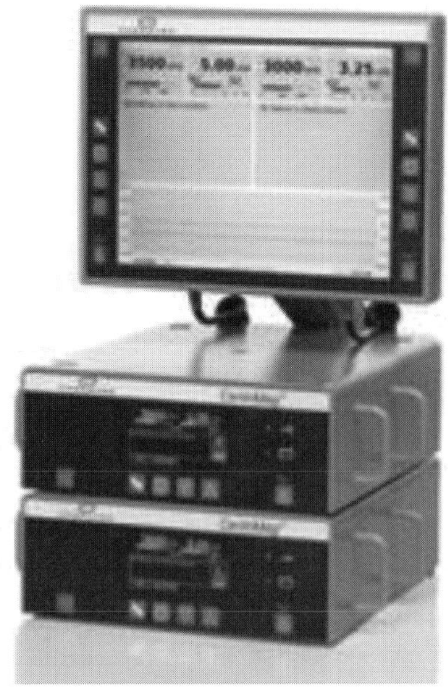

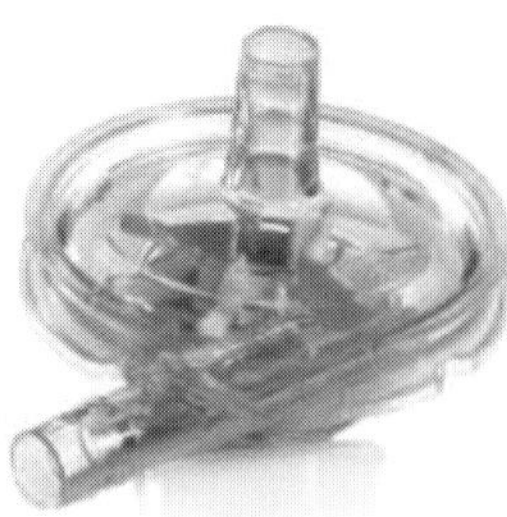

Figure 22.1 CentriMag primary console and centrifugal pump (courtesy of Thoratec Corporation, CA, USA). (A black and white version of this figure will appear in some formats. For the colour version, please refer to the plate section.)

Table 22.2 Types of Impella devices and characteristics

Device and function	Impella 2.5	Impella CP	Impella 5/LD	Impella RP
Access	Percutaneous femoral	Percutaneous femoral	Surgical, axillary, femoral or ascending aorta	Percutaneous femoral vein
Maximum output, litre per minute	2.5	4.0	5.0	4.6
Catheter size, F	9	9	9	11
Motor size, F	12	14	21	22
Maximum revolutions per minute (rpm)	51,000	46,000	33,000	33,000
EU approved duration of use, days	5	5	10	14

pulsatility. They include devices like the Thoratec HeartMate II and Jarvik 2000 amongst others.

- Third generation pumps use hydrodynamic and/or electromagnetic bearings to suspend the impeller inside the pump housing, thereby eliminating contact between moving parts and avoiding friction. Their smaller size allows intrathoracic placement (Figure 22.2) and obviates the need for an abdominal pump pocket. Examples of third generation devices include the HeartWare HVAD and the Thoratec HeartMate 3.

Indications and Patient Selection

Current indications for LVAD therapy can be broadly classified as follows.

1. Bridge to transplant (BTT): For patients eligible for heart transplant but deteriorating before a donor heart is available.
2. Bridge to candidacy (BTC): For patients with contraindication(s) to heart transplantation secondary to advanced heart failure, such as renal dysfunction or pulmonary hypertension, that is potentially reversible after a period of LVAD support.

Table 22.3 Contraindications and complications associated with temporary circulatory support

Device	Contraindications	Complications
All devices	Severe peripheral vascular disease Irreversible neurological disease Sepsis	Bleeding Vascular injury Infection Neurological injury
Impella	LV thrombus Moderate to severe aortic stenosis Moderate to severe aortic insufficiency Mechanical aortic valve Recent TIA or stroke Aortic abnormalities Contraindication to anticoagulation	Haemolysis Pump migration Aortic valve injury Aortic insufficiency Tamponade due to LV perforation Ventricular arrhythmia
TandemHeart	Ventricular septal defect Moderate to severe aortic insufficiency Contraindication to anticoagulation	Cannula migration Tamponade due to perforation Thromboembolism Air embolism during cannula insertion Interatrial shunt development
CentriMag	Contraindication to anticoagulation	Thromboembolic events Air embolism

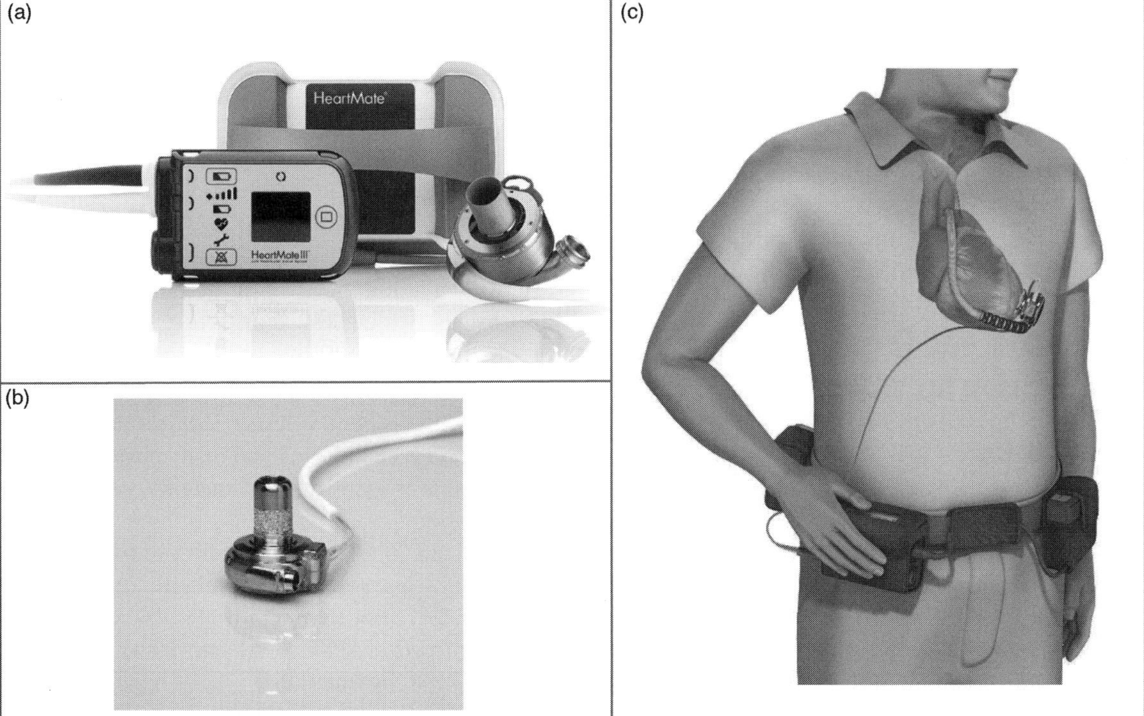

Figure 22.2 (a) HeartMate 3 with its controller. (b) HeartWare HVAD with driveline. (c) Diagram of a patient with a HeartWare HVAD sited in the left ventricular apex and a percutaneous driveline going to a wearable controller and batteries. (Courtesy of Thoratec Corporation, CA, USA and HeartWare Corporation, MA, USA). (A black and white version of this figure will appear in some formats. For the colour version, please refer to the plate section.)

Table 22.4 INTERMACS profile descriptions

INTERMACS level	Definition	Description
1: Critical cardiogenic shock	Crash and burn	Haemodynamic instability in spite of increasing doses of catecholamines and/or mechanical circulatory support with critical hypoperfusion of target organs (severe cardiogenic shock)
2: Progressive decline	Sliding on inotropes	Intravenous inotropic support with acceptable blood pressure but rapid deterioration of kidney function, nutritional state, or signs of congestion
3: Stable but inotrope dependent	Dependent stability	Patient with stable blood pressure, organ function, nutrition and symptoms on continuous intravenous inotropic support (or a temporary circulatory support device or both), but demonstrating repeated failure to wean from support due to recurrent symptomatic hypotension or renal dysfunction
4: Resting symptoms	Frequent fliers	Patient can be stabilised close to normal volume status but experiences daily symptoms of congestion at rest or during activities of daily living (ADL); doses of diuretics generally fluctuate at very high levels
5: Exertion intolerant	Housebound	Complete cessation of physical activity, stable at rest, but frequently with moderate water retention and some level of kidney dysfunction
6: Exertion limited	Walking wounded	Minor limitation on physical activity and absence of congestion while at rest; easily fatigued by light activity
7: Advanced NYHA III	Placeholder	Patient in NYHA functional class II or III with no current or recent unstable fluid balance

3. Destination therapy (DT): As a permanent treatment for patients who are not eligible for heart transplant.

The Interagency Registry for Mechanically Assisted Circulatory Support (INTERMACS) is a North American registry established in 2005 to collect clinical data on patients receiving mechanical circulatory support. The INTERMACS stratifies patients with advanced heart failure into seven profiles based on their clinical status as outlined in Table 22.4.

Risk Factors and Their Assessment for Implantation for VAD

Cardiac Factors

Right ventricular (RV) function is one of the most important parameters to consider before LVAD implantation. Adequacy of RV function after LVAD implantation is a balance between the intrinsic RV function and the RV afterload. During RV ejection, RV afterload is proportionate to pulmonary artery pressure, which is a sum of the impedance of the pulmonary vasculature and the left atrial pressure.

A number of risk prediction models for RV failure following LVAD insertion have been described. However, these have all been derived from retrospective studies on patients supported with pulsatile devices. A validation study on continuous-flow LVAD recipients showed that none of the described risk models reliably predicted the need for RVAD support post LVAD. In any case, preoperative risk models would not be able to take account of intraoperative events.

Echocardiographic Assessment

Numerous echocardiographic parameters for assessing RV function have been described and some are listed below. However, their usefulness in predicting RV failure after LVAD implant are still debated.

- Visual assessment: volumetric assessment of RV function is challenging and many physicians rely on visual assessment to estimate RV size and function.
- Tricuspid annular plane systolic excursion (TAPSE): assess RV systolic longitudinal function of RV. TAPSE < 16 mm indicates RV systolic dysfunction. TAPSE correlates well with RV global systolic function.
- Right ventricular index of myocardial performance (RIMP): RIMP > 0.40 by pulse Doppler indicates RV dysfunction; fractional area change (FAC) <35% indicates dysfunction.

- RV diastolic function can be assessed by tricuspid inflow velocities, pulsed Doppler imaging of hepatic veins and measurement of IVC size and collapsibility. Tricuspid E/A ratio <0.8 indicates impaired relaxation.
- Tricuspid valve regurgitation (TR) can help assessment of right atrial pressure in the absence of right ventricular outflow obstruction (RVOT). TR velocity >2.8 to 2.9 m/second corresponds to systolic pulmonary artery pressure (PAP) of approximately 36 mmHg assuming right atrial pressure (RAP) of 3–5 mmHg, and indicates elevated RV systolic and pulmonary artery pressures.

Invasive Monitoring

Transpulmonary gradient (TPG) is the difference between mean pulmonary artery pressure and left atrial pressure (estimated by pulmonary capillary wedge pressure (PCWP)). Assessment of the TPG is recommended for the detection of pulmonary vascular disease in left heart conditions associated with elevated pulmonary venous pressure. Elevated pulmonary vascular resistance (PVR) is present when PVR is ≥ 3 Wood units or TPG ≥ 12 mmHg.

The optimal haemodynamic parameters of preoperative RV function indicating a low likelihood of developing RV failure include:

- CVP ≤8 mmHg
- PCWP <18 mmHg
- CVP/PCWP ≤0.66
- PVR ≤2 Wood units
- RVSWI ≥400 l min^{-2} m^{-2}.

Right ventricular stroke work index (RVSWI) = CI/HR × 1000 × (mPAP – RAP), where CI is cardiac index in l m^{-2}; HR is heart rate in beats per minute; mPAP is mean pulmonary artery pressure in mmHg; RAP is right atrial pressure in mmHg.

Other intracardiac lesions such as aortic valve regurgitation or patent foramen ovale (PFO) will need to be corrected because after LVAD implantation, decompression of the left heart will increase the amount of aortic valve regurgitation and allow right to left shunt across a PFO, leading to significant oxygen desaturation. It will also increase the chance of paradoxical embolisation. Intracardiac repairs have an impact on the conduct of surgery since use of cardiopulmonary bypass will be required with or without a period of myocardial ischaemia.

Non-cardiac Factors

Presence of end organ dysfunction is a risk factor for poor outcome. Contraindication to LVAD implantation includes the following:

- Irreversible end organ failure, especially renal, hepatic and respiratory system. Parameters such as elevated bilirubin, elevated prothrombin time suggest an auto-anticoagulated state signifying reduced hepatic synthetic function and may be signs of underlying right heart dysfunction.
- Active and uncontrolled systemic infection.
- Irreversible neurological injury. Recent stroke will increase risk of bleeding.
- Contraindication to systemic anticoagulation or antiplatelet therapy.
- History of substance abuse or non-compliance.

Perioperative Management of Patients Undergoing VAD Implantation

Preoperative Preparations

The assessment of patients for LVAD therapy consists of detailed medical, physical and psychosocial assessment. Cardiovascular investigations including echocardiogram and right heart catheterisation are essential to assess right heart function. CT scan of the thorax may help identify underlying pulmonary disease and establishes the anatomy of the LV apex. Other investigations to assess kidney, liver and lung function are essential. Abnormal results will require further evaluation and efforts to optimise end organ functions must be undertaken. Active malignancy should be ruled out. Infection screen is essential to rule out any existing infection, hepatitis or HIV. Dental checks should be carried out prior to surgery. Psychosocial assessment is very important. Patients will need robust social support and a thorough understanding of possible complications.

It is important to educate the patient and their families about risks and benefits of LVAD therapy. The patient's understanding and expectations are important considerations before accepting the patient for long term LVAD therapy. In complex situations, psychiatric evaluation may be pivotal in decision making. Extensive teaching and training through multidisciplinary support staff is an integral part in preparing patients for LVAD implantation.

Table 22.5 Essential components of VAD care

- Exercise and physical therapy
- Nutrition
- VAD self-care
- Driveline site dressing changes
- System controller checks
- VAD log book
- Activity restrictions

Care in the ITU, Ward and Discharge Planning

Durable LVAD implantations are generally carried out using a median sternotomy incision and cardiopulmonary bypass. Some units adopt a minimally invasive approach using ministernotomy and small left anterior thoracotomy. Careful consideration is necessary whilst dressing and securing the drive line exit site right from theatre.

The early phase of patient return into the ITU requires careful monitoring and optimisation of pump speed, flows, filling status and attention to tissue perfusion status using various parameters such as mixed venous oxygen saturation. Any coagulopathy should be corrected to avoid bleeding. A pulmonary artery catheter is a valuable tool to assist with haemodynamic monitoring. Acidosis, hypoxia and hypercapnoea can potentially result in pulmonary vasoconstriction and therefore should be avoided. If inhaled nitric oxide was required during the implant procedure, early weaning may be facilitated by the use of nebulised iloprost at intervals. The latter could be transitioned to oral sildenafil after extubation if required.

After a period of stability has been achieved, early return to spontaneous respiration and extubation allows for early mobilisation and minimises the period on mechanical ventilation. Careful fluid balance monitoring and aggressive use of diuretic therapy helps optimise intravascular volume status. Renal, liver and other end organ function must be regularly assessed to make sure that they are recovering with improved end organ perfusion. The key issues are early mobilisation, good nutrition and meticulous wound care (see Table 22.5).

The VAD Team

Care of the patient with durable VAD necessitates a team approach (Figure 22.3). The VAD team consists of a multitude of specialties including cardiologists, surgeons, intensivists, physiotherapists, nutritionists, microbiologists, pharmacists and psychiatrists. VAD coordinators are central in organising various activities for these patients. They remain a constant point of contact in maintaining continuity of care when patients have been discharged into the community. VAD coordinators are usually specialist nurses or physician assistants with an in depth knowledge of all aspects of LVAD care, equipment and support. Once the decision to implant a durable LVAD is made, they are actively involved in education and training of the patient and family. They also work with other team members and arrange activities with patient and family in such a way that they are ready for self-care by the time of discharge. Following discharge, they help transition home visits to community nurses but remain a point of contact for the patient and their family for support or advice.

Chronic heart failure can lead to malnutrition and wasting which may have a negative impact on wound healing and immune resistance. The dietician monitors caloric intake and makes recommendations on nutritional supplements. Physiotherapists help with early mobilisation and restore patient confidence and independence.

There are some issues unique to the clinical management of LVAD supported patients.

- Measurement of blood pressure: Due to the continuous flow nature of modern LVADs, Korotkoff sounds cannot be heard with a stethoscope while measuring blood pressure. For the same reason, non-invasive blood pressure measurement devices are ineffective. A Doppler probe and a sphygmomanometer must be used to measure average blood pressure.
- High blood pressure: Hypertension is commonly observed after implantable LVAD therapy. This will have a negative impact on pump flow since LVAD output is preload dependent and afterload sensitive. Hypertension has also been shown to be associated with an increased risk of intracranial haemorrhage in LVAD supported patients. Therefore, careful control of blood pressure with vasodilator therapy is essential.
- Anticoagulation: Due to the contact of blood component to artificial surfaces, anticoagulation is necessary. Current International Society for Heart and Lung Transplantation (ISHLT) recommendation is to prescribe both antiplatelet

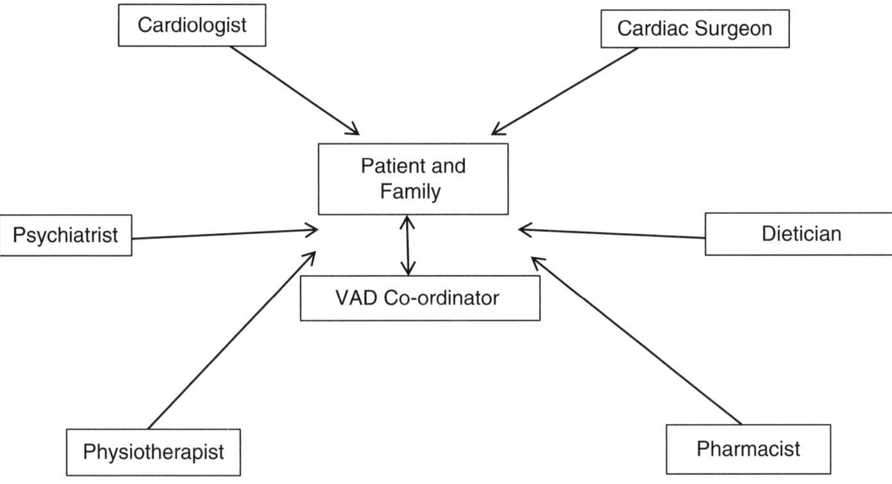

Figure 22.3 Configuration of multispecialty VAD team.

therapy and warfarin to maintain device specific INR.

- Arrhythmia and issues with ICD devices: One of the issues with excessive pump speed may be suction causing collapse of the LV cavity and ventricular arrhythmias. For patients who already have a pacemaker or automatic implantable cardioverter defibrillator (AICD) implanted preoperatively, the device may need to be checked for compatibility and may need readjustment to prevent unnecessary pacing or shocks.

VAD Self-Care

In addition to medical and physical fitness, discharge planning requires complete independence for VAD self-care. The main elements for self-care are:

- Once at home, patient and carer should be able to take care of the equipment and ensure regular cleaning.
- Drive line dressing needs meticulous attention to aseptic techniques since exit site infection remains one of the commonest complications and once established are very difficult to eradicate.
- Regular record of vital signs and LVAD parameters is essential.
- Shower is allowed with care of the console and batteries but bathing and swimming is not permitted. Similarly, contact sports and strenuous activities are discouraged due to fear of device damage or drive line trauma.

Postimplant Adverse Events

Bleeding

Early postoperative bleeding remains common after LVAD implantation. Immediately post implant, the patient may be coagulopathic due to preoperative hepatic congestion or antiplatelet therapy. A low threshold for re-exploration is required since tamponade is poorly tolerated in these patients. Haemodynamic instability, rising filling pressures and unexplained alterations in LVAD flows should raise suspicion of tamponade. Causes of such postoperative haemorrhage can be bleeding from anastomotic sites, leaky connections or generalised coagulopathy. Later onset bleeding may be caused by anticoagulation therapy in combination with development of acquired von Willebrand factor deficiency. Late bleeding may occur from mucosal surfaces, especially from the gastrointestinal tract through arteriovenous malformations. The HeartMate II destination therapy trial showed rates of bleeding requiring transfusion at 1.66 and 1.13 events per patient year in early and mid trial groups.

Right Heart Failure

LVAD causes geometric changes to the right ventricle and impairs global RV contractility with leftward septal shift. The RV performance following LVAD implantation depends on many factors including afterload, preload, ventriculoarterial coupling and ventricular interdependence. The INTERMACS registry defines the right ventricular failure based on the following diagnostic criteria:

- Symptoms and signs of persistent right ventricular dysfunction.
- Central venous pressure (CVP) >18 mmHg with a cardiac index (CI) < 2.0 l min^{-1} m^{-2} in the absence of elevated pulmonary capillary wedge pressure >18 mmHg, tamponade, ventricular arrhythmias or pneumothorax.
- Requiring RVAD implantation, or requiring inhaled nitric oxide or inotropic therapy for duration of more than 1 week at any time after LVAD implantation.

The severity of right heart failure has been classified based on the following criteria:

Severe: Need for RVAD.

Moderate: Need for inotrope or intravenous or inhaled pulmonary vasodilator (e.g. prostaglandin E or inhaled nitric oxide).

Mild: Meeting two of the four clinical criteria listed below:

- CVP > 18 mmHg or mean RA pressure >18 mmHg;
- CI < 2.3 l min^{-1} m^{-2};
- Ascites or evidence of moderate to worse peripheral oedema;
- Evidence of elevated CVP by echo (dilated inferior vena cava without collapse);
- physical exam (signs of increased jugular venous pressure).

In the HeartMate II destination therapy trial, 20% of patients received extended inotropic therapy for persistent heart failure and 4% required placement of RVAD. In the HeartWare ADVANCE BTT trial, 25% of patients were dependent on prolonged inotropes and 3% required RVAD. The 1-year mortality rate for patients requiring RVAD support following LVAD implantation increases significantly from 21% to 44%.

RV failure can be managed as follows:

- Preventive strategies include minimising fluid load, early extubation, maintaining sinus rhythm and high index of suspicion.
- Management strategies include inotropes, pulmonary vasodilators such as inhaled nitric oxide (up to 5 ppm) and nebulised iloprost (2.5–10.0 μg every 3 hours) or RVAD support.

Infection

Sepsis occurs in 11–26% of LVAD patients and accounts for 21–25% of LVAD deaths. The commonest area for infection is at the driveline exit site. The fifth annual report of INTERMACS reported a driveline infection rate of 8 per 100 patient months. Infections of device pocket, blood and endocarditis are some of the other complications. Left pleural collection and formation of empyema is a possible complication for a thoracotomy approach to implantation. High index of suspicion, prompt treatment and active involvement of the microbiology team in the day to day management of these patients yields better long term outcome. ISHLT has published guidelines for identification of specific MCSD related infections.

Thrombosis

Patients with LVAD are at risk of pump thrombosis and other thromboembolic events. Pump thrombosis can lead to pump obstruction, which can be fatal. It results from ingestion of debris into the LVAD or in situ thrombosis and can occur as an early or late complication. Risk factors for pump thrombosis include inadequate anticoagulation, atrial fibrillation, hypercoagulable state and coexistent infection. For continuous flow LVAD, the rate of pump thrombosis ranges from 0.01 to 0.11 per patient year. Patients may present with manifestations of heart failure and evidence of haemolysis in the form of red or reddish brown urine, worsening renal function, increased serum LDH level and/or increased free plasma haemoglobin. The LVAD power consumption is abnormally high with either power spikes or gradual increase in power requirement. Treatment of pump thrombosis includes augmentation of anticoagulation, thrombolytic therapy and pump exchange.

Neurological Complications

Neurological complication remains a leading cause of long term morbidity and mortality. Stroke in LVAD patients predominantly occurs in the right hemisphere. The fifth annual report of INTERMACS reports a stroke risk of 11% at 1 year and 17% at 2 years. The mechanism of stroke may be partial cannula obstruction, deformation of blood pathway within the pump, twisting or kinking of outflow graft, inadequate anticoagulation and infection.

Aortic Regurgitation

De novo aortic regurgitation has been observed in up to 25% of patients supported by continuous flow LVAD therapy. This complication is more commonly seen in patients in whom the aortic valve does not open during LVAD support. Regurgitant aortic flow reduces the overall effectiveness of LVAD support and leads to volume load of the left ventricle. Asymptomatic patients can be treated by optimisation of pump flow under echo guidance to allow intermittent aortic valve opening. Symptomatic patients will need higher pump flows in the initial phases and in late phases may require surgical intervention to replace the aortic valve with a bioprosthesis or urgent transplant.

Device Failure

This is generally a late complication. Failed external components can generally be replaced and hence may not be life threatening. Internal component failure is uncommon these days except for pump thrombosis. Third generation continuous flow LVAD pumps use magnetic levitation impellers, which do not have mechanical wear and are expected to be more durable than the earlier generation devices.

Other complications include ventricular arrhythmias, abdominal complications like device erosions or adhesions and haemolysis.

Outcomes

For patients with advanced heart failure, outcome with medical therapy is dismal. LVAD support provides marked improvement in quality of life, functional status and survival. Outcomes following treatment with continuous flow LVAD have continued to improve over the last decade. However, despite improvements in survival and symptoms of heart failure, LVAD therapy is still associated with a significant risk of major adverse events.

Survival

The HeartWare ADVANCE BTT trial reported a 1-year survival of 86%. The HeartMate II DT trial reported an actuarial survival of 58% at 2 years. The fifth annual report of INTERMACS reported 1, 2, 3 and 4 years survival at 80%, 70%, 59% and 47% respectively.

Quality of Life and Functional Status

One of the main objectives of LVAD therapy is to improve quality of life and functional status of patients with symptomatic heart failure. In the HeartMate II BTT and DT trials, approximately 80% of patients reported improvement in their functional status from NYHA class IIIb to IV at baseline to class I or II.

Between January 2007 and December 2013, there have been 10 industry funded trials and registries, 10 multicentre reports and multiple single centre observational experience. Using data from these studies, a single page pictogram (Figure 22.4) has been developed which provides patients, their families and clinicians a visual representation of the full spectrum of possible outcomes with LVAD therapy at 1 year. This serves as a useful tool to explain what could be expected with LVAD therapy and help guide the decision making process.

Future Directions

Third generation continuous flow LVADs have already paved the way for smaller devices that do not require an abdominal pump pocket. This allows LVAD implantation through less invasive approaches and obviates the need for full sternotomy incision or even the use of CPB. This may reduce some of the common early postimplant complications such as bleeding and right ventricular failure.

Driveline exit site infection remains the Achilles' heel of long term LVAD therapy at present. Device manufacturers have been developing fully implantable LVAD systems with internal batteries that could be recharged wirelessly. Such transcutaneous energy transfer systems (TETS) have already been tested in small clinical trials as a proof of concept and have shown promise.

With increasing experience of LVAD, it has become apparent that chronic low arterial pulsatility may contribute to complications such as arteriovenous malformations and aortic valve insufficiency. Pump speed modulation that allows for greater pulsatility is a focus of much research. Similarly, miniaturisation and remote monitoring are the other areas of active development.

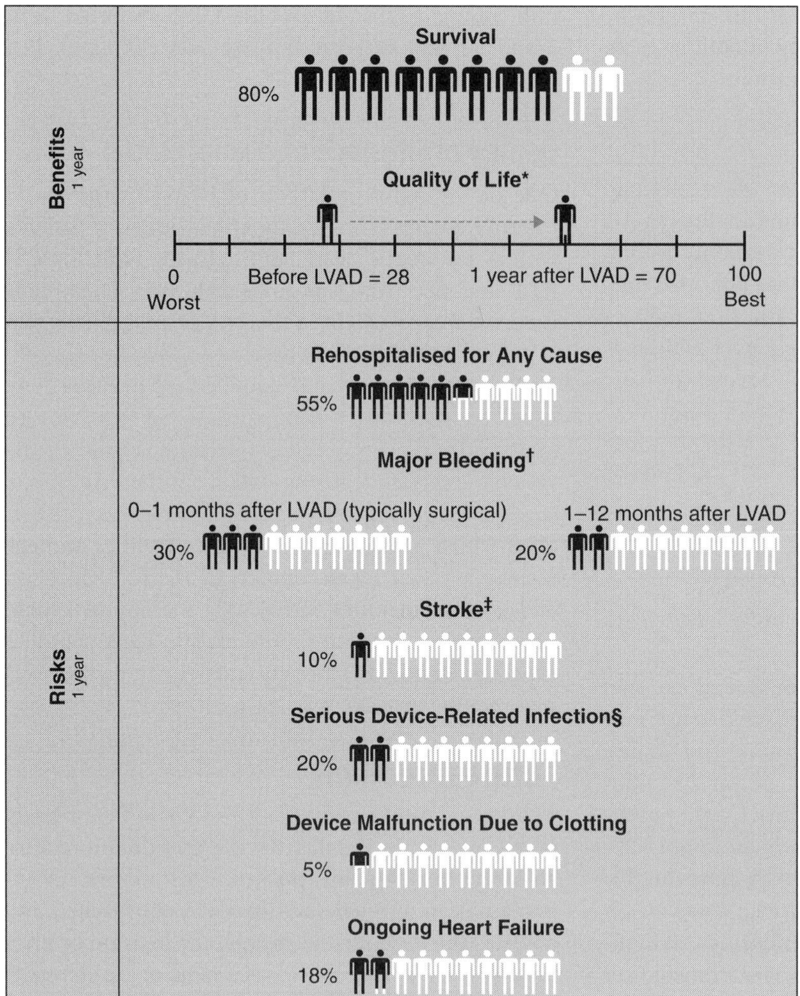

Figure 22.4 1 year outcomes using weighted averages from LVAD studies (combined BTT and DT therapies). Shaded area, affected; white areas, not affected. Quality of Life: Kansas City cardiomyopathy questionnaire score. Major bleeding: requiring transfusion or urgent medical attention. Stroke: ischaemic 5% ± 5, haemorrhagic 5% ±4. Serious device related infection: driveline 18% ± 2, pump pocket 2% ± 2. Device malfunction due to clotting: typically requiring surgery to replace the device. On-going heart failure: requiring inotropes >2 weeks after implant 15% ± 7, requiring right ventricular assist device 3% ± 2.

LVAD therapy is a rapidly evolving branch of medicine. As the demand for donor hearts continues to outstrip the limited supply, we shall have to increasingly rely on the development of devices with better durability and reduced long term complications.

Learning Points

- Heart transplantation remains the best treatment option for advanced heart failure patients with median survival of 11 years post transplant.
- However, with a rising incidence of heart failure and shortages of donor hearts, it is inevitable that more patients will require MCSD as a substitute.
- The experience of managing MCS has grown considerably leading to better patient selection and improved outcomes.
- For patients ineligible for transplantation, implantable LVAD can serve as an alternative treatment or destination therapy.
- Development of newer devices that enable less invasive implantation with lower adverse event

rates will further increase the adoption of this life saving therapy.

Further Reading

Cheng JM, Den Uil CA, Hoeks SE, et al. Percutaneous left ventricular assist devices vs intra-aortic balloon pump counterpulsation for treatment of cardiogenic shock: a meta analysis of controlled trials. *European Heart Journal*. 2009; 30: 2102–2108.

Gilotra NA, Stevens GR. Temporary mechanical circulatory support: a review of the options, indications, and outcomes. *Clinical Medical Insights: Cardiology*. 2014; 8(Suppl 1): 75–85.

Kirklin JK, Naftel DC, Kormos RL, et al. Fifth INTERMACS annual report: risk factor analysis from more than 6,000 mechanical circulatory support patients. *Journal of Heart and Lung Transplantation*. 2013; 32: 141–156.

Mancini D, Colombo PC. Left ventricular assist devices. a rapidly evolving alternative to transplant. *Journal of the American College of Cardiology*. 2015; 65: 2542–2555.

Park SJ, Milano CA, Tatooles AJ, et al. HeartMate II Clinical Investigators. Outcomes in advanced heart failure patients with left ventricular assist devices for destination therapy. *Circulation: Heart Failure*. 2012; 5: 241–248.

Patlolla B, Beygui R, Haddad F. Right-ventricular failure following left ventricle assist device implantation. *Current Opinion in Cardiology*. 2013; 28: 223–233.

Rose EA, Gelijns AC, Moskowitz AJ, et al. Randomized Evaluation of Mechanical Assistance for the Treatment of Congestive Heart Failure (REMATCH) Study Group. Long-term mechanical left ventricular assistance for end-stage heart failure. *New England Journal of Medicine*. 2001; 345: 1435–1443.

Slaughter MS, Pagani, FD, McGee EC, et al. HeartWare ventricular assist system for bridge to transplant: combined results of the bridge to transplant and continued access protocol trial. *Journal of Heart and Lung Transplantation*. 2013; 32: 675–683.

Stevenson LW, Pagani FD, Young JB, et al. INTERMACS profiles of advanced heart failure: the current picture. *Journal of Heart and Lung Transplantation*. 2009; 28: 535–540.

Uriel N, Han J, Morrison KA, et al. Device thrombosis in HeartMate II continuous-flow left ventricular assist devices: a multifactorial phenomenon. *Journal of Heart and Lung Transplantation*. 2014; 33: 51.

MCQs

1. **A 55 year old man with dilated cardiomyopathy presents with signs of advanced heart failure and severe left ventricular dysfunction. He is blood group O and has a body mass index of 26. His right heart catheter measured a transpulmonary gradient of 8 mmHg, pulmonary vascular resistance of 3 Wood units and cardiac index of 1.6 l m^{-2}. He has remained inotrope dependent despite several attempts at weaning and his renal function is normal. He does not have signs of sepsis. He has been on the urgent heart transplant waiting list for 10 weeks with no suitable offers. His best therapeutic option is:**
   (a) Continue on inotropic support indefinitely until a donor heart becomes available
   (b) Insert intra-aortic balloon pump and wait indefinitely until a donor heart becomes available
   (c) Consider implantation of long term LVAD, discharge him into the community and have an active life until a donor heart becomes available
   (d) Refer him to palliative care

2. **A 48 year old man presents with recent onset shortness of breath at rest and paroxysmal nocturnal dyspnoea. His blood group is A. His echocardiogram shows severe left ventricular systolic dysfunction with an ejection fraction of 16%, probably secondary to dilated cardiomyopathy. Pulmonary function tests and coronary angiogram were satisfactory. Right heart catheter showed normal pulmonary artery pressure and a transpulmonary gradient of 6 mmHg. His cardiopulmonary exercise test showed peak oxygen uptake (VO_2 max) of 12 ml kg^{-1} min^{-1} and his brain natriuretic peptide (BNP) is 4500 pg ml^{-1}. He has peripheral oedema and is on maximum diuretic therapy. His therapeutic best option is:**
   (a) Continue medical management and listing for heart transplantation
   (b) Consider intravenous inotropic therapy
   (c) Consider putting him on ECMO support
   (d) Consider putting him on short term Bi-VAD support

3. **A 44 year old male with a 2 week history of angina was admitted with an anterior ST elevation myocardial infarction (STEMI). He was taken to the cathlab for a percutaneous intervention to a lesion in his left main stem coronary artery. During this procedure, he developed severe hypotension and circulatory collapse, which was unresponsive to boluses of epinephrine or insertion of an intra-aortic balloon pump (IABP). He went on to have a cardiac arrest in the cathlab and external cardiac compressions were commenced to maintain circulation. His best therapeutic option is:**
   (a) Continue external cardiac massage to maintain circulation
   (b) No therapeutic options are available in such extreme situations
   (c) Emergency sternotomy and internal cardiac massage
   (d) Institution of extracorporeal life support (ECLS) as bridge to decision

4. **A 51 year old male, blood group O, previously fit and well, presents with a short history of breathlessness, right upper quadrant abdominal pain and gross peripheral oedema. On examination, he was clinically jaundiced. His echocardiogram shows severe biventricular dysfunction. His angiogram shows normal coronaries. A right heart catheter shows right atrial pressure of 18 mmHg, mean pulmonary artery pressure of 28 mmHg, a wedge pressure of 18 mmHg and PVR of 4.5 Wood units. Liver and renal functions are deranged with elevated prothrombin time and elevated serum creatinine. He is inotrope dependent and no further improvement is evident despite IABP insertion. The best therapeutic option is:**
   (a) Continue to optimise medical therapy and wait for him to improve
   (b) Insert long term LVAD
   (c) Urgently list for heart transplant
   (d) Insert Bi-VAD (LVAD and RVAD) as a bridge to candidacy and once his end organ function recovers, list him for urgent heart transplant

5. **A 68 year old female with type II diabetes presents with a history of angina, triple vessel coronary artery disease and severe left ventricular dysfunction. She underwent elective coronary artery bypass grafting using the left internal mammary artery and two long saphenous vein grafts on cardiopulmonary bypass. On coming off bypass, she became hypotensive and a transoesophageal echocardiogram demonstrated global left ventricular hypokinaesia. The bypass grafts are patent and she was started on inotropes with little effect. What should be the next line of action?**
   (a) Insertion of intra-aortic balloon pump
   (b) Short term LVAD
   (c) Long term LVAD
   (d) Institution of ECMO

Exercise answers are available on p.468. Alternatively, take the test online at www.cambridge.org/CardiothoracicMCQ

Chapter 23

Cardiac Extracorporeal Membrane Oxygenation

Jason M Ali and David P Jenkins

Extracorporeal membrane oxygenation (ECMO) is an advanced form of temporary life support to aid respiratory and/or cardiac function that has been in existence since the 1970s. ECMO evolved from cardiopulmonary bypass (CPB) technology and similarly involves diverting venous blood through an extracorporeal circuit, in which gaseous exchange occurs, and returning it to the body. Early experience with ECMO was plagued by high complication rates and an inability to demonstrate a survival benefit over conventional management, leading to it being reserved as a last-resort treatment, initiated when death was a near certainty. Significant advances in ECMO technology and experience have resulted in the technique becoming safer and therefore part of the advanced management of severe cardiopulmonary disease.

This chapter focuses on the use of ECMO in the management of severe cardiac or cardiorespiratory failure. This is distinguished from ECMO used in respiratory failure by the site that oxygenated blood is reinfused (which will be discussed in Chapter 24). When being used for the management of cardiac failure, oxygenated blood is reinfused into the systemic arterial circulation (venoarterial (VA) ECMO). In this situation, both the heart and lungs are bypassed by the ECMO circuit. In contrast, when managing respiratory failure alone, oxygenated blood is reinfused into a central vein (venovenous (VV) ECMO), bypassing only the function of the lungs, and the patient is still dependent on intrinsic cardiac function for developing cardiac output.

Indication for Cardiac ECMO

Cardiac (VA) ECMO may be indicated in patients with cardiogenic shock (impaired cardiac output resulting in end-organ dysfunction) that is refractory to maximal conventional therapy with inotropic drugs and less invasive mechanical support, for example intra-aortic balloon counterpulsation. Common causes of such cardiogenic shock are included in Table 23.1.

Table 23.1 Indications for cardiac ECMO

Indications for cardiac ECMO
Acute myocardial infarction
Dilated cardiomyopathy
Fulminant myocarditis
Cardiac failure due to intractable arrhythmias
Postcardiotomy cardiac failure
Primary graft failure following cardiac transplantation
Acute heart failure secondary to drug toxicity

Concomitant respiratory failure is not an absolute requirement for considering cardiac ECMO over alternative mechanical circulatory support devices. There have been no randomised controlled trials in adults that have compared VA ECMO against isolated ventricular support with a temporary ventricular assist device (VAD). However, the coexistence of respiratory indications such as severe refractory hypoxia, hypercapnic respiratory failure or symptomatic pulmonary hypertension is certainly persuasive in deciding to pursue cardiac ECMO instead of other circulatory support techniques. The advantages of ECMO over alternative mechanical circulatory support devices such as ventricular assist devices (VAD) include the rapidity of insertion, the ability to support biventricular failure at high flow rates and the potential to support patients with concomitant lung injury when required.

More recently, cardiac ECMO has also been used to restore circulation during cardiac arrest refractory to standard resuscitative management (termed 'extracorporeal cardiopulmonary resuscitation' (eCPR)). This may be beneficial when a witnessed arrest occurs in hospital, especially if the patient is in an intensive care or cardiac catheter laboratory setting and ECMO can be instituted rapidly. Evidence suggests that outcome is best with resuscitation periods of less than 30 minutes although there are case reports of survival with far longer arrests.

Contraindications for Cardiac ECMO

Deciding to commence ECMO is a major decision and ideally it should be multidisciplinary with involvement of cardiology (and respiratory) physicians, cardiothoracic surgeons and specialist intensivists. The difficulty is that the patient is often deteriorating rapidly in cardiogenic shock with an uncertain diagnosis and prognosis at the time the decision needs to be made. A delay in restoring blood pressure and flow can result in irrecoverable multiorgan failure despite adequate ECMO flow. In many cases in critically ill patients, at the time of cannulation it is uncertain whether organ function is recoverable and support is expectant. Cardiac ECMO is not a long-term therapy and should only be considered in patients with anticipated early recovery, or as a bridge to heart transplantation or implantation of a long-term VAD. Cardiac ECMO is therefore contraindicated in patients with irrecoverable cardiac failure who will not be candidates for transplantation or VAD implantation and in patients with established multiorgan failure.

The following are considered relative contraindications to cardiac ECMO: the presence of severe aortic regurgitation, aortic dissection, contraindications to therapeutic anticoagulation (such as active bleeding, a haemorrhagic intracranial event), pre-existent multiorgan failure and patients who have already been mechanically ventilated for >10–14 days.

Although there are no absolute guidelines on the indications and contraindications for cardiac ECMO, the Extracorporeal Life Support Organisation (ELSO) and the European Extracorporeal Life Support (ECLS) Working Group have published recommendations for the use of ECMO in critically ill patients.

Circuit Design and Considerations

The ECMO circuit is similar for VV and VA use and consists of vascular access cannulae, a pump, an oxygenator, a temperature control system, monitors and access points.

The vascular access cannulae and circuit tubing are made of a plastic, which therefore necessitates therapeutic anticoagulation to prevent activation of the clotting cascade and thrombosis of the circuit. Heparin bonding of the material aims to reduce this activation. Most commonly anticoagulation is with unfractionated heparin, although there are reports of utilising newer agents such as bivilirudin and argatroban in the context of antithrombin III deficiency and heparin induced thrombocytopenia. Efforts are focused on developing a truly biocompatible plastic, which will obviate the need for anticoagulation which is responsible for a significant proportion of ECMO complications.

Blood flow through the circuit is driven by an external pump. Two types exist: simple roller-pumps and constrained vortex centrifugal pumps.

ECMO oxygenators are usually polymethylpentene hollow-fibre devices, and modern devices have low resistance. Carbon dioxide is readily extracted via gradient-mediated mechanisms whilst the addition of oxygen is slower due to its reduced solubility and diffusion characteristics. An air/oxygen blender is used to achieve the desired FiO_2 and titrated based on arterial blood gases.

Cannulation Strategies

Peripheral Cannulation

Vascular access cannulae can be placed centrally, as for CPB, or peripherally to establish VA ECMO (Figure 23.1). They can be inserted by surgical cut-down under direct vision or percutaneously using the Seldinger technique under ultrasound guidance. The most common configuration in adults is placement of the venous drainage cannula in the femoral vein and reperfusion cannula into the femoral artery. The axillary/subclavian artery can also be utilised as an alternative arterial return vessel. Another strategy, commonly used in paediatric and neonatal ECMO, is the internal jugular vein–common carotid artery cannulation.

Each strategy has important considerations.

Femoral Artery Cannulation

This is associated with two main complications:

1. With this strategy, oxygenated blood is pumped in a retrograde direction up the descending aorta and into the ascending aorta to perfuse the coronary arteries and cerebral vessels. However, this assumes that there is no residual left ventricular cardiac output. If there is native cardiac output with the aortic valve opening, there will be a 'mixing zone' where ejected native anterograde and reinfused retrograde blood meet (Figure 23.2). This can cause a problem if, in the

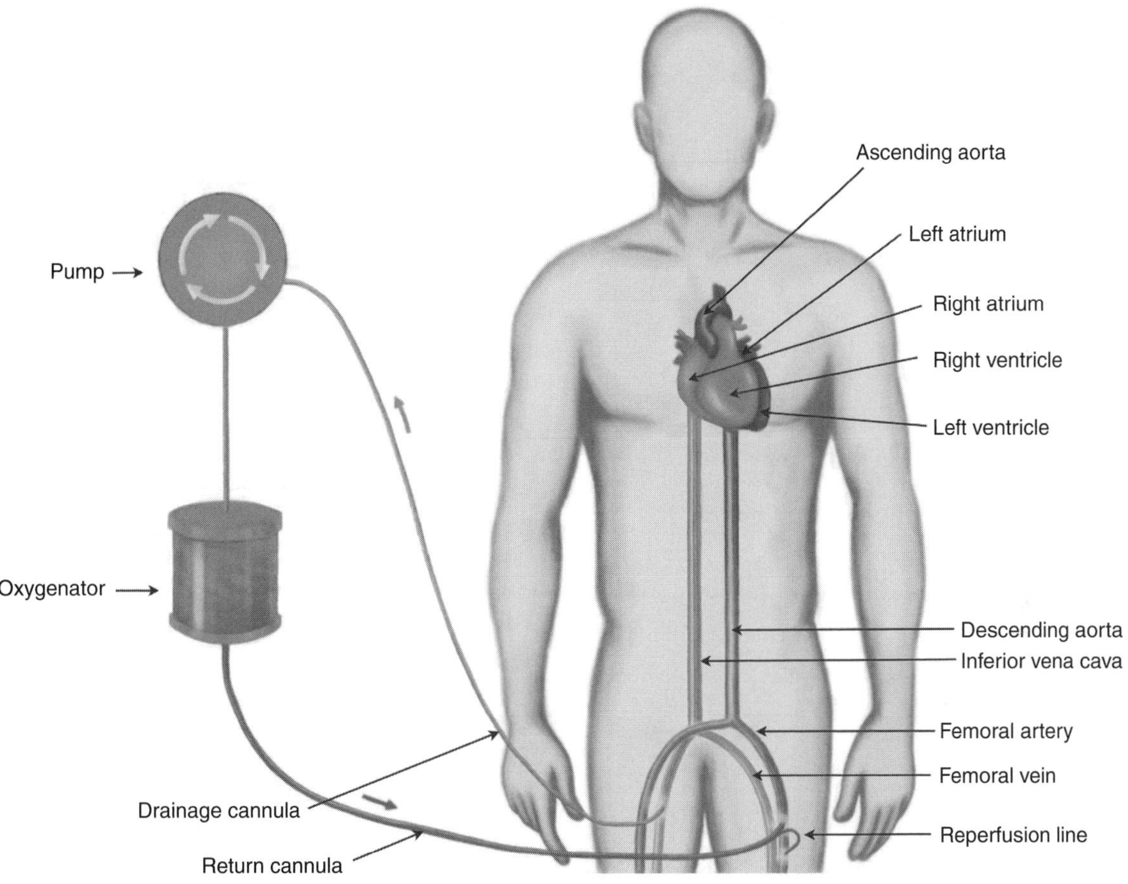

Figure 23.1 Peripheral ECMO. The blood is drained from a large vein, typically IVC, using femoral access. It is then pumped through an oxygenator and returned to the patient into the femoral artery in a retrograde fashion. A reperfusion line from the inflow cannula is inserted into the distal femoral artery to provide distal limb perfusion. Diagram drawn by Anna Valchanova. (A black and white version of this figure will appear in some formats. For the colour version, please refer to the plate section.)

context of respiratory failure, the blood exiting the left ventricle is deoxygenated. This situation is not infrequent when left ventricular failure is complicated by pulmonary oedema. As native cardiac function recovers and left ventricular ejection increases, if the mixing zone is within the descending aorta, the coronary and cerebral circulations may be exposed to deoxygenated blood. Monitoring of cerebral saturations and right radial artery blood gases can be indicative of this 'differential cyanosis' or Harlequin syndrome. Strategies to manage this complication include increasing ventilatory support in an attempt to improve oxygenation of the pulmonary venous blood, increasing the flow through the femoral arterial catheter with the aim of transferring the mixing zone to the ascending aorta, or placement of an additional reinfusion catheter into the internal jugular vein such that a proportion of the oxygenated blood is reinfused into the pulmonary circulation (increasing the saturation of antegrade ejected blood from the left ventricle). Alternatively, the femoral reinfusion cannula could be resited proximally to the subclavian, common carotid or ascending aorta.

2. The second complication of femoral arterial cannulation is ipsilateral ischaemic limb injury due to obstruction of distal femoral arterial blood flow that can lead to critical limb ischaemia necessitating fasciotomies or even amputation if not recognised. This can be avoided by placement of a small antegrade perfusion catheter into the superficial femoral artery distal to the ECMO cannula, to perfuse the leg.

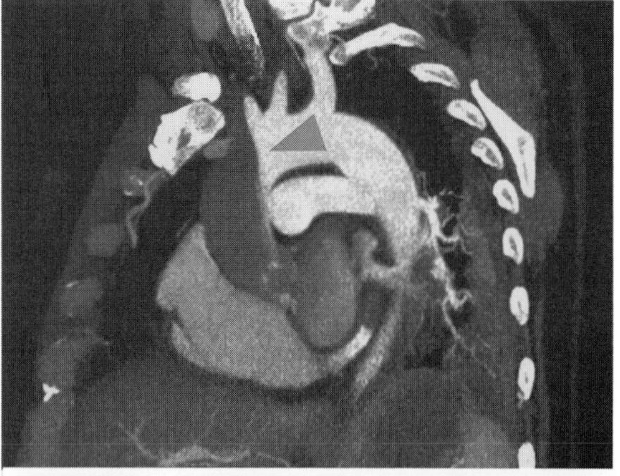

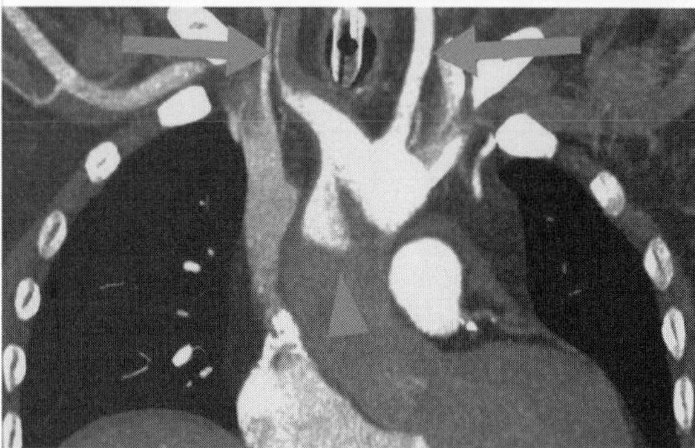

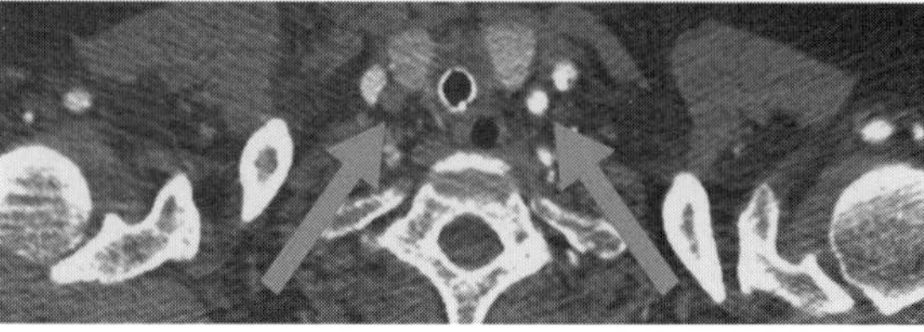

Figure 23.2 Watershed phenomenon during venoarterial ECMO visualised by computed tomography. Antegrade blood flow (low contrast) from the heart competes with retrograde blood flow (high contrast) from the ECMO in the aorta, resulting in a watershed phenomenon (arrowhead). Here computed tomography of a patient with pulmonary embolism and reduced cardiac output demonstrates a rather proximal watershed, leading to perfusion of the right carotid artery with 'heart blood' (dark) and the left carotid artery with 'ECMO blood' (bright, arrows). Upper panel, sagittal oblique maximum intensity projection (MIP); middle panel, coronal oblique MIP; lower panel, transverse plane. From Napp et al. (2016).

Axillary/Subclavian Cannulation

The main advantage of this strategy for arterial return is that the entry site for returned oxygenated blood is more central in the aorta, so that more of the flow is in the physiological antegrade direction, avoiding the potential for the first complication above. However, there are also disadvantages. A surgical cut-down is always needed, and it is usually necessary to sew a side graft onto the artery that is then cannulated. The latter allows flow to continue distally to perfuse the arm. Bleeding complications are relatively common from the suture lines and occasionally the arm can become hyperperfused with resulting severe swelling and damage if venous return is compromised.

Carotid Artery Cannulation

With ligation of the carotid artery, there is an increased risk of neurological injury, with dependence on a complete circle of Willis for collateral circulation to the brain.

Central Cannulation

Cardiac ECMO can also be instituted with central cannulation as for CPB (Figure 23.3). Central cannulation is performed by cardiothoracic surgeons via a median sternotomy. Larger catheters can be used which permit increased flow rates and maximal haemodynamic support with more certainty of the ECMO circuit taking over the whole of the patient's circulation. This approach is most commonly used if a sternotomy has already been made, for example in patients with postcardiotomy cardiac failure following cardiac surgery or primary graft failure at transplantation. It is occasionally necessary in patients where peripheral access is not possible. There are also reports of this strategy being used in cases of severe sepsis, taking advantage of the greater haemodynamic support possible; however the requirement for sternotomy adds to the potential complications and morbidity in these patients. This approach necessarily involves a major surgical incision and therefore bleeding is the most frequent problem. Usually institution of anticoagulation is delayed 6–12 hours until bleeding is controlled.

General Management of Patients on Cardiac ECMO

Patients supported by cardiac ECMO should be managed in an intensive care unit by multidisciplinary specialists. There are several important considerations that should be made when managing these patients, many of which are similar to patients supported by 'respiratory' (VV) ECMO.

The circulatory haemodynamics of patients must be closely monitored. ECMO support should be titrated to clinical targets, which may include:

- Arterial oxygen saturations >90%

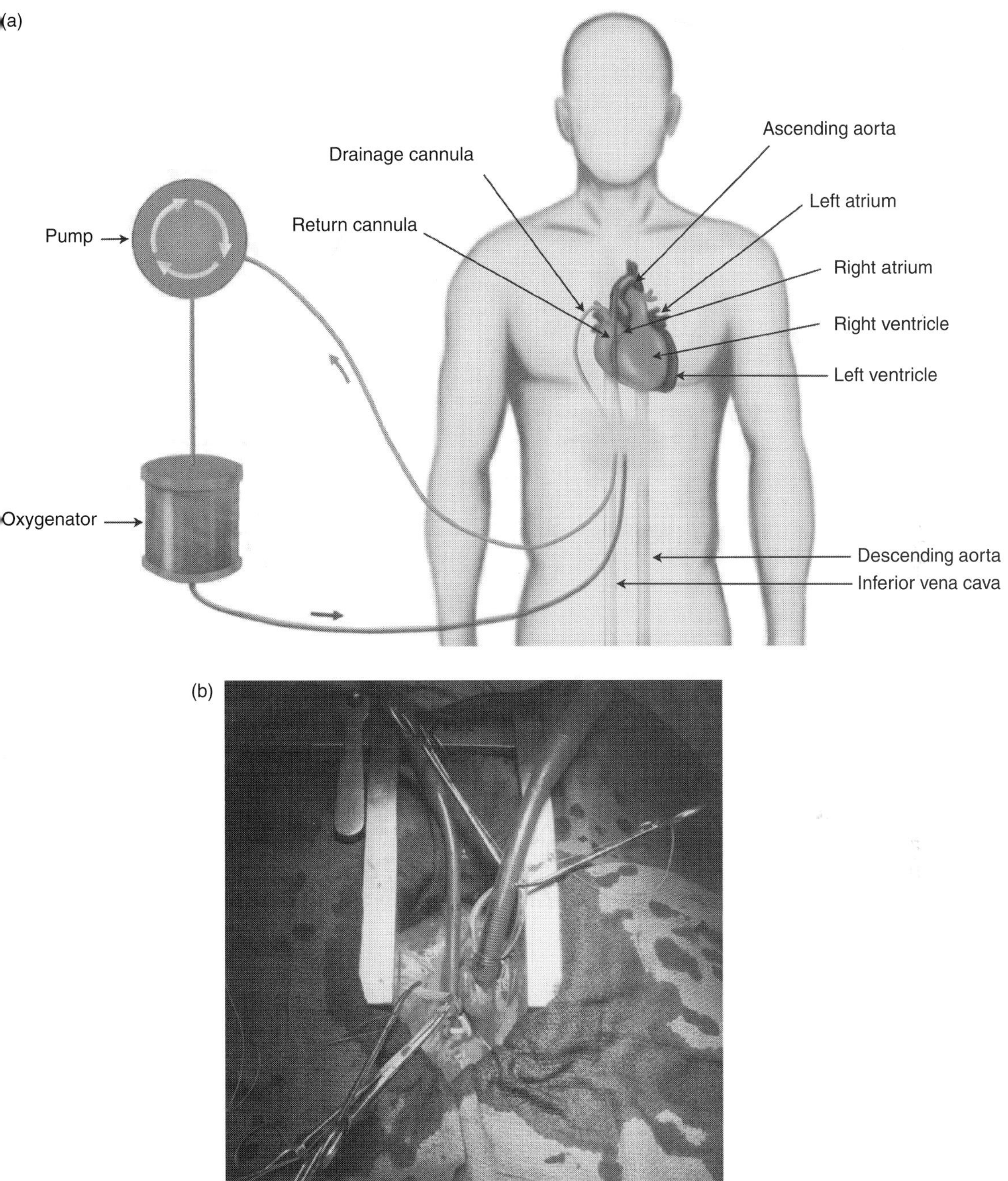

Figure 23.3 (a) Central ECMO diagram: using open chest, the blood is drained via a cannula from a central vein (IVC or SVC) or right atrium. It is pumped through an oxygenator and returned through an arterial cannula into the ascending aorta. The chest can be left open for a short while, or the cannulae can be tunnelled under the skin and chest closed. Diagram drawn by Anna Valchanova. (b) A photograph of the outflow and inflow cannulae secured with spigots. (A black and white version of this figure will appear in some formats. For the colour version, please refer to the plate section.)

- Venous oxygen saturations >70%
- Adequate tissue perfusion, as judged by end-organ function and lactate levels.

In most cases there is some residual ventricular function, and it is beneficial for some pulsatility to continue. This allows emptying of the ventricles and less chance of distension and stasis. Low dose inotropic support is sometimes required to achieve ventricular ejection and aortic valve opening; the latter can be confirmed by echocardiography. In cases of severe left ventricular dysfunction with no effective contraction, peripheral cardiac ECMO can lead to overdistension of the left ventricle and left atrium, worsening pulmonary oedema. This can also lead to further myocardial injury. Serial echocardiography should be performed to monitor for this complication. If identified, several strategies have been described to facilitate decompression, including addition of a vent cannula via the left ventricular apex, or transseptal via the atrium, increasing inotropic support, further mechanical support such as Impella I or IABP, conversion to central ECMO or alternative support modalities such as a percutaneous VAD.

Anticoagulation must be monitored to prevent circuit thrombosis and embolism, which could be fatal. For patients receiving unfractionated heparin, an activated clotting time (ACT) of 180–210 seconds is recommended, which is lower than the >400 seconds recommended for CPB.

Lung protective ventilation is usually adopted to minimise barotrauma and volutrauma. Positive end expiratory pressure is applied to the lungs to maintain alveolar recruitment, but the ventilator is usually set to low tidal volumes, low inspiratory pressures and a low inspired oxygen fraction. Reduction in the ventilator support is often accompanied by increased venous return and cardiac output. This strategy is found to help prevent ventilator induced lung injury, oxygen toxicity and ventilator associated haemodynamic compromise. Indeed, prevention of further lung injury in these patients is one of the major advantages of cardiac ECMO. However, it is important to remember that in patients with improving ventricular function, more blood will be ejected from the right ventricle into the pulmonary circulation and increased ventilation will be necessary to prevent deoxygenated blood reaching the left atrium.

The most comprehensive guidelines on the management of patients on ECMO are published by ELSO. These provide guidance on the use of ECMO including training, resources and quality assurance. They are not intended to represent a standard of care, however, and practice described in the literature often differs in parts from this guidance.

Weaning Cardiac ECMO

It is important to develop an individual strategy for all patients supported on VA ECMO. It will often be instituted as an emergency when the aetiology of circulatory collapse and diagnosis may be unclear at the time. Cardiac ECMO support will only be possible for 1–2 weeks and therefore ECMO in this situation is a temporary support to recovery of heart function or a bridge to another treatment. In some patients, weaning of support will not be possible, and after careful evaluation they may be candidates for urgent cardiac transplantation or if donors are not available a planned transfer to temporary or implantable ventricular assist.

Patients are monitored for recovery of intrinsic cardiac and respiratory function. Evidence of recovery of left ventricular function can be assessed by examining for pulsatility in the arterial line waveform and by echocardiography. In conjunction, for patients with concomitant respiratory failure, improvements in arterial oxygen saturation, pulmonary compliance and chest radiography can suggest recovery of respiratory function. Weaning of cardiac ECMO is more complicated than in the case of VV ECMO, where titration is against gas exchange alone, as in most cases both the heart and lungs have been supported and it is not safe to have a prolonged trial off support prior to decannulation.

Once adequate recovery is thought to have occurred, an attempt to wean off ECMO can be made. This is usually accomplished by successive reduction in flow of approximately 0.5 l on a daily basis, until the ECMO support is only 1.5–2.0 l/min. During this time, careful assessment of end-organ function is vital. Most patients will also require additional inotropic support. Final decannulation usually occurs in the operating room as formal vessel repair for peripheral cannulation, and chest closure for central cannulation is required. For circuits with a bridge between the inflow and outflow limbs, the arterial and venous catheters can be clamped, leaving blood circulating through the external circuit through the bridge. If a bridge is not present, flow through the circuit can be reduced to a minimal setting to prevent stasis. In both cases it is essential to ensure therapeutic anticoagulation due to the increased risk of thrombosis with reduced flow. During the final trial off ECMO completely, the patient is monitored for adequate cardiorespiratory function.

Should cardiac function begin to recover but respiratory failure persists, it is important to ensure adequate oxygenation of the coronary and cerebral circulation and such patients may need to be converted to respiratory ECMO.

Complications

Although cardiac ECMO can improve the survival of patients with advanced heart disease, these benefits must be weighed against the significant associated morbidity. The major complications are haemorrhagic or thrombotic, emphasising the importance of closely monitoring the level of anticoagulation – although there is no universally accepted anticoagulation protocol. Cardiac or major vascular perforation is a rare but potentially lethal complication of cannulation, and despite advances in equipment and technique, distal malperfusion remains a problem with peripheral cannulation. Mechanical equipment failure is now very uncommon with modern ECMO circuits.

Acute kidney injury (AKI) occurs in around half of patients supported by ECMO. This is important since AKI on ECMO is a marker of disease severity and is associated with increased mortality. As such, continuous renal replacement therapy has evolved into an adjunct support in patients on ECMO, with the advantage of permitting correction of metabolic and fluid disturbances, and it may also suppress inflammation by counteracting the systemic inflammatory response.

A recent meta-analysis summarised complications of cardiac ECMO from 20 studies reporting on outcomes in 1866 patients. The complication rates they reported are summarised in Table 23.2.

For survivors of ECMO, there has been the suggestion that there is an increase in neurological deficits and respiratory morbidities, and for the neonatal/paediatric population neurodevelopmental deficits and behavioural problems. However, more recent data comparing non-ECMO arms of randomised controlled trials have observed no between-group differences for these outcomes. Patients who survive ECMO require prolonged rehabilitation and multidisciplinary follow-up after discharge from hospital.

Outcomes and Evidence

There is a paucity of evidence demonstrating the absolute benefit of cardiac ECMO in improving survival or quality of life. This is partially due to the difficulty of designing randomised controlled trials of life support that are ethically acceptable. As such, evidence is primarily from case series, cohort studies and registry data.

Table 23.2 Complication rates of cardiac ECMO

Complication	Incidence (%)
Acute kidney injury	55.6
Renal replacement therapy	46.0
Rethoracotomy for bleeding or tamponade in postcardiotomy patients	41.9
Major or significant bleeding	40.8
Significant infection	30.4
Lower extremity ischaemia	16.9
Neurological complications	13.9
Fasciotomy or compartment syndrome	10.3
Stroke	5.9
Lower extremity amputation	4.7

Extracorporeal Life Support Organisation Registry

The Extracorporeal Life Support Organisation (ELSO) was founded in 1989. This organisation maintains an international registry of patients who have been treated with all types of extracorporeal life support. The results of the registry are published biannually and distributed to members. As of July 2015 a total of 69,114 patients (including neonatal, paediatric and adult) are included in the registry, with a total of 20,236 patients having been on cardiac ECMO and a further 5756 patients having eCPR. The registry data report that for cardiac ECMO, 62% of patients survived extracorporeal life support and 45% survived to discharge or transfer.

In general, the survival for cardiac ECMO in adults is inferior to the survival for respiratory ECMO. Patients supported postcardiotomy or as part of extended CPR have the worst survival. The chance of overall survival is determined by the diagnosis, state of end-organ damage at the time of initiation of support, and in the case of non-recovery the potential for cardiac transplantation or more permanent ventricular support.

Future Direction

The improvement in ECMO technology over the last 10 years has allowed greater adoption of cardiac

ECMO and use in expanding areas including accident and emergency, cardiac surgery, and PCI catheter labs. There has also been a steady increase in the use of ECMO during cardiopulmonary resuscitation (eCPR).

Although there are no randomised controlled trials, there is increasing evidence of efficacy. A prospective observational study of witnessed in-hospital cardiac arrest, with propensity matched controls, demonstrated significantly higher survival to discharge and at 1-year follow-up in the eCPR group. There is some evidence that combining eCPR with primary percutaneous coronary intervention for acute coronary syndromes improves likelihood of successful outcomes. Although data are supportive, overall survival is low with only 30% of adults surviving to discharge in the ELSO registry data. More research is required to define the patient population that will derive the greatest benefit from eCPR with an emphasis on survival with minimal neurological impairment.

Developments in the technology continue to be made with the goal of lowering complication rates, allowing more patients to benefit. The goal of developing antithrombogenic materials requiring no anticoagulation will be a big advance in ECMO technology that is likely to significantly reduce morbidity.

One challenge that remains with the management of patients on ECMO is discontinuation of support in patients with irreversible disease and no other option. As technology and experience increase, patients can be managed on ECMO for longer and so futility becomes more difficult to define. In order to facilitate use of this technology in an appropriate and cost effective manner, better predictors of outcome are necessary.

Despite the increasing use of ECMO for advanced cardiopulmonary disease, many questions remain unanswered and the benefit over conventional therapy has yet to be conclusively demonstrated. To date, the highest level of evidence for cardiac ECMO is limited to cohort studies. In view of this paucity of data supporting the benefit of ECMO, there is a need for large randomised controlled trials to better define the use of this advanced life support. Such studies would ideally include cost-benefit analyses to better quantify the economic impact of this resource intensive therapy.

Learning Points

- Cardiac ECMO is an advanced life support technique used in refractory cardiogenic shock in patients who have recoverable cardiac disease or who are candidates for transplantation or implantation of a ventricular assist device.
- In adults, most commonly, venous blood is drained via a catheter in the femoral vein and reinfused oxygenated via a catheter in the femoral artery, therefore bypassing both cardiac and respiratory function. Post cardiotomy, central cannulation is often utilised.
- Cannulation of the femoral artery can be complicated by ipsilateral ischaemic limb injury, and can also result in the phenomenon of 'differential cyanosis' with good oxygenation of the lower body, but with ejection of deoxygenated blood to the upper body.
- Complications of cardiac ECMO are largely related to the need for therapeutic anticoagulation, the major complications being thrombotic or haemorrhagic. Almost half of the patients on cardiac ECMO develop acute kidney injury, which is associated with a poorer outcome.
- Much of the evidence supporting the use of cardiac ECMO is based on small observational studies and the international registry held by the Extracorporeal Life Support Organisation (ELSO). Randomised controlled trials are required to expand the evidence base for this therapy. Overall survival is poor and reflects the severity of the disease state necessitating support.

Further Reading

Abrams D, Combes A, Brodie D. What's new in extracorporeal membrane oxygenation for cardiac failure and cardiac arrest in adults? *Intensive Care Medicine*. 2014; 40: 609–612.

Beckmann A, Benk C, Beyersdorf F, et al. Position article for the use of extracorporeal life support in adult patients. *European Journal of Cardio-Thoracic Surgery*. 2011; 40: 676–680.

Bembea MM, Annich G, Rycus P, et al. Variability in anticoagulation management of patients on extracorporeal membrane oxygenation: an international survey. *Pediatric Critical Care Medicine*. 2013; 14: e77–84.

Chen YS, Lin JW, Yu HY, et al. Cardiopulmonary resuscitation with assisted extracorporeal life-support versus conventional cardiopulmonary resuscitation in adults with in-hospital cardiac arrest: an observational study and propensity analysis. *Lancet*. 2008; 372: 554–561.

Cheng R, Hachamovitch R, Kittleson M, et al. Complications of extracorporeal membrane oxygenation for treatment of cardiogenic shock and cardiac arrest: a meta-analysis of 1,866 adult patients. *Annals of Thoracic Surgery*. 2014; 97: 610–616.

Extracorporeal Life Support Organisation. *General Guidelines for all Extracorporeal Life Support*, version 1.3. Ann Arbor MI, 2013.

Gaffney AM, Wildhirt SM, Griffin MJ, Annich GM, Radomski MW. Extracorporeal life support. *British Medical Journal*. 2010; 341: c5317.

Lawler PR, Silver DA, Scirica BM, Couper GS, Weinhouse GL, Camp (Jr) PC. Extracorporeal membrane oxygenation in adults with cardiogenic shock. *Circulation*. 2015; 131: 676–680.

Napp CL, Kühn C, Hoeper MM, Vogel-Claussen J, Haverich A, Schäfer A, et al. Cannulation strategies for percutaneous extracorporeal membrane oxygenation in adults. *Clinical Research in Cardiology*. 2016; 105: 283–296.

Tramm R, Ilic D, Davies AR, Pellegrino VA, Romero L, Hodgson C. Extracorporeal membrane oxygenation for critically ill adults. *Cochrane Database of Systematic Reviews*. 2015; 1: CD010381.

Werdan K, Gielen S, Ebelt H, Hochman JS. Mechanical circulatory support in cardiogenic shock. *European Heart Journal*. 2014; 35: 156–167.

MCQs

1. **When monitoring a patient supported on VA peripheral ECMO with cannulation of the femoral vessels, arterial blood gases should be taken from where to best reflect patient oxygenation?**
   (a) Contralateral femoral artery
   (b) Right radial artery
   (c) Left radial artery
   (d) ECMO circuit post oxygenator
   (e) ECMO circuit pre oxygenator

2. **Which of the following is not a strategy that can be used to manage 'differential cyanosis' due to return of native cardiac function?**
   (a) Increase ventilator support
   (b) Decrease the flow through the arterial reinfusion catheter
   (c) Insertion of an additional internal jugular venous reinfusion cannula
   (d) Re-site the reinfusion catheter into a more proximal artery
   (e) Vent the left heart to improve drainage

3. **Which of the following is considered a relative contraindication to commencement of cardiac ECMO?**
   (a) Aortic stenosis
   (b) Aortic dissection
   (c) Possible malignancy
   (d) Mechanical ventilation for 7 days
   (e) Recent cardiac surgery

4. **Compared with peripheral VA ECMO, central cannulation results in:**
   (a) Less drainage and emptying of the heart
   (b) Lower chance of left ventricular recovery
   (c) A lower risk of bleeding
   (d) More native flow in the pulmonary arteries
   (e) A more proximal mixing zone in the aorta

5. **According to the Extracorporeal Life Support Organisation (ELSO) registry, what percentage of patients receiving ECMO as part of cardiopulmonary resuscitation (eCPR) survive to discharge?**
   (a) 10%
   (b) 20%
   (c) 30%
   (d) 40%
   (e) 50%

Exercise answers are available on p.468. Alternatively, take the test online at www.cambridge.org/CardiothoracicMCQ

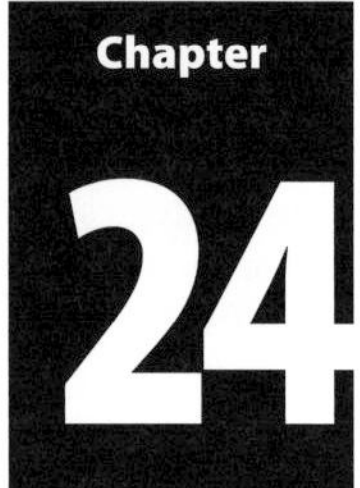

Respiratory Extracorporeal Membrane Oxygenation in the Cardiothoracic Intensive Care Unit

Darryl Abrams and Daniel Brodie

Introduction

Although extracorporeal membrane oxygenation (ECMO) was first introduced in the 1970s as a means of supporting severe impairments in gas exchange, original versions of the technology were associated with high device related and patient related complication rates, particularly thrombosis and haemorrhage, with no evidence of benefit over conventional management strategies at the time. Recent advances in ECMO technology have improved its risk-benefit profile, and a growing body of literature in the context of greater experience with its use has sparked a renewed interest in the use of ECMO for respiratory failure. This chapter will review the basic principles underlying the use of ECMO, cannulation strategies, indications and evidence for ECMO in the setting of respiratory failure, as it pertains to the cardiothoracic intensive care unit. Beyond the current considerations for ECMO, we will explore emerging indications that could change the approach to the management of respiratory failure in the intensive care unit in the future.

Basic Principles

ECMO refers to an extracorporeal circuit that directly oxygenates and removes carbon dioxide from the blood via an oxygenator, a device that consists of a semipermeable membrane that selectively permits oxygen and carbon dioxide to diffuse between blood and gas compartments. Deoxygenated blood is withdrawn through a drainage cannula via an external pump, typically a centrifugal pump, which creates negative pressure within the drainage cannula and tubing. The blood passes through the oxygenator, where gas exchange occurs, and is returned to the patient through a reinfusion cannula under positive pressure. When blood is both drained from and returned to a vein, it is referred to as venovenous ECMO and provides only gas exchange support. When blood is drained from a vein and returned to an artery, it is referred to as venoarterial ECMO, and the circuit is able to provide both respiratory and circulatory support. The amount of blood flow through the circuit (including the fraction of ECMO blood flow relative to the amount of native cardiac output), the fraction of oxygen delivered through the gas compartment of the oxygenator (referred to as the FDO_2), and native lung function are the main determinants of systemic oxygenation for patients supported with ECMO. The rate of gas flow through the oxygenator, known as the sweep gas flow rate, and, to a lesser degree, the blood flow rate are the major determinants of carbon dioxide removal. Extracorporeal circuits are more efficient at carbon dioxide removal than oxygenation, owing to the diffusion properties of the membrane and the manner in which oxygen and carbon dioxide are transported within the blood. Because carbon dioxide can be effectively removed at lower blood flow rates than those typically required for oxygenation, it may be possible to use smaller cannulae, which in turn may be easier and safer to insert. The technique of extracorporeal support for carbon dioxide removal at low blood flow rates is referred to as extracorporeal carbon dioxide removal ($ECCO_2R$). This approach has the potential to support patients with acute hypercapnic respiratory failure and to facilitate reductions in tidal volumes and airway pressures in the acute respiratory distress syndrome that would otherwise be limited by unacceptable levels of respiratory acidosis. An alternative, pumpless configuration that is less frequently employed is arteriovenous $ECCO_2R$ (blood drained from a femoral artery and returned to the contralateral femoral vein), in which the patient's native cardiac output generates blood flow through an oxygenator. Because extracorporeal blood flow tends to be lower, this approach is usually limited to the modulation of carbon dioxide.

Cannulation Configurations

Traditionally, venovenous ECMO is implemented by cannulation of a femoral vein for drainage and an internal jugular vein for reinfusion (Figure 24.1). This configuration may result in directing reinfused oxygenated blood toward the port of the drainage cannula. The phenomenon of drawing reinfused, oxygenated blood back into the circuit without passing through the systemic circulation is known as recirculation, which may negatively impact the effect of the ECMO circuit on systemic oxygenation. The development of the bicaval dual lumen cannula (Figure 24.2) has enabled the implementation of venovenous ECMO through a single vein, with the advantages – when positioned properly – of less recirculation and avoidance of femoral cannulation. In order to optimise blood flow and recirculation, cannulation typically requires imaging guidance to ensure that the tip of the cannula is properly positioned in the inferior vena cava and that the reinfusion jet is directed toward the tricuspid valve. The choice of cannula size is based on the physiological needs and size of the patient, and consideration should also be made for any history of chronic indwelling central venous catheters that may have led to stenosis within the venous system.

Indications and Evidence

Severe Acute Respiratory Distress Syndrome

The acute respiratory distress syndrome (ARDS) remains among the most common indications for ECMO for respiratory failure worldwide, although evidence supporting its use remains limited. Positive pressure ventilation, although often necessary for more severe forms of ARDS, is known to exacerbate lung injury, and a ventilation strategy that targets low tidal volumes and airway pressures has been established as one of the few interventions that improves outcomes in ARDS, along with prone ventilation. The potential role for ECMO in ARDS is two-fold. In patients with respiratory failure so severe that the ventilator is insufficient to support gas exchange (or can do so only at the expense of unacceptably high airway pressures), ECMO may serve as salvage therapy to manage refractory hypoxaemia or hypercapnia. Alternatively, in patients whose respiratory system compliance is so severely reduced that standard-of-care low tidal volume ventilation cannot be achieved due to unacceptable levels of respiratory acidosis, ECMO (or more specifically $ECCO_2R$) can facilitate reductions in tidal volumes by correcting the associated hypercapnia.

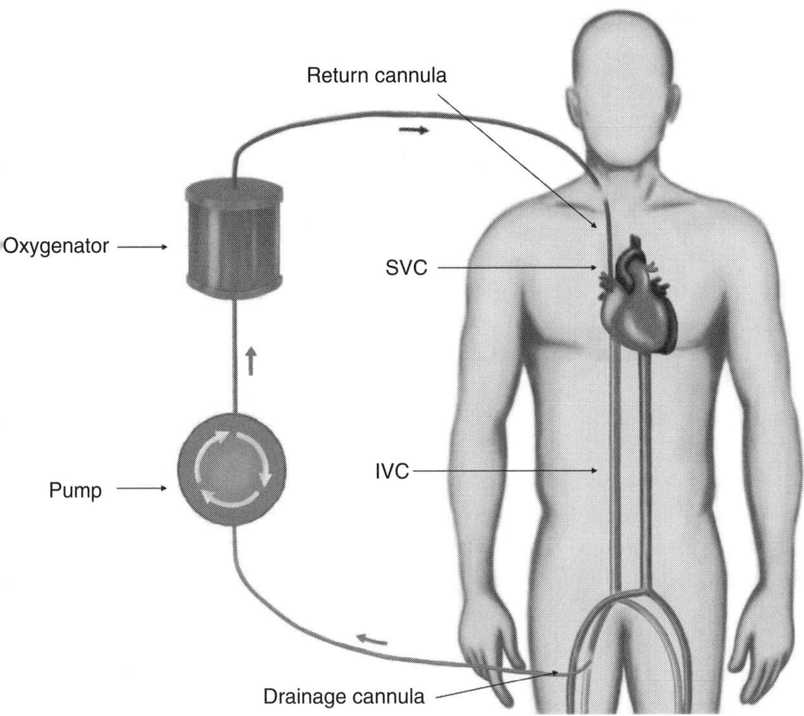

Figure 24.1 Peripheral VV ECMO using two cannulae. Blood is drained from the IVC using femoral approach. It is then pumped through an oxygenator and returned into the SVC through internal jugular approach. Diagram drawn by Anna Valchanova. (A black and white version of this figure will appear in some formats. For the colour version, please refer to the plate section.)

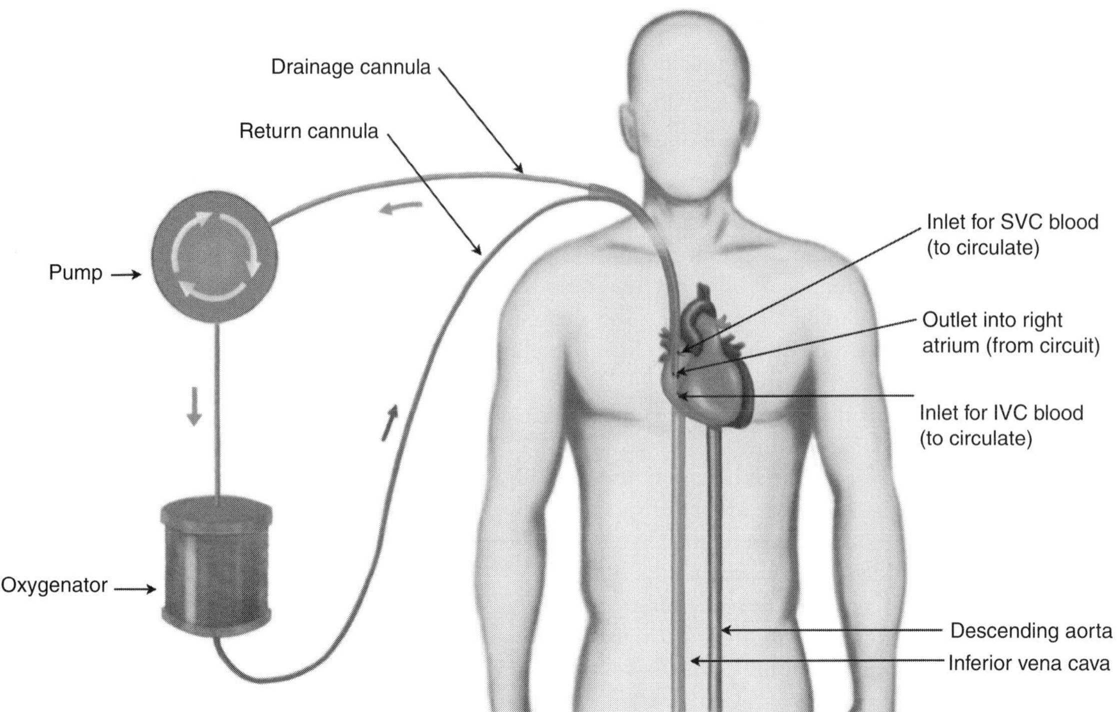

Figure 24.2 VVECMO using bicaval dual lumen cannula. Blood is drained from the IVC and SVC. It is pumped through an oxygenator and returned into the right atrium using the second lumen of the same cannula. Diagram drawn by Anna Valchanova. (A black and white version of this figure will appear in some formats. For the colour version, please refer to the plate section.)

As previously stated, the evidence supporting ECMO for ARDS has significant limitations. Prospective randomised controlled trials in the era of early device technology failed to show a benefit to ECMO in severe ARDS, with high mortality rates in both arms. In the first randomised trial with relatively modern ECMO technology for ARDS, entitled Conventional Ventilation or ECMO for Severe Adult Respiratory Failure (CESAR), 180 subjects with severe, potentially reversible respiratory failure were randomised to conventional mechanical ventilation or referral to a specialised centre for consideration of ECMO. Subjects referred for consideration of ECMO, compared to those receiving conventional management, had a significantly lower rate of death or severe disability at 6 months (37% versus 53%, RR 0.69, $p = 0.03$). These findings must be interpreted with caution given limitations in study design. Because it was designed as a pragmatic study, lung-protective ventilation was recommended but not mandated for the conventional arm, and only 70% of those subjects received such a strategy at any point in the study. Among those referred for consideration of ECMO, only 76% ultimately received ECMO, making it difficult to quantify the effect of ECMO itself on outcomes. One reasonable conclusion to draw from this study is that referral to an ECMO-capable centre may improve outcomes when compared with usual care in that setting. Non-randomised observational studies have shown conflicting results of the impact of ECMO on survival in severe ARDS, with a large amount of data derived from the influenza A (H1N1) epidemic. Propensity analysis of patients in the UK matched on their likelihood of receiving ECMO for severe ARDS due to influenza suggested a mortality benefit from ECMO (24% versus 47%, relative risk 0.51; 95% CI 0.31–0.84, $p = 0.008$). These findings contrast with other matched propensity analyses from a separate but similar French cohort, highlighting the limitations of non-randomised retrospective studies. To help address the role and impact of ECMO on patients with severe ARDS, the ECMO to Rescue Lung Injury in Severe ARDS (EOLIA) trial is being conducted; patients who remain in severe, refractory ARDS despite optimal standard of care ARDS management (including low tidal volume ventilation, with the option for prone positioning, neuromuscular blockade and other rescue therapies) are randomised to either ECMO or ongoing conventional support.

Several prognostic scores have been proposed in order to identify patients most likely to benefit from ECMO in ARDS. The Predicting Death for Severe ARDS on VV-ECMO (PRESERVE) score, which attempts to predict 6 month survival based on several pre-ECMO measurements (age, body mass index, immunocompromised status, prone position, days of mechanical ventilation, sepsis related organ failure assessment (SOFA), positive end-expiratory pressure (PEEP) and plateau pressure), was externally validated in a cohort of venovenous ECMO patients, with an AUC of 0.75 (95% CI 0.57 to 0.92; p = 0.01). A more recent prediction model that utilised a combination of pre-ECMO and ECMO day 1 data in a cohort of subjects receiving venovenous ECMO for severe ARDS demonstrated high discrimination with an area under curve of 0.79 (p = 0.03). With negative and positive predictive values of 81% and 82%, this model performed better than several other proposed scoring systems, including the PRESERVE score.

Beyond short-term mortality prediction modelling, little is known about the long-term functional, neurocognitive and psychiatric outcomes of ARDS survivors who received ECMO. Existing data suggest that such patients may have similar or potentially worse long-term neuropsychiatric sequelae compared with those who did not receive ECMO, though differences in severity of critical illness probably contribute to such findings.

Less Severe Forms of ARDS

Aside from its ability to support refractory hypoxaemic or hypercapnic respiratory failure in severe ARDS, ECMO may have the benefit of reducing lung injury even further than the current standard of care by facilitating the implementation of very low tidal volumes, airway pressures and respiratory rates through the use of $ECCO_2R$. This strategy, sometimes referred to as 'lung rest', or 'ultra-protective' ventilation, is already practised at many ECMO centres for patients with severe ARDS, and additional research is being conducted to systematically characterise current ventilation practices for these patients in order to help guide optimal management strategies. Data demonstrating the efficacy of such an approach, which may extend to less severe forms of ARDS, are limited but promising. Analysis of the ARDS Network's ARMA trial of conventional (12 ml per kg and plateau airway pressure <50 cmH_2O) versus low tidal volume ventilation (6 ml per kg, plateau airway pressure <30 cmH_2O) that established the current standard of care for ventilation strategies in ARDS suggests that subjects in the conventional group would have benefited from tidal volume reduction regardless of plateau pressure quartile. A prospective cohort study has demonstrated an independent linear relationship between lower tidal volume and decreased mortality that extends below 6 ml per kg. Reductions in tidal volumes (from 6.3 ml per kg to 4.2 ml per kg) and plateau airway pressures (from 29.1 to 25 cmH_2O) with the assistance of $ECCO_2R$ to manage hypercapnia and acidaemia have been shown to reduce inflammatory markers associated with lung injury in a single-centre cohort of patients with ARDS. In a more recent clinical trial comparing $ECCO_2R$ assisted very low tidal volume ventilation (approximately 3 ml per kg predicted body weight) to conventional low tidal volume ventilation (approximately 6 ml per kg) in patients with moderate to severe ARDS, those with more severe hypoxaemia were found in post hoc analysis to have a greater number of ventilator-free days when very low tidal volumes were used (40.9 versus 28.2, p = 0.033). Two prospective randomised trials comparing very lung protective ventilation to standard of care ventilation practices in less severe forms of ARDS or hypoxaemic respiratory failure are currently being designed and conducted, and may help to determine whether such a strategy translates into reductions in lung injury and improvement in clinical outcomes.

Acute Hypercapnic Respiratory Failure

Because of the relative ease with which $ECCO_2R$ can correct hypercapnia at lower blood flow rates than are needed to provide oxygenation, there is great promise in using $ECCO_2R$ for the management of acute hypercapnic respiratory failure, potentially eliminating the need for invasive mechanical ventilation in some patients. In COPD, the use of the ventilator is associated with multiple complications, including dynamic hyperinflation and elevations in intrinsic PEEP, ventilator associated pneumonia, and impaired delivery of aerosolised medications, and failure of non-invasive ventilation requiring invasive mechanical ventilation is associated with mortality as high as 30%. Several case series and cohort studies have demonstrated the feasibility of avoidance of or rapid weaning from invasive mechanical ventilation, with $ECCO_2R$ used to manage gas exchange. In a matched cohort study of acute exacerbations of COPD comparing the combination of non-invasive ventilation plus $ECCO_2R$ to historical controls receiving non-invasive ventilation alone, the $ECCO_2R$ group had a significantly lower risk of intubation (HR 0.27; 95% CI, 0.07–0.98, $p = 0.047$), though there was a high adverse event rate related to $ECCO_2R$. The rate of adverse events in this study may also have been related, in part, to the specific device used. Additional benefits of $ECCO_2R$ over mechanical ventilation may include increased success with early mobilisation. Although safety of early mobilisation during invasive mechanical ventilation has been well documented, it may have even greater success with $ECCO_2R$ because of better control of dyspnoea with $ECCO_2R$. Ultimately, more data are needed to identify patients most likely to benefit from this overall approach, as well as the cost effectiveness of such a strategy, before it should be implemented outside the research setting. The benefit of $ECCO_2R$ in hypercapnic respiratory failure may extend beyond COPD, particularly for patients with refractory status asthmaticus, where the avoidance of positive pressure ventilation is preferred.

Lung Transplantation and Primary Graft Dysfunction

ECMO had long been considered a relative contraindication to lung transplantation because of poor outcomes, especially when used as salvage therapy for patients failing invasive mechanical ventilation. However, in the era of improved technology and earlier implementation, recent studies have reported improved post-transplant survival, particularly when performed at centres with more extensive experience. In a systematic review of 441 patients across 14 studies supported with ECMO (the majority of whom were also receiving invasive mechanical ventilation) while awaiting transplantation, mortality and 1-year survival ranged from 10% to 50% and 50% to 90%, respectively. The heterogeneity of patients and outcomes suggests that patient selection and bridging technique are probably important factors in optimising post-transplant survival. Given the potential for complications from invasive mechanical ventilation, a non-intubated ECMO strategy may be considered for select transplant candidates who would otherwise be ventilator dependent. The combination of endotracheal extubation and early mobilisation may further improve outcomes and prevent loss of transplant eligibility due to deconditioning. A major limitation to the use of ECMO for end-stage respiratory failure remains the lack of a destination device therapy. Patients with severe, irreversible respiratory failure, who are not lung transplant candidates, should therefore not be offered ECMO.

Primary graft dysfunction (PGD) is a form of acute lung injury that is the leading cause of early death after lung transplantation. Similar to its ability to support gas exchange in ARDS, ECMO may be used to manage PGD while underlying causes are treated and the allograft recovers. ECMO supported severe PGD may have comparable survival to less severe PGD without ECMO support, particularly when instituted early though long-term effects on allograft function have not been reported.

Pulmonary Vascular Disease

ECMO is an emerging management option in decompensated pulmonary hypertension with concomitant right ventricular failure. In patients with an identifiable and reversible aetiology for decompensation, ECMO may offer an opportunity to correct gas exchange abnormalities and unload the right ventricle while the underlying process is treated and directed pulmonary hypertension therapies are initiated or optimised. In patients with irreversible decompensation who are transplant candidates, ECMO can serve as a bridge to lung transplantation. The configuration typically used for decompensated pulmonary hypertension is femoral venoarterial ECMO. A venoarterial approach decompresses the right ventricle and results in reinfusion flow bypassing the pulmonary vasculature. Alternative configurations include: the use of a bicaval dual lumen cannula in patients with pre-existing interatrial defects, where the reinfusion jet is directed across the defect, creating an oxygenated right-to-left shunt; an upper body venoarterial approach with the combination of internal jugular venous drainage and subclavian arterial reinfusion via a graft, as discussed above; and pumpless arteriovenous ECMO inserted between the main pulmonary artery and the left atrium, though this strategy typically requires a sternotomy.

Acute massive pulmonary embolism may likewise benefit from ECMO. Although there are no randomised controlled trials for ECMO in the management of massive pulmonary embolism, single centre cohort data from an experienced centre suggest reasonable outcomes (62% overall survival when combined with anticoagulation or surgical embolectomy, including patients in active cardiac arrest). Combining modalities, such as ECMO, thrombolysis, and catheter directed thrombectomy or embolus fragmentation, has also been reported with good outcomes (70% 30-day survival).

Chronic thromboembolic pulmonary hypertension may develop as a consequence of recurrent or unresolved acute pulmonary emboli, the treatment of choice for which remains pulmonary thromboendarterectomy (PTE). Residual pulmonary hypertension and reperfusion injury may complicate the post-PTE course, both of which may benefit from ECMO support. In cases of isolated reperfusion injury without haemodynamic compromise, venovenous ECMO may be sufficient, with earlier institution of ECMO support associated with better outcomes, though still worse than outcomes for those who never develop reperfusion injury. When PTE is complicated by an inability to wean off cardiopulmonary bypass or residual pulmonary hypertension with right ventricular failure in the postoperative period, venoarterial ECMO can offload the right ventricle and support gas exchange in a similar fashion to other ECMO supported forms of pulmonary hypertension, although this is a patient population with a high expected mortality.

Future Directions

Unlike cardiac failure in which destination device therapy exists in the form of ventricular assist devices, there is no destination device therapy for end-stage respiratory failure. Therefore, ECMO for respiratory failure in its current form may only serve as a bridge to recovery or to lung transplantation. There is hope that as ECMO technology evolves, including smaller, more durable circuits with more efficient gas exchange, there will come the development of destination therapy, effectively an artificial lung. With such advances, there would be the potential for significant alterations in the way we approach patients with both acute and chronic respiratory failure.

Conclusion

ECMO has the potential to support a broad spectrum of diseases that result in severe cardiopulmonary compromise. Although data remain limited, ongoing and future studies should help shed light on whether ECMO has benefits beyond the current standard of care and, if so, which patients are likely to derive the greatest benefit. Further technological advances have the potential to greatly alter the current paradigm in how we manage patients with severe respiratory and cardiac failure.

Learning Points

- For respiratory failure, ECMO is most commonly used as 'rescue therapy' in severe ARDS, in order to support patients with refractory hypoxaemia.
- Extracorporeal carbon dioxide removal ($ECCO_2R$) is a version of ECMO in which the primary intention of the device is to remove carbon dioxide from the blood. This technique is performed at lower blood flows than are traditionally required for oxygenation.
- $ECCO_2R$ may facilitate the application of standard of care low tidal volume ventilation when respiratory system compliance is reduced. It may also allow for the use of *very* low tidal volumes and airway pressures, though more data are needed before such a strategy can be recommended. $ECCO_2R$ may also have a role in patients with acute hypercapnic respiratory failure, such as acute exacerbations of COPD and severe status asthmaticus.
- Recent data suggest that ECMO can effectively serve as a bridge to either recovery or transplantation in select patients with decompensated pulmonary hypertension with right ventricular failure.
- In its current form, venovenous ECMO remains a temporary form of support. Ongoing technological advances hold the promise of the development of a destination device that would significantly alter the approach to severe, irreversible respiratory failure.

Further Reading

Abrams D, Bacchetta M, Brodie D. Recirculation in venovenous extracorporeal membrane oxygenation. *ASAIO Journal*. 2015; 61: 115–121.

Abrams DC, Brenner K, Burkart KM, et al. Pilot study of extracorporeal carbon dioxide removal to facilitate extubation and ambulation in exacerbations of chronic obstructive pulmonary disease. *Annals of the American Thoracic Society*. 2013; 10: 307–314.

Abrams D, Brodie D. Emerging indications for extracorporeal membrane oxygenation in adults with respiratory failure. *Annals of the American Thoracic Society*. 2013; 10: 371–377.

Abrams DC, Brodie D, Rosenzweig EB, et al. Upper-body extracorporeal membrane oxygenation as a strategy in decompensated pulmonary arterial hypertension. *Pulmonary Circulation*. 2013; 3: 432–435.

Abrams D, Javidfar J, Farrand E, et al. Early mobilization of patients receiving extracorporeal membrane oxygenation: a retrospective cohort study. *Critical Care*. 2014; 18: R38.

Berman M, Tsui S, Vuylsteke A, et al. Successful extracorporeal membrane oxygenation support after pulmonary thromboendarterectomy. *Annals of Thoracic Surgery*. 2008; 86: 1261–1267.

Brodie D, Bacchetta M. Extracorporeal membrane oxygenation for ARDS in adults. *New England Journal of Medicine*. 2011; 365: 1905–1914.

Chiumello D, Coppola S, Froio S, Colombo A, Del Sorbo L. Extracorporeal life support as bridge to lung transplantation: a systematic review. *Critical Care*. 2015; 19: 19.

Combes A, Bacchetta M, Brodie D, Muller T, Pellegrino V. Extracorporeal membrane oxygenation for respiratory failure in adults. *Current Opinion in Critical Care*. 2012; 18: 99–104.

MacLaren G, Combes A, Bartlett RH. Contemporary extracorporeal membrane oxygenation for adult respiratory failure: life support in the new era. *Intensive Care Medicine*. 2012; 38: 210–220.

Mikkelsen ME, Woo YJ, Sager JS, Fuchs BD, Christie JD. Outcomes using extracorporeal life support for adult respiratory failure due to status asthmaticus. *ASAIO Journal*. 2009; 55: 47–52.

Noah MA, Peek GJ, Finney SJ, et al. Referral to an extracorporeal membrane oxygenation center and mortality among patients with severe 2009 influenza A(H1N1). *Journal of the American Medical Association*. 2011; 306: 1659–1668.

Paden ML, Conrad SA, Rycus PT, Thiagarajan RR; ELSO Registry. Extracorporeal Life Support Organization Registry Report 2012. *ASAIO Journal*. 2013; 59: 202–210.

Peek GJ, Mugford M, Tiruvoipati R, et al. Efficacy and economic assessment of conventional ventilatory support versus extracorporeal membrane oxygenation for severe adult respiratory failure (CESAR): a multicentre randomised controlled trial. *Lancet*. 2009; 374: 1351–1363.

The Acute Respiratory Distress Syndrome Network. Ventilation with lower tidal volumes as compared with traditional tidal volumes for acute lung injury and the acute respiratory distress syndrome. *New England Journal of Medicine*. 2000; 342: 1301–1308.

Zapol WM, Snider MT, Hill JD, et al. Extracorporeal membrane oxygenation in severe acute respiratory failure. A randomized prospective study. *Journal of the American Medical Association*. 1979; 242: 2193–2196.

MCQs

1. **Major determinants of systemic oxygenation in venovenous ECMO include all of the following EXCEPT:**
   - (a) ECMO blood flow rate
   - (b) Fraction of delivered oxygen
   - (c) Sweep gas flow rate
   - (d) Native lung function
   - (e) Recirculation
2. **A patient receiving venovenous ECMO develops hypotension in the setting of sepsis. Which of the following is the most appropriate management option?**
   - (a) Increase blood flow rate
   - (b) Start vasopressors
   - (c) Decrease sweep gas flow rate
   - (d) Add additional venous drainage cannula
3. **Endotracheal extubation in awake patients receiving ECMO is:**
   - (a) Standard of care in all patients
   - (b) Standard of care in selected patients
   - (c) Reasonable but of unproven benefit in selected patients
   - (d) Never appropriate
4. **Prospective randomised controlled trials have demonstrated a mortality benefit for which of the following management strategies in ARDS?**
   - (a) Low tidal volume ventilation
   - (b) Prone positioning
   - (c) High frequency oscillatory ventilation
   - (d) (a) and (b)
   - (e) (a) and (c)

5. **Venovenous extracorporeal carbon dioxide removal is most likely to be effective at managing which of the following disease states?**

(a) Status asthmaticus

(b) Decompensated pulmonary hypertension

(c) Severe hypoxaemic respiratory failure

(d) Acute massive pulmonary embolism

Exercise answers are available on p.469. Alternatively, take the test online at www.cambridge.org/CardiothoracicMCQ

Chapter 25A

Resuscitation after Adult Cardiac Surgery

Jonathan H Mackay

Defibrillation, ventilation, pacing and resuscitation are essential components of cardiac surgical care. The 2015 European Resuscitation Council (ERC) guidelines report the incidence of resuscitation as 0.7–8% after adult cardiac surgery. This wide range is almost certainly due to resuscitation interventions frequently being undertaken *in house* on many cardiac surgical ICUs, and therefore going under the radar of the clinical audit. Prompt and effective basic life support (BLS) and early defibrillation for shockable rhythms are the two most important interventions after cardiac arrest. Chest reopening and extracorporeal membrane oxygenation (ECMO) for patients with refractory cardiogenic shock are additional therapeutic options. As patients undergoing cardiac surgery become older and sicker, quality of resuscitation will continue to increase in importance.

Resuscitation Guidelines

Conventional basic and advanced life support guidelines provide a useful framework but require modification in the cardiac surgical ICU setting. The European Association of Cardiothoracic Surgery (EACTS) guidelines summarise the key modifications that must be considered for adult patients in cardiac arrest after cardiac surgery. Although current resuscitation algorithms typically divide arrests into two (shockable and non-shockable) limbs, EACTS subdivide the non-shockable category and utilise a three-limb approach. The EACTS three-limb model emphasises important initial differences in management of patients presenting with severe bradycardia or asystole compared to those presenting with pulseless electrical activity (see Figure 25A.1). Important changes in the revised 2015 European Resuscitation Council guidelines are discussed below.

Adult Basic Life Support

Maintaining the circulation has been promoted ahead of airway management and breathing in recent adult basic life support (BLS) guidelines. The traditional Airway, Breathing, Circulation and Defibrillation (ABCD) algorithm described in previous guidelines has been replaced by Circulation, Airway and Breathing (i.e. CAB). In general, 30 chest compressions at a rate of 100–120 per minute should now be given before any attempt to deliver rescue breaths. The efficacy of chest compressions can usually be verified in the ICU by studying the arterial pressure waveform. Interruptions to chest compressions should be minimised and last less than 10 seconds.

In situations where BLS is undertaken, the recommended ratio of chest compressions to ventilations is now 30:2. More chest compressions and fewer interruptions are achieved with this ratio than with the previously recommended 15:2 ratio. In the presence of a patent airway, effective chest compressions are considered more important than ventilation in the first few minutes of resuscitation. It should be borne in mind that coronary perfusion pressure progressively rises during chest compressions and rapidly falls with each pause for ventilation. Following a witnessed collapse in a patient with oxygenated arterial blood, the initial emphasis should normally be on chest compressions.

Because chest compressions may be injurious immediately following cardiac surgery, external cardiac massage is frequently deferred in the cardiac ICU providing defibrillation or external pacing therapy can be delivered within 30–60 seconds. The rationale for this approach and modifications to the Advanced Life Support (ALS) algorithm are discussed later.

Adult Advanced Life Support

The new 2015 Advanced Life Support (ALS) algorithm for the management of cardiac arrest in adults retains the shockable and non-shockable limbs (Figure 25A.2). There are subtle but important differences in recommendations for defibrillation for

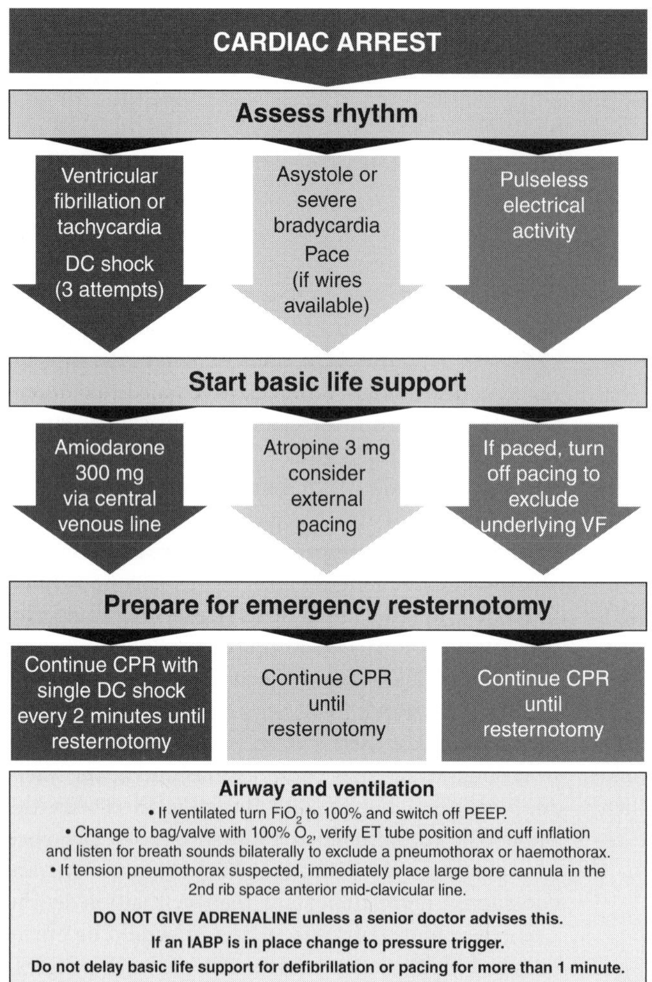

Figure 25A.1 EACTS guideline for resuscitation of a postoperative cardiac surgical ICU (or recovery) patient. From Dunning et al. (2009).

shockable rhythms in cardiothoracic ICU and the catheter laboratory. The EACTS guidelines include important advice on how to expedite the decision making and actual chest reopening process (see Figure 25A.1).

Pulseless VT/VF

Pulseless VT and VF account for the majority of underlying dysrhythmias in patients who survive cardiac arrest in hospitals. For every minute the chances of successful defibrillation decline by 7–10%. Specialist cardiothoracic units should be capable of early detection, rapid defibrillation and superior outcomes. In the setting of the cardiac ICU, when external cardiac massage may be injurious, immediate defibrillation (i.e. DCAB) should be the first line response for all monitored in-hospital VF arrests.

Since 2005, a single shock ($\geq$150 J biphasic or 360 J monophasic) has been recommended instead of three 'stacked' shocks, in general hospitals. Interruptions to CPR during delivery of three shocks and improved first shock efficacy of biphasic defibrillators were cited as reasons for the change. In practice, most cardiac surgical ICU and catheter laboratory staff were unconvinced by the evidence for single shocks and continued to deliver up to three stacked shocks in quick succession when treating VF. More recent EACTS and ERC guidelines recognised this and recommend three stacked shocks in quick succession for VF/VT arrests occurring in the cardiac catheter laboratory and cardiac surgical ICU. In addition, contrary to the latest guidelines, there is usually no need to commence chest compressions after a successful shock in invasively monitored cardiac surgical patients.

Table 25A.1 An aide memoire to the causes of pulseless electrical activity and asystole

The Four 'Hs'	The Five 'Ts'
Hypoxia	Tension pneumothorax
Hypovolaemia	Tamponade
Hyperkalaemia	Thromboembolic
Hypothermia	Therapeutic substances in overdose
	Toxic substances

Non-VF/VT Arrests

A heterogeneous group of conditions may present as non-VF/VT cardiac arrest (Table 25A.1). Outcome is generally poor unless a reversible cause can be found and treated effectively. In the cardiac surgical ICU – where bleeding, hypovolaemia and tamponade are all readily treatable, and where additional therapeutic options are available – outcomes are considerably better than in the general ICU population. Examination of trends in RA pressure, PAWP and airway pressure all provide useful pointers as to the likely aetiology. Cessation of drainage from mediastinal drains does not exclude haemorrhage or tamponade as the drains may have become blocked. Although TTE and TEE echocardiography is often very useful in the cardiac ICU, echocardiography may miss localised collections and thus delay reoperation. Patients with clinical signs suggestive of tamponade should be reopened even if echocardiography is inconclusive.

When faced with an arrest of this type, it is essential to:

- confirm that VF is not being missed and that ECG leads or pads are correctly attached,
- treat bradycardia with epicardial pacing if wires are present,
- exclude tension pneumothorax,
- exclude underlying VF in the presence of fixed rate pacing, and
- consider chest reopening if closed chest CPR is unsuccessful.

Symptomatic bradycardia is extremely common in the cardiac surgical ICU. ALS guidelines no longer recommend atropine as first line treatment. In the cardiac surgical ICU, where tachycardia is equally undesirable, pacing (when possible) is the preferred option. If pacing is not an option (e.g. no wires in situ or failure to capture), isoproterenol or dopamine are often used. Management of asystole that fails to respond to pacing is an indication for prompt chest reopening.

Suggested modifications to the standard ALS algorithm are shown in Figure 25A.2.

Drugs in Advanced Cardiac Life Support

Although the use of vasopressors at cardiac arrests has become standard practice, proof of efficacy is limited. Epinephrine 1 mg is recommended every 3 minutes to improve coronary and cerebral perfusion. The American Heart Association has suggested that vasopressin may be used as an alternative to epinephrine. Clinical studies, however, have failed to demonstrate that either vasopressin or high dose epinephrine (5 mg) offers any additional benefit.

On the cardiac surgical ICU it is entirely appropriate to modify the recommended pharmacological management of a monitored cardiac arrest. An α-agonist or smaller initial dosages of epinephrine (0.1–0.2 mg) may be administered to minimise the risk of hypertension and tachycardia following successful resuscitation. For patients with VF/VT arrests, it is standard practice to attempt at least three shocks before giving any epinephrine.

The evidence supporting the use of antiarrhythmic drugs in VF/VT is surprisingly weak. Two studies of out-of-hospital VF/VT arrest demonstrated that the administration of amiodarone after three unsuccessful shocks increased the likelihood of survival to hospital admission. Significantly, neither study demonstrated that amiodarone improved survival to discharge. Despite this latter finding, amiodarone has now been promoted ahead of lidocaine in the pulseless VF/VT algorithm. A bolus of amiodarone 300 mg is recommended for VF/VT arrests that persist after three shocks but this should not delay surgical reopening (see below). A further dose (150 mg) may be given for recurrent or refractory VF/VT, followed by an infusion of 900 mg over 24 hours. Lidocaine can still be given for VF/VT if the patient has received amiodarone but the evidence supporting its efficacy is weak. Magnesium should also be considered if there is clinical suspicion of hypomagnesaemia. Administration of sodium bicarbonate should be considered if arterial or mixed venous pH < 7.1.

Airway and Ventilation

The Fourth National Audit Project (NAP4) of the Royal College of Anaesthetists reported that 61% (22 of 36) of airway events in the ICU led to death or

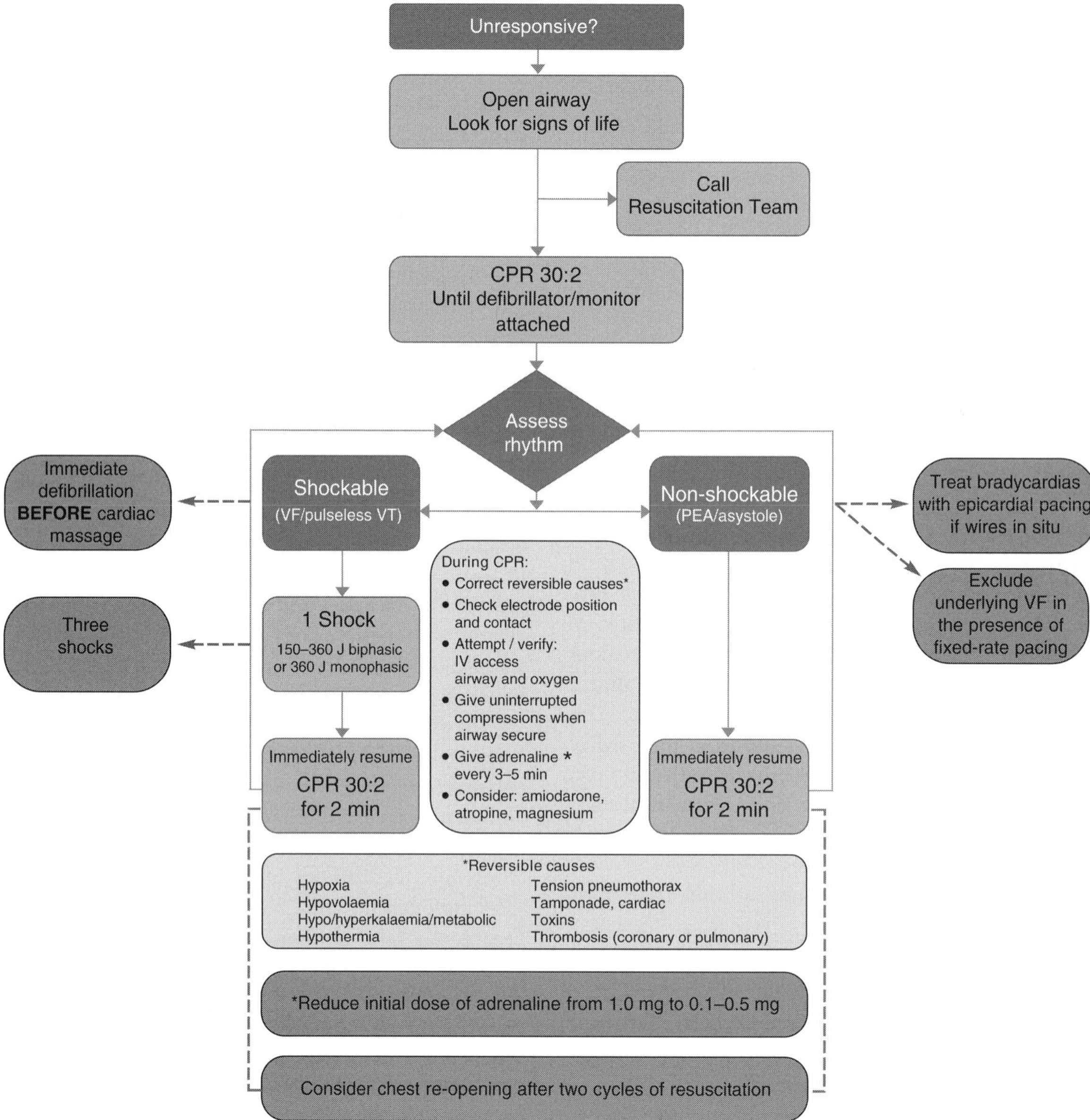

Figure 25A.2 Algorithm for resuscitation after adult cardiac surgery. Six suggested modifications to the standard ALS algorithm are highlighted in the six bright yellow boxes to the sides and below. Therapeutic hypothermia may be considered after successful resuscitation. Adapted from the Resuscitation Council (UK) 2010 ALS algorithm. (A black and white version of this figure will appear in some formats. For the colour version, please refer to the plate section.)

persistent neurological injury. Major risk factors for adverse events included anaesthetic experience of doctors, out-of-hours airway interventions, patient obesity and failure to use (or correctly interpret) capnography. A recurrent finding was the failure to consider the possibility of oesophageal intubation when presented with a flat capnograph trace. As well as providing valuable information about endotracheal tube position and patency, and ventilation, capnography also provides invaluable additional information about return of spontaneous circulation and cardiac output (see Table 25A.2). The introduction of mandatory waveform capnography in the CICU has arguably made the single biggest contribution to improved patient safety on the CICU since the publication of the first edition of CTiCICU 1e nearly a decade ago.

Table 25A.2 Waveform capnography during ALS

Confirmation of tracheal intubation
Monitoring ventilation rate
Monitoring quality chest compressions
Identifying ROSC during CPR
Prognostication during CPR: failure to achieve CO_2 value >1.33 kPa (10 mmHg) after 20 minutes CPR associated with poor outcome

Chest Reopening

Following surgery through a sternotomy, chest reopening is both a diagnostic and therapeutic option in the cardiac surgical ICU. In addition, chest reopening allows internal cardiac massage, which is considerably more effective than external chest compressions. Haemorrhage, tamponade, graft occlusion and graft avulsion are conditions likely to be remedied by this approach. Patients most likely to benefit are: those with a surgically remediable lesion, those who arrest within 24 hours of surgery and those in whom the chest is reopened within 10 minutes of arrest. Delayed reopening or the finding of a problem that is not amenable to surgery (e.g. global cardiac dysfunction) is associated with a poor prognosis. Recent resuscitation guidelines confirm that chest reopening should be triggered by:

- three failed shocks in VF/VT arrests (i.e. one resuscitation cycle);
- exclusion of reversible causes (e.g. tension pneumothorax) and failure of initial treatment for non-VF/VT arrest.

Chest reopening should not be used as a 'last ditch' manoeuvre after a prolonged period of unsuccessful resuscitation. Although some units advocate initially stopping all infusions and syringe drivers to exclude iatrogenic drug administration errors, the majority tend to continue infusions unless there is a clinical suspicion of inadvertent vasodilator flushing being responsible for loss of CO. Whichever policy is used, it is important to ensure that anaesthesia and analgesia are restored prior to chest reopening. The EACTS guidelines and Cardiac Advanced Life Support (CALS) courses recommend six key roles in the management of a cardiac surgical ICU arrest (Figure 25A.3).

Cardiopulmonary Bypass and ECMO

The reinstitution of cardiopulmonary bypass (CPB) following emergency chest reopening may allow the resuscitation of a patient who would otherwise die. Hypothermic CPB restores organ perfusion, decompresses the heart, and allows the surgeon to consider all possible options in a more controlled setting. Valve replacement, repair of bleeding cannulation sites, graft revision and additional grafting may be undertaken with often surprisingly successful clinical outcomes. Whenever possible the patient should be transferred to the operating room before emergency reinstitution of CPB.

VA ECMO is a therapeutic option for those who cannot be weaned from emergency bypass. The indications, methods and outcomes of postcardiotomy ECMO are discussed elsewhere.

Late Resuscitation on the ICU

Patients with greater preoperative surgical risk, adverse intraoperative events and poor physiological state at the time of ICU admission are less likely to survive to hospital discharge. Similarly, refractory multisystem organ failure and recurrent nosocomial infection have been shown to be important determinants of mortality. For some patients, there comes a point when aggressive resuscitation is inappropriate and cardiopulmonary arrest becomes a terminal event. It is the duty of a doctor to identify these patients and to ensure that they are spared the indignity of futile interventions.

DNAR directives should be instituted if it is believed that death is inevitable and that CPR is unlikely to be successful. Sensible guidelines on implementation of DNAR orders can be found on the UK Resuscitation Council's website (www.resus.org.uk/dnacpr).

Resuscitation Outside the ICU

General Ward or Surgical Floor

The management of a cardiac arrest outside the ICU differs little from a cardiac arrest on a general surgical or medical ward. Seemingly trivial symptoms and vague 'early warning' signs should be taken seriously as they may herald a more sinister event. Although some arrests are unheralded, the majority of patients who arrest in the general ward setting display signs of physiological deterioration long before the event.

Early intervention seems intuitive and may reduce the incidence of cardiac arrests in the surgical ward setting. Early warning scores (EWS) are used to 'track'

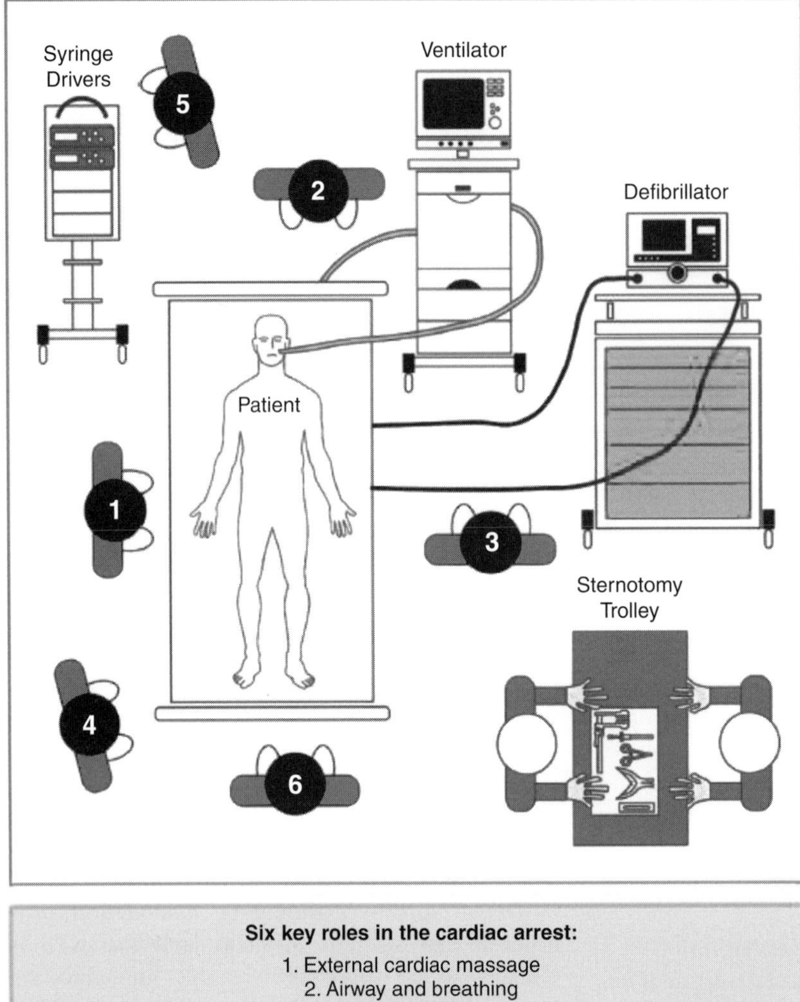

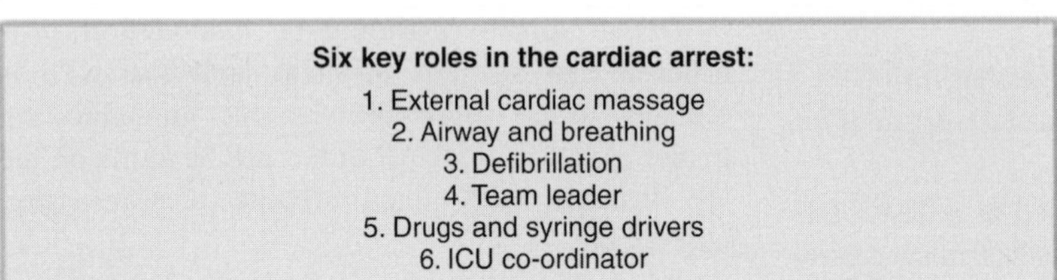

Figure 25A.3 Six key roles in cardiac surgical ICU arrest. From Dunning et al. (2009).

patients' physiological status and 'trigger' a response or intervention. Tracking the patient – the so-called 'afferent limb' – involves either a single or multiple parameter scoring system. Single parameter scoring systems have limitations. Many of the suggested criteria for triggering a response are actually relatively late markers of physiological deterioration (Table 25A.3). Aggregated weighted systems may provide earlier warning of deterioration and can be adapted for use in cardiothoracic wards (Table 25A.4).

The use of medical emergency teams (MET) has been shown to reduce both the incidence of and mortality from unexpected ward arrests in general hospitals. The effectiveness of the MET concept is significantly hampered by incomplete documentation of patient observations. Given the importance of respiratory rate and urinary output, recording of these values is often surprisingly poor.

The relative success of chest reopening following cardiac arrest on the ICU cannot be reproduced when chest reopening is undertaken on the ward or surgical floor. The proportion of surgically remediable causes of cardiac arrest decreases exponentially after surgery. As time passes, thromboembolic phenomena and cardiac failure become more common than surgical bleeding or tamponade. A small number of patients who sustain a *witnessed* arrest on the ward or surgical floor may benefit from chest reopening either locally with appropriate facilities or in the operating room. The decision to reopen a ward patient either locally or after 'scoop and run' is usually more difficult than the decision to reopen on the cardiac ICU. Whereas there is level-one evidence to support chest reopening in the cardiac ICU, the latest ERC guidelines do not specifically address the role of chest reopening for patients who arrest outside the cardiac ICU. A scoop and run approach should be considered following:

1. A witnessed arrest;
2. Unexpected arrest in a patient who had initially been making good progress;
3. Tension pneumothorax considered and excluded;
4. Close proximity to operating theatres;
5. Non-VF/VT arrest with a high index of suspicion of hypovolaemia (major bleeding), tamponade, acute thromboembolism or air embolism;
6. VF/VT arrests unresponsive to DC shocks that may have acute graft occlusion.

A patient's suitability for chest reopening and reinstitution of CPB should be considered after one cycle of CPR. The decision to scoop and run must be made early because time is of the essence. Good quality chest compressions and ventilation must be maintained during transfer. Epinephrine 1 mg (or an alternative vasopressor) should be given every 3–5 minutes as per standard ALS guidelines, rather than the reduced dosages recommended in cardiac surgical ICU for

Table 25A.3 Suggested criteria for calling the medical emergency team in a cardiothoracic hospital; oximetry is widely available and a potentially useful monitor in a cardiothoracic ward

Acute change	Physiology
Airway	Threatened
Breathing	All respiratory arrests Respiratory rate <5 or >36
Circulation	All cardiac arrests Pulse rate <40 or >140
Neurology	Fall in Glasgow coma scale (GCS) score >2 points
Renal	Urine output <0.5 ml/kg/hr for 2 consecutive hours
Oximetry	SpO_2 < 90% regardless of FiO_2
Other	Patients giving cause for concern who do not meet above criteria

Table 25A.4 Papworth Cardiothoracic Early Warning Score (CTEWS)

Score	Tem p(ºC)	Neuro AVPU or ACDU	Respiratory rate	pO_2/ FiO_2ratio	Heart rate	Systolic BP	Urine output catheter in situ *No catheter*
3	≤35.0	Unresponsive	≤8	<18	<40	≤75	<0.1 ml/kg/hr
2	35.1–35.5	Response to pain	9–10	18–24.9	40–44	76–85	≥0.1 ml/kg/hr <0.3 ml/kg/hr
1	35.6–36.0	Response to voice		25–34.9	45–50	86–100	≥0.3 ml/kg/hr <0.5 ml/kg/hr
0	36.1–38.0	Alert	11–19	≥35	51–104	101–199	≥0.5 ml/kg/hr *or PU* *<6 hr – day* *<10 hr – night*
1	38.1-38.4	Confused	20–24		105–134		*NPU* *≥6 hr day* *≥ 10 hr night*
2	≥38.5	Drowsy	25–29		≥135	≥200	*NPU* *≥ 12 hr*
3		Unresponsive	≥30				*NPU* *≥ 18 hr*

** pO_2/FiO_2 ratio = (kPa).
PU = passed urine; NPU = not passed urine.

patients in the immediate postoperative period. It needs to be emphasised that scoop and run will only be successful if both the heart and *brain* are successfully restored to normal or near-normal function.

Catheter Laboratory Arrests

VF/VT arrests during elective procedures in the catheter laboratory are invariably iatrogenic, typically amenable to very early defibrillation and associated with return of spontaneous circulation in >90% of cases, and have >80% chance of survival to discharge. As discussed earlier, recent ERC guidelines recommend administration of three stacked shocks in quick succession for VF/VT arrests occurring in the cardiac catheter laboratory. In cases of coronary dissection or other surgically amenable conditions, early consideration of transfer to the operating room and institution of CPB should be considered.

Patients undergoing primary percutaneous intervention who require airway intervention present similar challenges to those on the ICU albeit in a remote environment with potentially limited immediate anaesthetic support. As with the ICU, skilled anaesthetic assistance and waveform capnography are both mandatory.

ECMO assisted CPR, so-called E-CPR, is an additional therapeutic option for selected patients in ECMO centres. The CHEER trial recently reported that 14 of 26 (54%) patients with refractory in-hospital and out-of-hospital arrests survived to hospital discharge with full neurological recovery. Running a 24/7 catheter laboratory ECMO service mandates funding of:

1. Resident (or very close proximity) consultant cardiologist, intensivist and perfusion cover;
2. ICU costs associated with potentially prolonged ICU lengths of stay awaiting neurological prognostication in comatose survivors.

Conclusion

Patients sustaining cardiac arrests in a cardiothoracic surgical unit are twice as likely to survive to hospital discharge as patients who arrest in a general hospital. The essential requirements for a good clinical outcome are early detection, effective BLS and early defibrillation.

Learning Points

- ALS algorithms require modification in the cardiac surgical ICU.
- Consider the possibility of underlying VF in 'asystolic' arrests and paced patients with apparent pulseless electrical activity.
- Look for epicardial pacing wires in bradycardic arrests before giving atropine and epinephrine!
- The majority of cardiac arrests after cardiac surgery are heralded by symptoms and signs.

Further Reading

Cook TM, Woodall N, Harper J, Benger J; Fourth National Audit Project. Major complications of airway management in the UK: results of the Fourth National Audit Project of the Royal College of Anaesthetists and the Difficult Airway Society. Part 2: intensive care and emergency departments. *British Journal of Anaesthesia.* 2011; 106: 632–642.

Dunning J, Fabbri A, Kolh PH, et al. Guideline for resuscitation in cardiac arrest after cardiac surgery. *European Journal of Cardio-Thoracic Surgery.* 2009; 36: 3–28.

Mackay JH, Powell SJ, Osgathorp J, Rozario CJ. Six-year prospective audit of chest reopening after cardiac arrest. *European Journal of Cardio-Thoracic Surgery.* 2002; 22: 421–425.

Nielsen N, Wetterslev J, Cronberg T, et al. Targeted temperature management at 33°C versus 36°C after cardiac arrest. *New England Journal of Medicine.* 2013; 369: 2197–2206.

Sandroni C, Cariou A, Cavallaro F, et al. Prognostication in comatose survivors of cardiac arrest: an advisory statement from the European Resuscitation Council and the European Society of Intensive Care Medicine. *Intensive Care Medicine.* 2014; 40: 1816–1831.

Stub D, Bernard S, Pellegrino V, et al. Refractory cardiac arrest treated with mechanical CPR, hypothermia, ECMO and early reperfusion (the CHEER trial). *Resuscitation.* 2015; 86: 88–94.

Truhlar A, Deakin C, Soar J, et al. European Resuscitation Council Guidelines for Resuscitation 2015 Section 4. Cardiac arrest in special circumstances. *Resuscitation.* 2015; 95: 148–201.

MCQs

1. **Aetiology of arrests in the cardiac surgical ICU:**
   (a) Vast majority unheralded
   (b) Commonly due to mild hypothermia (temperature 34.0–35.0 °C)
   (c) Commonly due to moderate hyperkalaemia (K^+ 5.5–6.0)
   (d) Almost invariably due to unstable arrhythmias
   (e) Bleeding is the most common cause
2. **VF arrests in the cardiac surgical ICU:**
   (a) Immediate BLS 30:2 always
   (b) Prepare to restart chest compressions after single shock
   (c) Amiodarone (300 mg) and adrenaline (1 mg) should be given within 3 minutes of arrest
   (d) May be due to problems with intracardiac air or graft malfunction
   (e) Chest compressions are required after successful shock to reduce LV distension
3. **Chest reopening in the cardiac surgical ICU:**
   (a) Should only be undertaken by a surgeon
   (b) Should only be undertaken as a last resort
   (c) Can be undertaken by any member of the team
   (d) Is usually associated with poor outcomes
   (e) Is no longer necessary due to advances in AV ECMO
4. **PEA arrests due to tamponade:**
   (a) Are usually unheralded
   (b) External massage may be ineffective
   (c) A focused TTE is mandatory within 5 minutes of arrest
   (d) TTE has >90% sensitivity, >90% specificity
   (e) Can usually be managed by needle paracentesis
5. **Capnography in the cardiac ICU:**
   (a) Rarely provides useful information
   (b) Is desirable in spontaneously breathing patients
   (c) High $ETCO_2$ is a hallmark of deteriorating cardiac function
   (d) Is mandatory in all cardiac arrests requiring airway intervention
   (e) Failure to achieve CO_2 value >4 kPa (40 mmHg) after 20 minutes CPR is associated with a poor outcome

Exercise answers are available on p.469. Alternatively, take the test online at www.cambridge.org/CardiothoracicMCQ

Out-of-Hospital Cardiac Arrest Patients in the Cardiothoracic Intensive Care Unit

Lisen Hockings and Sophia Fisher

Introduction

Patients suffering from cardiac arrest in the community and surviving it are frequently transferred to a cardiothoracic centre where further investigations and treatment are possible. The majority of these patients have already been intubated and ventilated, and are transferred directly to an angiography laboratory where percutaneous interventions are performed. Once the investigations and treatment in the angiography laboratory are completed the patients are then transferred to the cardiothoracic intensive care unit for further management.

With the advent and increasing availability of mechanical circulatory support (MCS) devices (including mechanical chest compression devices (MCCD) and extracorporeal membrane oxygenation (ECMO)/extracorporeal CPR (ECPR)) there are likely to be increasing numbers of out-of-hospital cardiac arrest patients transported to hospitals whilst still in cardiac arrest. Critical care clinicians must be comfortable with continuing high quality CPR and ACLS and with the operation of MCS devices.

Survival

Survival after out-of-hospital cardiac arrest (OHCA) is increasing but remains low, and varies across geographic regions and institutions. Where outcomes have improved it appears to be in younger patients and in those who have an initial shockable rhythm. This has been attributed to a focused improvement in each of basic life support (BLS), advanced cardiac life support (ACLS) and post-resuscitation care (PRC) – the elements that form a continuum of links in the 'chain of survival' (Figure 25B.1) outlined by the International Liaison Committee on Resuscitation (ILCOR):

- early recognition and call for help to prevent cardiac arrest;
- early cardiopulmonary resuscitation (CPR) to buy time;
- early defibrillation to restart the heart;
- post-resuscitation care to restore quality of life.

ILCOR publishes a five yearly update to the International Consensus on cardiopulmonary resuscitation (CPR) and emergency cardiovascular care (ECC) Science with Treatment Recommendations (CoSTR). This document forms the basis for guidelines that are subsequently produced and endorsed by member organisations. An in-depth discussion of basic and advanced life support is beyond the scope of this chapter.

Strategies that have led to increased survival in a variety of settings have included systematic community based projects to enhance first responder CPR training, increased numbers of public access automated external defibrillators (AEDs) and protocolised in-hospital care pathways.

The Post-cardiac Arrest Syndrome

Overall survival and long-term outcomes after OHCA are related to the underlying cause of the arrest, the hypoxaemic/ischaemic insult to the brain and other organs during the period of circulatory arrest, and to the severity of the post-cardiac arrest syndrome (PCAS) that occurs with reperfusion – in the setting of a return of spontaneous circulation (ROSC) or with institution of MCS.

Post-cardiac arrest care begins immediately on reinstitution of circulation. Some patients with a readily reversible cause and short duration of cardiac arrest will suffer very little, if any, systemic insult. Immediate goals of treatment having achieved restoration of circulation (ROSC or MCS) include the diagnosis and management of the underlying cause of the cardiac arrest in order to prevent recurrence, minimising ongoing injury from both the cardiac arrest itself and the insults from reperfusion injury, and multiple organ support.

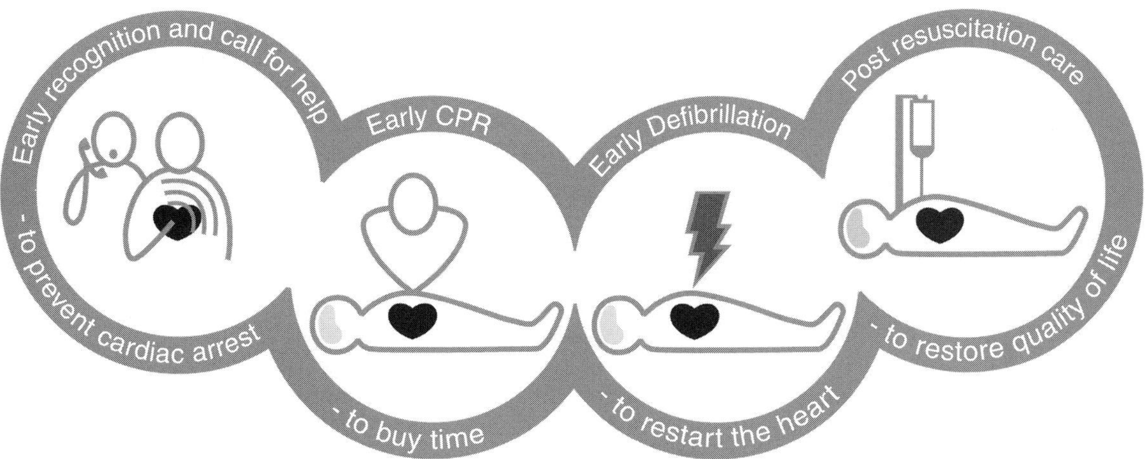

Figure 25B.1 Chain of survival, courtesy of the Adult Basic Life Support Guidelines of the Resuscitation Council. (A black and white version of this figure will appear in some formats. For the colour version, please refer to the plate section.)

Four key components of PCAS have been described:

- Post-cardiac arrest brain injury;
- Post-cardiac arrest myocardial dysfunction;
- Systemic ischaemia/reperfusion response;
- Persistent precipitating pathology.

Post-cardiac Arrest Brain Injury

The brain is particularly vulnerable to hypoxic ischaemic injury in the setting of circulatory arrest. Reperfusion is associated with an ongoing cascade of cerebral injury. Mechanisms are incompletely understood but are thought to include: disruptions to calcium homeostasis, excitotoxicity, alterations in membrane permeability with resultant cellular oedema, free radical generation, mitochondrial dysfunction and activation of apoptotic pathways. Cerebrovascular autoregulation may be impaired for an extended period of time following cardiac arrest.

Clinical findings in post-cardiac arrest brain injury include coma, seizures, myoclonus, neurocognitive dysfunction and in the most severe cases, brain death. Post-cardiac arrest brain injury is the leading cause of morbidity and mortality after cardiac arrest. The protracted pattern of neuronal cell death suggests a wide therapeutic window with multiple potential pharmacological and physiological interventions to optimise outcome. To date, only therapeutic temperature management has shown any likelihood of improved outcomes. Post-cardiac arrest brain injury may be compounded by the other features of PCAS (persistent cardiovascular instability, complications from systemic ischaemia-reperfusion (hypo/hypergycaemia, hyperthermia), and persistent precipitating pathology (hypoxaemia)) as well as potentially by therapeutic interventions (hypo/hypercarbia, hyperoxia).

Post-cardiac Arrest Myocardial Dysfunction

Haemodynamics in the immediate post-ROSC setting can be extremely labile, reflecting circulating endogenous and exogenous catecholamines, and an ischaemia-reperfusion injury to the myocardium (regardless of the initial cause of arrest). Following cardiac arrest there is a period of myocardial 'stunning' that occurs despite evidence of preserved coronary blood flow (where coronary ischaemia was not the primary cause of cardiac arrest) characterised by global hypokinesis and elevated filling pressures. Observational data and animal studies suggest that this reversible period of myocardial stunning lasts for up to 72 hours.

Clinically this can manifest as dysrhythmia, hypotension and evidence of a low cardiac output state with systemic hypoperfusion. Treatment is supportive and can include judicious fluid administration, inotropes, vasopressors, temporary pacing and MCS (intra-aortic balloon counterpulsation pump (IABP), venoarterial ECMO or left ventricular assist device (LVAD)). Cardiovascular instability and complications remain a leading cause of death in patients who survive an initial cardiac arrest.

Systemic Ischaemia-Reperfusion Response

Circulatory arrest prevents tissue oxygen and nutrient delivery and metabolic waste removal. Even with continuous CPR there is an accumulated systemic oxygen debt that causes endothelial activation and cellular (and subsequently organ) dysfunction and results in generalised activation of the inflammatory and coagulation cascades. The endothelial glycocalyx appears to play a central role in these processes. Systemic hypoperfusion may self-propagate and progress even with reinstitution of circulation due to post-cardiac arrest myocardial dysfunction, vasodilatation and microcirculatory failure. This 'systemic inflammatory response syndrome' (SIRS) shares many features with sepsis and can result in the clinical appearance of relative hypovolaemia (with interstitial oedema and capillary leak), abnormal circulatory autoregulation, impaired oxygen delivery and uptake, and an increased susceptibility to infection. The severity of the syndrome and markers of inflammation are associated with a poorer prognosis.

Persistent Precipitating Pathology

Primary myocardial disease is the most common cause of OHCA. However, circulatory arrest can be the presenting feature or final common pathway in any number (if not all) pathologies. More common etiologies can include the following:

Respiratory	pulmonary embolus; pneumothorax; hypoxaemia – drowning, aspiration, asphyxiation; end-stage chronic obstructive airways disease (COAD), asthma
Neurological	subarachnoid haemorrhage (SAH), cerebrovascular accident, prolonged seizures
Sepsis	
Metabolic	including electrolyte abnormalities and temperature derangement
Trauma	hypovolaemia (haemorrhage), tension pneumothorax, tamponade
Toxicology	envenomation and overdoses

Where cardiac arrest has occurred as a result of a systemic illness, the likelihood of sustained ROSC when the underlying pathology has not been treated is remote. Addressing potentially reversible causes remains a key component of ACLS resuscitation algorithms with the 4 Hs and 4 Ts mnemonic:

- Hypoxia
- Hypovolaemia
- Hypokalaemia/hyperkalaemia/other metabolic
- Hypothermia/hyperthermia
- Thrombosis – coronary or pulmonary
- Tension pneumothorax
- Tamponade – cardiac
- Toxins

Assessment of likely antecedent cause(s) for the cardiac arrest must occur contemporaneously with ACLS and post-resuscitation care. This involves collateral history from first responders, paramedics, family members and medical staff as well as a focused clinical examination and investigations where appropriate.

Persistent precipitating pathology can both confound and complicate management of the post-cardiac arrest patient. Asphyxiation is associated with more severe cerebral oedema and post-cardiac arrest brain injury than other causes of circulatory arrest. A SIRS response in the setting of sepsis may potentiate the haemodynamic instability and multiple organ dysfunction associated with systemic ischaemia-reperfusion. Acute coronary syndrome (ACS) as a cause for cardiac arrest will exacerbate post-arrest myocardial dysfunction, and early percutaneous coronary intervention has been associated with improved neurologically intact survival.

Intensive Care Management

The intensive care management of OHCA patients involves the diagnosis and treatment of the underlying cause for the arrest, managing subsequent cardiovascular dysfunction, minimising and managing any further organ damage, and prognostication. Critical care physicians are increasingly involved in the very early management of cardiac arrest patients – as part of rapid response teams (RRTs) attending in-hospital cardiac arrest (IHCA) and as an integral part of protocolised in-hospital care pathways for OHCA patients.

Due to a relative paucity of high quality research in post-resuscitative care, there are only limited data to support specific interventions. However, several hospital level critical care interventions have consistently been associated with improved outcomes after OHCA (see Figure 25B.2):

- Early percutaneous coronary intervention (PCI);
- Targeted temperature management (TTM);
- Delayed prognostication before withdrawal of cardiorespiratory supports.

Return of spontaneous circulation and comatose

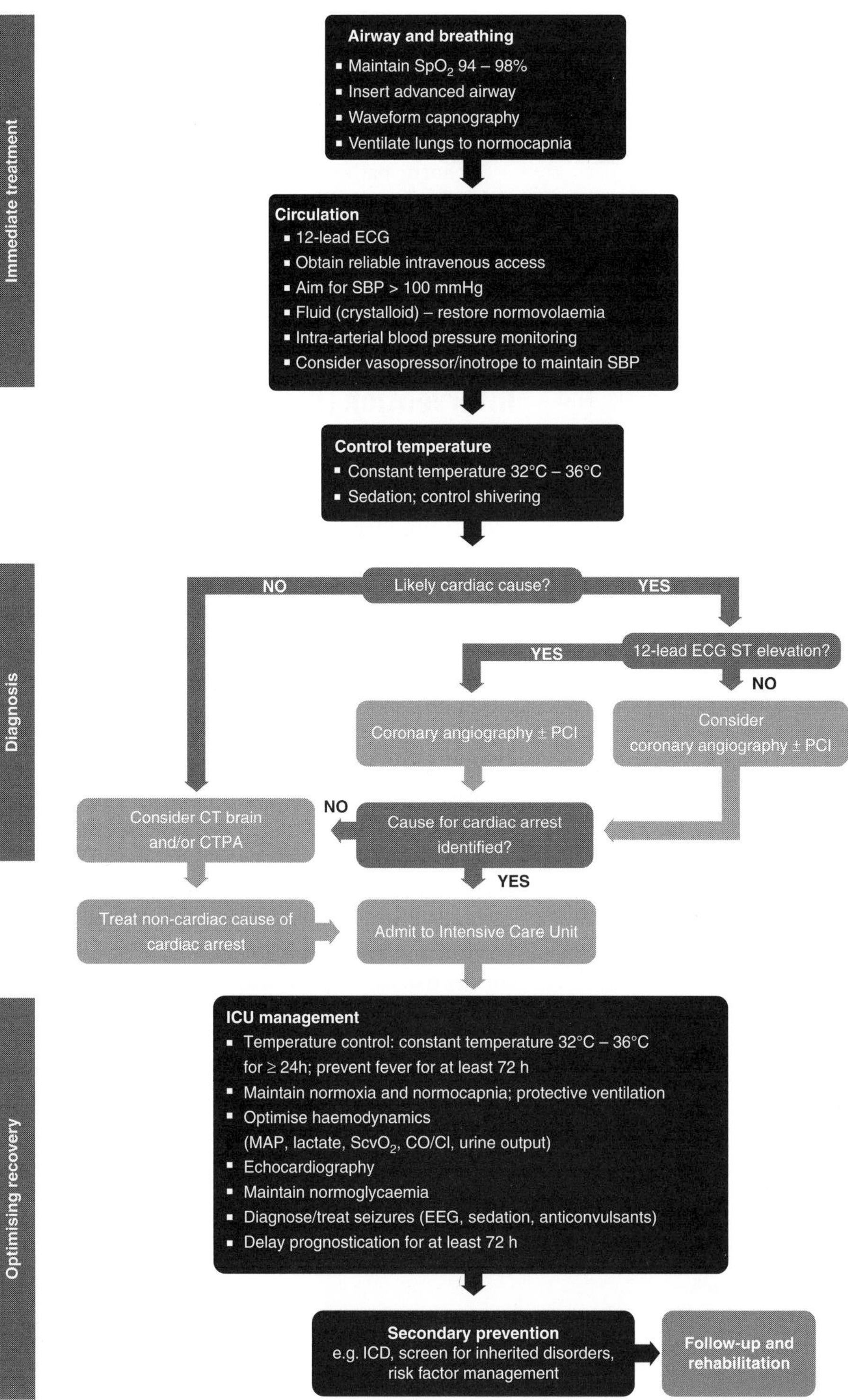

Figure 25B.2 Post-resuscitation care algorithm. SBP systolic blood pressure; PCI percutaneous coronary intervention; CTPA computerised tomography pulmonary angiogram; ICU intensive care unit; MAP mean arterial pressure; $ScvO_2$ central venous oxygenation; CO/CI cardiac output/cardiac index; EEG electroencephalography; ICD implanted cardioverter defibrillator.

Image courtesy of Elsevier Limited.

A Practical Approach

Assessment and management of the post-ROSC OHCA patient should occur simultaneously, using a team-based approach with an initial focus on the airway, breathing and circulation. History, examination, investigations and treatment should occur contemporaneously.

In the unconscious patient collateral **history** must be obtained from first responders, paramedic and emergency staff, medical records, and family members.

Physical examination should focus on excluding persistent precipitating pathologies and an assessment of the adequacy of circulation and end-organ perfusion.

Important **investigations** to aid diagnosis and subsequent management include the following:

12-lead electrocardiogram (ECG): to identify evidence of coronary ischaemia, abnormal conduction such as a prolonged QT interval, or right heart strain (suggestive of a pulmonary embolus).

Transthoracic echocardiography (TTE): ultrasound is playing an increasing role in emergency and critical care medicine and is now incorporated into ALS algorithms. Early focused and/or formal TTE may help to differentiate the aetiology of OHCA and guide treatment decisions.

Blood tests: these include a full blood count, a blood group and screen, electrolytes, urea and creatinine, troponin, and early arterial blood gas to help establish the cause of the arrest, assess the severity of insults and provide baseline information. Toxicology analysis may be considered.

Chest X-ray: evaluation of primary pulmonary pathology, potential injuries sustained during resuscitation and the correct position of an endotracheal tube and central vascular access.

Computerised tomography (CT) brain/chest: may reveal intracranial haemorrhage as the cause of the arrest, or cerebral oedema as a result of ischaemic-hypoxic injury. In selected patients a CT chest scan may reveal a pulmonary embolus or aortic pathology.

Treatment algorithms should include general management of the OHCA patient and specific interventions depending on the cause of the arrest.

Early Percutaneous Coronary Intervention (PCI)

In patients where there is not an obvious non-cardiac cause of arrest, early PCI is associated with improved overall survival, and improved neurological outcomes. This includes patients without obvious ST segment elevation myocardial infarction (STEMI).

However, routine PCI in OHCA involves significant resource utilisation and further randomised controlled trials are required to clearly define the optimum timing and role for PCI in this cohort (Table 25B.1).

Haemodynamics

Invasive arterial monitoring is recommended for continuous assessment of blood pressure, titration of fluids/vasoactive agents and to facilitate blood sampling. Large bore peripheral access may be used for fluid administration to correct any hypovolaemia. Where vasoactive agents (inotropes/vasopressors) are being considered, a central venous line should be inserted.

There is no evidence that defines an optimal target for mean arterial pressure (MAP). The aim should be to

Table 25B.1 Percutaneous coronary intervention

Emergency coronary angiography is reasonable for select (e.g. electrically or haemodynamically unstable) adult patients who are comatose after OHCA of suspected cardiac origin with ST elevation on ECG[b]
Emergency coronary angiography is reasonable for select (e.g. electrically or haemodynamically unstable) adult patients who are comatose after OHCA of suspected cardiac origin but without ST elevation on ECG[d]

[a] Class I, Level of Evidence B – randomised studies.
[b] Class I, Level of Evidence B – non-randomised studies.
[c] Class I, Level of Evidence C – expert opinion.
[d] Class IIa, Level of Evidence B – non-randomised studies.
[e] Class IIa, Level of Evidence C – limited data.
[f] Class IIa, Level of Evidence C – expert opinion.
[g] Class IIb, Level of Evidence B – non-randomised studies.
[h] Class IIb, Level of Evidence C – expert opinion.
[i] Class III, Level of Evidence B – non-randomised studies.
[j] Class III, Level of Evidence C – limited data.

deliver adequate coronary, cerebral and systemic organ perfusion that is balanced against increasing the metabolic demands of an already stressed heart through the use of fluids and vasoactive agents. A recent meta-analysis associated higher MAP with improved neurological outcome but it is not clear that improving MAP was responsible for the improved outcomes.

MCS theoretically offers improved systemic and coronary perfusion without necessarily increasing myocardial oxygen consumption. The role of the intra-aortic counterpulsation balloon pump (IABP) remains controversial; and newer devices including ECMO and left ventricular assist devices (LVADs) are being used in selected patients in some specialist centres.

Routine antiarrhythmic prophylaxis is not recommended in the absence of persistent dysrhythmia.

Oxygenation and Ventilation

Oxygen therapy after OHCA is controversial. There are conflicting retrospective data regarding whether hyperoxia is associated with an increased mortality in post-cardiac arrest patients. A prospective, multicentre, randomised controlled trial of air versus supplemental oxygen in STEMI patients who were not hypoxaemic demonstrated an increase in myocardial infarction size assessed at 6 months. In this context, it would seem prudent to titrate inspired oxygen levels to achieve saturations of 94–98%. Both hypoxaemia and hyperoxia should be avoided, but adequate peripheral perfusion and accurate saturation monitoring are imperative before considering reducing inspired oxygen concentrations.

In the comatose OHCA patient with ROSC an endotracheal tube (ETT) should be inserted if this was not done as part of the ALS resuscitation. Tube position should be confirmed with clinical examination, continuous (waveform) end-tidal carbon dioxide monitoring and imaging (CXR or on CT chest scan if this is performed).

Hyperventilation with subsequent hypocarbia has been associated with worse neurological outcome in observational studies of OHCA, presumably due to cerebral vasoconstriction. Where possible, patients should be ventilated to normocarbia with a $PaCO_2$ of 35–45 mmHg. This may need to be individualised in the patient with coexistent pathology where more definitive evidence exists for an alternative ventilation strategy – for example, permissive hypercarbia in the setting of acute respiratory distress syndrome (ARDS).

Targeted Temperature Management (TTM)

Post-cardiac arrest brain injury (as outlined above) is the major cause of morbidity and mortality in comatose patients who are initially resuscitated from OHCA. Multiple trials have demonstrated improved neurological outcomes with targeted temperature management to 32–36 °C in an attempt to mitigate the cascading cellular effects thought to be responsible for propagating neuronal cell death following ischaemia and reperfusion (see Table 25B.2). Benefits were most pronounced in patients with an initial shockable rhythm (ventricular fibrillation (VF) or pulseless ventricular tachycardia (VT)).

The practicalities of active TTM involve significant resource allocation – equipment, education and training – and are not without complexity and complications. Continuous temperature monitoring is required. Cooling strategies need to address the induction and maintenance of TTM, and rewarming. Options include infusion of ice cold fluid, simple surface cooling with ice packs, or more formal systems with fluid or air circulating blankets, vests and limb wraps that include integrated control from continuous temperature monitoring. More aggressive and invasive cooling strategies can include intravascular heat exchange catheters, body cavity lavage or the institution of MCS. The risk and benefit of each strategy need to be considered on an institutional and individual patient level.

Table 25B.2 Targeted temperature management

Comatose adult patients with ROSC after cardiac arrest should have TTM for VF/pulseless VT OHCA[a]; for non-VF/pulseless VT (i.e. 'non-shockable')[c] and in-hospital[a] cardiac arrest.
Select and maintain a constant temperature between 32 °C and 36 °C during TTM.[a]
It is reasonable that TTM be maintained for at least 24 hours after achieving target temperature.[f]
Whether certain subpopulations of cardiac arrest patients may benefit from lower (32–34 °C) or higher (36 °C) temperatures remains unknown, and further research may help elucidate this.

For footnotes see Table 25B.1.

The potential physiological responses to cooling need to be anticipated and addressed when they occur.

Shivering occurs as an autonomic response to hypothermia and can limit the effectiveness of TTM. Strategies to mitigate shivering include the use of short-acting sedative agents, opioid agonists and alpha-agonists but adequate temperature management often requires the use of short-acting non-depolarising neuromuscular blocking agents.

Bradycardia is common and can result in a reduced cardiac output. At lower temperatures systemic metabolic rate and oxygen consumption fall and the bradycardia is thought to be associated with improvements in diastolic function. Systemic vascular resistance may be increased where vasoconstriction predominates, but may be reduced in the setting of a significant SIRS response to systemic ischaemia-reperfusion. The net effect of the alterations to the adequacy of tissue oxygen delivery should be assessed on an individual basis.

A **cold diuresis** from renal tubular dysfunction may cause a relative hypovolaemia and significant electrolyte disturbance.

Insulin sensitivity is reduced at lower temperatures and blood glucose should be measured regularly. Where insulin is used in hypothermia, it is important to closely monitor blood glucose during rewarming as hypoglycaemia may occur.

Coagulation is impaired at lower temperatures but this does not appear to be associated with a clinically significant increase in bleeding rates.

Drug clearance is significantly reduced at lower temperatures and this must be taken into account when prognostication is being considered.

The perceived benefits of TTM have been demonstrated in a time where a focus on bundles of post-OHCA care has been instituted. It is unclear which component of these treatment bundles has been responsible for the greatest improvements in outcome. Although TTM is thought to be integral to these improved outcomes, the optimum temperature, timing and duration of TTM remain to be elucidated.

Delayed Prognostication before Withdrawal of Cardiorespiratory Supports

Post-cardiac arrest brain injury is the major cause of mortality in OHCA patients but the mode of death in these patients is invariably withdrawal of cardiorespiratory supports (WCRS) following prognostication of a poor neurological outcome. Where OHCA patients can be identified as having no prospect of meaningful neurological recovery, inappropriate treatments can be avoided. However, the gravity of the WCRS decision is such that prognostic assessment must be accurate and appropriate.

The self-fulfilling nature of a prognosis of poor neurological outcome leading to WCRS and death means that biases are inherent in many of the earlier studies of prognostication. This may have been further compounded by the use of sedative medications to facilitate TTM, from the effects of TTM on the pharmacokinetic and pharmacodynamic properties of the medications, and potentially from the TTM itself.

Various clinical examination findings, investigations and imaging methodologies have been examined for prognostic relevance in the pre-TTM and TTM eras (see Table 25B.3 and Figure 25B.3).

Mechanical Support

There is insufficient evidence to support routine use of MCS – mechanical chest compression devices (MCCD) and/or ECPR – in OHCA.

MCCDs have not been associated with improved survival to hospital discharge nor with improved neurological outcomes, and manual chest compression remains the standard of care. The use of MCCDs requires capital outlay for purchase and ongoing costs associated with education, training and maintenance. However, the appropriate use of MCCDs during patient transfer can facilitate staff safety whilst also minimising interruptions to chest compressions. This includes transport in emergency vehicles between health care facilities, and within hospitals for intervention in the angiography suite. Critical care practitioners should be familiar with the operation of these devices where they may be used in their centres. In accordance with current guidelines the focus should remain on minimising interruptions to chest compression.

ECPR is an area of growing interest and research. Preliminary reports from specialist ECMO centres with early institution of ECPR in selected patients have shown promising results when compared with conventional CPR – particularly in the setting of witnessed, in-hospital cardiac arrest (IHCA) with a short interval from arrest to starting ECMO. Results for

Table 25B.3 Timing of prognostication

The earliest time for prognostication using clinical examination in patients treated with TTM, where sedation or paralysis could be a confounder, may be 72 hours after return to normothermia.[h]
The earliest time to prognosticate a poor neurological outcome using clinical examination in patients not treated with TTM is 72 hours after cardiac arrest.[b]
This time until prognostication can be even longer than 72 hours after cardiac arrest if the residual effect of sedation or paralysis confounds the clinical examination.[e]
Prognostication clinical examination
In comatose patients who are not treated with TTM, the absence of pupillary reflex to light at 72 hours or more after cardiac arrest is a reasonable exam finding with which to predict poor neurological outcome (false positive rate (FPR), 0%; 95% CI, 0%–8%).[d]
In comatose patients who are treated with TTM, the absence of pupillary reflex to light at 72 hours or more after cardiac arrest is useful to predict poor neurological outcome (FPR, 1%; 95% CI, 0%–3%).[b]
The findings of either absent motor movements or extensor posturing should not be used alone for predicting a poor neurological outcome (FPR, 10%; 95% CI, 7%–15% to FPR, 15%; 95% CI, 5%–31%)[i]. The motor examination may be a reasonable means to identify the population who need further prognostic testing to predict poor outcome.[g]
The presence of myoclonus (as distinct from status myoclonus) should not be used to predict poor neurological outcomes because of the high FPR (FPR, 5%; 95% CI, 3%–8% to FPR, 11%; 95% CI, 3%–26%).[i]
In combination with other diagnostic tests at 72 or more hours after cardiac arrest, the presence of status myoclonus during the first 72 to 120 hours after cardiac arrest is a reasonable finding to help predict poor neurological outcomes (FPR, 0%; 95% CI, 0%–4%).[d]
Prognostication investigations
In patients who are comatose after resuscitation from cardiac arrest regardless of treatment with TTM, it is reasonable to consider the bilateral absence of the N20 SSEP wave 24 to 72 hours after cardiac arrest or after rewarming a predictor of poor outcome (FPR, 1%; 95% CI, 0%–3%).[d]
The persistent absence of EEG reactivity to external stimuli at 72 hours after cardiac arrest, and persistent burst suppression on EEG after rewarming, may be reasonable to predict a poor outcome (FPR, 0%; 95% CI, 0%–3%).[g]
Intractable and persistent (more than 72 hours) status epilepticus in the absence of EEG reactivity to external stimuli may be reasonable to predict a poor outcome.[g]
In comatose post-cardiac arrest patients who are not treated with TTM, it may be reasonable to consider the presence of burst suppression on EEG at 72 hours or more after cardiac arrest, in combination with other predictors, to predict a poor neurological outcome (FPR, 0%; 95% CI, 0%–11%).[g]
Given the possibility of high FPRs, blood levels of NSE and S-100B should not be used alone to predict a poor neurological outcome.[j]
Prognostication imaging
In patients who are comatose after resuscitation from cardiac arrest and not treated with TTM, it may be reasonable to use the presence of a marked reduction of the GWR on brain CT obtained within 2 hours after cardiac arrest to predict poor outcome.[g]
It may be reasonable to consider extensive restriction of diffusion on brain MRI at 2 to 6 days after cardiac arrest in combination with other established predictors to predict a poor neurological outcome.[g]

For footnotes see Table 25B.1.

OHCA have been less promising and this is thought to be related to the prolonged time between onset of cardiac arrest and institution of ECMO. Solutions currently being explored include the more rapid transport of patients with OHCA to ECMO centres and the role of pre-hospital ECPR. Further economic and ethical evaluation is required to establish the role of ECPR in OHCA and how these patients should subsequently be managed.

Organ Donation

Mortality rates in OHCA patients remain high even after survival to ICU admission. Where patients fulfil broader criteria for organ donation this should be discussed with their family members and organ donor coordinators in line with hospital and national guidelines. In the setting of severe post-cardiac arrest brain injury patients may progress to brain death. Where

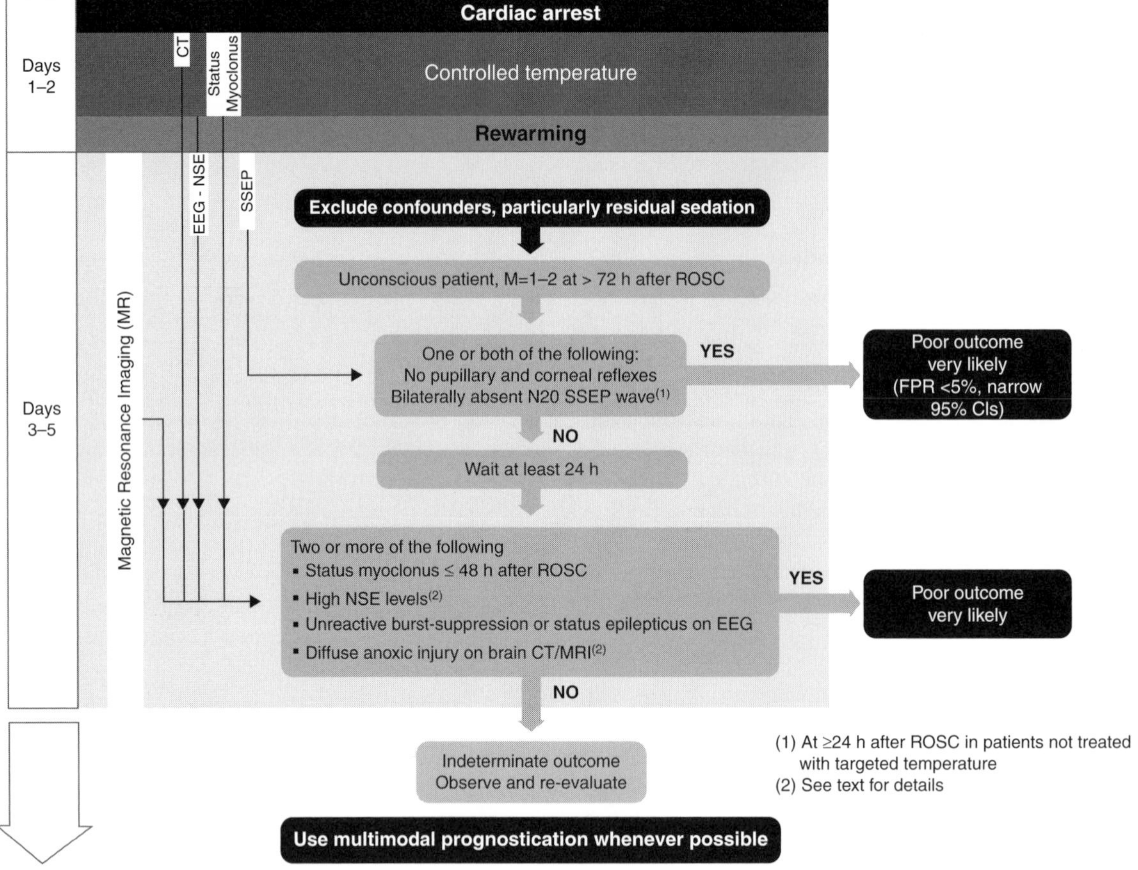

Figure 25B.3 Prognostication algorithm. EEG electroencephalography; NSE neuron-specific enolase; SSEP somatosensory evoked potentials; ROSC return of spontaneous circulation; FPR false positive rate; CI confidence interval.

cardiorespiratory supports are to be withdrawn, donation after circulatory death should be discussed.

Family Screening

Coronary ischaemia remains the leading cause of OHCA. Where OHCA occurs in younger patients or where investigations reveal no evidence of ischaemia, alternative diagnoses must be considered – including accelerated atherosclerotic disease, structural heart disease, and primary arrhythmias. Structural heart disease should be identified with imaging studies, and electrophysiological studies can help identify primary arrhythmias. In the event of death, a post mortem examination should be conducted. Where a heritable condition is identified as the cause of OHCA, screening should be offered to family members – including clinical examination, electrophysiological studies, cardiac imaging and potential genetic testing and counselling.

Learning Points

- Post-resuscitation care is one of the four essential links in the 'chain of survival' designed to improve survival in OHCA.
- Post-cardiac arrest syndrome comprises:
  - Post-cardiac arrest brain injury;
  - Post-cardiac arrest myocardial dysfunction;
  - Systemic ischaemia-reperfusion response;
  - Persistent precipitating pathology.
- The hospital interventions that have been consistently associated with improved outcomes after OHCA are:
  - Early percutaneous coronary intervention (PCI);
  - Targeted temperature management;
  - Delayed prognostication before withdrawal of cardiorespiratory supports.

- Prognostication should involve multiple assessment strategies, including examination, neurophysiological testing and neuroimaging.
- Mechanical support in cardiac arrest is an evolving area. Further clinical, economic and ethical evaluation is required to establish the role of ECPR in both IHCA and OHCA.

Further Reading

Brrooks SC, Anderson ML, Bruder E, et al. Part 6: Alternative Techniques and Ancillary Devices for Cardiopulmonary Resuscitation: 2015 American Heart Association Guidelines Update for Cardiopulmonary Resuscitation and Emergency Cardiovascular Care. *Circulation.* 2015; 132(18 Suppl 2): S436–443.

Callaway CW, Donnino MW, Fink EL, et al. Part 8: Post-Cardiac Arrest Care: 2015 American Heart Association Guidelines Update for Cardiopulmonary Resuscitation and Emergency Cardiovascular Care. *Circulation.* 2015; 132(18 Suppl 2): S465–482.

Dragancea I, Rundgren M, Englund E, Friberg H, Cronberg T. The influence of induced hypothermia and delayed prognostication on the mode of death after cardiac arrest. Resuscitation. European Resuscitation Council, American Heart Association, Inc., and International Liaison Committee on Resuscitation. Elsevier, 2013, 84: pp. 337–342.

Link MS, Berkow LC, Kudenchuk PJ, et al. Part 7: Adult Advanced Cardiovascular Life Support: 2015 American Heart Association Guidelines Update for Cardiopulmonary Resuscitation and Emergency Cardiovascular Care. Lippincott Williams & Wilkins, 2015, pp. S444–S464.

Neumar RW, Nolan JP, Adrie C, et al. Post-cardiac arrest syndrome: epidemiology, pathophysiology, treatment, and prognostication. A consensus statement from the International Liaison Committee on Resuscitation (American Heart Association, Australian and New Zealand Council on Resuscitation, European Resuscitation Council, Heart and Stroke Foundation of Canada, InterAmerican Heart Foundation, Resuscitation Council of Asia, and the Resuscitation Council of Southern Africa); the American Heart Association Emergency Cardiovascular Care Committee; the Council on Cardiovascular Surgery and Anesthesia; the Council on Cardiopulmonary, Perioperative, and Critical Care; the Council on Clinical Cardiology; and the Stroke Council. Lippincott Williams & Wilkins, 2008, pp. 2452–2483.

Nielsen N, Wetterslev J, Cronberg T, et al. Targeted temperature management at 33°C versus 36°C after cardiac arrest. *New England Journal of Medicine.* 2013; 369: 2197–2206.

Nolan JP, Soar J, Cariou A, et al. European Resuscitation Council and European Society of Intensive Care Medicine Guidelines for Post-resuscitation Care 2015: Section 5 of the European Resuscitation Council Guidelines for Resuscitation 2015. Resuscitation. European Resuscitation Council, American Heart Association, and International Liaison Committee on Resuscitation. Elsevier, 2015, 95: pp. 202–222.

Soar J, Nolan JP, Böttiger BW, et al. European Resuscitation Council Guidelines for Resuscitation 2015: Section 3. Adult advanced life support. Resuscitation. European Resuscitation Council, American Heart Association, Inc., and International Liaison Committee on Resuscitation. Elsevier, 2015, 95: pp. 100–147.

Stub D, Bernard S, Duffy SJ, Kaye DM. Post cardiac arrest syndrome: a review of therapeutic strategies. *Circulation.* 2011; 123: 1428–1435.

Stub D, Smith K, Bernard S, et al. Air versus oxygen in ST-segment-elevation myocardial infarction. *Circulation.* 2015; 131: 2143–2150.

MCQs

1. **The chain of survival does NOT include:**
   (a) Early CPR
   (b) Early defibrillation
   (c) E-CPR
   (d) Post-resuscitation care
2. **Regarding OHCA patients:**
   (a) Primary myocardial disease is an uncommon cause of arrest in this population
   (b) Hyperoxia post-ROSC is associated with improved neurological outcomes
   (c) Hypercarbia should never be allowed to occur in these patients
   (d) Invasive arterial monitoring is indicated in the post-resuscitation care phase
3. **Current ALS guidelines suggest:**
   (a) Defibrillation should be delayed until the airway is secured

(b) Interruptions to chest compression should be minimised

(c) E-CPR has shown particularly promising results in the OHCA population

(d) The use of MCCDs (compared to manual chest compressions) is associated with improved neurological outcomes

4. Regarding the ICU management of OHCA patients:

(a) Observational studies suggest that the reversible 'myocardial stunning' effect can last for up to 6 hours

(b) Routine arrhythmia prophylaxis with amiodarone is recommended in all patients

(c) Echocardiography may help to guide patient management

(d) Early percutaneous coronary intervention (PCI) should only be considered in patients with ST elevation on their ECG

5. Regarding neurological prognostication in OHCA patients:

(a) A Glasgow coma motor score of 1 or 2 is a good predictor of poor neurological outcome

(b) Clinical neurological examination should be performed at least 36 hours after ROSC

(c) Multiple assessment strategies should be used, including examination, neurophysiological testing and neuroimaging

(d) Serum biomarkers can be used in isolation during prognostication

Exercise answers are available on p.469. Alternatively, take the test online at www.cambridge.org/CardiothoracicMCQ

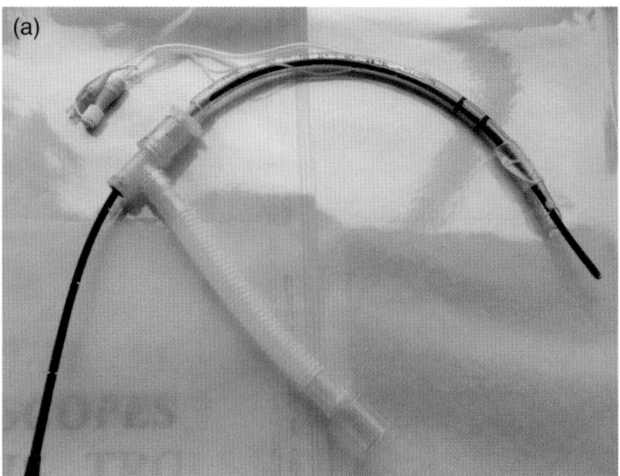

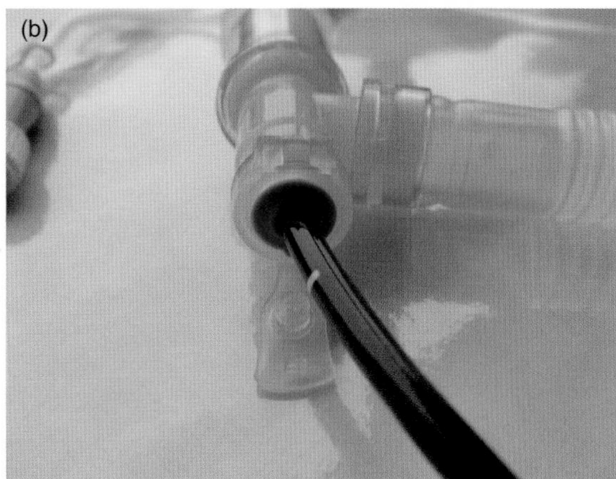

Figure 5.1 Bronchoscopy swivel catheter mount. (a) Close up image of the bronchoscope entering the catheter mount via a self-sealing soft rubber ring. This allows for reduced air leakage during bronchoscopy of an invasively ventilated patient. (b) Bronchoscope entering the catheter mount and passing via the endotracheal tube (ET). To ensure smooth passage down the ET tube, lubricant is applied to the outside of the bronchoscope.

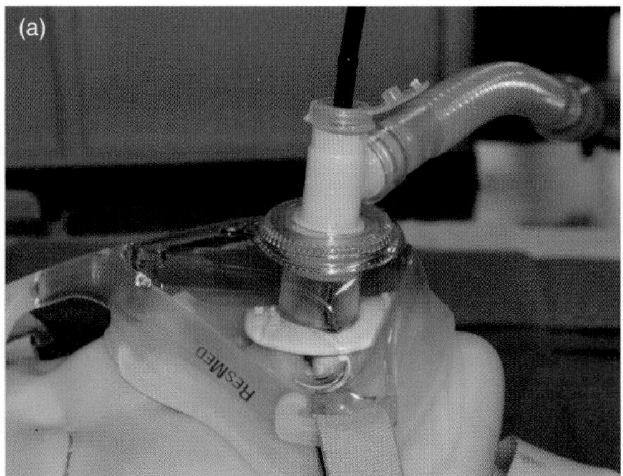

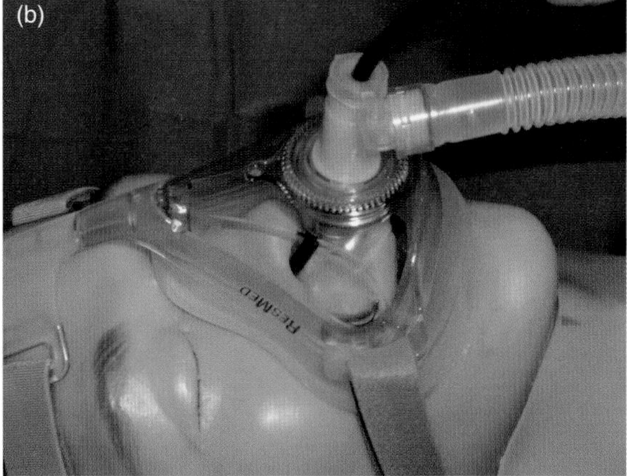

Figure 5.2 Bronchoscopy during non-invasive ventilation using modified full face masks (a) via the oral approach using a bite block and (b) via the nasal approach.

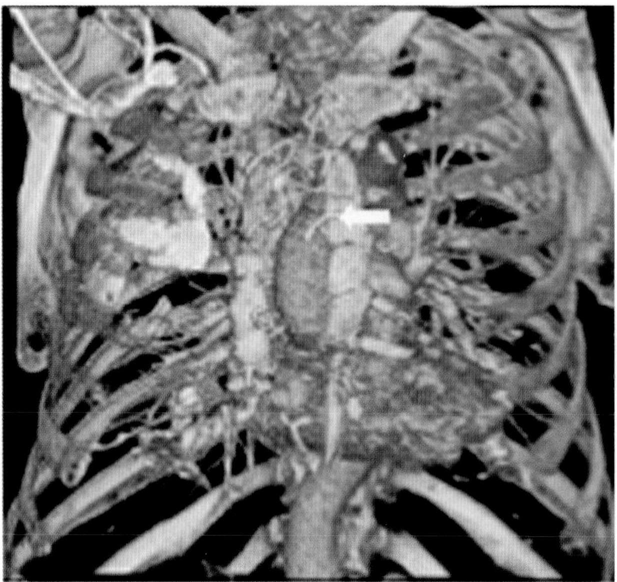

Figure 7.5 Empyema, lung abscess and sepsis. Top panel: CXR and CT demonstrate a loculated left pleural collection with (right image, white star) locules of free air secondary to empyema (right image, thin white arrow). Bottom panel: CXR of a cavitating lung abscess (left image, block black arrow) and left lower lobe collapse with a tiny effusion in an immunocompromised patient. Another profoundly septic patient with recent aortic valve replacement has sternal dehiscence due to osteomyelitis shown on CT (right image, block white arrow).

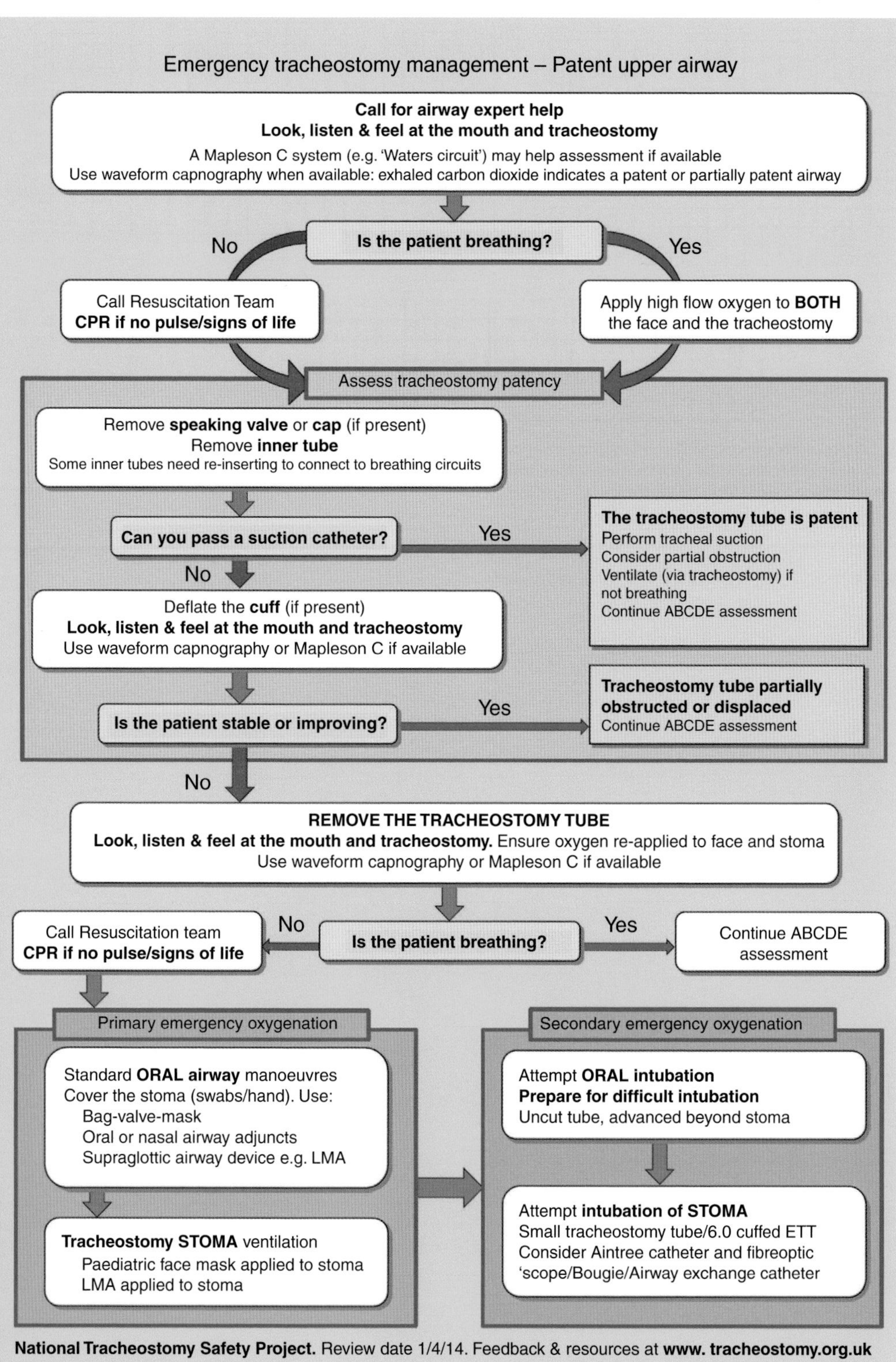

Figure 8.1 Emergency tracheostomy management. Reproduced from McGrath et al. (2012) with permission from the Association of Anaesthetists of Great Britain & Ireland/Blackwell Publishing Ltd.

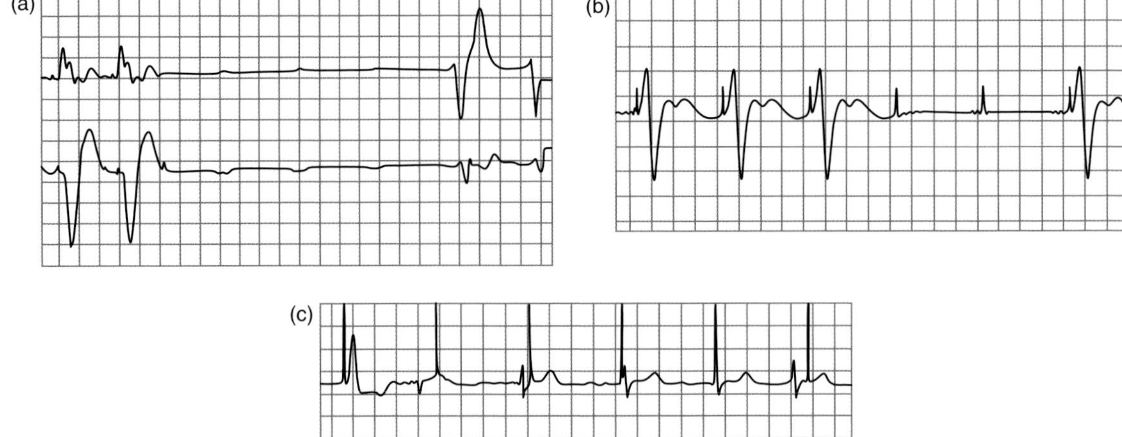

Figure 10.2 Pacemaker troubleshooting. (a) Failure to output (absence of pacing spikes causing a 3 second pause). (b) Failure to capture (4th and 5th pacing spikes are not followed by ventricular electrograms). (c) Undersensing (all but the first pacing spike are delivered inappropriately due to undersensing of electrical signals).

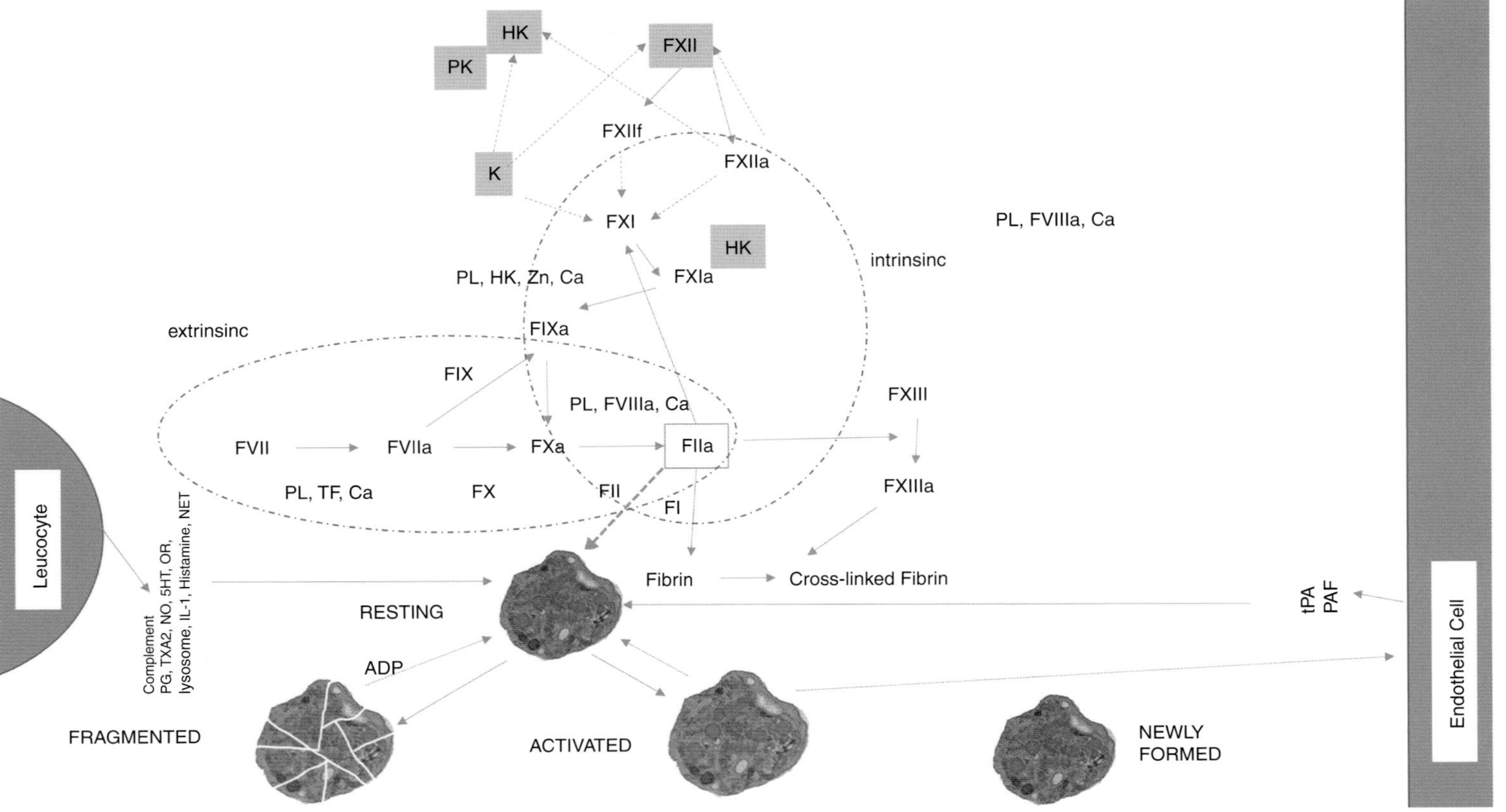

Figure 13.1 Cell based model of haemostasis.

Contact activation occurs with activation of the four contact factors: K, PK, HK and XII. This leads to activation of the intrinsic pathway and activated complement. Both the activation of the complement pathways and the formation of thrombin activate platelets and lead to platelet aggregation and fragmentation. Platelet activation, in turn, activates endothelial cells and causes release of tPA platelet activation.

K kallikrein, PK prekallikrein, HK high-molecular-kininogen, F factor, a activated form, f fragmented form, PG prostaglandin, LT leukotriene, NO nitrous oxide, TXA2 thromboxane A2, OR oxygen radicals, 5HT serotonin, IL1 interleukin 1, PAF platelet activating factor, tPA tissue plasminogen activator.

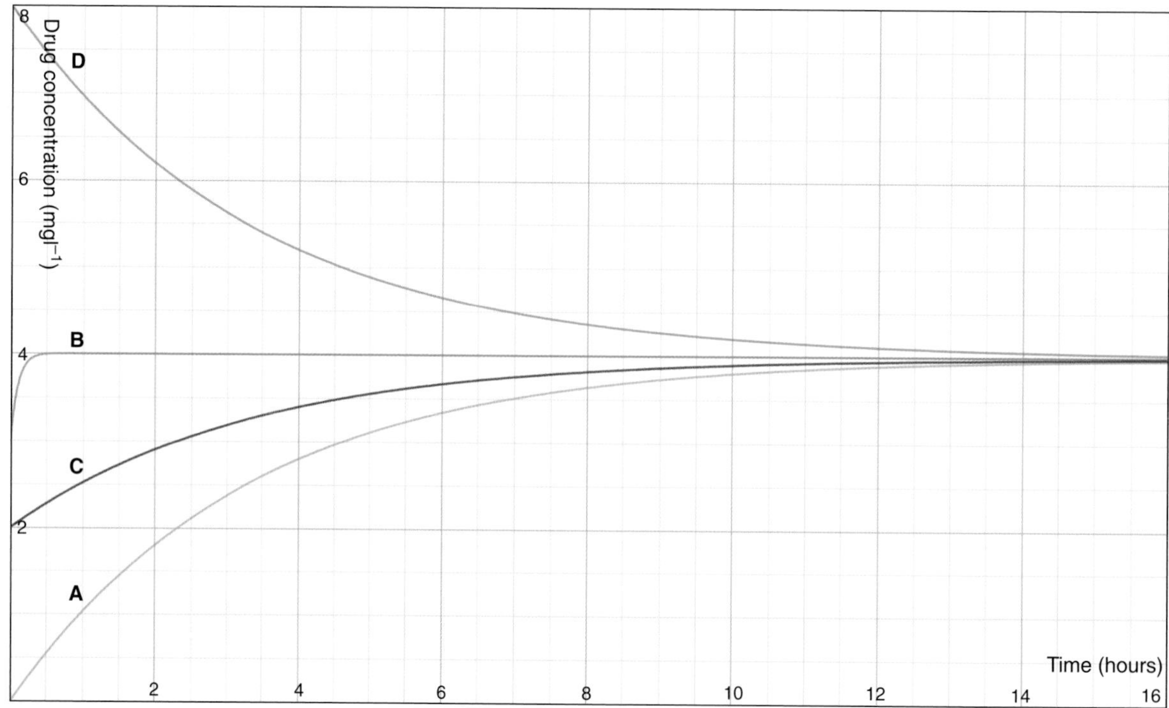

Figure 16.2 This graph demonstrates the effects of a loading dose for a hypothetical drug with a half-life of approximately 4 hours. Curve A demonstrates the effect of no loading dose, and the target steady state of 4 mg l^{-1} is reached after 4 half-lives. Curve B shows the effect of a perfectly calculated loading dose – the target steady state is reached immediately, and maintained by the infusion. Curve C shows the effect of a partial loading dose. The starting concentration is higher, but it still takes 4 half-lives until steady state is reached. Finally, curve D shows the effect of an excessive load. The starting concentration is extremely high, and takes 4 half-lives to fall to the target steady state concentration. Drug concentration in mg l^{-1}.

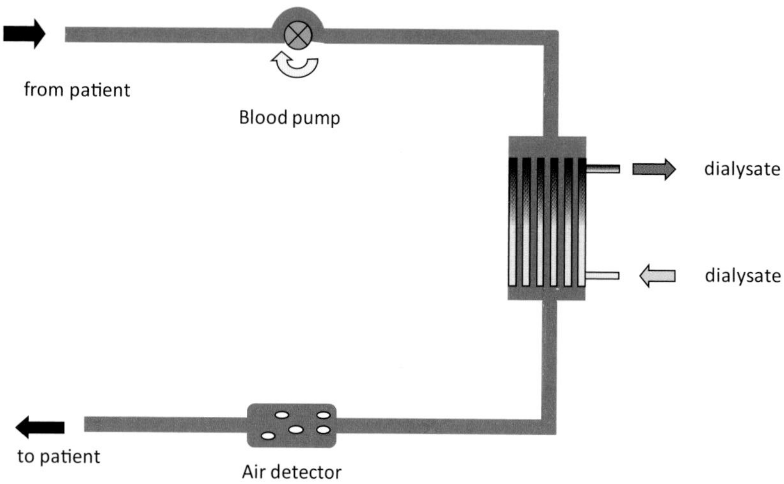

Figure 18.1 Haemodialysis.

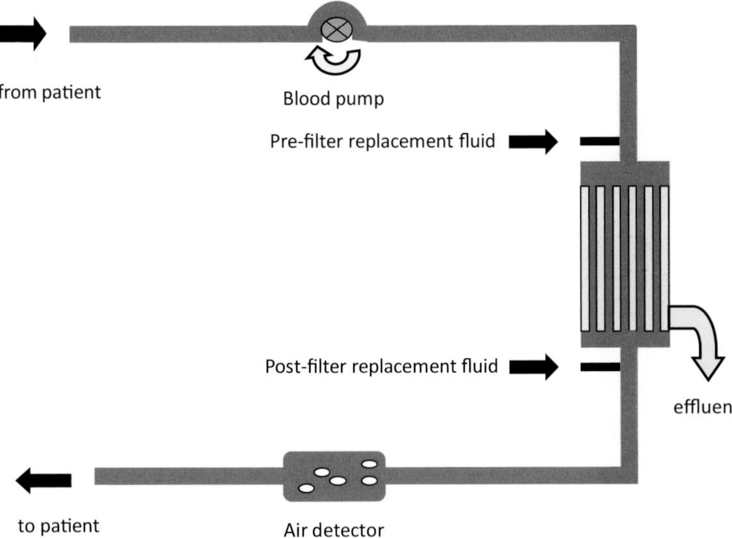

Figure 18.2 Haemofiltration.

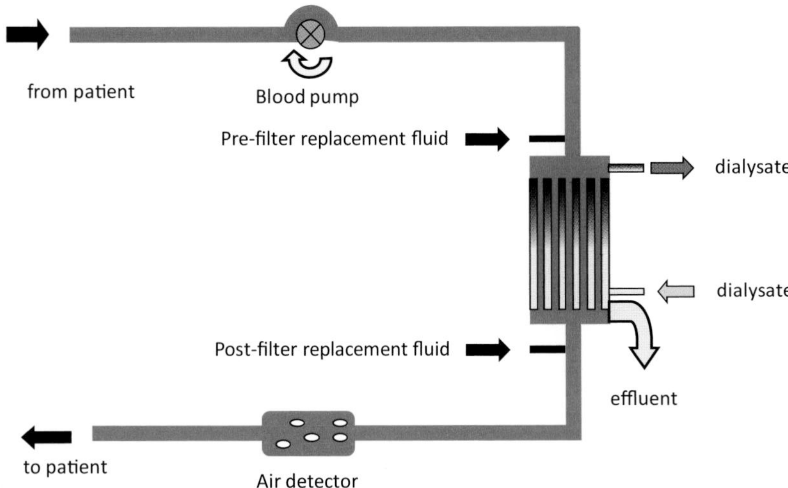

Figure 18.3 Haemodiafiltration.

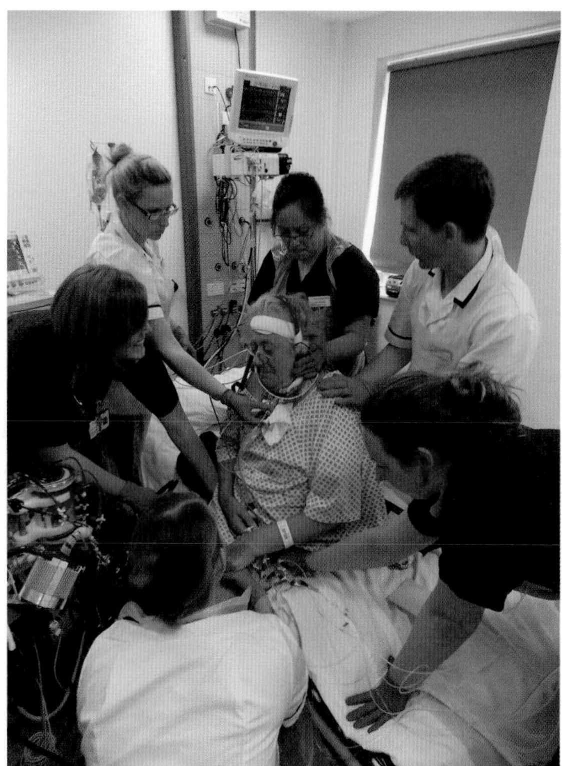

Figure 20.2 Example of ABCT: (b) Sitting on the edge of the bed rehabilitation with a patient on ECMO.

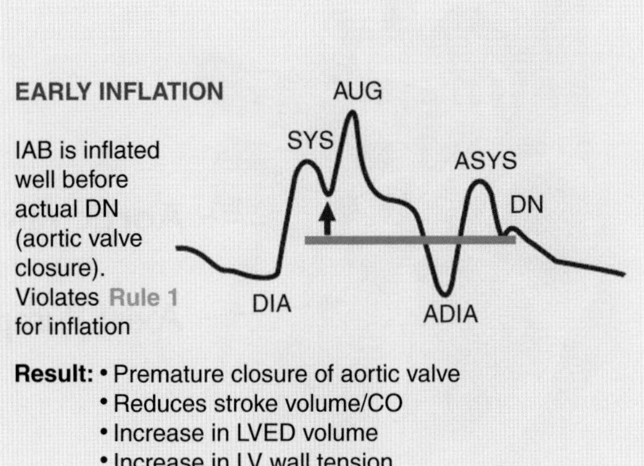

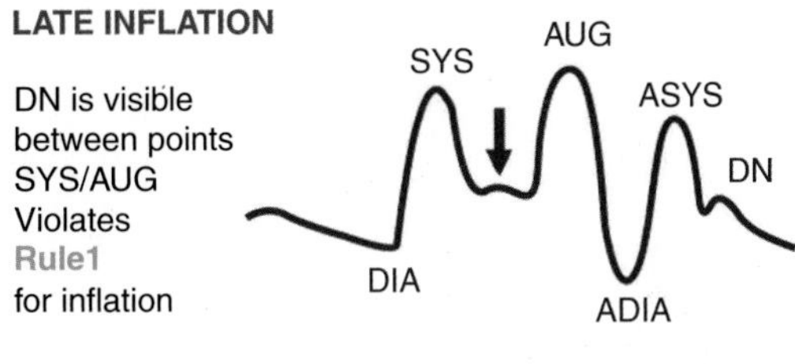

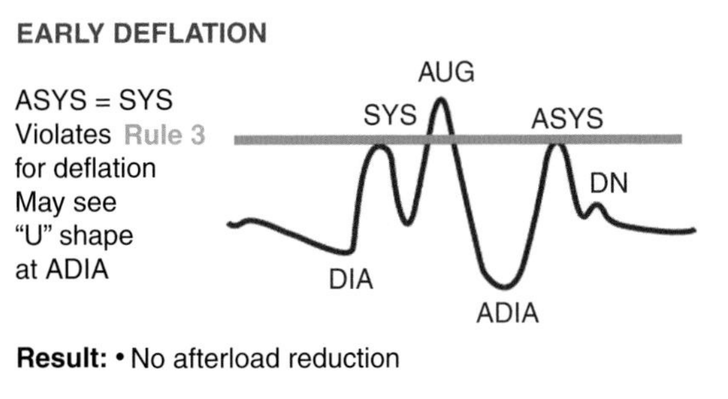

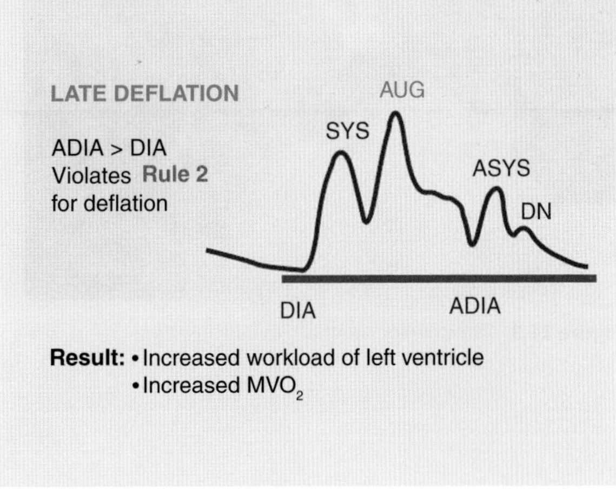

Figure 21.2 Timing problems with IABP.

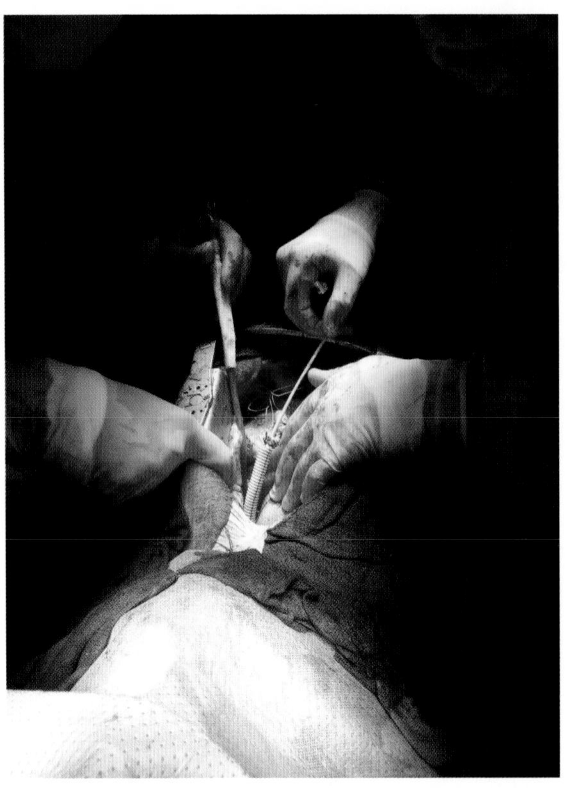

Figure 21.3. Transthoracic approach to IABP insertion.

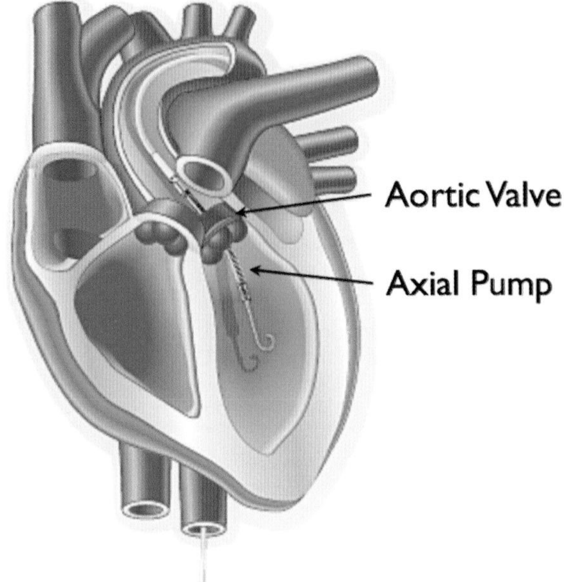

Figure 21.4 Diagram demonstrating the Impella LP2.5 axial flow left ventricular assist device sitting across the aortic valve. Reprinted with permission from Abiomed (Aachen, Germany), the manufacturer of this device.

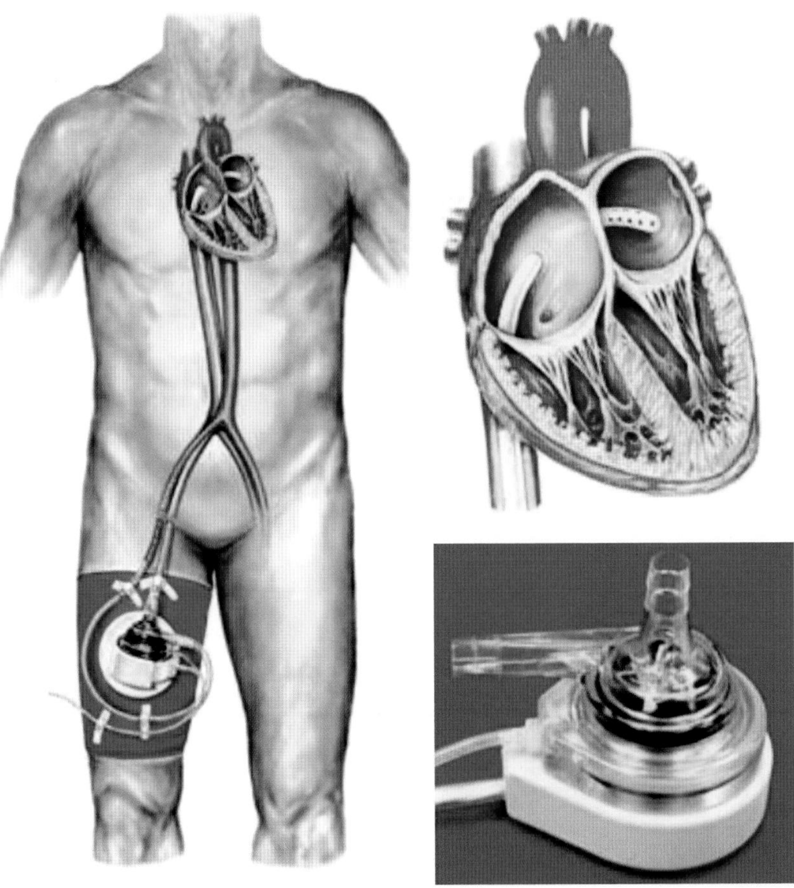

Figure 21.5 TandemHeart consists of a 21F inflow cannula in the left atrium after femoral venous access and transseptal puncture and a 15F to 17F arterial cannula in the iliac artery. Reproduced with permission from Naidu (2011).

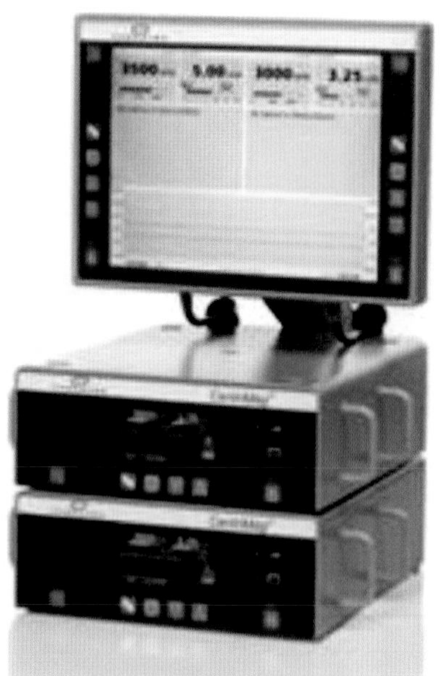

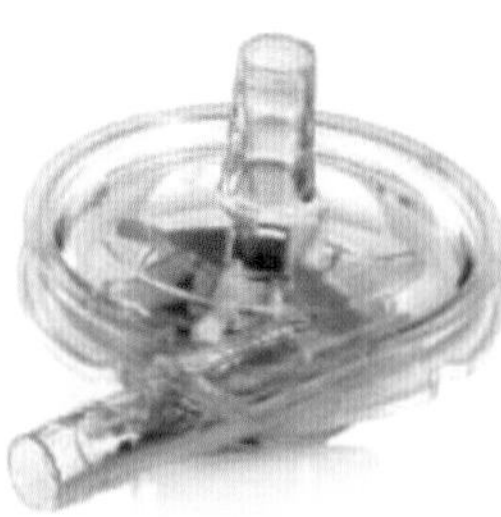

Figure 22.1 CentriMag primary console and centrifugal pump (courtesy of Thoratec Corporation, CA, USA).

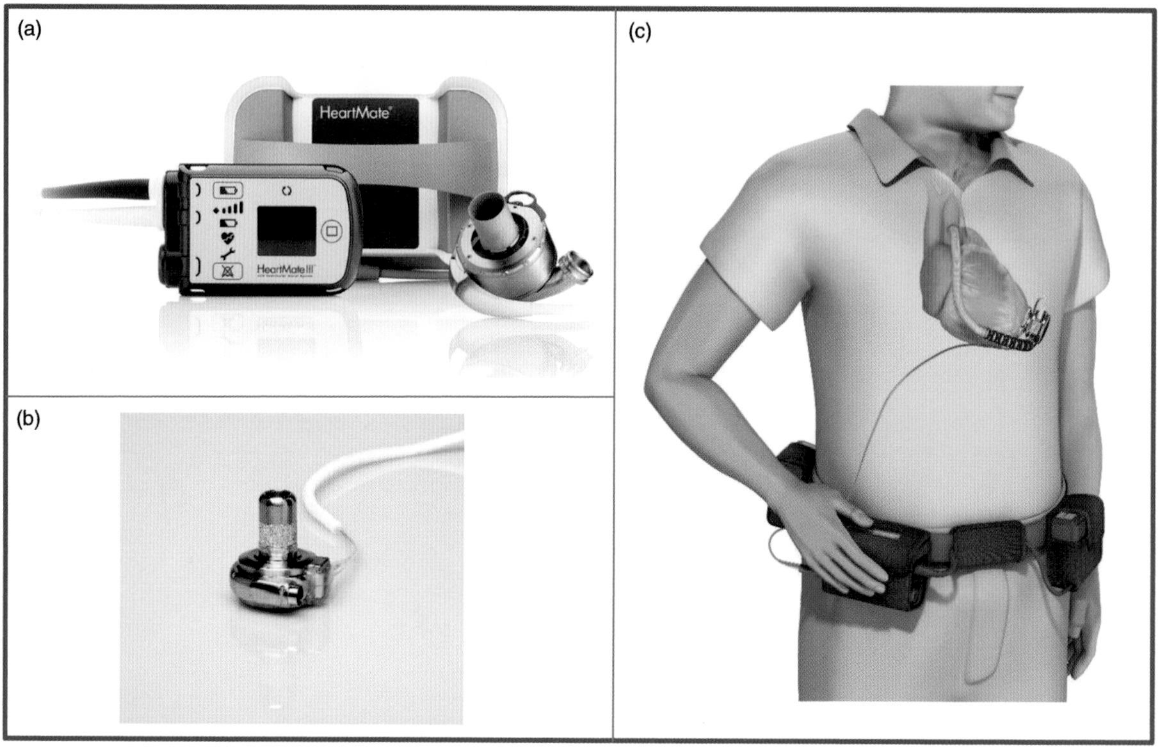

Figure 22.2 (a) HeartMate 3 with its controller. (b) HeartWare HVAD with driveline. (c) Diagram of a patient with a HeartWare HVAD sited in the left ventricular apex and a percutaneous driveline going to a wearable controller and batteries. (Courtesy of Thoratec Corporation, CA, USA and HeartWare Corporation, MA, USA).

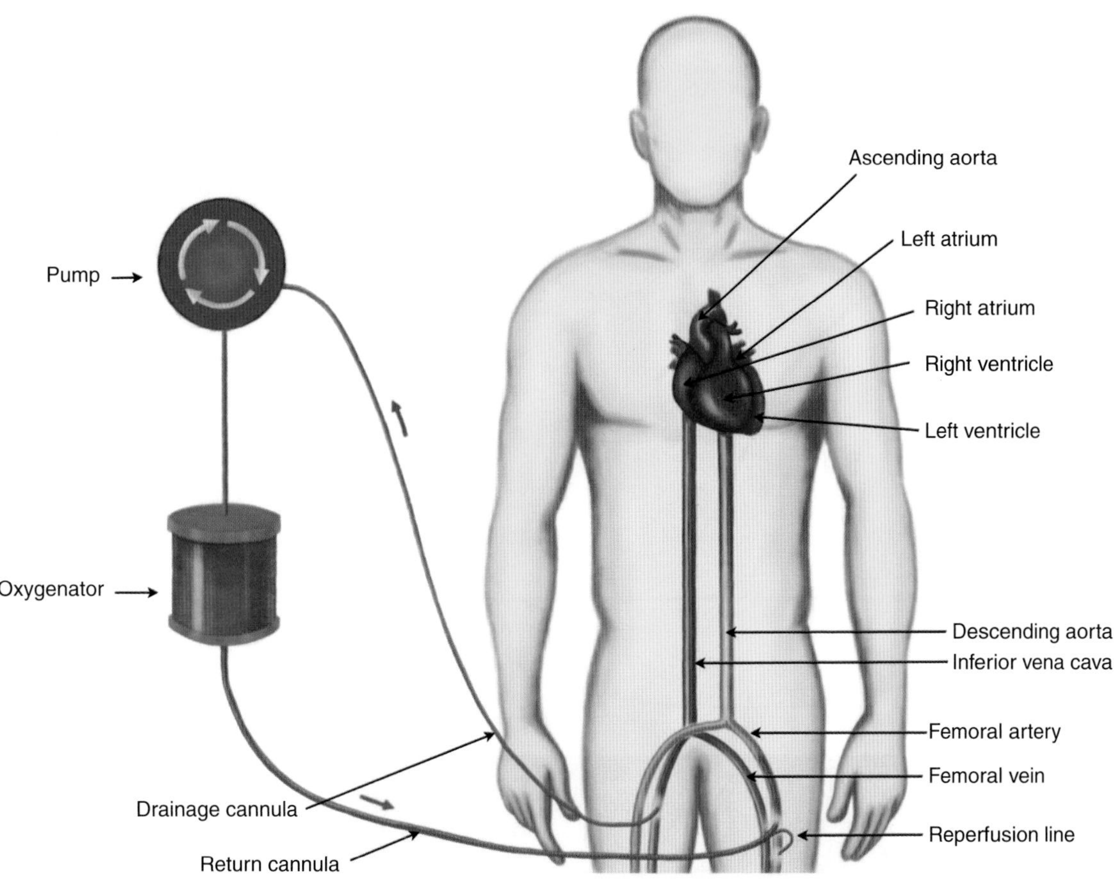

Figure 23.1 Peripheral ECMO. The blood is drained from a large vein, typically IVC, using femoral access. It is then pumped through an oxygenator and returned to the patient into the femoral artery in a retrograde fashion. A reperfusion line from the inflow cannula is inserted into the distal femoral artery to provide distal limb perfusion. Diagram drawn by Anna Valchanova.

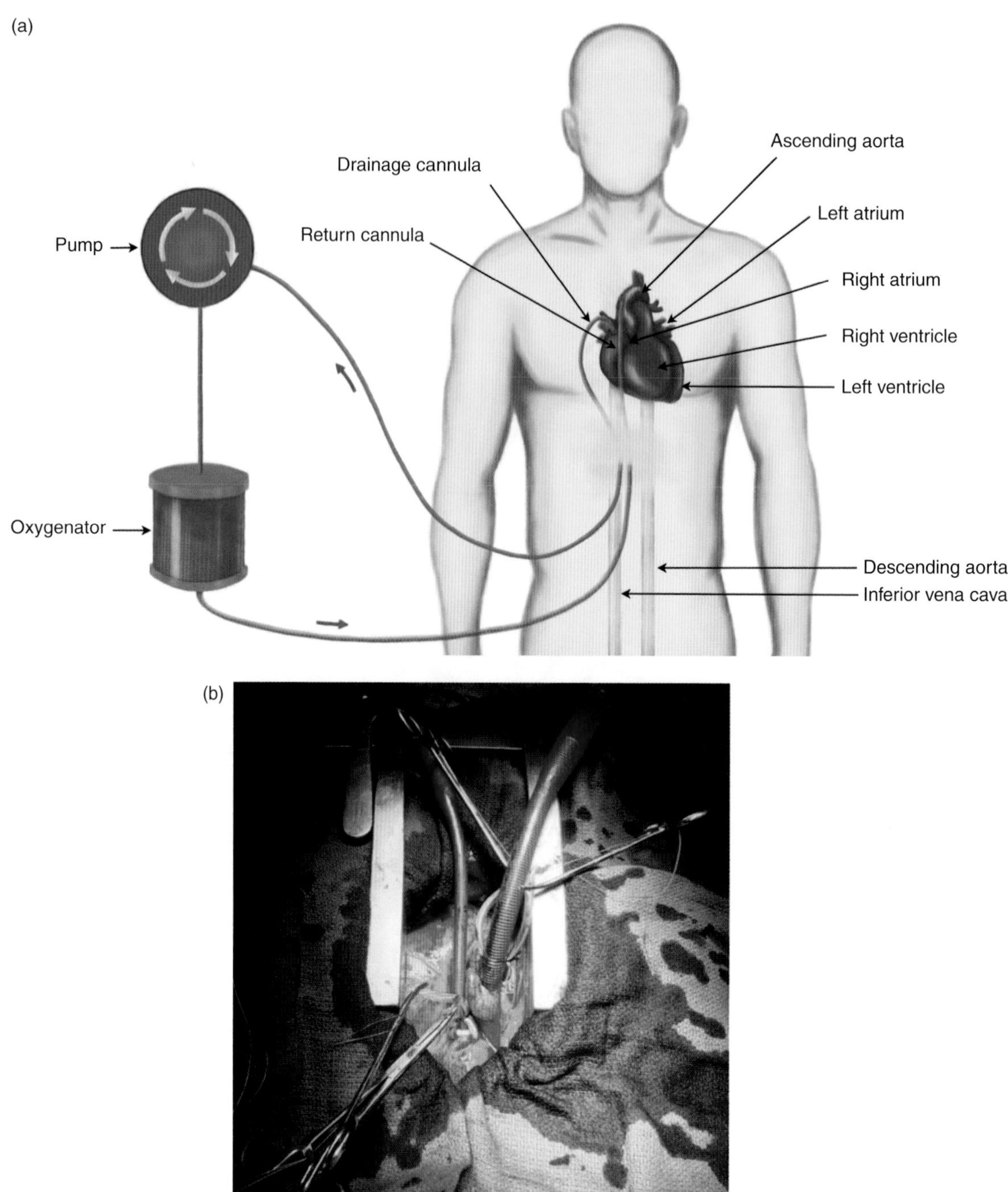

Figure 23.3 (a)Central ECMO diagram: using open chest, the blood is drained via a cannula from a central vein (IVC or SVC) or right atrium. It is pumped through an oxygenator and returned through an arterial cannula into the ascending aorta. The chest can be left open for a short while, or the cannulae can be tunnelled under the skin and chest closed. Diagram drawn by Anna Valchanova. (b) A photograph of the outflow and inflow cannulae secured with spigots.

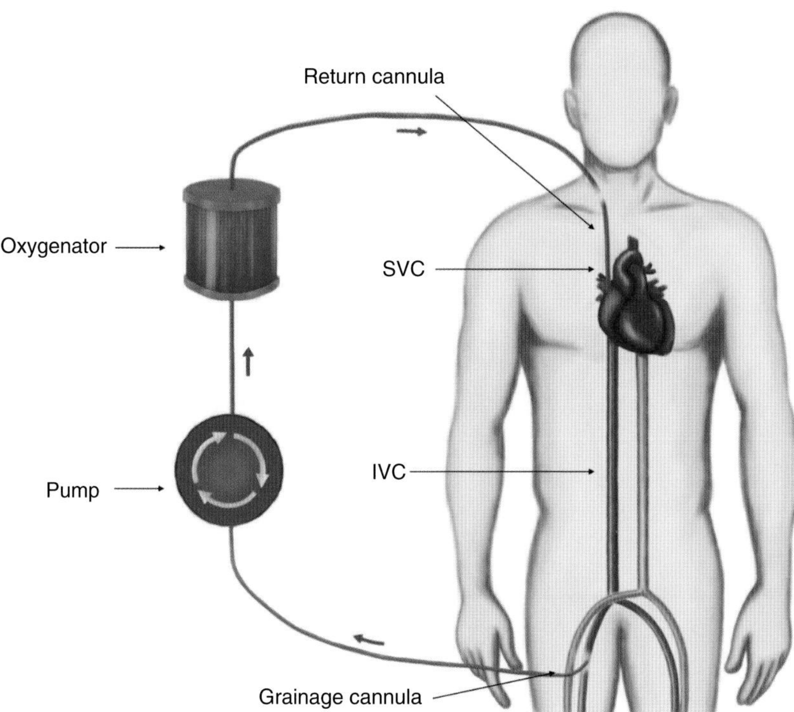

Figure 24.1 Peripheral VV ECMO using two cannulae. Blood is drained from the IVC using femoral approach. It is then pumped through an oxygenator and returned into the SVC through internal jugular approach. Diagram drawn by Anna Valchanova.

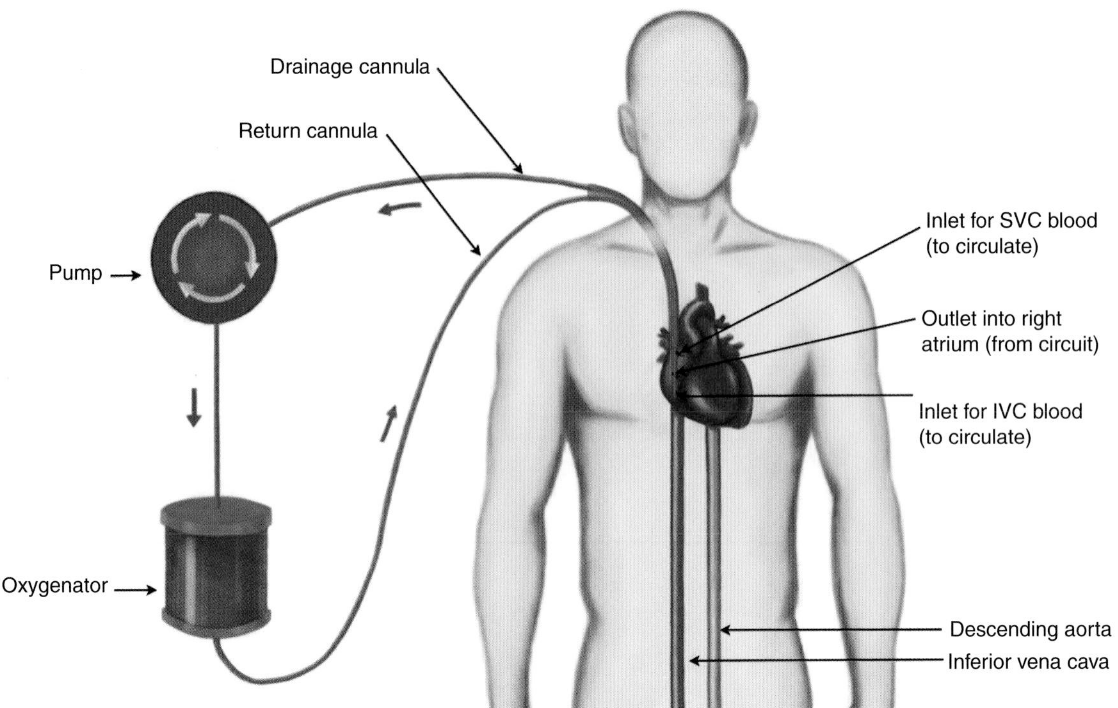

Figure 24.2 VV ECMO using bicaval dual lumen cannula. Blood is drained from the IVC and SVC. It is pumped through an oxygenator and returned into the right atrium using the second lumen of the same cannula. Diagram drawn by Anna Valchanova.

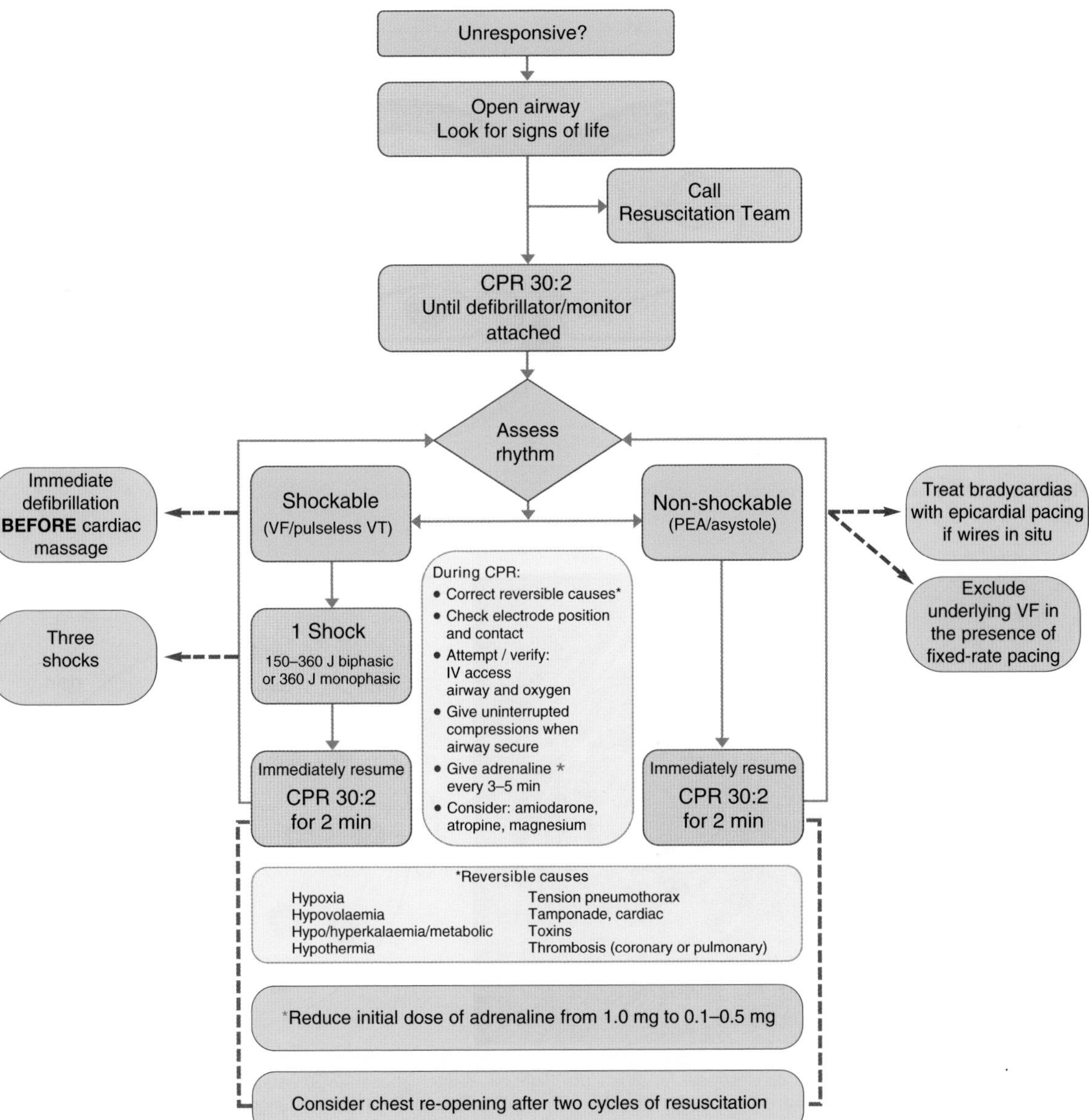

Figure 25A.2 Algorithm for resuscitation after adult cardiac surgery. Six suggested modifications to the standard ALS algorithm are highlighted in the six bright yellow boxes to the sides and below. Therapeutic hypothermia may be considered after successful resuscitation. Adapted from the Resuscitation Council (UK) 2010 ALS algorithm.

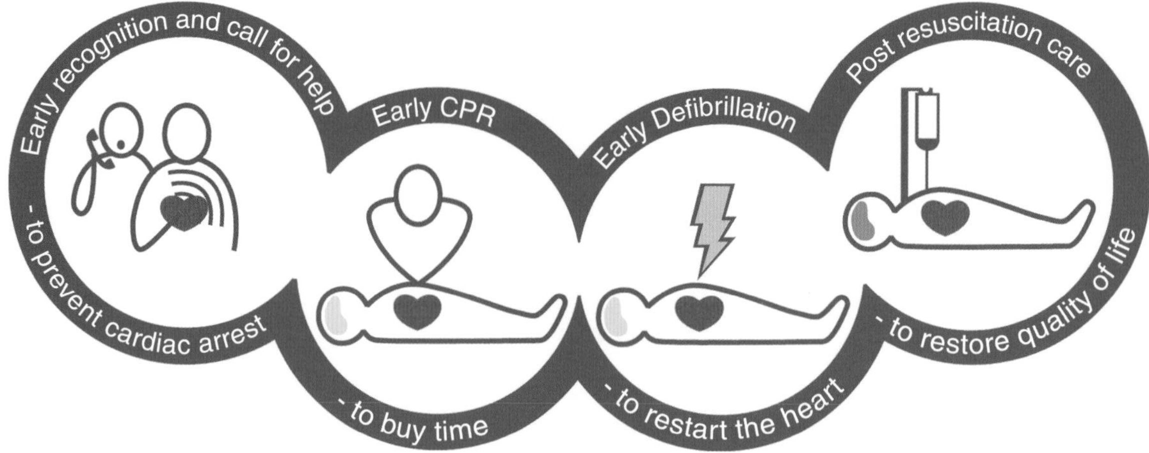

Figure 25B.1 Chain of survival, courtesy of the Adult Basic Life Support Guidelines of the Resuscitation Council.

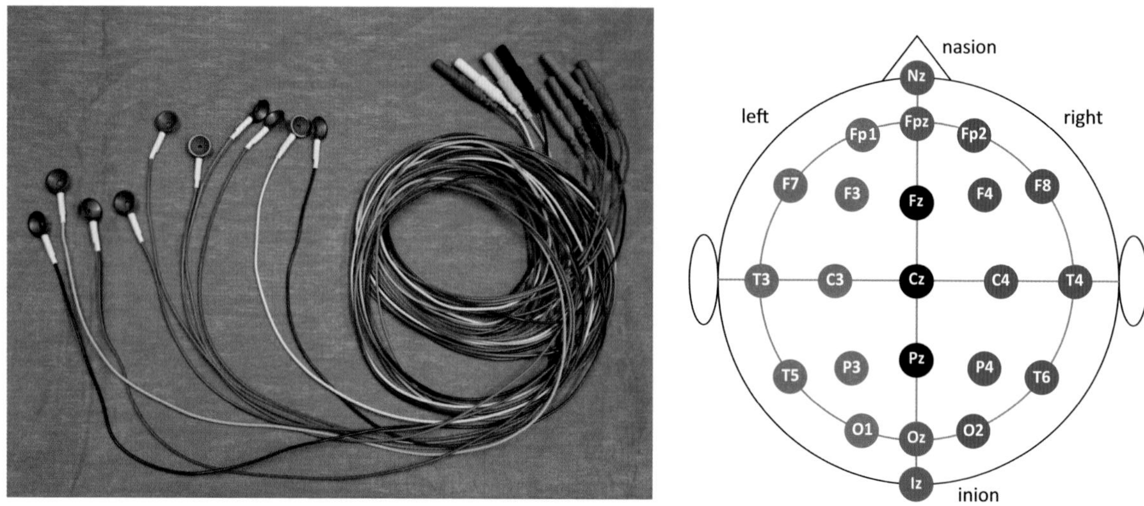

Figure 33.2 Left panel: typical EEG scalp electrodes for clinical use. Right panel: international 10–20 system for standard scalp electrode placement. The distances between adjacent electrodes are either 10% or 20% of the total anterior/posterior or left/right distance. Left and right are distinguished by odd and even numbers respectively. Each channel of the EEG is obtained by measuring the voltage between adjacent electrodes (bipolar montage, such as here) or of individual electrodes compared to a reference electrode or combination of electrodes (referential montage).

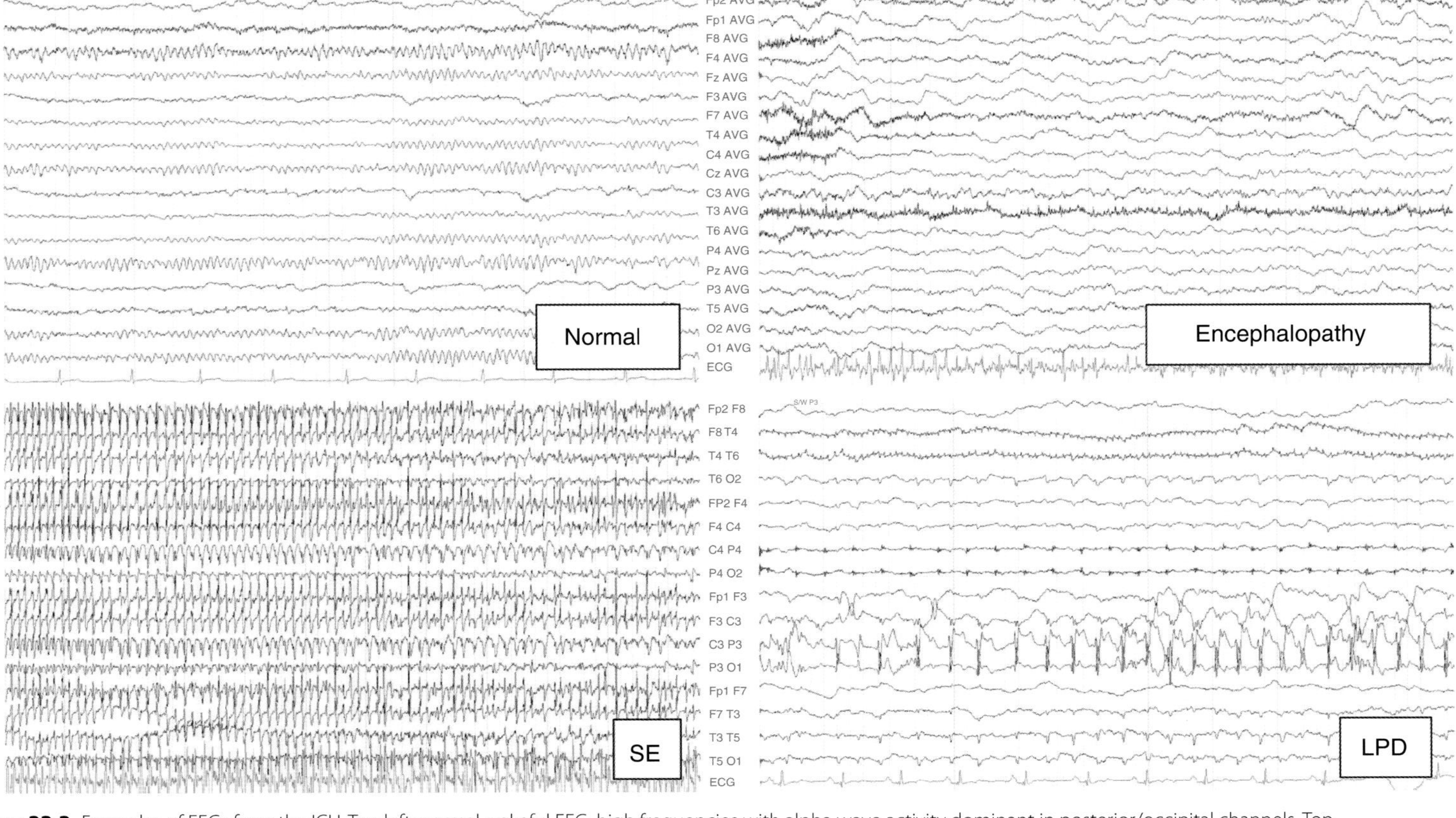

Figure 33.3 Examples of EEGs from the ICU. Top left: normal wakeful EEG, high frequencies with alpha wave activity dominant in posterior/occipital channels. Top right: encephalopathic EEG illustrating prominent slow (delta wave) activity. Bottom left: generalised seizure activity with sharp spikes and waves in all channels. Bottom right: LPDs, periodic spike discharges over the left hemisphere (odd numbered channels).

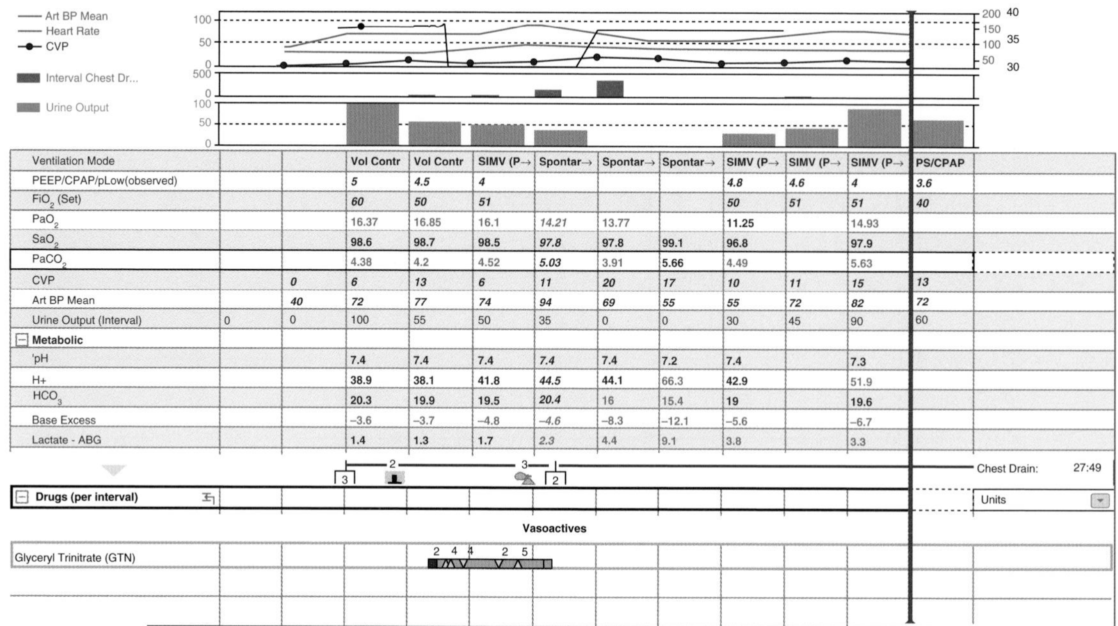

Ventilation Mode			Vol Contr	Vol Contr	SIMV (P→	Spontar→	Spontar→	Spontar→	SIMV (P→	SIMV (P→	SIMV (P→	PS/CPAP
PEEP/CPAP/pLow(observed)			5	4.5	4				4.8	4.6	4	3.6
FiO_2 (Set)			60	50	51				50	51	51	40
PaO_2			16.37	16.85	16.1	14.21	13.77		11.25		14.93	
SaO_2			98.6	98.7	98.5	97.8	97.8	99.1	96.8		97.9	
$PaCO_2$			4.38	4.2	4.52	5.03	3.91	5.66	4.49		5.63	
CVP		0	6	13	6	11	20	17	10	11	15	13
Art BP Mean		40	72	77	74	94	69	55	55	72	82	72
Urine Output (Interval)	0	0	100	55	50	35	0	0	30	45	90	60
Metabolic												
pH			7.4	7.4	7.4	7.4	7.4	7.2	7.4		7.3	
H+			38.9	38.1	41.8	44.5	44.1	66.3	42.9		51.9	
HCO_3			20.3	19.9	19.5	20.4	16	15.4	19		19.6	
Base Excess			−3.6	−3.7	−4.8	−4.6	−8.3	−12.1	−5.6		−6.7	
Lactate - ABG			1.4	1.3	1.7	2.3	4.4	9.1	3.8		3.3	

Figure 36.1 CIS illustration of reducing urine output, followed by reduction in blood pressure and increase in CVP and blood loss.

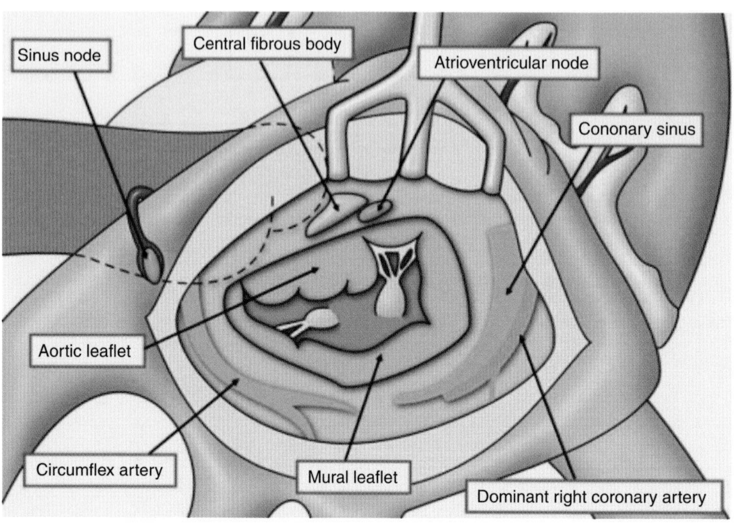

Figure 38.1 Mitral valve and its relation to various structures.

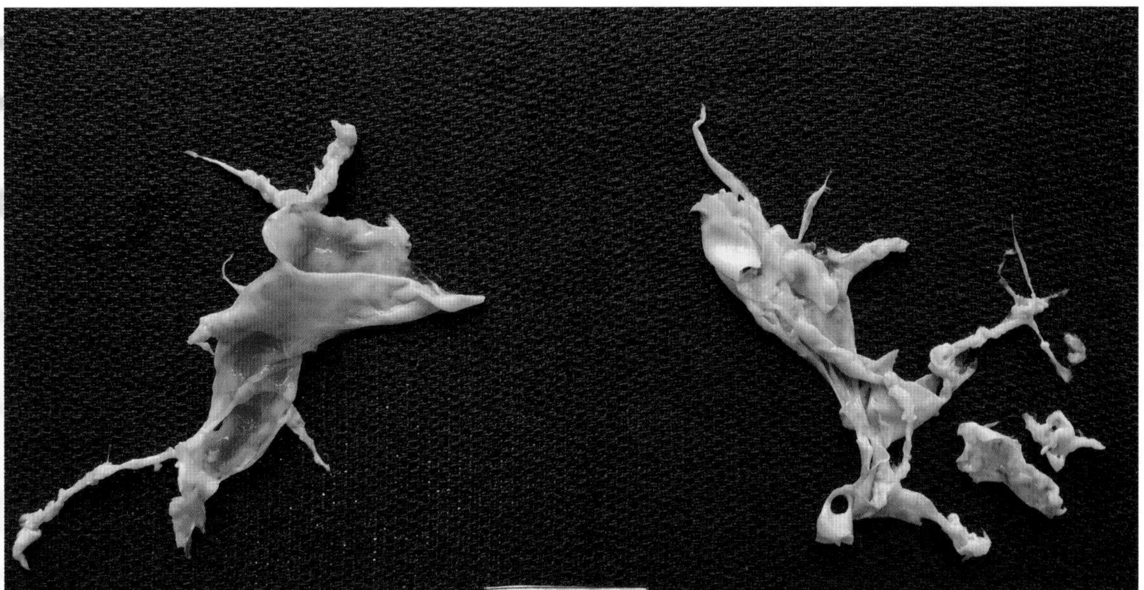

Figure 39.2 Endarterectomy casts from both pulmonary arteries of the same patient in Figure 39.1, demonstrating long tapering 'tails' which is a hallmark of good clearance.

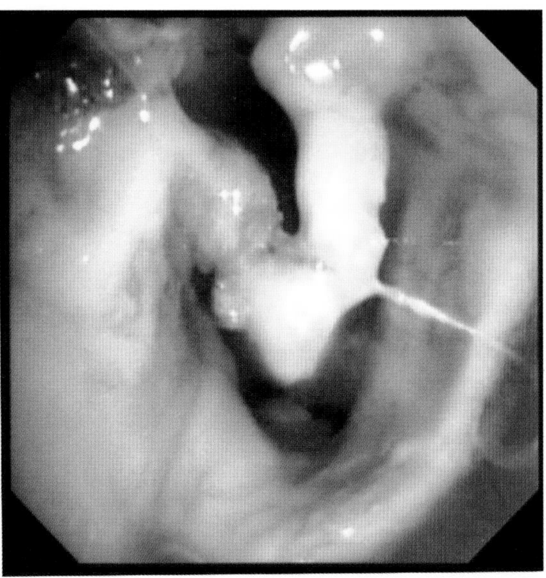

Figure 41.3 Bronchoscopic appearance of a right bronchial anastomosis, demonstrating a severely ischaemic airway with superadded *Aspergillus* infection.

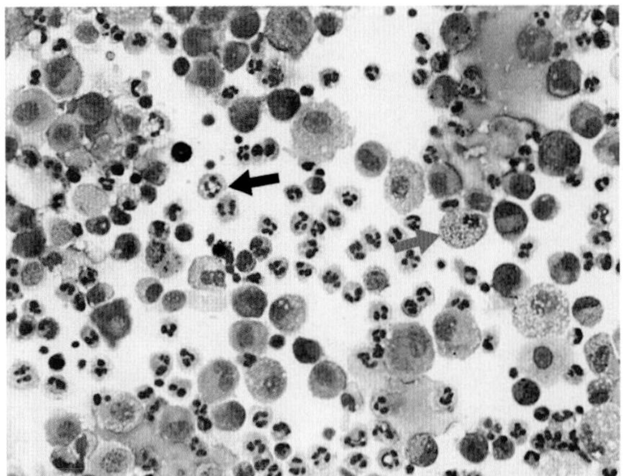

Figure 44.1 Bronchoalveolar lavage fluid from a patient with ARDS. Photomicrograph of modified Wright's stained cytospin. The white arrow denotes a hypersegmented neutrophil; the black arrow denotes a neutrophil which has been efferocytosed by a macrophage.

Chapter 26

Airway Emergencies

Tom P Sullivan and Guillermo Martinez

Introduction

The majority of patients admitted to an intensive care unit require mechanical ventilation and consequently they are vulnerable to a number of airway complications. In these circumstances, airway emergencies such as airway obstruction, failed airway instrumentation, airway device failure or postextubation problems are life threatening situations.

In general, the management of the airway in the intensive care unit is inherently more complex than in the operating theatre, and complications of airway management are disproportionately higher. There are multiple patient, staffing and environmental factors that contribute to the higher complication rate. These factors may include the following: (i) patients are physiologically compromised and frequently unstable; (ii) airway management is usually time critical; (iii) it often occurs out-of-hours; and (iv) it is initially managed by junior medical staff.

The recognition of a compromised airway is the crucial first step in managing an airway emergency. Clinical features of significant airway compromise often involve increased work of breathing, inspiratory stridor, obstructed breathing pattern, desaturation and agitation. Untreated, the rapid development of hypoxia, hypercapnia, acidosis and cardiovascular collapse may ensue.

Rapid assessment of the situation and prompt management is critical to achieve a successful outcome. Airway emergencies are dynamic and often complex situations. The initial treatment priorities are to seek help and establish adequate oxygenation, while preparation for deterioration or airway difficulty is being arranged. In this chapter we will overview the challenges associated with the instrumentation of the airway in critically ill patients, the prevention and management of their airway complications, and the organisational aspects of airway safety in intensive care.

The Obstructed Airway

Airway obstruction is a blockage of the airway resulting in reduced or impeded gas flow. The exact incidence of airway obstruction in the cardiothoracic ICU is unknown and it remains one of the most challenging clinical scenarios for anaesthetists and intensivists.

There are many causes of airway obstruction (see Table 26.1). Anatomically, the obstruction may be supraglottic, glottic or subglottic. The clinical presentation depends on both the location of the obstructing lesion and the time course of its development. Inspiratory stridor suggests a significant upper airway obstruction with a reduction in airway diameter of at least 50%, whilst an expiratory wheeze indicates lower airway pathology.

Clinical Presentation and Assessment

A focused history and examination allows rapid assessment of the patient. Important indicators of imminent airway compromise include hypoxia, agitation, inability to lie flat, failure to manage airway secretions and nocturnal symptoms. Importantly, any distress experienced by the patient may exacerbate the severity of the airway obstruction.

After initial assessment, the suspected site of the airway obstruction, the severity of the airway obstruction and the overall condition of the patient will guide further investigations. Initial tests may include a full blood count, inflammatory markers, blood cultures and a chest X-ray. In cases of suspected upper airway obstruction, computed tomography is ideal to delineate the lesion. However, in patients unable to lie flat, nasendoscopy exploration is the procedure of choice. In those with suspected lower airway obstruction due to a mass lesion, computed tomography of the chest and neck is indicated.

Table 26.1 Causes of airway obstruction

Supraglottic	Infection	Ludwigs angina Epiglottitis Retropharyngeal abscess Laryngotracheobronchitis
	Inflammatory	Angioedema Anaphylaxis
	Neurological	Bulbar palsy
	Obstructive sleep apnoea	
	Foreign body	
	Tumour	
Glottic	Tumour	Vocal cord polyp Vocal cord tumour
	Vocal cord palsy	
	Laryngospasm	
Subglottic	Tracheal stenosis	
	Tracheomalacia	
	External compression	Goitre Mediastinal mass
	Foreign body	

Initial Management of the Obstructed Airway

Acute or severe airway obstruction is a critical emergency. Initial supportive measures must include supplemental oxygen, sitting the patient upright and establishing intravenous access and appropriate monitoring. Deteriorating patients and those in extremis will need their airway secured. The definitive treatment should focus directly on the cause of the airway obstruction and is tailored to the individual patient. Antibiotics, corticosteroids and nebulised adrenaline may be effective for the treatment of upper airway swelling and infections, including epiglottitis or croup. Anaphylaxis should be managed with intravenous or intramuscular adrenaline in accordance with local and national guidelines. Foreign bodies may be dislodged by coughing or postural changes. Some patients can require urgent surgical assistance that may include ear, nose and throat, thoracic or cardiac surgery.

Advanced Airway Management

Airway management in patients with severe obstruction is a complex and high-risk process. All management decisions should be formulated after consultation between a senior anaesthetist and surgeon. The procedure is ideally performed in theatre and it is critical that the airway plan is well prepared and communicated, with all team members ready and the appropriate equipment in the room.

However, there is no universal management plan for securing the obstructed airway. Patients with upper airway obstruction should be assessed as to whether intubation is possible or a tracheostomy under local anaesthetic is required.

In patients who are considered possible to intubate, the airway plan may include awake fibreoptic intubation or gas induction. Caution should be exercised when using awake fibreoptic intubation – the procedure is often difficult and complete airway obstruction may be caused by the fibreoptic scope or loss of airway tone due to sedation or local anaesthesia. Regardless, an experienced surgeon, tracheostomy tray and rigid bronchoscope should be immediately available in the event of failure to intubate.

In patients with subglottic airway obstruction, the exact site of obstruction should be identified prior to embarking on intubation, unless the patient suffers an acute deterioration. The most important considerations are whether a tracheal tube can be safely passed beyond the obstruction and identification of an appropriate rescue plan. An awake fibreoptic intubation may be an appropriate plan A, allowing placement of the endotracheal tube beyond the site of obstruction. More distal tracheal obstruction precludes the use of tracheostomy as a rescue technique and requires the use of rigid bronchoscopy. In significant tracheobronchial obstruction, venovenous extracorporeal membrane oxygenation may be considered prior to securing the airway.

The Failed Airway

Failed airway management is a leading cause of morbidity and mortality in intensive care. The Fourth National Audit Project (NAP4) identified ten events in 2009 of failed endotracheal intubation in the intensive care unit and five of these deteriorated into a 'can't intubate, can't oxygenate' (CICO) situation, requiring cricothyroidotomy or emergency tracheostomy.

The incidence of a 'can't intubate, can't oxygenate' scenario was estimated to be less than 1/10,000 in 1991, and has probably fallen since then due to the advent of laryngeal masks. A thorough airway assessment will identify most patients with difficult airway, however, the positive predictive value of these tests is poor.

Factors identified in NAP4 as associated with failed intubation include patient obesity, known or predictable difficult airways, trainees with limited advanced airway experience, poor judgement and lack of equipment.

Prevention of a 'can't intubate, can't oxygenate' scenario requires proper airway assessment and planning. Every intubation should have a plan A, B, C and D as per the Difficult Airway Society (DAS) guidelines, with appropriate equipment ready, the patient position optimised and experienced personnel present.

Can't Intubate, Oxygenate (CICO)

'Can't intubate, can't oxygenate' exists when there have been failed attempts at intubation, failed attempts at oxygenation (facemask and supraglottic airway device) and low or falling oxygen saturations. Identification of a CICO situation is imperative to good outcomes. Repeated failed attempts at endotracheal intubation risk further airway trauma whilst delaying appropriate management. The reluctance to perform a surgical airway has been identified as a contributor to mortality in CICO situations.

The Difficult Airway Society published guidelines for management of unanticipated difficult intubation, including CICO. Failure to intubate necessitates that oxygenation, rather than intubation or ventilation, becomes the priority. Rapid development of severe hypoxaemia, hypoxic brain injury and cardiovascular collapse ensues if oxygenation is not re-established. Help should be sought as soon as intubation is recognised as difficult or failed.

Rescue Techniques for CICO

Oxygenation must be obtained emergently via front of neck access (FONA), usually through the cricothyroid membrane. The DAS guidelines recommend the scalpel-bougie technique as first-line approach for FONA. This technique uses a cricothyroid incision with a scalpel, insertion of a bougie and rail-roading of a small cuffed endotracheal tube. This technique has higher success rates than a cannula technique and may be more acceptable to anaesthetic and intensive care specialists.

Cannula cricothyroidotomy and surgical tracheostomy are alternative techniques for emergency tracheal access. Cannula cricothyroidotomy involves the insertion of a large-bore cannula through the cricothyroid membrane and use of a high pressure oxygen delivery device. This technique can provide rapid rescue oxygenation; however it is not appropriate for ventilation and clearance of CO_2. Further, the technique has reported high rates of failure, and inability to obtain a cannula cricothyroidotomy within five attempts requires an alternative technique. The risks of the technique include cannula displacement with potential to create significant surgical emphysema, barotrauma and volutrauma. A cannula cricothyroidotomy is an emergency and temporary oxygenation technique that allows stabilisation of the patient. A definitive airway should be established as a matter of priority by percutaneous or surgical tracheostomy.

Emergency surgical tracheostomy is less familiar to intensive care and anaesthetic specialists and risks inadvertent endobronchial intubation. It may be performed by those with suitable expertise and experience, particularly in failed FONA.

Percutaneous tracheostomy is a technique familiar to intensive care specialists, and presents a viable alternative to establishing an emergency surgical airway. The technique utilises a cannula cricothyroidotomy initially. A wire is then inserted into the trachea, followed by a dilator and then a tracheostomy tube. Various tracheostomy sets exist, including single dilation sets. Current guidelines recommend scalpel-bougie as the initial technique as it is fast, has few steps and it establishes a definitive airway. The alternative techniques may be considered when the scalpel-bougie approach has failed and suitable expertise is available.

Oxygen Delivery Techniques

A variety of oxygen delivery techniques are available, but a detailed discussion is included in Chapter 17. An established surgical airway utilising a cuffed endotracheal tube allows direct connection to most ventilators or bag-valve-mask devices via a 15 mm connector; however, the use of a cannula presents a number of limitations. In a CICO scenario, the upper airway is obstructed, and the main route of exhalation is via the cricothyroidotomy cannula. Many oxygen delivery techniques, including jet ventilation devices, fail to allow exhalation and continue to deliver oxygen to the patient, risking significant and rapid volutrauma. Specially designed devices have an adequate exhalation valve. In the absence of these devices, the oxygen

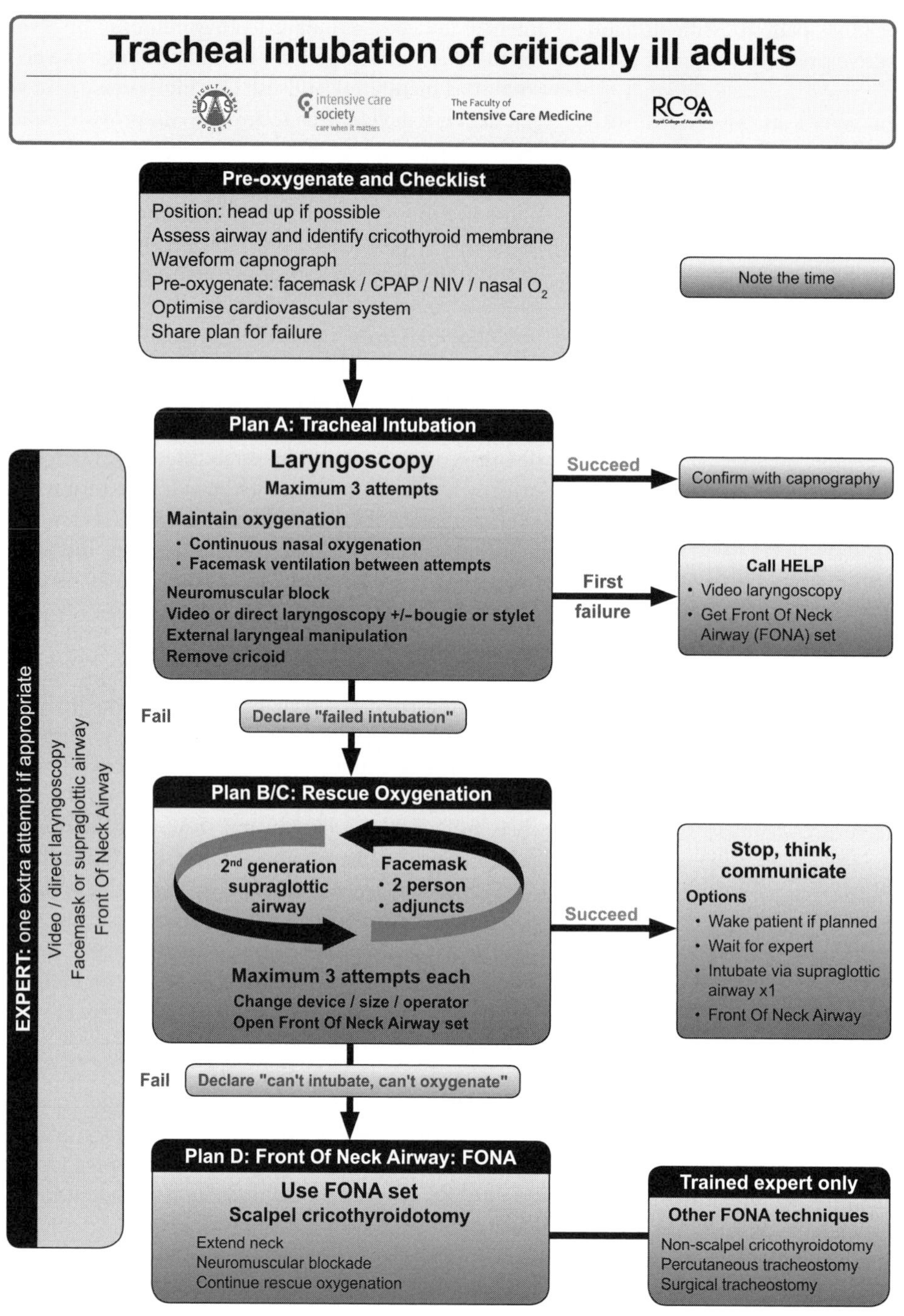

Figure 26.1 https://www.das.uk.com/guidelines/icu_guidelines2017. Reproduced from Guidelines for the management of tracheal intubation in critically ill adults, Higgs et al. (2017).

Table 26.2 Complications of tracheostomy

Immediate	Procedural complications	Hypoxia Hypercapnia Acidosis Loss of airway Haemorrhage Pneumothorax Surgical emphysema Oesophageal injury
	Cricoid cartilage damage	
	Tracheostomy obstruction	Cuff herniation Occlusion by tracheal wall
	Misplacement of tracheostomy	Endobronchial intubation False passage
	Tracheal tube complications	Puncture of tracheal tube cuff Dislodgement of tracheal tube
Early	Mechanical	Dislodgement
	Obstruction	Secretions Blood Cuff herniation
	Infection	Tracheostomy stoma site Tracheobronchial tree
Delayed	Mechanical	Dislodgement
	Obstruction	Secretions Blood Cuff herniation
	Infection	Tracheostomy site Tracheobronchial tree Ventilation associated pneumonia
	Fistula to surrounding structure	Tracheo-innominate artery fistula Tracheo-oesophageal fistula Persistent trachea-cutaneous fistula
	Tracheal injury	Tracheal and laryngeal stenosis Tracheomalacia

delivery device should be disconnected whenever the patient is not actively ventilated through the cannula cricothyroidotomy. Regular training and familiarisation with local cricothyroidotomy equipment is essential to maintain high standards for the rescue of CICO patients.

Tracheostomy Emergencies

Tracheostomy is commonly performed in the intensive care unit for prolonged mechanical ventilation, upper airway obstruction and management of respiratory tract secretions. It may also be performed for rescue airway management or electively in theatre for major airway surgery or laryngectomy. The EPIC study estimated approximately 16% of patients in UK intensive care units have a tracheostomy at any one time.

Tracheostomies accounted for 50% (18/36) airway events in the intensive care unit in NAP4. Fourteen patients had their tracheostomy dislodged, resulting in seven deaths and four hypoxic

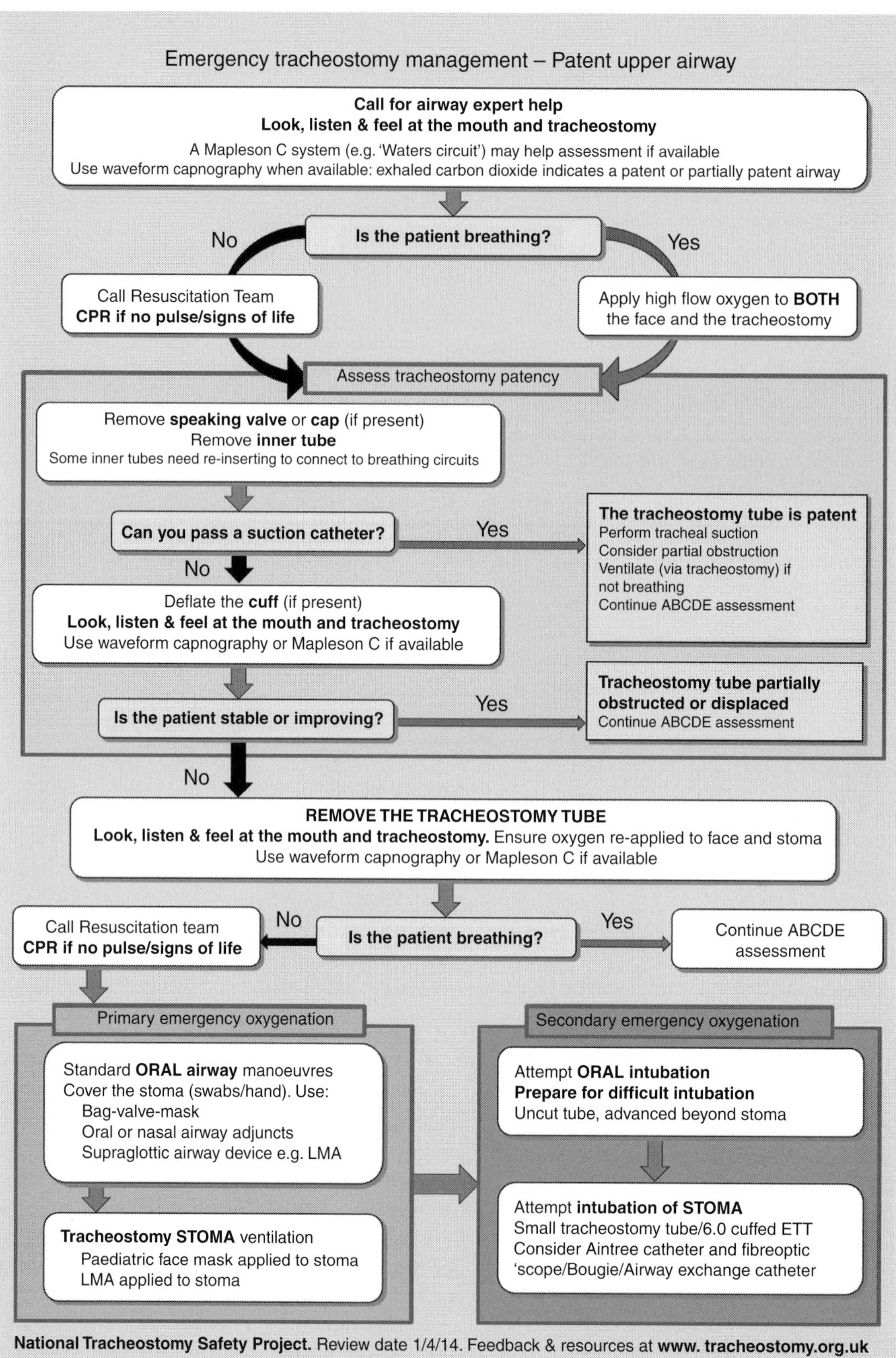

Figure 26.2 Management of tracheostomy and laryngectomy airway emergencies. Reproduced from McGrath et al. (2012), with permission from the Association of Anaesthetists of Great Britain & Ireland/Blackwell Publishing Ltd.

brain injuries (see Table 26.2). In two-thirds of these cases, the dislodgement occurred on moving or turning. Two further patients had failure to place an elective tracheostomy in intensive care and two had major haemorrhage post decannulation. Obesity was identified as a significant risk factor for tracheostomy complications and capnography was used infrequently. The high morbidity of tracheostomy complications led to the development of current national guidelines.

Dislodged Tracheostomy

Tracheostomy dislodgement is the most commonly lethal tracheostomy complication. Displacement occurs with all types of securement devices; however patient turning and obesity were associated with dislodgement. The infrequent use of capnography can lead to a delay in detection and worse outcomes.

A dislodged tracheostomy tube is an emergency and early recognition is crucial. Help and expert airway assistance should be sought. Assessment must be made immediately for airway, breathing and circulation (see Figure 26.2). Supplemental oxygen must be applied to both the face and neck stoma.

In those patients who require airway instrumentation, initial airway manoeuvres should be directed at the oral route, such as bag-mask ventilation and supraglottic airways, whilst sealing the neck stoma. Oxygenation may also be attempted via the stoma, using a small paediatric mask. Failure to oxygenate should lead to an attempt at oral intubation and advancing the tracheal tube beyond the stoma, followed by attempted intubation via the stoma, careful not to intubate the bronchus. Ideally, this is undertaken using fibreoptic bronchoscopy guidance. The use of capnography for the confirmation of a secured airway is mandatory.

Laryngectomy patients, however, have altered anatomy with no upper airway connection to the trachea. All attempts at oxygenation and airway instrumentation in these patients should be directed to the tracheostomy site.

Blocked Tracheostomy Tube

Tracheostomy tubes may become blocked at any stage due to blood, secretions, displacement or cuff herniation. Clinical presentation includes dyspnoea, increased work of breathing and desaturation.

Immediate assessment should be undertaken. The inner tube or speaking device can be removed, leaving the tracheostomy in situ. A suction catheter should be inserted to assess the patency of the tracheostomy. If a suction tube cannot be passed, the tracheostomy cuff should be deflated to relieve the obstruction. If the patient does not improve then the tracheostomy tube should be removed.

Airway Bleeding

Airway bleeding most commonly presents early post-tracheostomy insertion, but may also present postdecannulation. Bleeding or infection complicates 5% of percutaneous tracheostomies.

Tracheoinnominate artery fistula, caused by breaching of the tracheal wall into the innominate artery, is a rare but frequently fatal cause of airway haemorrhage, occurring days to weeks post tracheostomy insertion. It presents as massive airway haemorrhage, which requires immediate airway support. A tracheal tube may be advanced into the airway and the cuff inflated to tamponade the fistula before emergency surgery is performed.

Post Extubation Airway Emergencies

Extubation is an important but often neglected component of airway management. A stable airway is removed and remains unsecured until the patient is able to maintain airway patency and protective reflexes. Most complications post extubation are minor. However, airway emergencies may occur due either to airway obstruction or contamination.

The Difficult Airway Society published guidelines on extubation post anaesthesia, stratifying patients into 'low-risk' or 'at-risk' groups with corresponding extubation algorithms.

Unplanned Extubation

Inadvertent extubation is not uncommon, occurring at a rate of one per 100 ventilator days. However, only four cases were reported in the NAP4 audit. Three of these patients were obese, the fourth was a known difficult airway and two patients suffered aspiration as a result. Capnography was not utilised in any of these cases.

Accidental extubation typically occurred during patient movement, sedation breaks and minor airway manipulation. Risk factors for unplanned extubation include higher levels of arousal, agitation and less experienced nursing staff. Identification of inadvertent extubation is crucial to limit the risk of complications such as aspiration, hypotension, arrhythmias, airway injury and respiratory compromise.

Not all patients will require reintubation. Supplemental oxygen and supportive manoeuvres may be adequate. Reintubation is more likely to be required in patients with deeper levels of sedation, high oxygen requirements, high levels of pressure support or positive end-expiratory pressure and cardiovascular instability.

Airway Obstruction

Airway obstruction post extubation may occur secondary to reduced airway tone, laryngospasm or contamination of the airway. It is characterised by inspiratory stridor, respiratory efforts with reduced airflow and desaturation. The treatment depends on the cause.

Initial efforts should be focused on oxygenation. Jaw thrust and chin lift will frequently relieve obstruction due to drowsiness. An oropharyngeal or nasopharyngeal airway may help and bag-mask ventilation may be required. If the patient does not improve quickly, a secure airway should be re-established.

Laryngospasm causes either partial or complete airway obstruction. It often occurs in response to stimulation when patients are emerging from anaesthesia. Airway blood or mucus causing irritation of the vocal cords can result in laryngospasm. Initial management is supportive, with bag-mask ventilation utilising positive end-expiratory pressure. A strong jaw lift, known as Larson's manoeuvre, may break the spasm. If it continues, resedation and muscle relaxation will cause the laryngospasm to cease. The increased respiratory effort with the closed glottis may cause negative pressure pulmonary oedema.

Less common causes of airway obstruction postoperatively include recurrent laryngeal nerve injury and foreign body. Bilateral, rather than unilateral, recurrent laryngeal nerve injury will cause upper airway obstruction. Foreign bodies include swabs, teeth and dentures. Risk factors include surgery on the upper airway and traumatic intubation.

Airway Contamination

The airway may become contaminated with secretions, blood or foreign bodies. Airway contamination will present with coughing, gagging or airway obstruction. Initial management is supportive. The airway may need to be secured by intubation and plans for a difficult intubation need to be established. Care should be taken to suction out the airway prior to extubation.

Systemic and Organisational Considerations

Airway emergencies in the intensive care unit are associated with high morbidity and mortality. Recognition and diagnosis is often delayed, hindering effective management. They may occur at any time and are often managed by junior medical and nursing staff unfamiliar with airway equipment or management of complex airway emergencies. Numerous factors have been identified that may reduce the rate of these complications and improve outcomes.

Staff and Training

Intensive care skill-mix with variable experience in airway emergencies should be minimised. All junior medical staff should be familiar with basic airway management techniques and staff with experience in advanced airway support should be available at all hours.

Staff education should focus on identifying those with difficult airways, their assessment and management. Identification of potentially difficult airways allows a defined plan to be made in the event of an emergency, including seeking assistance early. Airway management education includes training in basic and advanced airway skills as well as management algorithms for difficult and failed airways. Maintenance of emergency airway skills, including 'can't intubate, can't oxygenate' scenarios, may be best achieved with simulation and skills sessions training.

Equipment

All intensive care units should have access to a difficult airway trolley and fibreoptic bronchoscopy. As specialists, it is important that intensivists are familiar with the contents and use of airway equipment available in their unit. Additionally, medical staff should be familiar and confident using a variety of different equipment.

Capnography is a crucial monitor for intubated and ventilated patients. Its use is universal in anaesthesia but variable in the intensive care unit. Capnography should be utilised for every intubation to confirm endotracheal tube position as well as throughout the period the patient is intubated and dependent on a ventilator.

Planning and Preparation

The early identification of patients at risk for airway complications and the recognition of an airway emergency is important for best outcomes. Identification of patients with potential airway difficulty allows the formulation and communication of an appropriate plan should trouble strike.

However, not all airway emergencies can be predicted and early recognition of an emergency remains crucial. A clearly formed management plan is critical; however all plans can fail and the back-up plans (B, C and D) are as important as the initial strategy. This must be communicated clearly with the team, experienced staff must be available and equipment ready.

Summary

Airway emergencies in the intensive care unit are complex situations associated with high rates of morbidity and mortality. Early identification of those at risk allows thorough planning and management in a controlled and timely manner. The nature of airway emergencies and complications necessitates that back-up plans with appropriately qualified staff and equipment are immediately available.

Learning Points

- Airway management in the intensive care unit is associated with disproportionately high rates of complications.
- Early recognition of emergencies allows preparation and planning.
- The initial airway management should focus on providing oxygenation.
- Securing the airway can be a complex process. Experienced personnel should be present and plans A, B, C and D ready in case of initial failure.
- All intubated and ventilator dependent patients should have continuous capnography monitoring.

Further Reading

Cook TM, Woodall N, Harper J, Benger J. On behalf of the Fourth National Audit Project. Major complications of airway management in the UK: results of the Fourth National Audit Project of the Royal College of Anaesthetists and the Difficult Airway Society. Part 2: intensive care and emergency departments. *British Journal of Anaesthesia*. 2011; 106: 632–642.

Da Silva PSL, Fonseca MCM. Unplanned endotracheal extubations in the intensive care unit. *Anesthesia & Analgesia*. 2012; 114: 1003–1014.

Flavell EM, Stacey MR, Hall JE. The clinical management of airway obstruction. *Current Anaesthesia and Critical Care*. 2009; 20: 102–112.

Greenland KB, Acott C, Segal R, Goulding G, Riley RH, Merry AF. Emergency surgical airway in life-threatening acute airway emergencies – why are we so reluctant to do it? *Anaesthesia and Intensive Care*. 2011; 39: 578–584.

Heard AMB, Green RJ, Eakins P. The formulation and introduction of a "can't intubate, can't ventilate" algorithm into clinical practice. *Anaesthesia*. 2009; 64: 601–608.

Henderson JJ, Popat MT, Latto IP, Pearce AC. Difficult Airway Society guidelines for management of the unanticipated difficult intubation. *Anaesthesia*. 2004; 59: 675–694.

Higgs BA, McGrath C, Goddard J. Rangasami G, Suntharalingam R, Gale, TM. Cook and on behalf of Difficult Airway Society, Intensive Care Society, Faculty of Intensive Care Medicine, Royal College of Anaesthetists. *British Journal of Anaesthesia*. 2017; In press. doi: 10.1016/j.bja.2017.10.021.

Huggs A, McGrath BA, Goddard C, et al. and on behalf of Difficult Airway Society, Intensive Care Society, Faculty of Intensive Care Medicine, Royal College of Anaesthetists. Guidelines for the management of tracheal intubation in critically ill adults. *British Journal of Anaesthesia*. In press.

Listello D, Sessler CN. Unplanned extubation. Clinical predictors for reintubation. *Chest*. 1994; 105: 1496–1503.

Mallick A, Bodenham AR. Tracheostomy in critically ill patients. *European Journal of Anaesthesiology*. 2010; 27: 676–682.

Mason RA, Fielder CP. The obstructed airway in head and neck surgery. *Anaesthesia*. 1999; 54: 625–628.

McGrath BA, Bates L, Atkinson D, Moore JA. Multidisciplinary guidelines for the management of tracheostomy and laryngectomy airway emergencies. *Anaesthesia*. 2012; 67: 1025–1041.

Mort TC. Emergency tracheal intubation: complications associated with repeated laryngoscopic attempts. *Anesthesia & Analgesia*. 2004; 99: 607–613.

Patel A, Pearce A. Progress in management of the obstructed airway. *Anaesthesia*. 2011; 66: 93–100.

Popat M, Mitchell V, Dravid R, et al. Difficult Airway Society Guidelines for the management of tracheal extubation. *Anaesthesia*. 2012; 67: 318–340.

Soar J, Pumphrey R, Cant A, et al. Emergency treatment of anaphylactic reactions – Guidelines for healthcare providers. *Resuscitation*. 2008; 77: 157–169.

Vincent JL, Suter P, Bihari D, Braining H. Organisation of intensive care units in Europe: lessons from the EPIC study. *Intensive Care Medicine*. 1997; 23: 1181–1184.

MCQs

1. **Time to desaturation following the onset of apnoea is influenced by:**
   (a) The muscle relaxant used
   (b) The adequacy of preoxygenation
   (c) The patient's age
   (d) Lying the patient supine
   (e) Insufflation of air

2. **Regarding patients with tracheostomy, which of the following is true?**
   (a) The use of capnography will prevent complications from tracheostomy displacement
   (b) In suspected airway blockage, the tracheostomy should be removed immediately
   (c) Oral endotracheal intubation is not possible in patients with tracheostomy
   (d) Capnography should be utilised in ventilator dependent tracheostomy patients
   (e) Laryngectomy patients may be oxygenated adequately by facemask oxygenation

3. **Regarding 'can't inubate, can't oxygenate' scenarios, which of the following is true?**
   (a) An emergency call for help should be made after failed intubation and inability to oxygenate with a supraglottic airway device
   (b) After three failed attempts at cannula cricothyroidotomy, emergency tracheostomy should be attempted
   (c) If a cannula cricothyroidotomy is successful and a laryngeal mask is in place, the laryngeal mask should be left in situ
   (d) Cannula cricothyroidotomy allows adequate exhalation
   (e) If rescue cannula cricothyroidotomy is successful, the patient should be woken up

4. **In the intensive care unit, which of the following is true regarding emergency airway management?**
   (a) Oesophageal injury is a recognised and unavoidable complication of airway management
   (b) Suxamethonium is the preferred muscle relaxant, due to its quick offset in case of a failed airway
   (c) Preoxygenation may be suboptimal
   (d) Capnography should be used if a difficult intubation is anticipated
   (e) Airway rescue with a laryngeal mask is not appropriate, as the patients are usually unfasted

5. **In postoperative patients after extubation, which of the following is true?**
   (a) Signs of airway obstruction require immediate attention and re-intubation
   (b) Laryngospasm may respond to positive end-expiratory pressure
   (c) A hoarse voice does not indicate an airway injury
   (d) Vomiting is unlikely to lead to pulmonary aspiration
   (e) If reintubation is required, it may be more difficult than previous attempts

Exercise answers are available on p.469. Alternatively, take the test online at www.cambridge.org/CardiothoracicMCQ

Chapter 27

Chest Pain as a Symptom on the Cardiothoracic Intensive Care Unit

Will Davies

Introduction

Chest pain as a symptom can lead to over 400 eventual diagnoses. Up to one third of those patients admitted to an acute medical unit may have chest pain as a component of their presenting complaint. Chest pain is almost ubiquitous in patients admitted to the cardiothoracic intensive care unit (CICU). For example, the preoperative patient with ischaemic heart disease may experience the full range of associated symptoms from central crushing pain with radiation, to the silent myocardial infarction of a long-term diabetic with associated neuropathy. Once these same patients have undergone surgical revascularisation, this ischaemic pain will probably be substituted for the dull, central tenderness of a median sternotomy, or the pleuritic pain of a residual pneumothorax irritated by the intercostal chest drains. The evaluation and subsequent treatment of chest pain on the CICU is vital to enhance the clinical outcome of this patient population.

In this chapter we will endeavour to discuss the rapid yet thorough assessment of chest pain as a symptom, the initial examination and investigation strategy required, and outline the emergent therapeutic options required for each differential diagnosis.

History

As with all clinical encounters the greatest aid to formulation of an accurate differential diagnosis is a thorough clinical history. Several confounding factors exist in the ICU patient that make the history less reliable. The spectrum of confounders ranges from those patients that are sedated and ventilated, through the heavily narcotised and disorientated, to the patient with 'distraction' pains who may under-report symptomatic changes. These challenges can result in important delays in the detection of the pathology underlying chest pain.

Given the above issues a focused approach to history taking is required. The mainstays of site, character, radiation, onset, severity, exacerbating factors and timing all still apply although many of these will be very dependent on the preceding interventions and current therapy that the patient is undergoing. The new onset of a complaint of chest pain, therefore, requires a flexible approach to clinical assessment to rule out the most important and potentially life threatening causes in a systematic fashion.

Clinical Examination

The role of clinical examination in the CICU can often be overlooked. With all the intensive monitoring and real time data that are now available, including bedside transthoracic echocardiography and easy access computerised tomography, the stethoscope can become a vestigial appendage. However, this patient population with positive pressure ventilation and invasive procedures is particularly prone to complications such as tension pneumothorax that need to be rapidly assessed, diagnosed and treated to avoid unnecessary morbidity and potential mortality. Indeed, the CICU patient is at particular risk when transferred from the controlled environment of the unit to other departments for investigation, and the role of clinical assessment must not be forgotten.

Differential Diagnosis

The elective patient recovering on the CICU is likely to have been thoroughly investigated prior to admission. Many of the emergent admissions will also have a diagnosis underlying their chest pain by the time they arrive. However, these critically unwell and increasingly aged patients are prone to further, sometimes unrelated, pathologies. Thus a physician must have a widespread understanding of those conditions that most commonly occur in the CICU patient.

It is beyond the scope of this chapter to cover all of the differential diagnoses the CICU staff may encounter in the patient with chest pain. However, we will aim to discuss those that are most common, those that are less common but life threatening, and those that are rare but need highlighting to ensure they are not overlooked.

Myocardial Ischaemia

Most of the patients that arrive on the CICU are likely to have undergone some investigation into their coronary vasculature, be it an invasive coronary angiography or some form of non-invasive functional or anatomical test. In fact, the majority of such patients will be admitted to the CICU to recover from a procedure, performed either percutaneously or surgically, to improve the vascular supply of the myocardial bed. These patients are not, however, immune from further myocardial ischaemia.

Postpercutaneous Coronary Intervention

Primary percutaneous coronary intervention is now the revascularisation method of choice for patients presenting with an ST elevation myocardial infarction. The admission rate to the CICU following this procedure is around 5% and has been rising steadily year on year. The majority of these patients are intubated and ventilated in the periarrest period in the community, although some will require ventilation during the PPCI procedure itself. If the cardiac arrest is prolonged then these patients will undergo a period of cooling, or at least avoidance of hyperthermia, to aid neurological recovery.

A particular challenge in the ventilated patient post PPCI is the administration and absorption of dual antiplatelet medication. The risk of acute stent thrombosis in this population is tenfold that of the spontaneously ventilating patient, with a mortality approaching 40%. It is, therefore, important to ensure that patients receive and are absorbing the dual antiplatelets as prescribed by the interventional cardiology team, and that premature cessation is avoided in all but life threatening bleeding. In those patients who are unable to absorb enterically, alternatives include administration per rectum or substitution for an intravenous agent, for example the glycoprotein IIb/IIIa inhibitors such as abciximab, eptifibatide and tirofiban.

Any chest pain with concomitant ECG changes in the post PCI cohort of patients should trigger an emergent cardiology consultation to rule out acute stent thrombosis requiring repeat intervention. The second most common cause of postprocedural chest pain in this group is a technical problem with the stent placement, either an inflow or outflow coronary artery dissection, or perhaps the obstruction of a side branch. Finally, the role of untreated bystander disease is important as lesions that remain in other vessels may well become symptomatic in the high catecholamine milieu that exists post PPCI.

Postsurgical Revascularisation

The rate of postoperative myocardial infarction following coronary artery bypass grafting is estimated to be between 5 and 10%. The incidence of graft related ischaemia is thought to be approximately 3%. In the intubated patient the clues to infarction and ischaemia are persistent low cardiac output state, dysrhythmia, evolving ECG changes and new regional wall motion abnormalities on echocardiographic imaging. The routine use of biochemical markers of myocardial damage is unlikely to be useful in the diagnosis in this population. In the awake patient, the chest pain of myocardial ischaemia can be difficult to differentiate from the postoperative sternal wound pain although any patient describing their usual angina should be investigated further. Patients in whom early graft failure is suspected have a significant adverse outcome unless treated promptly.

A second form of postprocedural cardiac ischaemia is that induced by poor myocardial protection. This is difficult to diagnose and may present as a global reduction in left or right ventricular function with associated haemodynamic compromise requiring inotropic support.

Even in the patient with apparently unobstructed coronary arteries who undergoes cardiac surgery, for example for a valve replacement, there is a risk of both plaque rupture and importantly embolic obstruction of the coronaries. This is particularly prevalent in those patients with dilated atria and preoperative atrial fibrillation. One final consideration is the occlusion of the coronary ostia by the stent struts on a prosthetic aortic valve.

A further mechanism of potential coronary flow limitation is the phenomenon of coronary vasospasm. This is often difficult to diagnose and is particularly prevalent at the time of high catecholamine drive, such as during extubation. Intravenous vasodilators usually allow rapid resolution and prevent the lasting damage of infarction.

Aortic Dissection

Acute aortic dissection is the most common life threatening pathology of the thoracic aorta and carries a mortality of 1% per hour in the early stages. In the simplest Stanford classification, type A aortic dissection involves the ascending aorta, whereas type B dissections are those that do not involve the ascending aorta. This classification is useful, as type A dissections benefit from emergent surgical repair, whereas type B aortic dissections are best managed medically unless they become complicated. Type A aortic dissections are more common in patients in their sixth and seventh decades, whereas type B dissections typically affect the elderly.

Although traditionally thought to be associated with the connective tissue disorders such as Marfan, Loeys–Dietz and Ehlers–Danlos syndromes, more common predisposing factors include hypertension and bicuspid aortic valve anatomy. In the CICU setting, the physician must always be cognisant of the postsurgical patient with sudden onset of intrascapular pain and haemodynamic instability. Any instrumentation of the ascending aorta, be that percutaneously with ostial coronary stent placement, or surgically during aortic cannulation for cardiopulmonary bypass or during aortic valve replacement, may subsequently cause separation of the layers of the aortic wall. Rarely, reports have been published of aortic dissection following cocaine use, during heavy lifting and during systemic inflammatory vasculopathy. Although perhaps the most feared complication of pregnancy, dissection during pregnancy is relatively uncommon.

The typical chest pain associated with aortic dissection is said to be a searing or tearing pain that starts in the chest and rapidly radiates to the intrascapular region. Immediate complications include right coronary artery occlusion and associated inferior ST elevation, cardiac tamponade, acute aortic valve insufficiency and neurological deficit. Atypical presentations include renal failure of uncertain aetiology due to loss of the renal arterial supply, and mesenteric ischaemia manifest by rising serum lactate, abdominal pain and frequently loose stools. The loss of a peripheral pulse was only present in 19% of patients recorded in the International Registry of Acute Aortic Dissection series. In 15% of patients with an acute aortic dissection the chest radiograph will fail to show the classic widened mediastinum, and contrast enhanced computed tomography has become the first line in investigation. In those centres with expertise in transoesophageal echocardiography, this imaging modality has the advantage of being both sensitive and specific, and also relatively rapidly performed.

Once diagnosed, type A aortic dissection is initially treated by stabilisation of the patient using intravenous beta blockade. Thereafter, emergent surgery to obliterate the false lumen and repair the ascending aorta using an interposition graft is required.

Postprocedural management requires tight blood pressure control with beta-blocker therapy providing the pharmacological mainstay. Various authors have reported survival rates of between 50 and 90% 1 year following acute type A aortic dissection.

Superior Vena Cava Syndrome

Although originally described as occurring in conjunction with an infective cause, the most common cause of superior vena cava syndrome (SVCS) worldwide is now malignancy of the lung, breast or mediastinal nodes. Of particular concern to the patients under consideration in this chapter, is the increasing incidence of iatrogenic SVCS secondary to device insertion, be those permanent pacemakers, implantable cardiac defibrillators or vascular access catheters. Although most commonly diagnosed due to the presence of distended neck and chest wall veins, cough, dyspnoea and facial swelling, several authors report the presence of a dull chest ache, mimicking that of cardiac ischaemia. Treatment very much depends on the underlying aetiology, with external neoplastic compression being best treated with debulking therapies be those chemotherapeutic or surgical. Thrombosis can be successfully reversed with thrombolysis and anticoagulation, and some cases require stenting to secure long-term patency.

Vascular Air Embolism

The CICU has evolved over the last few decades such that the average unit has a plethora of patients undergoing various stages of organ support. Wide-bore vascular access catheters can be connected to continuous venovenous haemofiltration machines, extracorporeal membranous oxygenators, rapid infusers and ventricular assist devices. All of these life support technologies have the potential to allow the accidental entrainment of air into the circulation. Clinically, this often manifests as chest pain, dysrhythmia, right sided heart failure and dyspnoea. A venous air embolus can sometimes manifest as an arterial issue, such as stroke or myocardial infarction due to the passage from the right atrium to the left atrium through a patent foramen ovale or atrial septal defect.

The immediate management of vascular air embolus is to identify the source and eliminate further entrainment. In the case of the patient in cardiac arrest then vigorous cardiopulmonary massage has been shown to be beneficial. As with all iatrogenic complications, vigilant prevention is always better than the cure.

Pericarditis and Myocarditis

Both myocarditis and pericarditis are usually caused by an acute inflammatory process that may be secondary to a viral infection, an autoimmune inflammation or the presence of a toxin, either exogenous or from the accumulation of a metabolite. They may occur synchronously or can be seen as separate diagnoses. In Western countries most cases of myocarditis in previously healthy individuals are caused by enteroviruses, especially Coxsackie B. Other less prevalent causes include Lyme disease, caused by *Borrelia burgdorferi*, Chagas' disease, caused by *Trypanosoma cruzi* (common in South America), and Kawasaki disease.

The prevalence is difficult to determine, as many cases are mild and may be subclinical. Patients usually present with myalgia, malaise, cough or GI upset, and fever. The risk of fatal arrhythmia may persist for several weeks after the onset of symptoms, and appears to be linked to strenuous exercise. The chest pain of both myocarditis and pericarditis may mimic that of acute myocardial infarction, and in the early stages of the illness the ECG may also be suggestive of an ST elevation MI. The typically scooped ST segment elevation and PR depression classically reported in pericarditis may take several hours to develop. Both echocardiography (which may show a regional wall motion abnormality in focal myocarditis) and troponin levels (which are frequently raised) are also poor differentiators. Many of these patients who present to the cardiologist will, therefore, be investigated with an invasive coronary angiogram.

Once recognised, the treatment of both myocarditis and pericarditis is largely supportive. Complications of cardiac failure are relatively rare and bridging to recovery is seldom necessary. Even in cases of acute cardiac decompensation, the majority of patients make a full recovery and preserve their myocardial function long term.

Cardiac Tamponade and Myocardial Rupture

Cardiac tamponade is defined as the compression of the cardiac chambers due to the accumulation of fluid, pus, blood clots or gas in the pericardial space. In the CICU environment the most common causes are the accumulation of blood post cardiac surgery, following percutaneous coronary intervention complicated by coronary artery perforation or myocardial rupture. The triad of high venous pressure, low systemic arterial pressure and muffled heart sounds is often observed. The presence of pulsus paradoxus, defined as a fall in arterial pressure of greater than 10 mmHg during inspiration, can often be determined by observing the respiratory variation of the arterial line trace during the ventilatory cycle. However, this clinical sign is not pathognomonic, and can also be seen in haemorrhagic shock, massive pulmonary embolus and severe obstructive pulmonary disease.

The most useful and immediate bedside test in the CICU environment is the echocardiogram, which typically confirms a pericardial collection, diastolic compromise of the right ventricle, the loss of respiratory variation in the IVC diameter, and greater than 25% respiratory variation in the transmitral and transtricuspid Doppler parameters. The treatment of cardiac tamponade is drainage of the pericardial collection, either percutaneously using CT or echo guided pericardiocentesis, or by re-exploration of the median sternotomy post cardiac surgery.

Myocardial rupture is an infrequent complication of myocardial infarction, occurring in approximately 2% of patients who have had unsuccessful or delayed revascularisation, but carries a high mortality due to cardiac tamponade. Clinical features that aid the diagnosis are a sudden onset of cardiovascular collapse, chest pain and jugular venous distension. Surgical repair is often fraught with the difficulty of very friable tissues.

Tension Pneumothorax

Pneumothorax is particularly common in the postoperative patient on the CICU. However, the onset of a tension pneumothorax may be insidious, and must be recognised and treated swiftly to avoid potentially fatal consequences. More details of its management will be discussed in Chapter 28.

Gastrointestinal Causes of Chest Pain

There are several well-recognised gastrointestinal causes of chest pain that are often overlooked in the initial assessment of the patient on the CICU. In the postoperative period the presence of a ruptured oesophagus secondary to transoesophageal echocardiography may be difficult to differentiate from a pneumothorax caused by the inadvertent opening of the pleural space. The leakage of gastric contents into the thorax can be insidious, and the subsequent sepsis difficult to manage unless a high clinical suspicion is maintained.

Cholecystitis is another mimic of acute myocardial infarction, with right upper quadrant or epigastric pain, symptoms of sympathetic overdrive and even inferior ST elevation on the 12-lead ECG. A complication of a common bile duct stone, pancreatitis is also seen in the critically unwell patient and serum or urinary amylase assays can aid in the diagnosis. The stress response to critical illness also raises the acidity of the contents of the upper gastrointestinal tract and can lead to gastric ulceration and haemorrhage and the subsequent chest pain.

Wound Pain and Sternal Dehiscence

Although sternal wound dehiscence is a rare complication of cardiac surgery, it is associated with significant morbidity and mortality. Preoperative risk factors include diabetes mellitus, obesity, chronic obstructive pulmonary disease and smoking. Operative factors include a long cardiopulmonary bypass time, postoperative haemorrhage, re-exploration of the wound, prolonged ventilation and the need for tracheostomy. The conscious patient often complains of sternal pain, and CT scanning of the thorax can reveal the sternal dehiscence, even in patients with little evidence of skin breakdown. Treatment varies from intravenous antibiotics through to complete sternotomy and reconstruction.

Takotsubo Cardiomyopathy

Takotsubo cardiomyopathy was first described in the early 1990s and is a reversible left ventricular apical ballooning that may mimic acute myocardial infarction. It is typically precipitated by acute emotional distress, especially in postmenopausal female patients with unobstructed coronary arteries. The Japanese term takotsubo means octopus pot, as the shape of the left ventricle with the typical apical ballooning is said to resemble the pot used by fishermen for catching octopodes. The syndrome often presents with severe chest pain, anterior ST elevation and a raise in cardiac biomarkers. It can, on occasion, cause cardiac arrest. The course is usually self-limiting with supportive care, but it can recur in up to one third of cases. Various pathogenic mechanisms have been proposed including vasospasm of the coronary vasculature secondary to a high catecholamine drive, although a neurogenic mechanism of myocardial stunning, as seen during acute neurological events, has also been considered.

Conclusion

Chest pain as a symptom is almost ubiquitous amongst patients on the cardiothoracic ICU. Without a broad understanding of the myriad of underlying diagnoses the ICU clinician may not be able to rapidly identify those that are life threatening versus those that are benign. The role of clinical examination must not be forgotten in these days of sophisticated monitoring and the easy availability of diagnostic imaging.

Learning Points

- A broad understanding of the differential diagnoses underlying chest pain as a symptom is vital to rapid assessment and diagnosis in the CICU.
- The mortality of an intubated and ventilated patient post primary PCI is tenfold that of a spontaneously ventilating patient.
- The survival following type A aortic dissection is directly related to the time taken to diagnosis and subsequent initiation of definitive treatment.
- Several gastrointestinal causes of chest pain are commonly seen in patients on the CICU and these diagnoses can be easily overlooked by the unwary.

Further Reading

Braverman AC. Acute aortic dissection. *Circulation.* 2010; 122: 184–188.

Figueras J, Alcalde O, Barrabés JA, et al. Changes in hospital mortality rates in 425 patients with acute ST-elevation myocardial infarction and cardiac rupture over a 30-year period. *Circulation*. 2008; 118: 2783–2789.

Oakley CM. Myocarditis, pericarditis and other pericardial diseases. *Heart*. 2000; 84: 449–454.

Spodick DH. Acute cardiac tamponade. *New England Journal of Medicine*. 2003; 349: 684–690.

Virani SS, Khan AN, Mendoza CE, et al. Takotsubo cardiomyopathy or broken heart syndrome. *Texas Heart Institute Journal*. 2007; 34: 76–79.

MCQs

1. **Following primary PCI, dual antiplatelet therapy can be:**
   (a) Safely withheld for 48 hours post procedure
   (b) Substituted for a glycoprotein IIb/IIIa inhibitor in those patients who are not absorbing orally
   (c) Discontinued with signs of non-life-threatening bleeding
   (d) A significant cause of a low platelet count
   (e) Omitted until the patient is spontaneously ventilating

2. **Type A aortic dissection:**
   (a) Typically results in a loss of a peripheral pulse
   (b) Is reliably diagnosed on chest radiography
   (c) Is more common in the elderly
   (d) Can be effectively treated medically
   (e) May present with chest pain and diarrhoea

3. **Superior vena cava syndrome:**
   (a) Is declining in incidence
   (b) Is unlikely to be iatrogenic
   (c) Is most commonly caused by intrathoracic malignancy
   (d) Does not cause chest pain
   (e) Should not be treated with thrombolysis

4. **In the absence of a pathological communication between the right and left heart, an air embolus should not present with:**
   (a) Dysrhythmia
   (b) Chest pain
   (c) Stroke
   (d) Right sided cardiac failure
   (e) Dyspnoea

5. **Takotsubo cardiomyopathy is uncommonly associated with:**
   (a) Postmenopausal women
   (b) Cardiac arrest
   (c) Severe coronary artery disease
   (d) Left ventricular apical ballooning
   (e) Long-term cardiac failure

Exercise answers are available on p.469. Alternatively, take the test online at www.cambridge.org/CardiothoracicMCQ

Chapter 28

Acute Dyspnoea and Respiratory Failure

Ken Kuljit Parhar

Introduction

Respiration is a complex process during which gas exchange occurs between the respiratory system of the patient and the surrounding atmosphere. The two major functions of the respiratory system are to oxygenate the blood and to clear carbon dioxide (CO_2) through ventilation of the lungs. Appropriate respiration requires several intact physiological pathways including the central and peripheral nervous systems, the respiratory muscles, the cardiopulmonary system, and an appropriate oxygen carrying capability with red blood cells. Pathological disruption of any of these systems can result in respiratory dysfunction.

Dyspnoea (breathlessness) is a symptom and sign. It is described by patients as difficulty with either inspiration, expiration or both. As a sign dyspnoea presents with involvement of accessory respiratory muscles and general distress. Dyspnoea is frequently but not exclusively associated with respiratory failure. Dyspnoea can be caused by both physical and psychological stimuli.

Dyspnoea as a sign is frequently obvious and most often associated with tachypnoea. Use of accessory respiratory muscles is a common sign. Acute dyspnoea leads to fatigue due to increased work of breathing.

Acute respiratory failure (ARF) is defined as the inability to meet the metabolic requirements of the patient through a failure of either oxygenation or ventilation. ARF can therefore be divided into two distinct subtypes including hypoxaemic respiratory failure (type 1) resulting in low arterial oxygen (PaO_2) or hypercarbic respiratory failure (type 2) resulting in elevated arterial CO_2 ($PaCO_2$).

ARF is a common indication for admission to the intensive care unit (ICU), and can account for 17–56% of all admissions.

The relationship between dyspnoea and acute respiratory failure is variable. Some patients suffer and display dyspnoea without respiratory failure, and vice versa, some patients can be hypoxic or hypercarbic without the symptoms and signs of dyspnoea. The match of the two entities can give a clue to the duration of the problem, adaptive mechanisms and homeostatic control of the patients.

Hypoxaemic Respiratory Failure

There are several pathophysiological mechanisms through which hypoxaemic ARF can occur, including inadequate alveolar oxygen concentration (PAO_2), ventilation-perfusion mismatch (V/Q), shunt, diffusion abnormalities and increased venous admixture (Figure 28.1). The most common cause of hypoxaemia in ICU patients is V/Q mismatch.

Inadequate Alveolar Oxygen (PAO_2)

Inadequate alveolar oxygen is most often caused by either hypoventilation or a low partial pressure of inspired oxygen.

Hypoventilation results in hypoxaemia through two mechanisms: a reduction in the PAO_2–PaO_2 gradient that causes a fall in PaO_2 due to acidosis from inadequately cleared CO_2, resulting in a rightward shift of the oxyhaemoglobin dissociation curve and lower affinity of haemoglobin for O_2.

The second mechanism of low alveolar oxygen is uncommon in the ICU population. It more commonly occurs at high altitudes where the partial pressure of the atmosphere is much lower than at sea level. It may also happen in an airplane where the cabin pressure is not pressurised to sea level but to a higher elevation (6000–10,000 feet).

The alveolar–arterial (A–a) gradient calculation is a measure of the efficiency of alveolar gas exchange and can be used to determine whether hypoventilation is the cause of a low PaO_2 (Figure 28.2). The normal A–a gradient is 10–20 mmHg; it is influenced by age

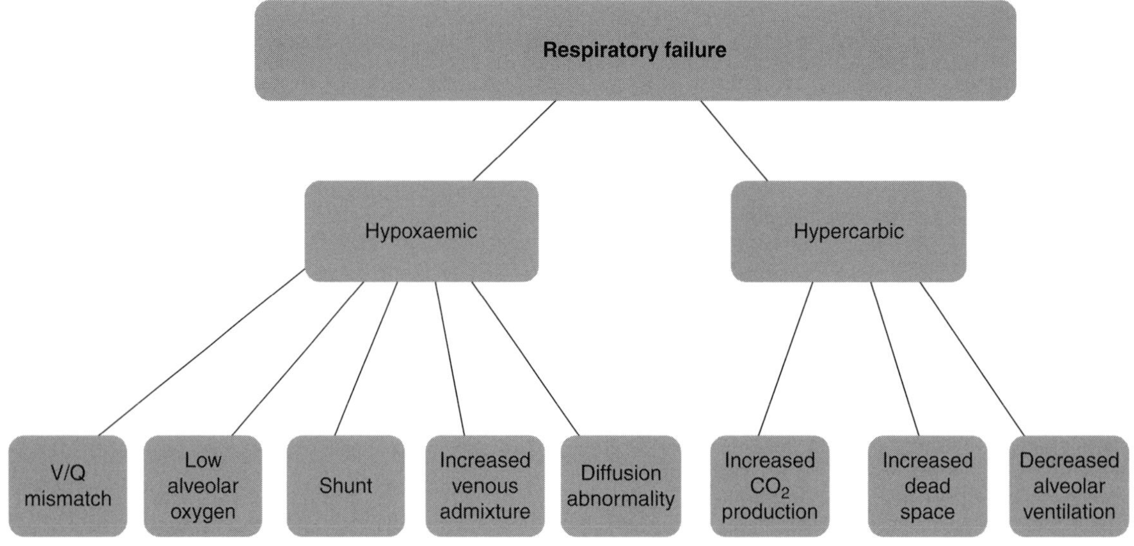

Figure 28.1 Common aetiologies of respiratory failure within the ICU.

$$\textbf{Alveolar–Arterial (A–a) oxygen gradient} = PiO_2 - \frac{PaCO_2}{R} - PaO_2$$

$$\textbf{Partial pressure of inspired oxygen } (\mathbf{PiO_2}) = FiO_2\ (P_B - \text{water vapour pressure})$$

Thus:

$$\textbf{Alveolar–Arterial (A–a) oxygen gradient} = FiO_2\ (760 - \text{water vapour pressure}) - \frac{PaCO_2}{R} - PaCO_2$$

Figure 28.2 Calculation of an alveolar–arterial (A–a) oxygen gradient. R respiratory quotient (VCO_2/VO_2) = 0.8, PaO_2 arterial oxygen concentration, FiO_2 fraction of inspired oxygen, $PaCO_2$ arterial CO_2 concentration, P_B (barometric pressure) = 760 mmHg at sea level, water vapour pressure = 47 mmHg.

and increases with each decade of life. Hypoxaemia with a normal A–a gradient is suggestive of hypoventilation. The patient's history can be used to rule out low inspired partial pressure of O_2 in most cases, and the A–a gradient in this situation should be normal as well.

Ventilation and Perfusion Mismatch

Ventilation and perfusion (V/Q) mismatch is the most common mechanism for hypoxaemia within the ICU. In a normal upright lung there is a degree of regional V/Q mismatch as the apices of the lung are ventilated more than perfused (high V/Q), in contrast to the bases of the lungs, which are perfused much more than ventilated (low V/Q). In aggregate the lung has an overall matched V/Q ratio of approximately 1. Body position, posture and lung volumes, as well as age, can influence V/Q ratios in normal lungs.

Any disease process that affects the lung parenchyma can influence V/Q ratios (Figure 28.3). For example low V/Q ratios are associated with processes that impair ventilation such as bronchoconstriction, or secretions from pneumonia. High V/Q ratios are associated with processes that impair perfusion such as pulmonary embolism, or that lead to increased ventilation due to large tidal volumes such as emphysema. The lung vasculature has mechanisms to attempt to match V/Q and maintain an equal ratio such as

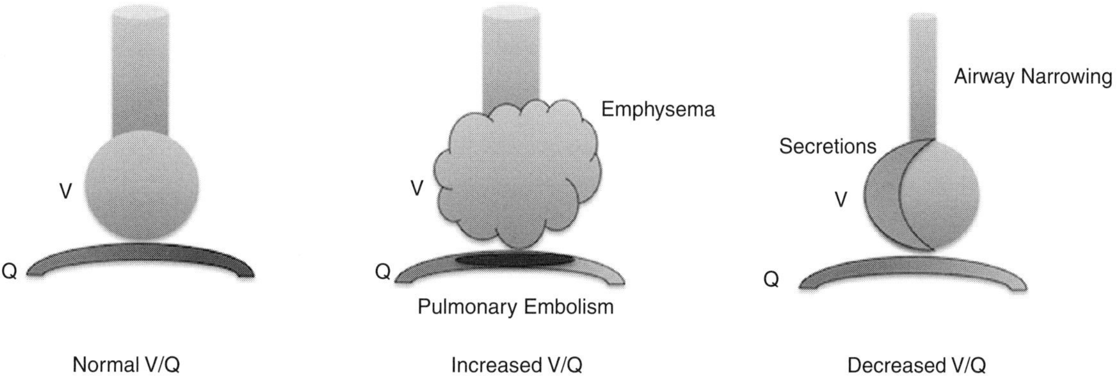

Figure 28.3 Pathophysiological mechanisms of V/Q mismatch.

hypoxaemic pulmonary vasoconstriction, which results in reduced perfusion to those areas of the lungs which are poorly ventilated.

Shunt

There are two types of shunts that may cause significant hypoxaemia: intrapulmonary and intracardiac.

Intracardiac shunts include such aetiologies as a patent foramen ovale or an atrial septal defect. These shunts will cause hypoxaemia as venous blood bypasses the lungs and travels from the right side of the heart directly to the systemic side.

Intrapulmonary shunt is an extreme V/Q mismatch where there is no ventilation of the associated lung unit despite being fully perfused. The most common cause of intrapulmonary shunt is atelectasis, and fluid filled alveoli due to cardiogenic or noncardiogenic pulmonary oedema. In non-diseased states there is a small physiological degree of intrapulmonary shunt (up to 3% or the systemic cardiac output), which is due to circulation from the Thebesian and bronchial circulation.

Severe shunts (greater than 30% of systemic cardiac output) due to the lack of ventilation do not respond to supplemental oxygen therapy. This can be used as a diagnostic feature when assessing a patient suspected to have a shunt.

Diffusion Abnormalities

Diffusion of oxygen and CO_2 across the alveolar-capillary membrane is an extremely efficient process. The ability of gases to diffuse efficiently is dependent upon several key features of the capillary-alveolar membrane including its total surface area, thickness, diffusability and the solubility of the gases. Conditions that can cause diffusion abnormalities include end stage pulmonary fibrosis or fibroproliferative acute respiratory distress syndrome (ARDS).

Increased Venous Admixture

Low oxygen content returning to the pulmonary circulation can be a cause of hypoxaemia. This is often in the context of poor cardiac function or very high tissue consumption and extraction of oxygen. When this is suspected as a primary cause of hypoxaemia, detailed evaluation of cardiac function is required.

Hypercarbic Respiratory Failure

Hypercarbic respiratory failure, also known as type 2 respiratory failure or acute ventilatory failure, results in a rise in $PaCO_2$ above the patient's baseline. In most patients the normal CO_2 is between 35 and 40 mmHg.

CO_2 production is matched by CO_2 elimination in steady state conditions. Hypercarbia can result from three major pathophysiological mechanisms: increased CO_2 production, decreased tidal ventilation or increased dead space.

Increased CO_2 Production

This can occur in both physiological and disease state conditions such as exercise, fever, major trauma, sepsis and hyperthyroid states. The compensatory response to an increase in CO_2 production is to increase alveolar minute ventilation by increasing both tidal volumes and respiratory rate, with the objective both of maintaining a normal CO_2 and of preventing acidosis. Patients who do not have the ability or reserve to increase their alveolar minute ventilation (i.e.

pre-existing neuromuscular disease) can develop hypercarbic respiratory failure.

Decreased Tidal Ventilation

Decreased tidal volume ventilation resulting in reduced alveolar ventilation can be caused by pathology anywhere from central or peripheral nervous system to the respiratory muscles, chest wall, pleural space and parenchyma. Common conditions in the ICU which may cause this include CNS depressant medications such as narcotics and intravenous sedation, brainstem strokes, neuromuscular disorders like myasthenia gravis, critical illness neuropathy and myopathy, circumferential chest burns with significant eschar, rib fractures with a flail segment, airflow obstruction due to severe emphysema, and central sleep disordered breathing.

Increased Dead Space

Increased dead space results from disease processes that increase areas of the lung that do not participate in gas exchange, despite being ventilated. Dead space can be both anatomical and alveolar.

Anatomical dead space comprises the trachea, main bronchi and the conducting airways that do not participate in gas exchange. An average adult has approximately 150 ml of anatomical dead space. In mechanically ventilated patients this is also increased due to the ventilator circuitry, endotracheal tube and heat-moisture exchanger. Tracheostomy can significantly reduce the amount of anatomical dead space in comparison to an endotracheal tube.

Alveolar dead space results when non-perfused alveoli are ventilated. This is often the sequelae of disease processes such as chronic obstructive pulmonary disease, pulmonary emboli or fibroproliferative ARDS.

Illustrative Clinical Scenarios in the ICU

Acute Respiratory Distress Syndrome

Acute respiratory distress syndrome (ARDS) is characterised by the acute onset of severe hypoxaemic respiratory failure with associated bilateral infiltrates on chest X-ray in the absence of significant left ventricular dysfunction (see Table 28.1). Initially described in 1967 in a series of 12 patients, ARDS has been the subject of significant clinical and research investigation due to the significant morbidity and mortality associated with the diagnosis. By most recent estimates, mortality for patients diagnosed with severe ARDS is over 40%.

The details of ARDS diagnosis and treatment will be discussed in Chapter 44. However, an important part of the diagnosis of this condition is to exclude a cardiogenic cause of pulmonary oedema.

Pneumothorax

A pneumothorax is the accumulation of air within the pleural space. It is most often caused by an acquired defect in either the parietal or visceral pleura. Pneumothoraces can be classified as either spontaneous or non-spontaneous. Spontaneous pneumothoraces are less common within the ICU in comparison to non-spontaneous pneumothoraces.

Spontaneous pneumothoraces most often occur in healthy young adults. Certain risk factors can increase the risk of a spontaneous pneumothorax such as underlying lung disease (i.e. emphysema), familial history, drug abuse or more rare causes such as catamenial pneumothorax.

Most pneumothoraces that are encountered in the ICU are not spontaneous and are trauma induced or iatrogenic. Iatrogenic pneumothoraces can be due to barotrauma from mechanical ventilation, or they can be procedure related (such as central venous catheter insertion, thoracentesis, transbronchial lung biopsy, percutaneous tracheostomy).

Mechanical ventilation induced pneumothoraces are often the result of barotrauma. Tissue disruption allows the passage of air along the bronchovascular bundle back to the hilum and into the pleural and pericardial spaces, as well as into other interstitial tissues such as subcutaneous chest, neck and abdominal tissues. Insufficient decompression via one of these routes can lead to rupture of the pleural space and subsequent pneumothorax.

Clinically, a pneumothorax should be suspected if a mechanically ventilated patient has an acute increase in peak and plateau airway pressures. If the pneumothorax is significant or causes obstruction to cardiac inflow or outflow via tension, there may be associated hypotension. Hypoxaemia is common as the pneumothorax results in collapse of the underlying lung. The chest X-ray can reveal a pneumothorax with evidence of a visceral pleural line and no lung markings beyond this. Radiography

Table 28.1 Berlin definition of acute respiratory distress syndrome

Timing	Within 1 week of known clinical insult or worsening respiratory symptoms
Chest X-ray	Bilateral opacities (not due to effusions, collapse or nodules)
Origin of oedema	Not primarily due to cardiac failure or fluid overload (use echo or pulmonary artery catheter)
Severity	
Mild	PaO_2:FiO_2 ratio 200–300 mmHg with PEEP/CPAP ≥ 5 cmH_2O
Moderate	PaO_2:FiO_2 ratio 100–300 mmHg with PEEP ≥ 5 cmH_2O
Severe	PaO_2:FiO_2 ratio < 100 mmHg with PEEP ≥ 5 cmH_2O

in the upright position and at end expiration may improve the successful diagnosis of pneumothorax by chest X-ray. Patients with a pneumothorax may have chest X-rays supine and as a result pleural air rises to the anterior costophrenic sulcus resulting in a deep visible costophrenic angle and double diaphragm, known as a deep sulcus sign.

Treatment of pneumothorax varies depending on the severity and may include expectant management, supplemental high concentration oxygen, aspiration and tube thoracostomy. High concentration supplemental oxygen increases the rate of pneumothorax resolution. An increase in the partial pressure of oxygen in the pleural space results in a reduction in partial pressure of nitrogen in the pleural space. Oxygen is more readily absorbed and results in increased reabsorption of pleural gas. In large or unresolving pneumothoraces, tube thoracostomy can be performed either with a large bore chest tube, or via percutaneous small bore chest tube.

Cardiogenic Pulmonary Oedema

Pulmonary oedema is a much more common cause for dyspnoea in the cardiothoracic ICU. The causes of pulmonary oedema can be multifactorial but involve three main categories:

- Increased preload: Increased circulatory volume due to chronic conditions (congestive cardiac failure); excessive fluid administration; position allowing increased venous return; removal of a venous return obstruction.
- Reduced left atrial emptying: Mitral stenosis; change of sinus rhythm to atrial fibrillation; worsening of mitral regurgitation (papillary muscle rupture); sudden onset of severe AR; cardiogenic shock; severe bradycardia (complete heart block); diastolic heart failure.
- Increased afterload: Left ventricular outflow tract obstruction (systolic anterior mitral leaflet prolapsing in the left ventricular outflow following mitral valve repair); tamponade; severe vasoconstriction; peripheral VA ECMO counterflow in the descending aorta.

In each case of pulmonary oedema the main cause needs to be identified and treated. However, basic principles for all patients include oxygenation, maintenance of adequate perfusion and patient comfort. The timing and magnitude of response are variable. Some patients respond to a single dose diuretic, others need CPAP or IPPV, and in some ECMO may be required to stabilise the situation.

Congestive heart failure can lead to significant hypoxaemia via the development of pulmonary oedema. It most often occurs in patients with left ventricular systolic dysfunction related to a history of myocardial infarction or diastolic dysfunction from hypertension. There are several other aetiologies of cardiogenic origin that may lead to pulmonary oedema, including inherited and acquired cardiomyopathies, valvular abnormalities (such as severe mitral regurgitation or severe aortic stenosis) and long standing dysrhythmias.

Diagnosis of cardiogenic pulmonary oedema can be made in a variety of ways. Chest X-ray findings include pleural effusions, peribronchial cuffing and Kerley-B lines, as well as vascular redistribution. There may be evidence of cardiomegaly on the X-ray if the process is chronic. Serum B-type natriuretic peptide (BNP) can be elevated; however, this can be non-specific in ICU patients. Echocardiography can be used to assess cardiac function and rule out valvular abnormalities. Pulmonary artery catheters can be diagnostic as an elevated pulmonary capillary wedge pressure suggests elevated filling pressures and likely venous capillary hypertension.

Cardiogenic pulmonary oedema, due to its hydrostatic aetiology, is amenable to treatment with positive pressure ventilation (PPV). Application of either non-invasive positive pressure ventilation or intubation and invasive mechanical ventilation can counteract elevated venous pressures. Benefits of PPV include reduction of both left and right ventricular preload as well as reduction of left ventricular afterload.

Pneumonia

Pneumonia is a common aetiology for the development of hypoxaemic respiratory failure. For patients admitted to hospital with a community acquired pneumonia (CAP), up to 20% may require ICU admission. In one study in the UK, 6% of all ICU admissions were due to pneumonia.

Several risk factors can predispose patients to develop CAP such as advanced age, chronic respiratory insufficiency (e.g. COPD), smoking, alcohol abuse, immunosuppression and multiple comorbid illnesses.

The most common aetiologies for CAP include the bacteria *Streptococcus pneumoniae*, *Haemophilus influenzae*, *Klebsiella pneumoniae*, *Chlamydia pneumoniae*, and the viruses influenza A/B, adenovirus, respiratory syncytial virus, and parainfluenza. Nosocomial pneumonias that develop while in hospital (hospital acquired pneumonia) or whilst on the ventilator (ventilator associated pneumonia) are more commonly caused by Gram-negative bacteria such as *Pseudomonas aeruginosa*, *Acinetobacter* spp., and Enterobacteriaceae spp., as well as Gram-positive bacteria such as *Staphylococcus aureus*. Antibiotic resistance is much more common with nosocomial pneumonias as Gram-negative bacilli are often extended spectrum beta lactamase producing and *Staphylococcus aureus* is methicillin resistant (MRSA).

Sputum and blood cultures can aid in stepping down antibiotics based on sensitivities. Chest X-ray findings of a lobar pneumonia include silhouetting of the diaphragm or heart borders without signs of associated volume loss (silhouette sign). In addition, air bronchograms are highly suggestive of a consolidative process.

There are several pathophysiological mechanisms associated with pneumonia that cause hypoxaemia. Secretions and inflammatory infiltrates can lead to both shunt physiology as well as V/Q mismatch. Progressively consolidated lungs have poor compliance that can result in significant alveolar collapse, which can also contribute to intrapulmonary shunting. Bacterial pneumonias in particular can be associated with a hyperdynamic state, which can lead to increased venous admixture.

COPD

Exacerbations of chronic obstructive pulmonary disease (COPD) resulting in acute respiratory failure are a common indication for admission to ICU. These patients often present with hypercarbic respiratory failure. COPD patients have either chronic bronchitis or emphysema as a dominant phenotype of their disease. The primary issue in patients with COPD is expiratory flow limitation. Several mechanisms are responsible for this including impaired ciliary function, excess mucus production and narrowing of the peripheral airways, as well as decreased elastic recoil from tissue destruction of the airway elastic support. Chronic CO_2 retention is due to the increase in dead space and reduction in alveolar minute ventilation. Patients often have clinical signs of hyperinflation and airway obstruction including pursed lip breathing, presence of a barrel chest and the use of accessory respiratory muscles such as intercostals.

Acute exacerbations of COPD are commonly triggered by respiratory infections, usually viral in nature. Other less common causes of acute exacerbations include bacterial community acquired pneumonias, environmental exposures or medication non-compliance.

During an acute exacerbation, expiratory airflow obstruction is worsened by increased mucus production and bronchoconstriction. This leads to worsening hyperinflation and reduced alveolar minute ventilation, ultimately resulting in a rise in CO_2 and a respiratory acidosis. Concomitant hypoxaemia is often related to reduced alveolar minute ventilation and not V/Q mismatch.

In addition to standard medical management of acute exacerbations with bronchodilators, steroids and antibiotics, non-invasive positive pressure ventilation is an important therapeutic option to consider, as it can significantly reduce the work of breathing. By allowing the respiratory muscles to rest, it improves alveolar minute ventilation and reduces hyperinflation. With less hyperinflation, the diaphragm can restore its normal conformation and operate at a more favourable position on the length-tension relationship curve. Clinical benefits of NIPPV use in COPD include potentially reducing nosocomial infections, ICU length of stay and mortality, as well as rates of primary intubation.

Treatment of Acute Respiratory Failure

Several strategies can be used to improve oxygenation and help CO_2 clearance. Most importantly, the primary pathological process driving respiratory failure must be addressed and treated appropriately. For example, pneumonia must be treated with appropriate empirical antibiotics, or heart failure treated with inotropes and diuretics. In addition to this several adjunctive strategies can be used.

Supplemental Oxygen

Supplemental oxygen delivered via nasal cannula or facemask is very simple to apply to patients, and is a good starting point for mild to moderate hypoxaemia. More recently, high flow humidified oxygen has become more readily available, and offers certain advantageous features. High flow humidified oxygen can deliver high concentrations of oxygen without the need for intubation. In addition the heated air improves secretion mobilisation. The high rates of oxygen flow can also provide a small amount of positive end-expiratory pressure (PEEP) that may help improve atelectasis and shunt.

Non-invasive Positive Pressure Ventilation (NIPPV)

There are two common indications for the use of NIPPV including pulmonary oedema causing hypoxaemic respiratory failure and acute exacerbations of COPD leading to hypercarbic respiratory failure. For pulmonary oedema the use of continuous positive airway pressure (CPAP) is sufficient to reduce right and left ventricular preload as well as left ventricular afterload, which can result in improvement in hypoxaemia. Patients with COPD induced hypercarbic respiratory failure should be treated with bilevel positive airway pressure (BIPAP). This will provide assistance in both oxygenation and ventilation.

General contraindications to the use of NIPPV include decreased level of consciousness due to reasons other than CO_2 narcosis, inability to clear secretions, recent facial trauma or surgery precluding the application of an oronasal mask, active myocardial ischaemia, and haemodynamic instability. Details of NIPPV are discussed in Chapter 17.

Endotracheal Intubation with Mechanical Ventilation

In patients for whom supplemental oxygen techniques are insufficient and for whom NIPPV has failed or is contraindicated, endotracheal intubation and invasive mechanical ventilation is an important therapeutic option.

There are several ways in which invasive mechanical ventilation can improve oxygenation. High inspired fractions of oxygen can be delivered directly to the lungs. The ventilator allows a much more sophisticated manipulation of the respiratory cycle. The primary determinant of oxygenation is the mean airway pressure (mean Paw) and significant manipulation of the mean Paw can be accomplished while on the ventilator. By increasing the inspiratory cycle length time, the inspiratory pressure or the pulmonary end-expiratory pressure (PEEP), the mean Paw can be elevated to improve oxygenation. In order to avoid damaging the lungs further, however, a lung protective ventilation strategy which limits both volume and pressure should be applied. Appropriate application of PEEP to optimise compliance and/or oxygenation will also prevent the development of atelectrauma. Details of endotracheal intubation with mechanical ventilation are discussed in Chapter 17.

Prone Positioning

Prone positioning of a patient with severe hypoxaemic respiratory failure has been shown to improve oxygenation and also to potentially reduce mortality. The primary mechanism for improvement of oxygenation is improved V/Q matching and reduced shunt. In the supine position, dependent lung zones that are well perfused do not ventilate well due to atelectasis from lung injury, secretions and the weight of the heart. Dorsal lung segments benefit from increased perfusion in the prone position. In addition, secretion clearance is improved while in the prone position.

Inhaled Pulmonary Vasodilators

The use of inhaled pulmonary vasodilators, such as inhaled nitric oxide and prostaglandins, can improve oxygenation. Despite an improvement in oxygenation, no studies to date have shown a definitive mortality benefit. The primary mechanism through which oxygenation is improved is by better V/Q matching.

Restrictive Fluid Strategy

In many conditions such as sepsis, trauma or pancreatitis it is very easy to acquire a significant positive fluid balance during the process of being resuscitated. Studies demonstrating a restrictive fluid strategy approach have shown a reduced duration of mechanical ventilation.

Extracorporeal Membrane Oxygenation

Extracorporeal membrane oxygenation can potentially be considered should all other less invasive methods of improving oxygenation and CO_2 clearance fail. This is reviewed in detail in Chapter 24.

Learning Points

- There are two major types of respiratory failure: hypoxaemic and hypercarbic.
- Hypoxaemic respiratory failure can be caused by five mechanisms: low alveolar oxygen, V/Q mismatch, shunt, diffusion impairment and increased venous admixture.
- Hypercarbic respiratory failure can be caused by three mechanisms: reduced alveolar ventilation, increased dead space and increased CO_2 production.
- V/Q mismatch is the most common mechanism of hypoxaemia within the ICU.
- Using the correct therapy for the underlying aetiology of respiratory failure is crucial. For example, NIV is very efficacious for exacerbations of COPD and cardiogenic pulmonary oedema.

Further Reading

Ashbaugh DG, Bigelow DB, Petty TL, et al. Acute respiratory distress in adults. *Lancet.* 1967; 2: 319–323.

Force ADT, Ranieri VM, Rubenfeld GD, et al. Acute respiratory distress syndrome: the Berlin definition. *Journal of the American Medical Association.* 2012; 307: 2526–2533.

Girou E, Schortgen F, Delclaux C, et al. Association of noninvasive ventilation with nosocomial infections and survival in critically ill patients. *Journal of the American Medical Association.* 2000; 284: 2361–1267.

Keenan SP, Sinuff T, Burns KE, et al. Clinical practice guidelines for the use of noninvasive positive-pressure ventilation and noninvasive continuous positive airway pressure in the acute care setting. *Canadian Medical Association Journal.* 2011; 183: E195–E214.

Rubenfeld GD, Caldwell E, Peabody E, et al. Incidence and outcomes of acute lung injury. *New England Journal of Medicine.* 2005; 353: 1685–1693.

Slutsky AS, Ranieri VM. Ventilator-induced lung injury. *New England Journal of Medicine.* 2013; 369: 2126–2136.

The Acute Respiratory Distress Syndrome Network. Ventilation with lower tidal volumes as compared with traditional tidal volumes for acute lung injury and the acute respiratory distress syndrome. *New England Journal of Medicine.* 2000; 342: 1301–1308.

Vincent JL, Akca S, De Mendonca A, et al. The epidemiology of acute respiratory failure in critically ill patients. *Chest.* 2002; 121: 1602–1609.

Ware LB, Matthay MA. Clinical practice. Acute pulmonary edema. *New England Journal of Medicine.* 2005; 353: 2788–2796.

Woodhead M, Welch CA, Harrison DA, et al. Community-acquired pneumonia on the intensive care unit: secondary analysis of 17,869 cases in the ICNARC Case Mix Programme Database. *Critical Care.* 2006; 10(Suppl 2): S1.

MCQs

1. **A 78 year old female is currently postoperative day 1 following an elective cholecystectomy. Her pain control following surgery has been poor and she was getting regular intravenous morphine. She develops progressive hypoxaemia and an arterial blood gas is performed on room air. The results are as follows: pH 7.20, $PaCO_2$ 75 mmHg and PaO_2 46 mmHg. Assume she is at sea level (atmospheric pressure 760 mmHg). Based on this arterial blood gas her A–a gradient is:**

   (a) 10
   (b) 17
   (c) 20
   (d) 29

2. **In the previous question the most likely cause of her hypoxaemia is:**

   (a) Hypoventilation

(b) V/Q mismatch

(c) Shunt

(d) Diffusion abnormality

3. Which of the following clinical scenarios does not meet the Berlin criteria for ARDS?

(a) 5 day history of bilateral pneumonia with P/F ratio of 250 while intubated and on mechanical ventilation with PEEP of 10 cmH_20.

(b) 5 day history of bilateral pneumonia with P/F ratio of 250 while on non-invasive positive pressure ventilation with CPAP of 5 cmH_20.

(c) 5 day history of unilateral pneumonia with P/F ratio of 100 while intubated and on mechanical ventilation with PEEP of 10 cmH_20.

(d) 5 day history of bilateral opacities following aspiration with P/F ratio of 100 while intubated and on mechanical ventilation with PEEP 10 cmH_20.

4. Which of the following is a contraindication to the use of non-invasive positive pressure ventilation?

(a) Hypercarbic respiratory failure due to COPD exacerbation

(b) Hypoxaemic respiratory failure due to cardiogenic pulmonary oedema

(c) Somnolence due to hypercarbia

(d) Poor secretion clearance

5. Which of the following statements about pneumothoraces is correct?

(a) The presence of a deep sulcus sign on chest X-ray will rule out a pneumothorax

(b) Barotrauma induced pneumothoraces are the result of air travelling along the bronchovascular bundle towards the hilum

(c) Most pneumothoraces in the intensive care unit are spontaneous

(d) Small bore percutaneous chest tubes should not be used to drain pneumothoraces

Exercise answers are available on p.469. Alternatively, take the test online at www.cambridge.org/CardiothoracicMCQ

Chapter 29

Shock in the Cardiothoracic Intensive Care Unit

Fabio Guarracino and Rubia Baldassarri

Definition

Shock may be defined as acute circulatory failure characterised by inadequate tissue perfusion and cellular damage. The inability of the circulatory system to deliver adequate quantities of oxygen to meet cellular demand is called cellular dysoxia. Therefore, the pathophysiological feature of shock is the imbalance between oxygen delivery (DO_2) and cellular oxygen consumption (VO_2).

Pathophysiology

It should be considered that although the mismatch between oxygen supply and demand is the main pathophysiological determinant of shock, the acute circulatory decompensation responsible for the altered perfusion of shock can be induced by four main mechanisms.

Circulatory insufficiency in shock can result from one or a combination of these mechanisms, leading to four main patterns of shock: hypovolaemic, cardiogenic, obstructive and distributive shock.

Hypovolaemic Shock

Acute loss of circulating volume (haemorrhage, loss of fluids) reduces venous return, which leads to severe hypovolaemia and consequent circulatory impairment.

Cardiogenic Shock

Acute cardiac failure, as occurs in acute myocardial infarction, myocardial ischaemia, cardiomyopathies and arrhythmias, is the main cause of cardiogenic shock. Dysfunction of heart pumping leads to low cardiac output (CO) and circulatory failure. Although the underlying mechanisms of hypovolaemic and cardiogenic shock are different, circulation is impaired, and oxygen delivery is decreased, with consequent tissue hypoperfusion.

Obstructive Shock

The main cause of circulatory failure is obstruction of circulation, as occurs in pulmonary embolism, pneumothorax and cardiac tamponade. Mechanical obstructions of ventricular ejection render the heart unable to pump adequate stroke volume (SV), resulting in low CO and tissue hypoperfusion.

Despite the different underlying pathophysiological mechanisms, in each of these three shock states (hypovolaemic, cardiogenic and obstructive), blood flow is significantly decreased, and oxygen delivery to peripheral tissues by the circulation is surpassed by cellular oxygen consumption.

Distributive Shock

Loss of vascular tone and consequent reductions in systemic vascular resistance (SVR) alter the distribution of blood flow, as in severe sepsis, major trauma and anaphylaxis. In this pattern of shock, the cause of circulatory failure is misdistribution of blood flow.

The macrocirculation is defined at a haemodynamic level in terms of CO and DO_2, where, at stable concentrations of haemoglobin, CO is the main determinant of DO_2.

The microcirculation regulates blood flow and cellular oxygen supply according to cellular metabolic requests. This regulation consists of increased tissue perfusion and increased cellular metabolism, which occur in response to long-term signals from cells under different metabolic conditions. Microcirculatory dysfunction is responsible for tissue damage and organ failure despite adequate systemic blood flow and optimisation of the macrocirculation.

In septic shock, the microcirculation is profoundly affected, and tissue perfusion is consequently altered. Vasoplegia and vascular hyporeactivity are the most important features of the haemodynamic impairment of septic shock. The loss of control of vascular tone seems to be related to an imbalance between vasodilators and vasoconstrictors and is associated with high mortality rates. The loss of vascular tone is induced by inflammatory mediators and endogenous vasodilatory mediators produced by cells under oxidative stress conditions and increased metabolic activity. Markers of both systemic inflammation and cellular oxidative metabolism (pCO_2, lactate, K^+, H^+, nitric oxide (NO), prostaglandins, interleukin-1, adenosine, inorganic phosphate) can be commonly detected in patients with altered cardiovascular function and shock. The actions of these products result in endothelial dysfunction and altered microvascular perfusion. The altered modulation between vasodilating and vasocostricting agents is responsible for vasoplegia and for hyporeactivity of arterial vessels to vasoconstriction, which is common in septic shock patients. The predictive value of these mediators as biomarkers is lower than that of the concentration of plasma lactate; therefore, their routine use as biomarkers is not recommended.

Ventriculoarterial (VA) Coupling

VA coupling reflects the interaction between cardiac function and the vascular system. When the two components of the cardiovascular system, the heart and the arterial tree, are coupled, maximal efficiency is achieved. VA coupling can be defined as the ratio of arterial elastance (Ea) to ventricular elastance (Ees) (Ea/Ees), as proposed by Suga in 1969. When the heart pumps a quantity of blood that matches the capability of the arteries to receive it, the system is optimised. Under different physiological and pathological conditions, the heart provides adequate flow and pressure to ensure tissue perfusion. The arterial system adapts to match the continuous variations in blood flow. VA decoupling occurs in most acute altered haemodynamic states. This means that cardiovascular function is impaired and that global perfusion is suboptimal. Both increased and decreased arterial tone negatively affect VA coupling in shock. Loss of vascular tone due to septic shock and vasoconstriction imposed by either autoregulatory mechanisms induced by hypotension or the use of vasopressors are the main causes of changes in Ea. Ees can be decreased by alterations in LV contractility, which occurs in both cardiogenic shock and septic shock when myocardial depression occurs.

Epidemiology

All types of shock can occur in critically ill patients admitted to the cardiothoracic intensive care unit (CT ICU), and two or more patterns of shock may be present in the same patient. It is not uncommon for cardiogenic shock to be complicated by septic shock, and cardiogenic shock can complicate pre-existing septic shock. It should be considered that haemodynamic instability is one of the most common causes of admission to the ICU.

Diagnosis

Circulatory shock is commonly associated with haemodynamic instability characterised by moderate to severe arterial hypotension and signs of tissue hypoperfusion. Arterial hypotension, which is defined as a systolic blood pressure less than 90 mmHg, a mean arterial pressure (MAP) <65 mmHg, or a decrease ≥40 mmHg from baseline, is commonly present in patients with shock. However, hypotension is not required to diagnose shock, as recently emphasised by the revision of the recommendations of the 2006 guidelines for the management of patients with shock. Signs of peripheral hypoperfusion are more suggestive in the diagnostic evaluation of shock, along with increased plasma levels of lactate and decreased central oxygen saturation. The three sites that can be easily evaluated and most commonly reveal tissue hypoperfusion are the skin, kidneys and brain (Table 29.1). Patients with cardiovascular impairment generally present with non-specific symptoms, such as moderate to severe arterial hypotension associated with clinical signs of tissue hypoperfusion, such as increased concentrations of blood lactate, decreased central venous oxygen saturation ($ScvO_2$), reduced urine output, cold skin and neurological symptoms, such as mental confusion or agitation. As recently reported in the literature, hyperlactataemia is so strongly associated with shock that it is assumed to be part of the definition of shock. Increased blood concentrations of lactate above the cut-off of 2 mEq/l represent severe metabolic alterations due to inadequate utilisation of oxygen carried to cells via the circulation (DO_2/VO_2 mismatch). Although lactate levels can also increase with normal tissue perfusion and adequate oxygenation, in most cases, especially in cases of acute circulatory failure, hyperlactataemia is associated with cellular dysfunction, and it negatively affects the outcomes of patients with all types of shock. Recently,

Table 29.1 Signs of systemic hypoperfusion at three levels

Skin	Inspection	Cold Pale Mottled Cyanotic Slow capillary refill time
Kidney	Urine output	≤0.5 ml/kg/hr
Brain	Mental status	Obtunded Disorientation Confusion

lactate-guided therapy was proposed for patients with shock. Some authors have reported that this reduces hospital mortality by 20% every 2 hours for the first 8 hours of therapy. Plasma lactate levels should be routinely evaluated in patients exhibiting acute haemodynamic changes to assess peripheral organ perfusion; lactate values can also be helpful in determining the effectiveness of therapeutic strategies as normalisation of plasma lactate concentrations is correlated with improvements in tissue perfusion.

$ScvO_2$ may reflect DO_2/VO_2 mismatches in acute circulatory failure. Low $ScvO_2$ (<70%) is assumed to reflect inadequate oxygen delivery to peripheral tissues. Nevertheless, normal or even high values of $ScvO_2$ do not seem to be correlated with adequate oxygen transport.

Another indicator of adequate blood flow and tissue perfusion is the venoarterial carbon dioxide difference (pCO_2 gap), the difference between central or mixed venous carbon dioxide partial pressure (pCO_2) and arterial pCO_2. A value ≥6 mmHg indicates low peripheral perfusion despite normal $ScvO_2$ levels.

It should be considered that some patients have normal systolic blood pressure despite evident cardiovascular decompensation because of activation of compensatory mechanisms of autoregulation. Arterial vasoconstriction is the primary mechanism of immediate compensation in cases of circulatory failure. Increased SVR induced by arterial vasoconstriction allows systemic blood pressure to be maintained within a normal range, even in cases of large volume loss or severe cardiac dysfunction. This autoregulation mechanism also counteracts the loss of vascular tone, which is present in maldistributive shock, ensuring normal arterial blood pressure in the early phase of cardiovascular decompensation.

Autoregulation mechanisms ensure adequate blood flow and DO_2 to tissues and organs at different systemic blood pressure levels; when blood pressure falls below the limits of autoregulation, haemodynamic instability manifests, and cellular injury occurs. Ultimately, the mismatch between DO_2 and VO_2 results from an imbalance between the macrocirculation and microcirculation.

Patients with cardiogenic shock should be further investigated with respect to cardiac function, and the use of inotropes is recommended to improve contractility and SV in severe heart dysfunction.

The use of vasopressors is indicated in cases of insufficient responsiveness to fluid administration.

Monitoring Cardiac Function and Haemodynamics in Patients with Shock

Cardiac function should be accurately evaluated in cases of acute circulatory dysfunction to define the type of shock, first distinguishing among cardiogenic, hypovolaemic and obstructive shock, which are all characterised by low CO. In addition, in patients with suspected septic shock, investigations of cardiac performance may provide information about global haemodynamic impairment and the eventual myocardial depression that frequently complicates septic shock.

Advanced haemodynamic monitoring may be required in patients with severe cardiovascular instability either to categorise shock or to evaluate responsiveness to therapy.

In this context, echocardiography has been recognised as the most useful tool to either evaluate cardiac function or allow haemodynamic assessments in patients with shock. Echocardiography is a non-invasive and reliable bedside method of detecting cardiac function, CO and preload in acute circulatory decompensation or in follow-up of patients with shock. Assessment of cardiac function is also recommended to determine either therapeutic strategies or the need for adjunctive haemodynamic monitoring. The main limitation of echocardiography is that it cannot be continuously performed; therefore, haemodynamic monitoring should be performed in critical patients for whom continuous information about haemodynamics is required.

Fluid Responsiveness

For these reasons, therapeutic interventions to restore adequate circulation and global perfusion should be

Table 29.2 Static and dynamic methods for the evaluation of fluid responsiveness

Static methods	Pressures	• Central venous pressure (CVP) • Pulmonary artery occlusion pressure (PAOP)
	Areas and volumes	• Left ventricular end diastolic area (LVEDA) • Left ventricular end diastolic volumes (LVEDV)
	Diameters	• Inferior vena cava (IVC)
Dynamic methods		• Systolic pressure variation (SPV) • Pulse pressure variation (PPV) • Stroke volume variation (SVV) • IVC respiratory variation • Subaortic velocity time integral (VTI) variation • SVC respiratory variation • Internal jugular vein (IJV) and subclavian vein respiratory variation • Aortic velocity variation • Carotid artery peak velocity variation

based on preload, afterload and cardiac function. Although fluid resuscitation is the first line therapy in patients with shock, the risks associated with unnecessary fluid administration have recently been demonstrated. In this context, in cases of acute circulatory failure, appropriate fluid administration and the response of the patient to an increased preload should be adequately investigated. The role of fluid responsiveness (FR) as a guide for fluid resuscitation in shock has been progressively emphasised. FR represents the ability of the left ventricle to increase SV after administration of fluids. An increase of 15% in SV or CO after administration of a bolus of fluid indicates the so-called fluid response. FR can be evaluated either by static or by dynamic methods, as reported in Table 29.2. Although central venous pressure (CVP) and pulmonary artery occlusion pressure (PAOP) are commonly employed to assess left ventricle (LV) and right ventricle (RV) preload, respectively, their prognostic value is poor. Measurements of cardiac chamber area and volumes detected by echocardiographic assessments and the thermodilution method are good indicators of preload but have poor prognostic value. The static diameter of the inferior vena cava (IVC) has been proposed as an index of volaemia because it is reduced in hypovolaemic patients. Its use is not recommended in the detection of FR. While static measures indicate preload with more or less accuracy, depending on the method employed, dynamic measures evaluate the ability of the LV to increase preload after fluid administration. Dynamic measures are based on the physiological interaction between the heart and lungs in patients under positive pressure mechanical ventilation (MV). The effects of positive pressure ventilation on RV ventricle preload and afterload have been well demonstrated. During the respiratory cycle, RV preload decreases (reduction in the venous return), and RV afterload increases because of an increase in transpulmonary pressure. The decrease in RV preload negatively affects LV filling and LV SV. The changes induced on LV SV by positive pressure ventilation and arterial pulse pressure can be used to detect FR.

Dynamic measures of preload in patients with acute circulatory decompensation have been increasingly used in recent years because they have been recognised as accurate and reliable. These methods evaluate the dynamic response to fluid administration by measuring variations in LV SV. Several methods to assess FR with dynamic measurements have been proposed in recent years. Evaluations of changes in internal jugular venous (IJV) pressures, as assessed by echocardiographic measures of changes in IJV diameter, have also been reported to be effective in FR detection.

Echocardiography

In cases of shock, evaluation of the haemodynamic profile in terms of CO, LV filling pressure and flow is fundamental to defining the type of shock and to assessing the adequacy of therapy. Because cardiovascular impairment may be due to different underlying mechanisms, the availability of a diagnostic instrument that allows complete assessments of haemodynamic variables in shock is of paramount importance. In this context, echocardiography has been largely recognised as the best diagnostic tool in acute altered haemodynamic states. Echocardiographic examinations allow direct visualisation of the heart and cardiac structures that support the diagnoses of different types of shock. In addition to its well-known ability to investigate both LV and RV function, echocardiography allows estimation of the most useful haemodynamic parameters to categorise the haemodynamic profile of shock. Application of various echocardiographic techniques (two-dimensional imaging, Doppler and colour-Doppler, tissue Doppler and, more recently, three-dimensional echocardiography) permits the study of myocardial contractility and cardiac performance. Evaluation of the haemodynamic profile of shock is primarily achieved via evaluations of SV and CO. Application of pulse wave Doppler at the level of the mitral valve allows evaluations of transmitral flow. The two peak velocities of diastolic flow through the mitral valve are the E wave (early filling) and A wave (atrial contraction). The E/A ratio is a good index of LV diastolic function. The use of tissue Doppler imaging at the level of the annulus of the mitral valve measures early diastolic mitral annular peak velocity (E'). E/E' has been considered the best echocardiographic index of LV filling pressure and is a preload-independent measure of diastolic function. Although values of E/E' <8 and >15 are suggestive of low and high filling pressures, respectively, it should be considered that calculation of this ratio (E/E') provides semiquantitative estimations of intracardiac filling pressure and that in a range between 8 and 15, LV filling pressure is not necessarily adequate.

Echocardiography allows evaluation of RV morphology and performance with regard to the interaction between the LV and RV. In cases of obstructive shock, when pulmonary embolism or cardiac tamponade occur, direct visualisation of a dilated RV as well as of the loss of the normal shape of the interventricular septum are good indicators of increased pulmonary vascular resistance.

In this context, non-invasive evaluations of ventricular and arterial elastances allow detailed pathophysiological assessments of patients with shock, which promotes tailoring of treatments for VA uncoupling profiles.

Therapeutic Strategies

Restoration of adequate circulation and optimisation of tissue perfusion are the goals of therapeutic management in all pathophysiological patterns of shock.

It should be considered that there is no evidence of an optimal value of arterial blood pressure. Therefore, an individualised approach is recommended, even if a mean arterial pressure ≥ 65 mmHg is considered sufficient to maintain adequate tissue perfusion in most cases. It should be kept in mind that patients suffering from arterial hypertension may require higher levels of systemic pressure to ensure organ perfusion.

However, although early therapeutic strategies can be applied in all patients with haemodynamic instability and circulatory failure, early diagnosis of the specific type of shock is strongly recommended for targeting therapeutic interventions. Although the diagnosis of shock is easily achieved via clinical examination, differentiating among the various types of shock (Table 29.3) is neither simple nor immediate in most cases. Arterial hypotension is commonly

Table 29.3 Variation of haemodynamic parameters in the different patterns of shock

Type of shock	HR	BP	CVP	PAP	PAOP	CO	$ScvO_2$	SVR	PVR
Hypovolaemic	⇧	⇩	⇩	⇩	⇩	⇩	⇩	⇧	⇧
Cardiogenic	⇧	⇩	⇧	⇧	⇧	⇩	⇩	⇧	⇧
Obstructive	⇧	⇩	⇧	= ⇧ ⇩	= ⇧ ⇩	⇩	⇩	⇩	⇧
Distributive	⇧	⇩	⇧	= ⇧ ⇩	⇩	= ⇧ ⇩	= ⇧ ⇩	⇩	= ⇧

HR heart rate; BP blood pressure; CVP central venous pressure; PAP pulmonary artery pressure; PAOP pulmonary artery occlusion pressure; CO cardiac output; $ScvO_2$ central venous oxygen saturation; SVR systemic vascular resistances; PVR pulmonary vascular resistances.
⇧ increased; ⇩ decreased; = no change.

present in hypovolaemic shock, but normal or even higher values of arterial blood pressure can be found in patients with cardiogenic shock. Low CO is the main marker of cardiogenic and hypovolaemic shock, while septic shock patients can have hyperkinetic circulation. Obstructive shock can result in systemic hypotension and high pulmonary pressures and intracardiac filling pressures. Moreover, different pathophysiological patterns of shock can coexist in the same patient. For this reason, the diagnosis of the type of shock can be achieved only with an advanced haemodynamic investigation.

Conclusion

Shock is a complex, life threatening state in which tissue hypoperfusion and cellular injury induced by acute circulatory insufficiency can lead to organ failure and death. For this reason, restoring adequate tissue perfusion and DO_2/VO_2 balance is the primary objective of treatment. The role of the microcirculation, the site at which effective oxygen exchange between capillaries and cells occurs, has become a topic of interest in recent years. Therapeutic strategies that target restoration of normal microcirculatory efficiency have been proposed, although further investigations are required.

Because the peripheral organs have a different response to hypoxia and tissue damage can quickly worsen, early diagnosis and immediate treatment are mandatory in patients with shock. It should be considered that diagnosis of the type of shock is necessary to provide adequate therapy, including the removal of the underlying cause, to ensure haemodynamic stabilisation. It should be kept in mind that either inadequate or excessive therapy can be detrimental in shock. Haemodynamic monitoring is required to evaluate the haemodynamic profile of shock and to assess the effectiveness of therapy. Echocardiography has been recognised as the best tool to investigate both cardiac function and haemodynamics, particularly ventricular and arterial elastances. Optimisation of VA coupling may play a pivotal role in the therapeutic approach to altered haemodynamic states.

Learning Points

- Shock can be defined at a cellular level when the circulation becomes unable to deliver sufficient oxygen to meet the cellular demand. Either macrocirculation or microcirculation impairment induces the cellular dysfunction and organ failure in shock.
- Although arterial hypotension is commonly present in the states of circulatory decompensation and despite it being the main feature of the haemodynamic instability in shock, the presence of hypotension is not required to make a diagnosis of shock. The signs of tissue hypoperfusion are more suggestive for shock than arterial hypotension.
- Fluid resuscitation is the first intervention to restore volaemia and to improve arterial blood pressure in the majority of the patients with septic shock and hypovolaemic shock.
- The evaluation of the Ea/Ees ratio can be helpful for understanding the pathophysiology of altered haemodynamic states, and for guiding therapy and testing the effectiveness of treatments.
- The manipulation of the preload with fluid administration should be adequately monitored in the light of both diastolic and systolic function affecting the preload reserve. The increase of the preload can improve the CO and global perfusion in the majority of patients with circulatory failure, but not in all of them.

Further Reading

Antonelli M, Levy M, Andrews PJ, et al. Hemodynamic monitoring in shock and implications for management. International Consensus Conference, Paris, France, 27–28 April 2006. *Intensive Care Medicine*. 2007; 33: 575–590.

Aya HD, Carsetti A, Bazurro S, et al. From cardiac output to blood flow auto-regulation in shock. *Anaesthesiology Intensive Therapy*. 2015; 47: s56-s62.

Cecconi M, De Backer D, Antonelli M, et al. Consensus on circulatory shock and hemodynamic monitoring. Task force of the European Society of Intensive Care Medicine. *Intensive Care Medicine*. 2014; 40: 1795–1815.

Guarracino F, Baldassarri R, Pinsky MR. Ventriculo-arterial decoupling in acutely altered hemodynamic states. *Critical Care*. 2013; 17: 213.

Guarracino F, Bertini P. Use of echocardiography in critically ill patients: the intensivist's point of view. *Giornale Italiano di Cardiologia (Rome)*. 2015; 16: 341–343.

Guarracino F, Ferro B, Forfori F, et al. Jugular vein distensibility predicts fluid responsiveness in septic patients. *Critical Care*. 2014; 18: 647.

Pinsky MR. Both perfusion pressure and flow are essential for adequate resuscitation. *Sepsis*. 2000; 4: 143–146.

Sakr Y, Reinhart K, Vincent JL, et al. Does dopamine administration in shock influence outcome? Results of the Sepsis Occurrence in Acutely Ill Patients (SOAP) Study. *Critical Care Medicine*. 2006; 34: 589–597.

Suga H. Time course of left ventricular pressure-volume relationship under various end-diastolic volume. *Japanese Heart Journal*. 1969; 10: 509–515.

MCQs

1. **What is shock?**
   (a) Shock is presented as a low blood pressure
   (b) Shock is always a result of low cardiac output
   (c) Shock is acute circulatory failure characterised by inadequate tissue perfusion and cellular damage
   (d) Shock is always characterised by hypovolaemia
   (e) Shock is septic if it has high systemic vascular resistance

2. **Cardiogenic shock:**
   (a) Is always a result of lower pump function
   (b) Hypoperfusion is not always present
   (c) Hypotension is necessary for the diagnosis
   (d) Tachycardia is a necessary feature for diagnosis
   (e) Often presents with high preload

3. **Monitoring in cardiogenic shock:**
   (a) Patients must have arterial line for the diagnosis
   (b) CVP measure is mandatory for diagnosis
   (c) Pulmonary capillary wedge pressure is necessary for diagnosis
   (d) Can be diagnosed clinically
   (e) High mixed venous oxygenation rules out cardiogenic shock

4. **Treatment of shock:**
   (a) Fluid bolus is always the first step
   (b) Reduction of preload is appropriate in cardiogenic shock
   (c) ADH is the first line treatment for anaphylaxis
   (d) Increasing cardiac output is a treatment strategy in septic shock
   (e) Fluid bolus is appropriate for cardiogenic shock

Exercise answers are available on p.469. Alternatively, take the test online at www.cambridge.org/CardiothoracicMCQ

Chapter 30

Systemic Hypertension in Cardiothoracic Critical Care

Antonio Rubino and Susan Stevenson

Introduction

Hypertension is a commonly encountered clinical problem in the cardiothoracic critical care unit in both its chronic and acute forms. It is estimated that over one billion of the world's population are affected by hypertension, many of whom may be undiagnosed or inadequately managed. Chronic hypertension is a risk factor for cardiovascular disease and is therefore seen with greater prevalence in the cardiothoracic patient population. Such patients are at greater risk of pre-existing left ventricular dysfunction, cerebrovascular disease and chronic kidney disease, factors which are independently associated with poorer outcomes. Acute hypertension in cardiothoracic critical care may represent undiagnosed chronic hypertension or arise as a complication of the presenting complaint. Acute hypertension can complicate cardiac surgery, leading to haemorrhage, end-organ damage, prolonged length of stay and poorer outcomes.

Aetiology and Pathophysiology

The aetiology of hypertension in the cardiothoracic critical care unit is often multifactorial and may resolve with management of the underlying precipitant alone. Identification of the exact cause requires a systematic approach as seen in Table 30.1.

Before initiation of anti-hypertensive therapy, an underlying cause should be sought and corrected. This is particularly true in the case of raised intracranial pressure whereby mean arterial pressure is raised in order to maintain cerebral perfusion pressure.

Blood pressure or mean arterial pressure (MAP) is considered in simple terms as the product of the cardiac output (CO) and systemic vascular resistance (SVR). The cardiac output itself is determined by the product of the heart rate (HR) and stroke volume (SV) and can be summarised as follows:

$$\text{MAP (mmHg)} = (\text{HR} \times \text{SV}) \times \text{SVR}.$$

This simplification diminishes the contribution of other haemodynamic variables. For example, the stroke volume depends on the contractility of the left ventricle which itself depends on multiple factors including preload, afterload and sympathetic activation. Systemic vascular resistance is also influenced by the autonomic nervous system as well as precapillary sphincter tone. Hypertension can occur acutely with an increase in any of the above variables.

In chronic primary or essential hypertension, decreases in vascular compliance and endothelial cell dysfunction result in sustained elevations in blood pressure, which generally develop slowly over time. This is accompanied by compensatory changes in physiology which themselves have implications in managing chronically hypertensive patients on the cardiothoracic critical care unit.

In health, acute changes or swings in mean arterial pressure are sensed by baroreceptors found in the carotid sinus and aortic arch. An increase in blood pressure results in activation of a negative feedback reflex loop whereby both heart rate and systemic vascular resistance fall in response to increased parasympathetic tone. This results in a lowering of blood pressure. In chronic hypertension baroreceptors reset over time to a higher level of mean arterial pressure, a process which is reversed with initiation of anti-hypertensive therapy.

Additionally, organ blood flow, which is maintained at a near constant level by the process of autoregulation, is also adjusted to a higher level of perfusion pressure. Autoregulation allows blood vessels to adjust their calibre in response to metabolic, mechanical and neurogenic factors, and is particularly important in the maintenance of blood flow in cerebral, coronary and renal perfusion. Mechanical factors refer to changes in arterial pressure transmitted transmurally. Increases in arterial pressure lead to the compensatory response of vasoconstriction thereby

Table 30.1 Aetiology of hypertension in the cardiothoracic critical care unit

System	Cause
Central nervous system	Cerebrovascular accident
	Inadequate analgesia
	Postoperative cognitive dysfunction or delirium
	Raised intracranial pressure
	Anxiety
Cardiovascular	Preoperative hypertension
	Alleviation of obstructed outflow with hypertrophied LV
	Postbypass hypervolaemia
	Inappropriate or excessive vasopressor or inotropic support
Respiratory	Hypercapnia
	Hypoxaemia
Renal	Acute kidney injury
	Urinary retention
	Blocked urinary catheter
Other	Hypoglycaemia
	Acute alcohol or nicotine withdrawal
	Steroids
	Failure to reinitiate anti-hypertensive medication

preventing a sudden increase in flow. Autoregulation protects from the deleterious effects of acute hypoperfusion or hyperperfusion. However, this only occurs within a certain range of mean arterial pressures. The lower range of the autoregulation curve varies markedly between individuals and depending on acute care setting. Traditionally the lower limit is thought to be 60 to 70 mmHg in most individuals. The upper limit has never been clearly defined but it certainly is <110 mmHg in many individuals. Outside this range, blood vessels are either maximally dilated or constricted and flow therefore becomes directly dependent on perfusion pressure. In chronic hypertension, the autoregulation curve is shifted to the right for a given mean arterial pressure as shown in Figure 30.1. This explains why organ ischaemia may occur with rapid lowering of mean arterial pressure in patients with established chronic hypertension.

Chronic hypertension results in an increase in afterload, which leads to an increase in myocardial work. Over time this is maintained or compensated for by ventricular hypertrophy. In terms of coronary blood flow, unless the increase in demand can be met by an increase in supply, ischaemia may occur. Additionally, chronically elevated mean arterial pressure can lead to diastolic dysfunction due to failure of adequate ventricular relaxation and subsequent congestive heart failure can supervene.

Diagnosis

The diagnosis and management of hypertension must be taken in the context of its presentation. The spectrum of hypertension includes an incidental finding in an asymptomatic patient to hypertensive crises with associated organ damage. In the context of the cardiothoracic unit this ranges from cautious reintroduction of preoperative anti-hypertensive medication postoperatively to rapid lowering of blood pressure in the situation of aortic dissection to limit further extension of the false lumen.

Preoperative hypertension is typically diagnosed in the primary care setting through routine screening. The traditional cut-off blood pressure is 140/90 mmHg or more. The blood pressure must be measured in both arms and replicated on two separate occasions. Further confirmation requires ambulatory or home blood pressure monitoring. Hypertension can be classified based on the severity of blood pressure.

- Stage 1: Blood pressure of 140/90 mmHg or more AND an average blood pressure of 135/85 mmHg or more on home or ambulatory monitoring.

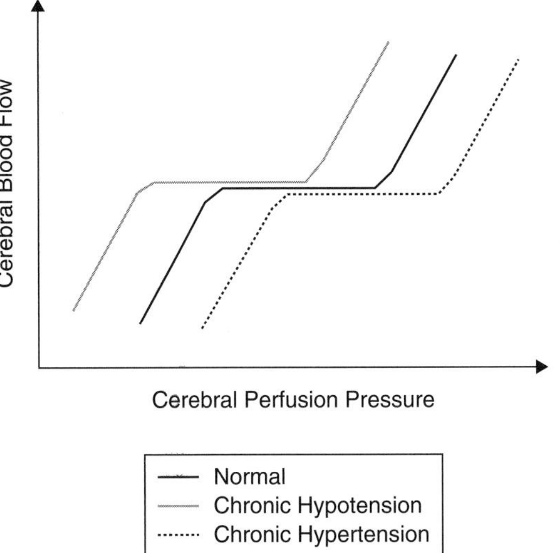

Figure 30.1 Cerebral blood flow autoregulation curve.

- Stage 2: Blood pressure of 160/100 mmHg or more AND an average blood pressure of 150/ 95 mmHg or more on home or ambulatory monitoring.
- Stage 3: Systolic blood pressure of ≥180 mmHg OR diastolic blood pressure ≥110 mmHg.

Whilst awaiting confirmation, further investigations looking for evidence of target organ damage should be performed. This includes fundoscopy, biochemistry for renal function and lipid profile, urinary protein levels and an electrocardiograph.

Stage 3 hypertension is also referred to as severe hypertension and is considered a hypertensive urgency. In these circumstances immediate initiation of treatment should be considered. In addition for patients with suspected accelerated hypertension, defined as severe hypertension with signs on fundoscopy of hypertensive retinopathy or papilloedema, a referral for immediate specialist advice and treatment should be made.

Hypertension can also be classified based on its aetiology. Primary or essential hypertension describes hypertension which occurs without an underlying identifiable cause. This represents over 90% of all cases. It typically arises in the elderly. The exact aetiology is unclear but is likely to be an interaction of environmental and genetic factors resulting in age-related decline in vessel compliance. Secondary hypertension on the other hand is hypertension as a consequence of an underlying disease process. This includes pathologies affecting the adrenal gland such as excess catecholamines as seen in phaeochromocytoma and aldosterone in Conn's syndrome. Secondary hypertension is more common in the younger population and treatment targets the underlying disease in addition to traditional anti-hypertensive medication.

Acute hypertension can present in the critical care setting, the emergency department or primary care. Acute severe elevations in blood pressure are often classified based on the presence or absence of end-organ damage. End-organ damage has been quoted as being present in 19% of all presentations of acute severe hypertension. A *hypertensive emergency* describes when severe hypertension as defined by BP >180/110 is associated with end-organ damage. Examples of end-organ damage can be seen in Table 30.2. Under these circumstances, anti-hypertensive treatment should be initiated as a priority in a monitored environment. Severe hypertension in the absence of end-organ damage is considered a *hypertensive urgency*. Treatment should be offered immediately but does necessitate hospitalisation.

Management

Preoperative Management

The guidelines for the management of chronic hypertension are outlined by NICE. Patients with hypertension requiring cardiothoracic surgery should ideally be established on effective anti-hypertensive therapy in primary care. Current targets suggest an optimal BP of below 140/90 mmHg in those aged less than 80 years and below 150/90 mmHg in people aged over

Table 30.2 System based examples of end-organ damage

System	End-organ damage
Central nervous system	Cerebrovascular accident
	Hypertensive encephalopathy
	Hypertensive retinopathy
Cardiovascular	Left ventricular hypertrophy
	Heart failure
	Myocardial ischaemia
	Aortic dissection
Renal	Hypertensive nephropathy
Respiratory	Pulmonary oedema

80 years. Poorly managed or undiagnosed hypertension should be identified at surgical pre-assessment and appropriate treatment instigated. No specific cut-off values exist above which surgery should be cancelled based on the presence of hypertension alone. For non-cardiac elective surgery, a blood pressure above 180/110 mmHg would be an indication for cancellation and optimisation of blood pressure control prior to surgery.

Initiation of anti-hypertensive therapy is indicated in the following situations:

- Stage 1 hypertension, less than 80 years of age and one of the following:
  - Target organ damage
  - Any cardiovascular disease
  - Renal disease
  - Diabetes
  - Predicted 10 year cardiovascular risk of more than 20%.
- Stage 1 and less than 40 years of age.
- Stage 2 or 3.

The choice of treatment subsequently depends on age, ethnicity and response to treatment. This is outlined in Table 30.3.

Before moving on to each step, compliance and optimal dosing should be ensured before the addition of a further agent. Additionally, hypertension which persists despite triple therapy is considered resistant hypertension and expert advice at this stage should be sought.

Presently beta-blockers are not recommended as initial therapy for hypertension except in certain circumstances such as women of child-bearing age and those intolerant of ACE inhibitors and ARBs. Extreme caution should be exercised with all of these agents in patients with aortic stenosis, impaired ventricular function or pulmonary hypertension.

Guidance on Pre-existing Anti-hypertensive Therapy in the Perioperative Period

The nature of cardiac surgery dictates that optimal blood pressure control should be ensured throughout the perioperative and postoperative period. For example, dehiscence of coronary grafts can result in life threatening haemorrhage, cardiac tamponade, return to theatre with resternotomy, use of blood products and therefore potentially death. Patients on established therapy should therefore continue up until the day of surgery unless specifically contraindicated.

Current practice advocates the continuation of both beta-blockers and calcium channel blockers on the day of surgery. Significant work has looked specifically at the cardioprotective effects of beta-blockers in the perioperative period. Withdrawal of beta-blockers on those taking them chronically is

Table 30.3 NICE recommendations for management of hypertension

Treatment step	Patient	Recommended therapy
1	• Less than 55 years	ACE inhibitor or ARB
	• Over 55 years • Black people of African or Caribbean origin of any age	CCB or thiazide-like diuretic
2	• Any patient not controlled on step 1	Combined ACE inhibitor and CCB
	• Black people of African or Caribbean origin or any age not controlled on step 1	ARB (in preference to ACE inhibitor) combined with CCB
3	• Any patient of any origin not controlled on step 2	Triple therapy: combination of ACE inhibitor or ARB with CCB and diuretic therapy
4	• Any patient of any origin not controlled on step 3 and blood potassium level of 4.5 mmol/l or less	Addition of spironolactone to step 3 treatment
	• Any patient of any origin not controlled on step 3 and blood potassium level of more than 4.5 mmol/l	High-dose diuretic therapy in addition to step 3 treatment

ACE angiotensin converting enzyme, ARB angiotensin II receptor blocker, CCB calcium channel blocker.

associated with significant adverse cardiac outcomes and they should therefore be continued. Controversy however exists over their introduction in the perioperative period due to evidence demonstrating an increase in risk of stroke and all-cause mortality despite a reduction in adverse cardiovascular outcomes.

In the case of diuretics, including thiazides and thiazide-like diuretics, concerns exist over the potential for diuretic induced volume depletion and electrolyte imbalances, specifically potassium. Hypovolaemia and hypokalaemia are associated with haemodynamic instability during induction of anaesthesia and should therefore be avoided. Patients taking diuretics who present to pre-assessment should have their serum electrolytes measured and advised to omit medication on the day of surgery.

ACE inhibitors should also be discontinued the day before surgery. The renin-angiotensin-aldosterone system is involved in maintenance of normotension during anaesthesia. Inhibition is therefore associated with refractory hypotension in the perioperative period and omission is recommended. Refractory hypotension may still occur with angiotensin II receptor blockers and they should be discontinued for 2 days prior to surgery.

Hypertension is not uncommon in the anaesthetic room prior to induction. In most cases there is a significant contribution from patient anxiety and reference should be made to the patient's preoperative blood pressure as assessed at admission. During induction for cardiac surgery, efforts are made to avoid a dramatic reduction in arterial pressure whilst also preventing the pressor response associated with laryngoscopy. Traditionally, this has led to the use of induction agent dose-sparing approaches such as the use of high dose opiates and local anaesthetics. Intraoperatively, anaesthesia can be maintained by a total intravenous or volatile approach. Volatiles, specifically isoflurane and to a lesser extent sevoflurane, have the additional advantage of being associated with myocardial preconditioning. Additionally, during stimulating periods such as sternotomy, volatiles can be used to rapidly deepen anaesthesia whilst also preventing the associated hypertensive response. Other agents used specifically for their hypotensive effects include boluses of intravenous magnesium sulphate and fast acting beta-blockers such as esmolol. Ideally, the blood pressure should be kept within 20% of the baseline blood pressure.

Postoperative Management

Any invasive surgery to the thorax is associated with a significant acute phase response mediated by activation of the sympathetic nervous system and renin-angiotensin-aldosterone system, both of which serve to promote an increase in cardiac output and therefore tissue oxygen delivery but may in doing so increase blood pressure. Hypertension is therefore a common finding in the initial hyperdynamic postoperative period. Postoperative hypertension has previously been described as systolic blood pressure greater than 190 mmHg and/or diastolic greater than 100 mmHg.

The initial approach should focus on identification and treatment of any underlying cause, for example, providing appropriate analgesia. Once precipitants have been addressed, subsequent measures should focus on a targeted approach to the pathophysiology of hypertension, for example, identifying increases in the cardiac output or systemic vascular resistance or both.

Cardiac output may be raised in cases of good left ventricular function and in the presence of hypervolaemia and sympathetic activation. An associated tachycardia may be observed. In these instances, diuretics can be used to off-load the intravascular volume and beta-blockers to provide sympatholysis. Alternatively, dihydropyridine calcium channel blockers or centrally acting alpha-agonists such as clonidine can be used with less negative inotropic effects. If hypertension is driven by raised vascular tone, a vasodilating agent would be an appropriate treatment. In circumstances where vascular tone has been chronically high, replacement of the intravascular volume may also be required with vasodilation.

Specific Medications used in the Management of Acute and Chronic Hypertension

There are several agents available for the management of chronic hypertension. However, it is more challenging to achieve an effective and sustained control of blood pressure in the acute care setting. In fact, if many anti-hypertensive agents effectively lower blood pressure, only few have the capacity to achieve strict control of hypertension in the acute setting.

The most commonly used anti-hypertensive agents, with their advantages and disadvantages, are outlined in Table 30.4.

Table 30.4 Commonly used anti-hypertensive agents

Class	Drug name	Mechanism of action	Indications	Contraindications	Significant side effects
Beta-blockers	Labetalol	Mixed alpha- and beta-AR antagonist	Acute hypertension Pregnancy Maintaining cerebral perfusion Rate control in SVTs	Asthma Acute heart failure Peripheral vascular disease	Hypotension Heart block Bronchospasm
	Esmolol	Selective beta-1-AR antagonist	Acute hypertension Aortic dissection Pregnancy	Acute heart failure	
Alpha-blockers	Phentolamine	Non-selective alpha-AR antagonist	Acute hypertension Phaeochromocytoma Cocaine intoxication	Pulmonary hypertension	Orthostatic hypotension Headache Tachycardia
	Urapidil	Selective alpha$_1$-AR antagonist	Acute hypertension	Aortic stenosis Major AV shunt	
Alpha$_2$-blockers	Clonidine	Central alpha$_2$-AR agonist	Acute hypertension Sedation weaning Analgesia	AV node disease Sinoatrial node disease	Drowsiness Dizziness Headache Fever
	Dexmedetomidine		Acute hypertension Sedation weaning	No absolute contraindication	Hypotension Vomiting Fever
	Methyldopa		Acute hypertension Pregnancy	Active hepatic disease Depression	Drowsiness Headache Muscle pain
Arterial vasodilators	Hydralazine	Direct arteriolar vasodilator	Essential hypertension Hypertensive crisis Congestive heart failure	Aortic or mitral stenosis Pulmonary hypertension Lupus	Headache Tachycardia Muscle pain
	Fenoldopam	Selective dopamine receptor 1 agonist	Hypertensive crisis Severe hypertension	Glaucoma Concomitant use of beta-blocker	Headache Nausea Flushing

Calcium channel blockers	Nicardipine	L-type calcium channel blocker (dihydropyridines)	Short-term treatment of hypertension	Aortic stenosis	Headache Flushing Muscle pain
	Diltiazem	L-type calcium channel blocker (non-dihydropyridines)	Chronic hypertension Chronic stable angina	Sick sinus syndrome AV block Acute MI	Headache Flushing Muscle pain Cough
Nitrites and nitrates	Nitroprusside	Nitric oxide donor	Hypertensive crisis	Vitamin B12 deficiency Active hepatic disease	Headache Flushing Reduced platelet aggregation Ileus Metabolic acidosis
	ISMN		Stable angina	Acute heart failure Aortic/mitral stenosis	Headache Nausea Dizziness
Diuretics	Furosemide	Inhibition of Na/Cl/K cotransporter	Congestive heart failure Cirrhosis Renal disease	Anuria	Hearing loss Itching Jaundice Nausea Vomiting
	Bumetanide	Inhibition of Na/Cl/K cotransporter	Congestive heart failure Cirrhosis Renal disease	Anuria	Nausea Vomiting Itching Dizziness

Special Circumstances

Hypertensive Crises

Severe or stage 3 hypertension associated with end-organ damage is a medical emergency and patients should be closely monitored with invasive monitoring and managed in a high dependency area. Ideally diastolic pressure should be reduced by no more than 10–15% or less than 110 mmHg within an hour. More dramatic reductions may result in hypoperfusion due to altered autoregulation of organ blood. This reduction typically requires the use of a short-acting intravenous agent by continuous infusion. In the absence of end-organ damage there is less urgency and blood pressure can be lowered over a period of 1–2 days.

Aortic Dissection

Aortic dissection itself is considered a hypertensive crisis due to the associated end-organ damage. Pressure related damage to the aortic intima results in a tear and passage of blood into the potential space between the intimal and medial layer. High arterial pressure promotes passage of blood into the false lumen and extension of tear both distally and proximally. Under these circumstances, aggressive blood control is required and ideally should be achieved within minutes. Whilst such patients are likely to be chronic hypertensives and therefore at risk of hypoperfusion and ischaemia, the benefits of preventing or avoiding further dissection of the aorta outweigh these risks.

Key Points

- The aetiology of hypertension in the cardiothoracic critical care unit is often multifactorial and may resolve with management of the underlying precipitant alone.
- Patients on established therapy, except for ACE inhibitors, should continue up until the day of surgery unless specifically contraindicated.
- The initial approach of postoperative management should focus on identification and treatment of any possible underlying cause, for example, providing appropriate analgesia.
- It is challenging to achieve an effective and sustained control of blood pressure in the acute care setting.
- Reintroduction of preoperative anti-hypertensive medication postoperatively should be cautiously considered in the context of the cardiothoracic unit.

Further Reading

Chobanian AV. The Seventh Report of the Joint National Committee on Prevention, Detection, Evaluation, and Treatment of High Blood Pressure: the JNC 7 report. *Journal of the American Medical Association*. 2003; 289: 2560–2572.

Devereaux PJ, Yang H, Guyatt GH. Rationale, design, and organization of Perioperative Ischemic Evaluation (POISE) trial: a randomised controlled trial of metoprolol versus placebo in patients undergoing noncardiac surgery. *American Heart Journal*. 2006; 152: 223–230.

Gal TJ, Cooperman LH. Hypertension in the immediate post-operative period. *British Journal of Anaesthesia*. 1975; 47: 70–74.

Lewington S, Clakre R, Qizilbash N, Peto R, Collins R. Prospective Studies Collaboration: age-specific relevance of usual blood pressure to vascular mortality: a meta-analysis of individual data for one million adults in 61 prospective studies. *Lancet*. 2002; 361: 106Q.

National Institute for Health and Care Excellence. Guideline CG127. Hypertension: Clinical Management of Hypertension in Adults. August 2011.

Rajgopal R, Rajan S, Paul J. Effect of pre-operative discontinuation of angiotensin-converting enzyme inhibitors or angiotensin II receptor antagonists on intra-operative arterial pressures after induction of anaesthesia. *Anethesia, Essays and Researches*. 2014; 8: 32–35.

Stevens RD, Burri H, Tramer MR. Pharmacologic myocardial protection in patients undergoing non-cardiac surgery: a quantitative systemic review. *Anesthesia & Analgesia*. 2003; 97: 623–633.

Valchanov K, Arrowsmith JE. Do venodilators have a role in the perioperative management of heart failure? *European Journal of Anesthesia*. 2012; 29: 121–128.

Vuylsteke A, Vincent JL, de la Payen GD, et al. Characteristics, practise patterns and outcomes in patients with acute hypertension: European registry for Studying the Treatment of Acute Hypertension (Euro-STAT). *Critical Care*. 2011; 15: R271.

MCQs

1. **Which of the following statements regarding hypertension are true?**

   (a) Blood pressure or mean arterial pressure (MAP) is considered the product of the stroke volume (SV) and systemic vascular resistance (SVR)

   (b) Blood pressure or mean arterial pressure (MAP) is considered the product of the cardiac output (CO) and systemic vascular resistance (SVR) and can be summarised as

   $$\text{MAP (mmHg)} = (\text{HR} \times \text{SV}) \times \text{SVR}$$

   (c) Blood pressure or mean arterial pressure (MAP) is considered the product of the heart rate (HR) and stroke volume (SV)

   (d) Hypertension can occur acutely only with an increase in systemic vascular resistance (SVR)

   (e) Blood pressure or mean arterial pressure (MAP) is considered the product of the cardiac output (CO) and heart rate (HR)

2. **Which of the following statements regarding hypertension are true?**

   (a) In chronic primary or essential hypertension, decreases in vascular resistance and endothelial cell dysfunction result in sustained elevations in blood pressure

   (b) Acute changes or swings in mean arterial pressure are sensed by baroreceptors found in the carotid sinus and aortic arch. An increase in blood pressure results in activation of a positive feedback reflex loop whereby both heart rate and systemic vascular resistance increase

   (c) Autoregulation protects from the deleterious effects of acute hypoperfusion or hyperperfusion. However this only occurs within a range of mean arterial pressures typically of 60–110 mmHg

   (d) In chronic hypertension, baroreceptors reset over time to a lower level of mean arterial pressure

   (e) In chronic hypertension, the autoregulation curve is shifted to the left for a given mean arterial pressure

3. **Which of the following statements regarding hypertension are true?**

   (a) Grade 2 hypertension is characterised by a diastolic pressure of 100–109 mmHg and a systolic pressure of 160–170 mmHg

   (b) A blood pressure of 135/95 would be considered normal

   (c) Hypertension seen in renal disease is classified as primary hypertension

   (d) Acute severe elevations in blood pressure are often caused by the presence of end-organ damage

   (e) Secondary hypertension is less common in the younger population

4. **Which of the following statements regarding hypertension management are true?**

   (a) Poorly managed or undiagnosed hypertension should be identified at surgical pre-assessment and appropriate treatment instigated in the immediate postoperative period

   (b) Presently beta-blockers are never recommended as initial therapy for hypertension

   (c) Current practice advocates the discontinuation of both beta-blockers and calcium channel blockers on the day of surgery

   (d) ACE inhibitors should be continued the day before surgery

   (e) Patients taking diuretics should be advised to omit medication on the day of surgery

5. **Which of the following statements regarding perioperative management of hypertension are true?**

   (a) At the time of surgery, ideally, the blood pressure should be kept within 20% of the baseline blood pressure

   (b) Both hypervolaemia and hypokalaemia are associated with haemodynamic instability during induction of anaesthesia and should therefore be avoided

   (c) Use of vasodilating agents is generally avoided in postoperative patients

   (d) In case of hypertensive crisis, in the absence of end-organ damage there is less urgency and blood pressure can be lowered over a period of 1–2 days

   (e) Calcium channel blockers or centrally acting alpha-agonists such as clonidine cannot be used because of their negative inotropic effects

Exercise answers are available on p.469. Alternatively, take the test online at www.cambridge.org/CardiothoracicMCQ

Chapter 31

Pulmonary Hypertension in the Cardiothoracic Intensive Care Unit

Mark Toshner and Joanna Pepke-Zaba

Introduction

Pulmonary hypertension (PH) represents a group of conditions which share the haemodynamic definition of a mean pulmonary artery pressure equal or greater than 25 mmHg at rest. Acute pulmonary hypertension in critical care may often be secondary to acute respiratory failure, left heart failure and pulmonary thromboembolism or due to decompensated chronic pulmonary hypertension by concurrent comorbid conditions. Pulmonary hypertension can complicate perioperative management in patients admitted for elective surgical procedures to treat their underlying pulmonary hypertension (e.g. pulmonary endarterectomy, lung transplantation).

In the assessment of patients with PH, the pulmonary capillary wedge pressure (PCWP) is of importance in discriminating between pulmonary arterial (precapillary) and venous hypertension (postcapillary). Current guidelines use the cut-off of 15 mmHg to differentiate but it is important to acknowledge the preload dependent nature of the PCWP, which can be affected in particular by fluid status. Pulmonary hypertension is commonly thought of as a rare disease but in reality is commonly associated with varied pathophysiological processes. This is reflected in current classification systems, which highlight just how many diseases can result in PH. Evidence from primary care suggests that up to 13% of all-comers to open access breathlessness clinics may have echocardiographic evidence of PH, and many of these patients remain essentially undiagnosed either due to lack of awareness of the managing physicians or fatalistic attitudes about prognosis. A particular problem lies in the classification categories where treatment with targeting PH therapies has not been of proven benefit, especially groups 2 and 3, pulmonary venous hypertension and hypoxic lung disease. Additionally the current classification system does not consider causes of transient PH in acutely ill patients. There are therefore three distinct patient populations when considering managing PH in the ITU: (1) those with recognised PH, (2) those with occult or unrecognised PH and (3) those who develop PH as a consequence of their acute illness. Compounding this challenge is the paucity of evidence of how to manage any of these differing groups and often the same evidence-free treatment approaches are trialed regardless of aetiology.

Patients with PH most commonly die of right ventricular (RV) failure and its consequences, regardless of whether it is acute or chronic. Any rise in pulmonary vascular resistance (PVR) triggers RV dysfunction, and impaired RV adaptation to rapid increases in afterload results in 'ventriculoarterial uncoupling', RV distension, myocardial oxygen consumption/delivery imbalance and heart failure. It is important to recognise that the right and left ventricles (LV) are not separate organs and functionally impact on each other. Not only do they share an interventricular septum, but 25% of the cross-fibres in the RV are common to the LV. Significant RV–LV interdependence exists in the setting of RV pressure and/or volume overload, reduced RV stroke volume, reduced LV venous return leading to impaired LV filling contributing to the fall in cardiac output and heart failure. In acute causes of PH the RV is unprepared to cope with a resultant inability to generate very high pressures and there is an easily breached contractile reserve. In chronic PH the RV ability to 'cope' will partly rely on its coupling to the pulmonary circuit. This will be dependent on the degree of disease but also varies between disease processes. More explicitly, how the RV copes is not linearly linked to simple pressure and resistance. This was elegantly demonstrated in a mechanical animal model of chronic progressive RV pressure overload (pulmonary artery banding). Despite identical pressure profiles to an established model of angioproliferative pulmonary hypertension (sugen/hypoxia), the banding model does not develop RV failure but the sugen/hypoxia does. This is borne out clinically most notably in congenital heart disease where suprasystemic pressures can develop but long-term outcomes are generally better than for other forms of PH. Added to this is the recognition that although pulmonary arterial hypertension (PAH) traditionally is thought of as affecting the small precapillary vessels, there is heterogeneity of vascular compartments affected across the spectrum of causes of PH (involving both precapillary and postcapillary compartments). This heterogeneity may in part explain the difficulty translating the success of treating PAH with pulmonary vasodilators to most of the other causes. Therefore all 'PH' is not the same from a biomechanical or treatment response perspective.

In this chapter we will clarify what evidence-based medicine and expert consensus is available and the impact on management and treatment strategies in the intensive care unit (ICU). Explicitly we will discuss managing the patient with known PH, and how to approach patient populations at risk.

Supportive Care and General Management of PH in the ICU

Acutely unwell patients need to be moved to a critical care environment. Appropriate investigations and monitoring should aim to identify and reverse precipitating factors, especially those associated with a high mortality.

Optimal fluid balance is paramount, as both hypovolaemia and hypervolaemia may be detrimental to cardiac output. In hypervolaemic patients, reducing RV preload through diuresis will improve RV function, RV-LV interdependence and LV diastolic compliance. Patients with decompensated RV failure develop secondary hyperaldosteronism and addition of an aldosterone antagonist, such as spironolactone, to a loop diuretic can be useful. In the critically ill patient with PH and right heart failure it is a constant and delicate balancing act getting the fluid balance right. The most common mistake is overfilling patients who are already fluid overloaded in an attempt to bolster systemic blood pressure. In the context of right heart failure it is likely that patients will be overfilled and therefore maintaining a negative balance is critical in the majority of cases. Underfilling, however, will affect LV output and systemic blood pressure. We are therefore often left in a situation considering vasopressors whilst trying to offload. Control of pulmonary artery pressure could be improved by treatment with high flow oxygen as a selective pulmonary vasodilator in patients with pulmonary hypertension, regardless of the underlying diagnosis, baseline oxygenation or RV function. Anticoagulation may be desirable due to the low cardiac output states usually seen, and should be considered. There is however no evidence basis for this. Mechanical ventilatory support may be considered depending on the underlying pathology, in particular if there is an identifiable and reversible cause of the PH. If the patient is a potential transplant candidate this should be considered. ECMO is largely currently restricted to bridging patients to transplantation; however its role may evolve.

Treatment of Underlying Causes

The underlying disease process should be improved or optimised. For example, with left heart failure, therapy needs to be optimised, ventilation in lung diseases needs to be optimised and antibiotics used if an infective process is suspected. Specific attention should be paid to avoiding respiratory acidosis and metabolic acidosis. This can be limited by maximisation of recruitment of lung alveoli and optimisation of ventilation-perfusion matching by patient positioning and optimisation of ventilation and positive end expiratory pressure. All attempts should be made to reduce PVR in PAH patients presenting with heart failure. An excellent example of successful management of patients in the ICU with significant pulmonary hypertension is chronic thromboembolic pulmonary hypertension (CTEPH) patients treated with pulmonary endarterectomy (PEA). This represents the largest cohort of PH patients successfully managed in the ICU. Mortality rates in high-volume centres are now down as low as 2–5%. Despite this, these patients are often not considered when assessing the evidence on how to manage patients with established PH. This is understandable as the majority of patients have significant early reduction in pulmonary pressure and resistance, and therefore are not comparable from this perspective to other groups of PH patients. The clearest lesson from PEA is that patients with PH can be successfully managed in the ICU but most notably when the cause of the increased resistance is treatable. In patients where the cause of the PH is unknown or unclear, consideration should be given to rarer causes of PH and investigations tailored to identify potentially reversible causes. The current classification of PH aetiology is delineated in Table 31.1.

Table 31.1 NICE classification of pulmonary hypertension

1. Pulmonary arterial hypertension

- 1 Idiopathic
- 1.2 Heritable
  - 1.2.1 BMPR2 mutation
  - 1.2.2 ALK-1, ENG, SMAD9, CAV1, KCNK3
  - 1.2.3 Unknown
- 1.3 Drugs and toxins induced
- 1.4 Associated with:
  - 1.4.1 Connective tissue disease
  - 1.4.2 HIV infection
  - 1.4.3 Portal hypertension
  - 1.4.4 Congenital heart disease
  - 1.4.5 Schistosomiasis

1′ Pulmonary veno-occlusive disease and/or pulmonary capillary haemangiomatosis

1″ Persistent pulmonary hypertension of the newborn

2. Pulmonary hypertension due to left heart disease

- 2.1 Left ventricular systolic dysfunction
- 2.2 Left ventricular diastolic dysfunction
- 2.3 Valvular disease
- 2.4 Congenital/acquired left heart inflow/outflow tract obstruction and congenital cardiomyopathies
- 2.5 Congenital /acquired pulmonary veins stenosis

3. Pulmonary hypertension due to lung diseases and/or hypoxia

- 3.1 Chronic obstructive pulmonary disease
- 3.2 Interstitial lung disease
- 3.3 Other pulmonary diseases with mixed restrictive and obstructive pattern
- 3.4 Sleep disordered breathing
- 3.5 Alveolar hypoventilation disorders
- 3.6 Chronic exposure to high altitude
- 3.7 Developmental lung diseases

4. Chronic thromboembolic pulmonary hypertension and other pulmonary artery obstructions

- 4.1 Chronic thromboembolic pulmonary hypertension
- 4.2 Other pulmonary artery obstructions
  - 4.2.1 Angiosarcoma
  - 4.2.2 Other intravascular tumours
  - 4.2.3 Arteritis
  - 4.2.4 Congenital pulmonary artery stenois
  - 4.2.5 Parasites (hydatidosis)

5. Pulmonary hypertension with unclear and/or multifactorial mechanisms

- 5.1 Haematological disorders: chronic haemolytic anaemia, myeloproliferative disorders, splenectomy
- 5.2 Systemic disorders, sarcoidosis, pulmonary histiocytosis, lymphangioleiomyomatosis
- 5.3 Metabolic disorders: glycogen storage disease, Gaucher disease, thyroid disorders
- 5.4 Others: pulmonary tumour thrombotic microangiopathy, fibrosing mediastinitis, chronic renal failure (with/without dialysis), segmental pulmonary hypertension

To Monitor or Not To Monitor?

The standard assessment of non-invasive haemodynamic and renal, hepatic and neurological function will provide direct and surrogate information on cardiac status, but beyond this there is no good evidence for or against additional monitoring. Echocardiography will potentially be diagnostically useful and can give extra information such as the presence of pericardial effusions but has no clear role in monitoring. This is largely due to the complicated physical nature of the RV, which makes bedside echo assessment of function crude at best. Invasive cardiac monitoring is no longer in vogue in the ICU having proven of no benefit in the management of critically ill general ICU patients or in high-risk postoperative cohorts. There is a lack of trials looking specifically at PH and therefore any advice is based on theory and opinion. However, most expert reviews still recommend invasive monitoring by pulmonary artery catheter (PAC) of PA pressure, cardiac output and PCWP, though not unambiguously. There are non-invasive methods for measuring cardiac output on its own, such as bioimpedance, bioreactance and pulse wave analysis, though again there are no data strongly supporting a role in guiding treatment decisions. Monitoring and basic investigations are outlined in Table 31.2.

Resuscitation In and Outside of the ICU

Patients with PH have been demonstrated to have very poor outcomes in a large but retrospective analysis of tertiary care centres. This included all comers but reflected the nature of specialist centres with 49% of

Table 31.2 Monitoring and investigations for pulmonary hypertensive patients

Monitoring	Investigations
Weight and fluid balance	WCC/CRP/blood and urine cultures
BP/pulse ± non-invasive CO	CXR
O_2 sats and ABGs	Troponin
Lactate	HRCT PA
Invasive haemodynamics • CVP • MPAP • PACWP • CO/mixed venous O_2	Right ventricular assessment • 12-lead ECG and continuous monitoring • Echocardiography • NT-proBNP • Non-invasive CO

the patients reported having a diagnosis of idiopathic PAH and the majority of the rest being either group 1 PAH or CTEPH. Only eight patients (6% of the survey) survived to 90 days without significant neurological damage. This was despite the very high proportion of 63% of the patients already being located in the ICU. Of these patients, all but one had an identifiable reversible cause for their arrest such as vasovagal reactions, digitalis toxicity or pericardial tamponade. The mean pulmonary vascular resistance in this cohort was very high at 1694 dyne s/cm^5 and it is probably extremely difficult to achieve effective pulmonary blood flow and left ventricular filling with chest compressions in this context. Therefore in the ICU it is appropriate in all PH patients, and specifically those with PAH, to address early the plans for escalation in the event of an arrest, with a clear understanding that in the absence of reversible causes, success is unlikely.

Acute Medical Therapy

Vasopressors in PH

It is facile to state the importance of maintaining systemic blood pressure in the context of critically unwell populations, however in PH there is the additional challenge of making sure systemic pressure exceeds PA pressure and therefore maintaining right coronary artery perfusion. The right coronary perfusion cycle differs from the left in that it occurs more diffusely and peaks in systole. To do this using vasopressors presents a number of challenges. The first is the inability to selectively spare the pulmonary circulation from the vasopressor effect. The second is the effect on heart rate and rhythm, cardiac function and output.

Animal studies are limited. In an experimental dog model of acute RV failure by pulmonary artery constriction, the administration of phenylephrine decreasing RV afterload, increasing aortic pressure and hence myocardial perfusion pressure increases myocardial blood flow, reverses ischaemia and improves RV function. Despite this potentially positive effect of vasopressors on RV function, in human studies the effects are more complex and potentially antagonistic. There are effectively no high quality large randomised controlled data for vasopressors and inotropes in PH ICU patients. Care therefore needs to be taken in interpreting the available data and also note made of the heterogeneity of the studied populations.

Catecholamines

In a study of 27 patients undergoing surgery for left-sided valvular replacement and congenital heart disease, there were increases in systemic pressure and pulmonary artery pressure with both phenylephrine and noradrenaline. Nineteen of the 27 patients were postcapillary PH with mitral valve replacement (MVR). Of interest there were no significant changes in cardiac output and surprisingly heart rate did not change.

There are conflicting data on the effects of dopamine, possibly attributable to the mixed populations studied. Initial studies in stable patients and healthy controls suggested heart rate, mPAP, aortic mean pressure and CI increased, while SVR reduced. PVR did not change significantly. In studies in over 1600 patients in the ICU (not however stratified by PH), dopamine caused an excess of arrhythmias when compared with noradrenaline and in subanalyses of patients with cardiogenic shock, an excess of deaths. When using dopamine in PH patients, who are prone to arrhythmias, physicians should be particularly alert to this possibility.

Vasopressin

In a case series of nine valve replacement patients who presented with postoperative refractory vasodilatory hypotension concomitant with PH, vasopressin increased mean systemic arterial pressure but at the expense of reduced cardiac output. Changes in PVR did not reach significance.

Dobutamine

In nine cirrhotic patients with mild PH undergoing liver transplantation, there was an increase in RV contractility and decrease in afterload when dobutamine was infused in the anhepatic phase. Mean pulmonary arterial pressure (mPAP) went up by 4 mmHg and cardiac index (CI) doubled from 2.3 to 5.1 l/min/m^2 with an overall reduction in pulmonary vascular resistance (PVR). In acute studies in patients with mixed lung diseases being assessed for lung transplantation, dobutamine also increased CI and mPAP (though not statistically significant). Again this appeared to result in an overall reduction in PVR, suggesting that there may be some recruitment of vessels given the absence of any reduction in pressure.

Levosimendan

Levosimendan sensitises calcium and acts as a vasodilator in addition to putative inotropic effects, which have been suggested to be of potential benefit. The evidence for levisomendan is however weak. A small placebo randomised clinical trial (RCT) in 28 patients with mixed aetiology PH was undertaken using levosimendan. This was in stable patients, not in the ICU, and administered using short-term infusions 4 times at 2-week intervals. There were only significant changes in PVR demonstrable acutely at 24 hours and not at 8 weeks, and surprisingly there was 25% deterioration in the PVR in the placebo group, which is difficult to explain. Hypotension was a significant side effect.

Pulmonary Vasodilators

We will not attempt to summarise the literature on pulmonary vasodilators in PH but restrict ourselves to the limited data and expert opinion on their use in ICU populations. Inhaled NO has been most widely used because of its selective action on the pulmonary circulation. The occurrence of rebound pulmonary hypertension when administration is interrupted has limited its use. The inhaled prostacyclin analogue iloprost is a valuable alternative, inducing more pronounced haemodynamic improvement acutely. The only randomised blind trial of nitric oxide in PH was in cardiopulmonary bypass patients undergoing mitral valve surgery with a PVR of over 200 dynes s/cm^5. This trial of inhaled NO at 20 ppm enrolled 58 patients but was a comparator trial to nitroprusside and inhaled prostacyclin. Prostacyclin and NO both reduced mPAP and consequently PVR (by 50 and 45% respectively) but with no significant effect on other haemodynamic parameters. The converse was also seen in a small and uncontrolled trial in seven patients with PH post left ventricular assisted device (LVAD) insertion where withdrawal of NO resulted in a significant increase in PVR. Post cardiac transplantation, both NO and prostacyclin decrease PVR with no change in SVR with NO but a decrease in SVR with prostacyclin administered intravenously. Thirteen patients post inferior myocardial infarct with cardiogenic shock behaved broadly the same in an uncontrolled study with an additional increase in CI of 24%. There is a cost implication as NO is considerably more expensive. In 18 consecutive heart transplant patients, 9 with PH, there was a modest 5 mmHg drop in mPAP with nebulised milnirone. Sildenafil (oral or intravenous) has no good quality data in the ICU setting but is often considered largely because of the reasonable side effect profile. It can still cause systemic vasodilatation. Endothelin receptor antagonists are not often considered as it takes time to establish their action.

Conclusions

Pulmonary hypertension is complicated and difficult to manage in the ICU. Usually it is complicated by right ventricular failure. The first question that should be asked is related to the aetiology of pulmonary hypertension – *Is this pre-existing PH, occult PH or PH associated with the acute illness*? As is often the case, identifying the cause will dictate treatment. Medical management relies on the attention to volume status and contractile state of the right ventricle and requires complex decision making on risk/benefit considerations in the absence of a definitively correct evidence-based approach. There is a need for well-controlled and well-designed prospective research in PH in the ICU to clarify best practice.

Learning Points

- Patients with pulmonary hypertension present with right ventricle failure due to different disease states. Determining the underlying aetiology can be critical to treatment.
- Management should concentrate on maximal reduction of RV afterload based on underlying pathophysiology including adequate coupling of RV contractility to vascular load.
- Haemodynamic monitoring can be essential to provide adequate data on which to base management decisions.
- Optimal fluid balance is paramount.
- There is a paucity of evidence for the therapies used for LV failure and PAH for management of pulmonary hypertension and right ventricular failure in the ICU settings.

Further Reading

Bogaard HJ, Natarajan R, Henderson SC, et al. Chronic pulmonary artery pressure elevation is insufficient to explain right heart failure. *Circulation*. 2009; 120: 1951–1960.

Cannon JE, Su L, Kiely DG, Page K. Dynamic risk stratification of patient long-term outcome after pulmonary endarterectomy: results from the United Kingdom national cohort. *Circulation*. 2016; 133: 1761–1771.

De Backer D, Biston P, Devriendt J, et al. Comparison of dopamine and norepinephrine in the treatment of shock. *New England Journal of Medicine*. 2010; 362: 779–789.

Fattouch K, Sbraga F, Bianco G. Inhaled prostacyclin, nitric oxide, and nitroprusside in pulmonary hypertension after mitral valve replacement. *Journal of Cardiac Surgery*. 2005; 20: 171–176.

Friedberg MK, Redington AN. Right versus left ventricular failure: differences, similarities, and interactions. *Circulation*. 2014; 129: 1033–1044.

Galie N, Humbert M, Vachiery JL. 2015 ESC/ERS Guidelines for the diagnosis and treatment of pulmonary hypertension: The Joint Task Force for the Diagnosis and Treatment of Pulmonary Hypertension of the European Society of Cardiology (ESC) and the European Respiratory Society (ERS): Endorsed by: Association for European Paediatric and Congenital Cardiology (AEPC), International Society for Heart and Lung Transplantation (ISHLT). *European Heart Journal*. 2016; 37: 67–119.

Gaynor SL, Maniar HS, Bloch JB. Right atrial and ventricular adaptation to chronic right ventricular pressure overload. *Circulation*. 2005; 112: I212–I218.

Harvey S, Harrison DA, Singer M. Assessment of the clinical effectiveness of pulmonary artery catheters in management of patients in intensive care (PAC-Man): a randomised controlled trial. *Lancet*. 2005; 366: 472–477.

Hoeper MM, Granton J. Intensive care unit management of patients with severe pulmonary hypertension and right heart failure. *American Journal of Respiratory and Critical Care Medicine*. 2011; 184: 1114–1124.

Hoeper MM, Olschewski H, et al A comparison of the acute hemodynamic effects of inhaled nitric oxide and aerosolized iloprost in primary pulmonary hypertension. German PPH study group. *Journal of the American College of Cardiology*. 2000; **35**: 176–182.

Hoffman D, Sisto D, Frater RW. Left-to-right ventricular interaction with a noncontracting right ventricle. *Journal of Thoracic and Cardiovascular Surgery*. 1994; 107: 1496–1502.

Kwak YL, Lee CS, Park YH. The effect of phenylephrine and norepinephrine in patients with chronic pulmonary hypertension. *Anaesthesia*. 2002; 57: 9–14.

Sandham JD, Hull RD, Brant RF. A randomized, controlled trial of the use of pulmonary-artery catheters in high-risk surgical patients. *New England Journal of Medicine*. 2003; 348: 5–14.

Sibbald WJ, et al. Pulmonary hypertension in sepsis: measurement by the pulmonary arterial diastolic-pulmonary wedge pressure gradient and the influence of passive and active factors. *Chest*. 1978; 73: 583–591.

MCQs

1. **Best general medical supportive care of PH patients on ICU includes:**
   (a) Oxygen therapy
   (b) Optimisation of fluid balance
   (c) Anticoagulation
   (d) ECMO
   (e) All except ECMO
2. **Appropriate volume management may involve:**
   (a) Intravenous loop diuretics (bolus, continuous infusion)
   (b) Addition of thiazide diuretic
   (c) Maintenance of a negative fluid balance
   (d) Addition of inotropes if low cardiac output
   (e) All of the above
3. **Treatment of underlying causes of PH involves:**
   (a) Steroids if coexisting asthma suspected
   (b) Optimisation of gas exchange in lung diseases
   (c) Antibiotics if an infective process is suspected
   (d) Pulmonary vasodilators
   (e) All of the above
4. **The best way of monitoring pulmonary arterial pressure is by using:**
   (a) Central venous pressure
   (b) Mean PAP
   (c) Pulmonary capillary wedge pressure
   (d) Cardiac output/mixed venous O_2
   (e) Arterial blood gases
5. **The most commonly used pulmonary vasodilator which avoids significant systemic vascular side effects in PH patients on the ICU is:**
   (a) NO
   (b) Prostacyclin
   (c) Phosphodiesterase 5 inhibitors
   (d) Endothelin receptor antagonist
   (e) GTN

Exercise answers are available on p.469. Alternatively, take the test online at www.cambridge.org/CardiothoracicMCQ

Chapter 32

The Infected Patient

Simon J Finney

Infection is a common problem for patients in cardiothoracic intensive care units (CT ICUs) and although it may be the primary reason for admission, many more infections are acquired on the ICU. Estimates of incidence rates vary but are at least 5%. Undoubtedly, infection increases morbidity, the length of ICU admission and mortality.

This chapter considers infected patients in general along with specific infections of particular importance to patients admitted to the cardiothoracic ICU. Antibiotic therapy is considered in Chapter 12. Patients undergoing thoracic transplantation (Chapter 40 and Chapter 41) are particularly prone to infections and susceptible to a wider range of pathogens.

Identification of Infected Patients

Many patients develop systemic inflammation following major surgery and cardiopulmonary bypass. It can be difficult to distinguish those in whom infection is the aetiology from the signs and symptoms of inflammation.

The identification of patients with sepsis and septic shock used to be based on heart rate, temperature, respiratory rate and the leucocyte count in the context of suspected infection. These criteria have poor predictive value of organ dysfunction and outcome in patients following cardiac surgery, maybe in part because they can be modified by recent cardiopulmonary bypass or concomitant therapies such as mechanical ventilation, pacing and renal replacement therapy. Recently, the consensus definition of sepsis has been modified and examines changes in the sequential organ failure score (SOFA) from baseline (see Table 32.1). This new system has not been validated specifically in the cardiothoracic patient but may be more useful. However, since organ dysfunction can be the result of an inadequate cardiac output, patients may have elevations in their SOFA score for an alternative reason.

Clinicians often use laboratory investigations to guide their assessment of the presence of infection. However, it is normal for the C-reactive protein (CRP) and white cell count to increase following cardiac surgery even in the absence of infection; whether the magnitudes of these changes are greater in the setting of concomitant infection is not clear. Procalcitonin (PCT) is a peptide biomarker that has greater sensitivity and specificity for bacterial sepsis, and its resolution, than other cytokines or CRP. It has been employed in general populations of critically ill patients to limit the initiation or duration of antibiotic therapy. PCT rises following cardiopulmonary bypass with levels exceeding thresholds used in other populations to define bacterial infection. Even higher levels of PCT are observed with infection following cardiac surgery, but whether modifying antimicrobial practices based on these higher thresholds impacts on patient outcomes has never been tested. Moreover, in one study over half of patients with mediastinal infections did not have increased PCT levels.

The nature of the infecting organisms may be revealed by standard microbiological investigations of samples from normally sterile sites. Frequently these investigations are negative in the context of prior initiation of antibiotic therapy. Molecular techniques such as 16S RNA sequencing of tissues and fluids can be invaluable in settings such as infective endocarditis where standard techniques fail due to the presence of antibiotics or fastidious organisms. Similarly, PCR based assays of respiratory samples can identify pathogenic viruses and *Pneumocystis jirovecii* rapidly. 1,3 beta-D-glucan assay, mannan and anti-mannan antibody assays may help diagnose invasive fungal infection. Close liaison with a clinical microbiologist or infectious disease specialist is important.

Therefore, ultimately the diagnosis of an infected patient is based on clinical judgement of the clinical

Table 32.1 SOFA (sequential organ failure assessment) score

Variables	0	1	2	3	4
Respiratory PaO$_2$/FiO$_2$ mmHg	>400	<400	<300	<200	<100
Coagulation Platelets × 10^3/µl	>150	<150	<100	<50	<20
Cardiovascular Hypotension	No hypotension	MAP <70 mmHg	Dopamine <5 µg/kg/min	Dopamine >5 µg/kg/min Epinephrine <0.1 µg/kg/min, or Norepinephrine <0.1 µg/kg/min	Dopamine >15 µg/kg/min Epinephrine >0.1 µg/kg/min Norepinephrine >0.1 µg/kg/min
Central nervous system Glasgow coma scale	15	13–14	10–12	6–9	<6
Renal Creatinine µg/dl OR Urine output ml/dl	<1.2	1.2–1.9	2.0–3.4	3.5–4.9	>5.0 or <200
Liver Bilirubin mg/dl	<1.2	1.2–1.9	2.0–5.9	6.0–11.9	>12

setting, laboratory results cogniscent that they may change for other reasons, microbiological data available and other investigations such as the chest radiograph.

General Clinical Management

The Surviving Sepsis Campaign has done much to educate clinicians about sepsis. It has created evidence-based guidelines for the management of patients with sepsis which are wide ranging and cover many aspects of care including antibiotic therapy, processes of care, management of concomitant respiratory failure and fluid resuscitation. Protocolisation of aspects of care has been associated with improved outcomes. Some of the key recommendations are highlighted in Table 32.2 and these are equally applicable to patients with cardiothoracic illness.

The guidelines published in 2012 have been modified recently to remove specific goals of initial fluid resuscitation based on the central venous pressure and venous oxygen saturations. Three well-conducted large multicentre randomised trials – ProMISe, ProCess and ARISE – did not demonstrate a benefit of targeting these parameters during initial fluid resuscitation. Moreover, it is likely that optimal fluid resuscitation strategies may differ in patients with intrinsic cardiac dysfunction.

The hallmark circulatory changes associated with severe infection are arterial and venous vasodilatation and increased vascular permeability resulting in tissue oedema. This causes systemic hypotension that is mitigated normally by the physiological response of an increased cardiac output. Healthy adults can increase their cardiac index to well in excess of 4–5 l/min/m^2. This may not be possible in those with heart failure, valvular heart disease or with therapies such as beta-adrenoreceptor blockade. Typically, clinicians administer considerable volumes of intravascular fluid to combat the increased venous compliance and hypotension. However, consideration should be given to the effects of further fluid administration on stroke volume (the primary goal of fluid administration) and the balance between the need to increase cardiac output versus the need to increase vascular tone with drugs such as noradrenaline and vasopressin. Consideration of these factors is ever more important in those with cardiac disease. For example, excessive fluid administration may adversely affect right ventricular dysfunction, which may be exacerbated by the increase in pulmonary vascular resistance that can occur during sepsis and systemic inflammation. Hypotension can be exacerbated further by the myocardial dysfunction related to systemic sepsis per se. In some settings inotrope therapy may be indicated.

Table 32.2 Excerpt from Surviving Sepsis (2012) recommendations

Recommendation	Grade of recommendation*
Give antibiotics early	1B (septic shock) 1C (severe sepsis)
Identify (e.g. take microbiological cultures) and control the source of infection early, for example drain an abscess	1C
Crystalloids are the first choice for intravascular fluid replacement	1B
Human albumin solution can be considered in patients requiring considerable amounts of crystalloid; avoid starch solutions	1C
Noradrenaline is the first choice vasopressor	1B
Protocolised blood sugar management should aim for a blood glucose <180 mg/dl (10 mM)	1A
Hydrocortisone (200 mg/day) should only be considered if fluids and vasopressors do not restore haemodynamic stability	2C

* Grade 1 recommendations are strong; Grade 2 are weak. The quality of the evidence is indicated as high (A, based on randomised controlled trials), moderate (B, downgraded RCTs or upgraded observational studies), low (C, well conducted observational studies with control RCTs) or very low (D, downgraded controlled studies or expert opinion).

No study demonstrates a specific inotrope to be superior, but anecdotally milrinone is often associated with worsening vasoplegia and many prefer dobutamine or small to moderate doses of adrenaline. A recent study of levosimendan, a myocardial calcium sensitiser, showed no advantage in preventing organ dysfunction or mortality in sepsis.

Corticosteroids have been demonstrated to reduce the duration of hypotension in a general critical care population whilst not impacting on mortality. Restoration of the shock state may beneficially enhance coronary perfusion in those with coronary artery disease or significant right heart failure due to pulmonary hypertension.

Management of Specific Infections

Endocarditis

Infective endocarditis (IE) is a challenging condition with poor outcomes for patients. In hospital mortality rates are as high as 30%. Its incidence is increasing at least in part due to the increasing number of patients at risk, for example those with intracardiac prosthetic material.

The management of infective endocarditis is complex and best undertaken by teams. Critical care physicians are often involved either following valvular interventions or if patients present with complications such as heart failure, uncontrolled infection or embolisation. Right sided endocarditis is less common and more often associated with intravenous drug abuse, congenital heart disease or invasive vascular devices such as central lines or pacing systems. It is generally tolerated better haemodynamically than left sided disease. Right sided endocarditis presents typically with multiple pulmonary septic emboli which may be manifested by breathlessness, chest pain and haemoptysis.

Antimicrobial therapy is the cornerstone of therapy in IE and choice of antibiotic is influenced by whether the endocarditis is on a native valve or prosthetic valve, the organism and the minimum inhibitory concentration (MIC) for a particular organism/antibiotic combination. There is less emphasis on aminoglycosides in recent guidelines due to renal toxicity. Rifampicin should not be instituted immediately as it probably has an antagonistic effect against other antibiotics with respect to replicating bacteria.

Heart failure may occur due to severe valvular regurgitation, a fistula (e.g. an acquired Gerbode ventriculoatrial defect) or rarely valvular obstruction. Severe heart failure refractory to medical therapies is an indication for expedited surgery.

Uncontrolled infection must be considered when fever persists or there is progressive perivalvular extension of infection as manifest by complications such as an aortic root abscess, fistula or pseudoaneurysms. Typically blood cultures become negative in a few days. New prolongation of the PR interval should raise suspicion of aortic root abscesses.

Cerebral embolisation from left sided endocarditis is a concern and can be associated with haemorrhagic transformation too. The risks of embolisation fall progressively following institution of antimicrobial therapy.

Surgery during the active phase of endocarditis has high risks and in general it is deferred until 4–6 weeks. Nevertheless it may be expedited in the setting of severe heart failure, uncontrolled infection or prevention of emboli.

Infections of Implanted Devices

Infection of implanted pacing systems or cardioverter defibrillators is increasing as more devices are inserted. It can be difficult to manage and may be associated with mortality as high as 10–22%. Infection can be in one or more of the endocardium, leads, or device and its pocket. Estimates of the incidence range from 0.5% to 2.2%. Risk factors for infection include inexperienced operators, low frequency of air changes in the operating environment, diabetes mellitus and renal failure. Management strategies include antibiotics and device removal. Device removal may be complex in those who are dependent on a device and if leads have been present for some time when they may become adherent to vascular structures. Device and lead removal may be complicated by bleeding, tamponade, pulmonary embolism and death.

Infection is a frequent complication of long term durable ventricular assist devices. Driveline infection is the most common and usually occurs at the exit site but infections may occur anywhere along the driveline up to the device pocket, or in the device or cannulae. Typically there is local trauma at the exit site or an inadvertent tug on the line. This underpins the careful initial surgical placement of the driveline and dressings that stabilise the line. Management strategies include the simultaneous use of antibiotics, fastidious exit site cleaning and source control with debridement of infected tissue and drainage of collections. Rarely, device exchange or cardiac transplantation may be considered.

Ventilator Associated Pneumonia

Ventilator associated pneumonia (VAP) is common following cardiac surgery, with an estimated incidence of 21–27 cases per 1000 ventilator days. It is more common in those undergoing emergency surgery, prolonged cardiopulmonary bypass and those with underlying lung disease, pulmonary hypertension, renal disease or New York Heart Associate (NYHA) class IV heart failure. It is associated with a prolonged ICU stay and increased mortality. It is felt that prolonged anaesthesia, hypothermia and underlying pulmonary pathology are key factors underpinning these increased risks.

Several interventions can lower the incidence of VAP (see Table 32.3). They are often bundled together with other interventions that ventilated patients may benefit from in a quality improvement strategy. Most aim to prevent contamination of the respiratory tract by colonised oral secretions or reflux of gastric contents.

Caring for patients in a semi-recumbent position rather than supine reduces VAP rates. The optimal position is not known, but most aim for an angle of over 30°.

Whilst peptic ulcer prophylaxis reduces the morbidity related to stress ulceration, it does so at the expense of increasing the incidence of VAP. Thus H2 antagonists and proton pump inhibitors should be discontinued in those at low risk of stress ulceration such as those that are fully fed enterally, do not have low cardiac output states, are not systemically anticoagulated and with no prior history of peptic ulcer disease.

Studies of oral decontamination with chlorhexidine have had mixed results in the general critical care population. Two meta-analyses suggest that patients who have undergone cardiac surgery particularly benefit from this strategy. It has an unpleasant taste for patients and does not obviate the use of fluoride containing toothpaste too.

Daily interruptions or retitration of sedative medications reduced the duration of mechanical ventilation and thus the exposure of individual patients to the risk of acquiring a VAP. It may reduce the incidence of VAP per se.

The benefits of subglottic suctioning on endotracheal tubes have been demonstrated in two meta-analyses. Suctioning reduces the pool of oral sections that collect above the endotracheal cuff and thus may reduce the contamination of the lower respiratory tract. The cost of the endotracheal tubes may act as a barrier for their use in all cardiothoracic surgical procedures, and the value of routine changes in patients who stay over a defined period of time has not been investigated. Nevertheless, it would seem prudent to use them in all patients who are reintubated following cardiac surgery as many of these patients stay on the ICU for prolonged periods of time.

Selective digestive decontamination (SDD) is the administration of broad spectrum antimicrobials

Table 32.3 Possible strategies to reduce ventilator associated pneumonia

Semi-recumbent patient positioning
Appropriate stress ulcer prophylaxis
Oral decontamination with chlorhexidine
Sedation interruptions
Subglottic suctioning
Selective digestive decontamination

enterally to reduce the pathogenic flora of the intestinal tract. Aerobic Gram-negative organisms are targeted particularly. Enteral agents include polymixin, colistin, tobramycin, nystatin and amphotericin that are poorly absorbed. They are combined with a short course of broad spectrum systemic antimicrobials such as ciprofloxacin or a cephalosporin. Meta-analyses have demonstrated reduced rates of VAP but concerns about the generation of multiantibiotic resistant infections have limited the adoption of SDD into clinical practice. Two large international studies are planned (SuDDICO – clinicaltrials.gov reference NCT02389036; RGNOSIS – clinical trials.gov reference NCY02208154) which may redress this clinical equipoise.

Monitoring rates of VAP on an individual ICU are complicated by difficulties in the commonly used definition. Many rely on clinical signs and changes in the chest radiograph which are subjective and not specific. The Centers for Disease Control and Prevention (CDC) has recently described a clinical entity of ventilator associated events using objective data that are relatively easy to collect electronically. In the setting of data suggesting infection then this may be upgraded to a diagnosis of VAP. The tools may be useful for surveillance within a specific unit. Local practices in ventilator setting can influence the rates, making inter-hospital comparisons difficult, although others have reported little inter-hospital variation (Table 32.3).

Central Line Associated Blood Stream Infections (CLABSI)

Central venous access is frequently required in the cardiothoracic ICU for the administration of vasoactive agents, renal replacement therapy and the measurement of cardiac output. Central line associated blood stream infections are associated with increased mortality in patients. The consequences may be worse in patients on cardiothoracic ICUs as it may result in endocarditis, infection of prosthetic valves and pacing systems.

Table 32.4 Strategies recommended to reduce CLABSI

Hand hygiene prior to catheter insertion or manipulation
2% chlorhexidine skin preparation prior to line insertion
Strict maximal aseptic technique during line insertion
Avoid femoral access
Remove all non-essential central lines
Disinfect hubs and injection ports prior to accessing the line

Many consider CLABSIs to be preventable. Multiple strategies (Table 32.4) can reduce the incidence of infection. The role of chlorhexidine impregnated dressings and patches or antibiotic/chlorhexidine/silver impregnated catheters is not clear. These strategies are often bundled together as a quality improvement initiative. In Pronovost's landmark study, this approach caused a sustained reduction in rates by 66%, which was confirmed subsequently in a randomised study. Globally, many countries have adopted this bundled approach.

Continuous monitoring of infection rates is important for any ICU. A typical target would be less than 1 infection per 1000 catheter days, although data collection is difficult and can vary between centres. The CDC has strict definitions of laboratory confirmed infection but does not define the scenario of suspected infection that could not be confirmed in the laboratory. In practice many central lines are replaced due to concerns about infection, although this is not subsequently proven even when the original concerns, such as elevated biomarkers of infection, are subsequently allayed. Monitoring of suspected infection rates would probably be an additional metric in any quality improvement process.

Surgical Site Infections

Sternal wound infections are a serious complication following cardiac surgery. Whilst superficial infections often increase length of stay in hospital, deep infections are associated with substantial morbidity and mortality. Deep infections are defined as those that are associated with sternal dehiscence or infections down to the sternum even if the sternum is stable. Risk factors include diabetes mellitus, bilateral mammary artery harvest, obesity, chronic obstructive pulmonary disease, prolonged surgery, surgical re-exploration and delayed sternal closure for haemodynamic compromise

Strategies to prevent deep sternal infection include preoperative skin care, prophylactic antibiotics prior to the surgical incision and aseptic surgical technique. Gentamicin impregnated sponges and beads have not been shown conclusively to reduce deep sternal infections and have not been adopted into routine practice.

The management of deep sternal wound infections requires liaison between the cardiac surgeon, plastic surgeon and microbiologist. Coagulase negative staphylococci (usually *Staphylococcus epidermidis*) are the most common aetiological organisms. Prolonged courses of antibiotics are often required and following surgical debridement it is often necessary to fill the defect with a myocutaneous flap such as a latissimus dorsi flap.

Conclusions

Infection impacts on our patients. Avoiding healthcare associated infections is probably the greatest benefit that we can afford our patients. Ventilator associated pneumonia and central line associated blood stream infection are frequent and are avoided through processes of care.

Broad spectrum antibiotics administered to patients for prolonged periods of time promote the development of multidrug resistant organisms and *Clostridium difficile* diarrhoea. Management of infected patients centres around appropriate early antibiotic therapy, source control and preservation of organ perfusion through the administration of intravenous fluids, intropes and vasoconstrictors.

Learning Points

- Many patients display significant systemic inflammation which manifests as vasoplegia, raised biomarkers and organ dysfunction following cardiothoracic surgery. It can be difficult to determine whether concomitant infection is a significant driver.
- The Surviving Sepsis Campaign guides clinicians in the evidence-based management of patients with sepsis and is usually equally applicable to patients with cardiorespiratory disease.
- Patients with cardiac dysfunction may not be able to increase their cardiac outputs to counter vasoplegia. Their response to intravascular fluid replacement may be different.
- Healthcare associated infections are common following cardiothoracic surgery, particularly ventilator associated pneumonia, central line associated blood stream infections and surgical site infections. Clinicians can prevent many of these infections and should measure their incidence as part of a quality assurance strategy.
- Endocarditis is a challenging condition best managed by a team of surgeons, cardiologists, microbiologists, intensivists and imaging experts.

Further Reading

Dellinger RP, Levy MM, Rhodes A, et al. Surviving Sepsis Campaign: international guidelines for management of severe sepsis and septic shock: 2012. *Critical Care Medicine*. 2013; 41: 580–637.

Epstein AE, DiMarco JP, Ellenbogen KA, et al. ACC/AHA/HRS 2008 Guidelines for Device-Based Therapy of Cardiac Rhythm Abnormalities: a report of the American College of Cardiology/American Heart Association Task Force on Practice Guidelines (Writing Committee to Revise the ACC/AHA/NASPE 2002 Guideline Update for Implantation of Cardiac Pacemakers and Antiarrhythmia Devices): developed in collaboration with the American Association for Thoracic Surgery and Society of Thoracic Surgeons. *Circulation*. 2008; 117: e350–408.

Habib G, Lancellotti P, Antunes MJ, et al. 2015 ESC Guidelines for the Management of Infective Endocarditis: The Task Force for the Management of Infective Endocarditis of the European Society of Cardiology (ESC). Endorsed by: European Association for Cardio-Thoracic Surgery (EACTS), the European Association of Nuclear Medicine (EANM). *European Heart Journal*. 2015; 36: 3075–3128.

He S, Chen B, Li W, et al. Ventilator-associated pneumonia after cardiac surgery: a meta-analysis and systematic review. *Journal of Thoracic and Cardiovascular Surgery*. 2014; 148: 3148–3155, e3141–3145.

Michalopoulos A, Geroulanos S, Rosmarakis ES, Falagas ME. Frequency, characteristics, and predictors of microbiologically documented nosocomial infections after cardiac surgery. *European Journal of Cardiothoracic Surgery*. 2006; 29: 456–460.

Pronovost P, Needham D, Berenholtz S, et al. An intervention to decrease catheter-related bloodstream infections in the ICU. *New England Journal of Medicine*. 2006; 355: 2725–2732.

Romero-Bermejo FJ, Ruiz-Bailen M, Gil-Cebrian J, Huertos-Ranchal MJ. Sepsis-induced cardiomyopathy. *Current Cardiology Reviews*. 2011; 7: 163–183.

Siempos II, Kopterides P, Tsangaris I, Dimopoulou I, Armaganidis AE. Impact of catheter-related bloodstream infections on the mortality of critically ill patients: a meta-analysis. *Critical Care Medicine*. 2009; 37: 2283–2289.

Singer M, Deutschman CS, Seymour CW, et al. The Third International Consensus Definitions for Sepsis and Septic Shock (Sepsis-3). *Journal of the American Medical Association*. 2016; 315: 801–810.

Thuny F, Grisoli D, Collart F, Habib G, Raoult D. Management of infective endocarditis: challenges and perspectives. *Lancet*. 2012; 379: 965–975.

MCQs

1. **Which of the following parameters have high sensitivity for infection in the first few days following cardiac surgery?**
   (a) White blood cell count
   (b) C-reactive protein
   (c) Pro-calcitonin
   (d) All of the above ((a)–(c))
   (e) None of the above ((a)–(c))

2. **Regarding ventilator associated pneumonias, which of the following interventions has NOT been shown to reduce the incidence in patients who have undergone cardiac surgery?**
   (a) Semi-recumbent patient positioning
   (b) Daily change of ventilator circuit
   (c) Oral hygiene with 2% w/v chlorhexidine
   (d) Avoidance of acid suppression therapies
   (e) None of the above

3. **Which one of the following is NOT an indication for expediting surgery in infective endocarditis?**
   (a) Mitral regurgitation
   (b) Heart failure, refractory to diuretics
   (c) Uncontrolled infection
   (d) Prosthetic valve whose sewing ring is loose on TOE
   (e) Repeated cerebral emboli

4. **Which is the best parameter to target during intravenous fluid resuscitation of patients with cardiac disease and proven septic shock?**
   (a) Central venous/right atrial pressure
   (b) Stroke volume
   (c) Central venous oxygen saturations
   (d) Urine output
   (e) Arterial lactate

5. **Which of the following parameters should be assessed in infective endocarditis of the aortic valve?**
   (a) MIC of antibiotics for the organism
   (b) PR interval
   (c) Blood cultures after a few days
   (d) Only (a) and (b)
   (e) All of the above ((a)–(c))

Exercise answers are available on p.469. Alternatively, take the test online at www.cambridge.org/CardiothoracicMCQ

Chapter 33 Seizures

Ari Ercole and Lara Prisco

Introduction

Seizures are common in intensive care patients generally and cardiac surgery or post-cardiac arrest patients are at particular risk. Seizures are an important and potentially reversible cause of prolonged unconsciousness as well as being associated with poorer ICU outcome, although the latter may be multifactorial. Cerebral metabolic rate is greatly increased during seizure activity, which may lead to energetic crisis and neuronal injury. Non-convulsive seizures are particularly common in ICU patients and are under-recognised. Electroencephalography (EEG) is therefore an essential ICU investigation for the diagnosis of seizures or epileptiform activity and for distinguishing these from other disorders of consciousness, which may have characteristic EEG signatures. Continuous EEG (cEEG) is particularly sensitive for clinically occult seizures and is also helpful for managing seizures refractory to simple treatment. However, EEG requires specific expertise to perform and interpret which can be a barrier to its use in the cardiothoracic intensive care unit.

The Burden and Characteristics of Seizures in Intensive Care

Seizures are common but under-recognised in the ICU. Subclinical electrographic seizure activity is common in neurosciences patients but may also occur in critically ill patients without a history of seizures. Most studies show a prevalence of seizures of 15–40% and identify the presence of seizures and status epilepticus as independent predictors of poorer outcome. To what extent this represents a modifiable pathology or an epiphenomenon of worse underlying neurological injury is uncertain. However, prolonged seizure activity is associated with neuronal energetic failure and injury. Therefore recognition and treatment of seizures is important. Furthermore, seizures are also an important reversible cause of unconsciousness and should be considered in the differential diagnosis of a patient who does not wake appropriately from sedation or anaesthesia.

Clinically apparent seizures are due to focal or global disorganised brain electrical activity and may be manifest as changes in behaviour/level of consciousness or abnormal movements. However, in sedated or critically ill patients, none of these findings may be clinically obvious or apparent. The diagnosis of true seizures is complicated by other types of abnormal movements that may be seen in intensive care patients (such as shivering, myoclonus, tremor, emergence from neuromuscular blockade). A systematic approach to distinguishing seizures from non-seizure movements is helpful (Figure 33.1).

Most clinical seizures are self-limiting. Patients will regain consciousness although a postictal period of altered mental state is common due to neurotransmitter depletion, changes in receptor concentration/inhibition or altered cerebral blood flow. Sometimes clinical seizures may be prolonged or repeated. Status epilepticus (SE) is defined as 'an acute epileptic condition characterised by continuous generalised convulsive seizures for at least five minutes, or by two seizures without full recovery of consciousness between them'. Electrographic seizure activity may also occur without movement, and this is particularly important in ICU patients. Such non-convulsive seizures (NCS) are a more elusive diagnosis that is frequently unrecognised. Its incidence after cardiac surgery is probably particularly high due to exposure of the patient to some degree of subclinical embolic phenomena, metabolic derangement, hypotension or proconvulsive drugs. Non-convulsive SE (NCSE) is further defined as an electrographic diagnosis of 'continuous or intermittent ictal discharges without the patient regaining consciousness, and no overt clinical signs of convulsive activity'. NCSE is often suspected in patients who

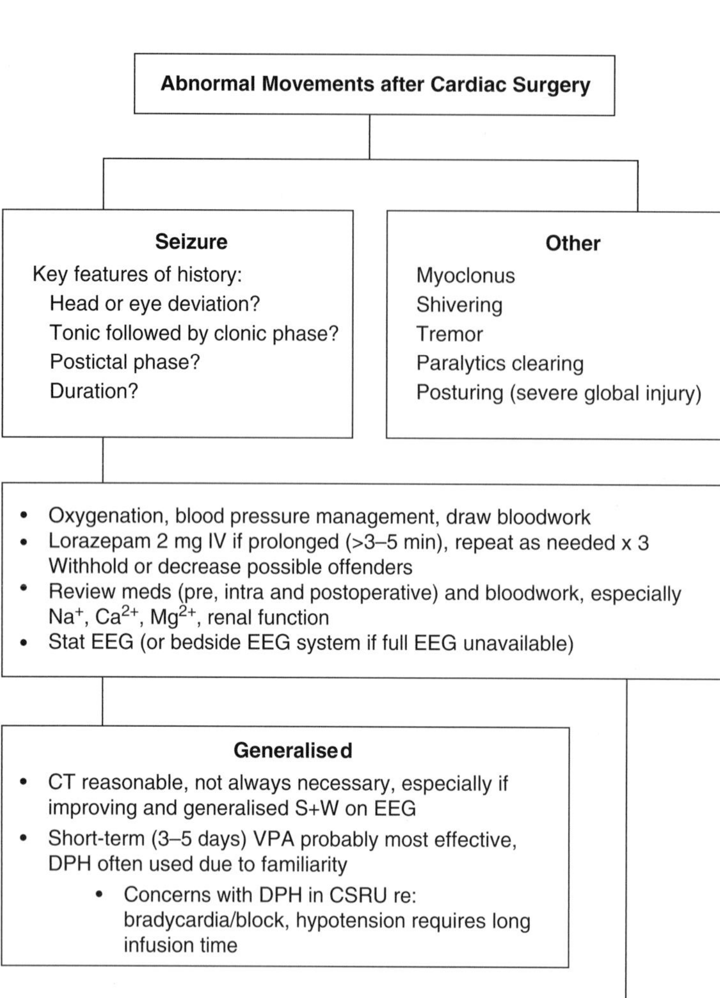

Figure 33.1 The diagnosis and initial management of seizures after cardiac surgery. After Hunter and Young (2011), with permission. VPA valproate; DPH phenytoin; SRU seizures after cardiac surgery; LOC NYD altered level of consciousness not yet diagnosed.

were in convulsive SE and subsequently do not fully regain consciousness. Hence, if coma persists after SE, EEG is necessary to identify the cause of unconsciousness (NCSE or a postictal state). However, it may occur de novo in ICU patients and this represents a particular diagnostic challenge.

NCS have been reported in up to 37% of critically ill patients undergoing cEEG monitoring. The highest proportion of NCS is seen in patients who underwent emergency EEGs for altered mental status and clinically suspected NCSE. Studies prospectively performing EEGs in unselected comatose patients without clinical signs of seizures found either NCS or NCSE in up to 8% of cases.

Electroencephalography

Given the diagnostic difficulties presented by critically ill patients, the unequivocal detection/exclusion of seizures often requires EEG. This is a technique that measures the spatial distribution of voltage fields on

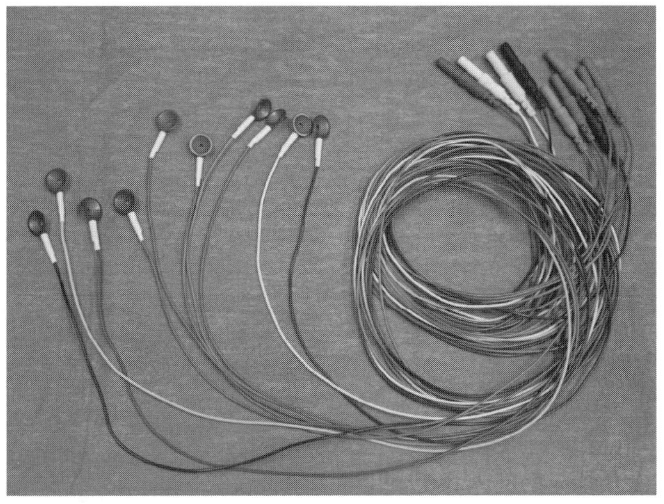

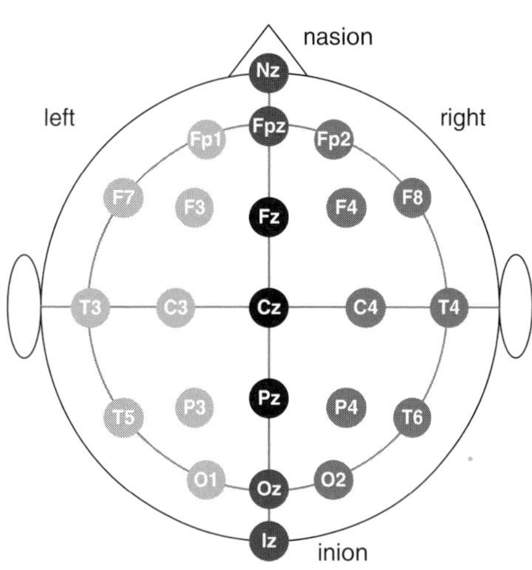

Figure 33.2 Left panel: typical EEG scalp electrodes for clinical use. Right panel: international 10–20 system for standard scalp electrode placement. The distances between adjacent electrodes are either 10% or 20% of the total anterior/posterior or left/right distance. Left and right are distinguished by odd and even numbers respectively. Each channel of the EEG is obtained by measuring the voltage between adjacent electrodes (bipolar montage, such as here) or of individual electrodes compared to a reference electrode or combination of electrodes (referential montage). (A black and white version of this figure will appear in some formats. For the colour version, please refer to the plate section.)

the scalp and their variation over time. The origin of this activity is thought to reflect the fluctuating sum of excitatory and inhibitory postsynaptic potentials that arise primarily from apical dendrites of pyramidal cells in the outer layer of the cerebral cortex under the input from subcortical structures.

The potentials recorded by the EEG are very small (of the order of microvolts) and are therefore easily contaminated by electrical noise and other artefacts such as the electromyogram when trying to record from areas with larger underlying muscles. Furthermore, EEG changes may be relatively localised, meaning that an array of electrodes is needed to cover the whole scalp adequately. Finally, seizures may occur intermittently and so continuous recordings (cEEG) over 12–24 hours or even longer are needed to realise the highest diagnostic sensitivity. Such considerations make recording a clinically useful EEG much more complex and involved than, say, an ECG. The American Clinical Neurophysiology Society has published recommendations for recording ICU cEEG. Equipment, length of recording and electrode montages should meet the technical standards defined in these consensus statements (Figure 33.2).

Even in the absence of seizures, the EEG shows stereotypical changes with consciousness, which can be diagnostically useful. EEG activity can be classified by frequency, amplitude, distribution or location, symmetry, synchrony, reactivity (to external stimulation), morphology, rhythmicity and regulation. The signal frequencies detected by a standard clinical EEG are divided into four standard frequency ranges or 'bands': alpha (8 to <13 Hz, usually occipital), beta (>13 to 25 Hz, usually frontal and central), theta (4 to <8 Hz, usually central or diffuse) and delta (<4 Hz, focal or diffuse).

The most important EEG pattern of wakefulness is a posterior dominant rhythm (PDR). The PDR is located predominantly at the occipital poles but becomes anterior as the patient becomes drowsy (normal sleep). This activity is normally in the alpha range and is symmetrical. Slower rhythms such as generalised continuous delta are always abnormal and are usually associated with diffuse or multifocal cortical injury or metabolic derangement. Intermittent slowing, such as intermittent rhythmic delta activity (IRDA) and frontal IRDA (FIRDA) or occipital IRDA (OIRDA) are thought to be caused by dysfunction in subcortical centres influencing cortical activation and may represent a manifestation of a more generalised process not limited to the frontal or occipital lobes.

Reactivity refers to a clinical (electromyographic activity, respiratory pattern change) and/or EEG response (increased continuity, amplitude reduction, frequency change) to external stimulation (pain, passive eyes opening, auditory stimuli). In cardiac arrest patients, a non-reactive EEG background after rewarming is associated with poor neurological outcome. However, the association is complex: this pattern is still compatible with good recovery when observed during therapeutic hypothermia and patients with myoclonus and no EEG reactivity within 72 hours from cardiac arrest have occasionally gone on to have good outcomes.

Electrographic seizures are characterised by repetitive or rhythmic focal or generalised epileptiform discharges at greater than 3 Hz, and lasting more than 10 seconds or at less than 3 Hz but with clear evolution in frequency, location, waveform or field or clinical manifestation. They usually resolve or improve after administration of rapid acting intravenous antiepileptic drugs such as benzodiazepines. The electrographic features of SE are highly variable, including rhythmic, generalised and symmetric spike-and-waves or polyspikes-and-waves at 2 to 3.5 Hz, or atypical spike-and-wave with lower frequency and less symmetry, or multiple spike-and-wave, or high voltage, repetitive, rhythmic (focal or generalised) delta activity with interspersed spikes, sharp waves or sharp components (Figure 33.3).

If continuous EEG is not available, multiple intermittent serial recordings are desirable as seizures may otherwise be missed, especially as high dose anaesthetics are weaned. Whilst the EEG does not change significantly at body temperatures between 32 and 34°C, sedative drugs commonly used during therapeutic hypothermia can markedly affect the EEG background.

Regular electrode maintenance, scalp inspections, keeping the scalp dry and reducing pressure on the scalp from the electrodes is important to avoid scalp injuries. Sweating and scalp breakdown are more common in patients with fever, sepsis and prolonged systemic disease requiring frequent changes of electrodes. Hypothermia presents a theoretically increased risk of coagulopathy. However, scalp breakdown with bleeding or infection has not been reported among postarrest patients treated with therapeutic hypothermia (even up to several days of cEEG with either disposable or reusable versions of disc electrodes, Figure 33.2).

The EEG is typically recorded for later off-line analysis by a neurophysiologist. To this end the use of simultaneous video recording is recommended to identify sources of artefact and must be correctly repositioned when the staff moves either the patient or the camera of the EEG acquisition unit. Routine ICU care such as physiotherapy, suctioning and oral care can create rhythmic artefacts that mimic electrographic seizures but are easily identified with video analysis.

EEG electrode technology is sophisticated. The low voltages involved mean that very low electrical impedances are required. Poor contact renders the electrodes susceptible to electrical interference. Electrical noise from intravenous pumps, electrical beds, dialysis machines and other medical devices can obscure the EEG recording and requires proper identification and trouble-shooting.

Specialised hardware and software increase the utility of cEEG for monitoring at the bedside. Options include the ability to enter nursing notes, pushbuttons for seizures and other clinical events, software to integrate physiological data, and quantitative EEG software for graphical display of quantitative EEG trends.

Causes and Prognostic Significance of Seizures in Intensive Care

The dominant aetiology and prognostic significance of seizures in the cardiothoracic intensive care unit varies from patient to patient. Three distinct patient populations are of particular importance in the cardiac ICU: those who are post cardiac surgery (where embolic phenomena are likely to be important), patients successfully resuscitated from cardiac arrest (where hypoxic-ischaemic injury dominates) and those patients suffering from general critical illness.

Postcardiac Surgery

Postoperative seizures are known to complicate cardiac surgery with an incidence of up to 7% and recurrence rates of around 50%. This is almost certainly an underestimate, with NCS probably frequently missed and not necessarily benign. The manifestations and causes of seizures in the context of cardiac surgery are diverse, as are the expected outcomes. Both convulsive and non-convulsive seizures may contribute to prolonged reduced levels of consciousness, an increased length of stay in the ICU, and a possible increase in morbidity and mortality. Furthermore, convulsive seizures lead to cardiovascular strain and metabolic derangement in patients already in a fragile state.

Perioperative seizures may be caused by thromboembolic ischaemic stroke, cerebral air embolism, antibiotic toxicity or other perioperative drugs such as

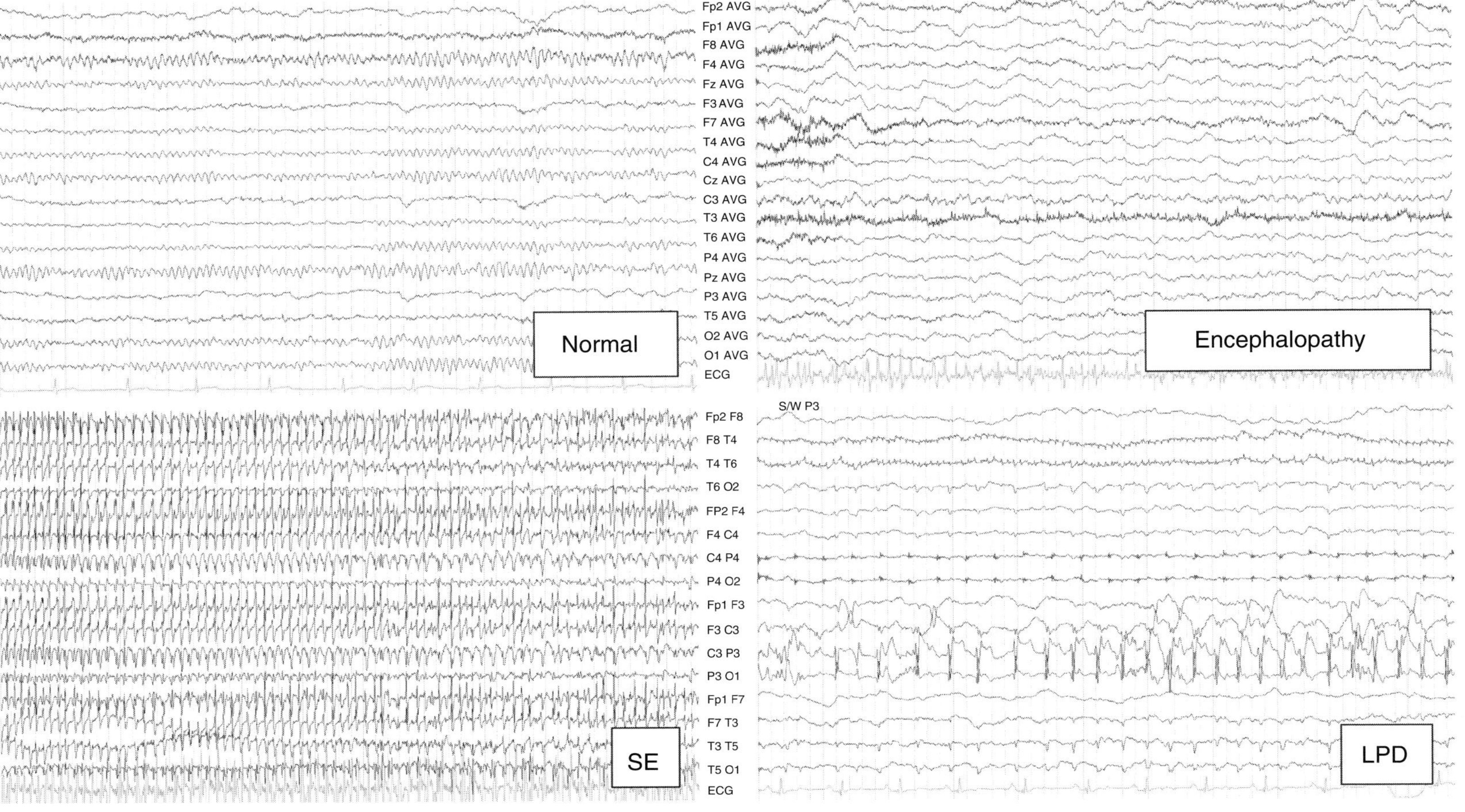

Figure 33.3 Examples of EEGs from the ICU. Top left: normal wakeful EEG, high frequencies with alpha wave activity dominant in posterior/occipital channels. Top right: encephalopathic EEG illustrating prominent slow (delta wave) activity. Bottom left: generalised seizure activity with sharp spikes and waves in all channels. Bottom right: LPDs, periodic spike discharges over the left hemisphere (odd numbered channels). (A black and white version of this figure will appear in some formats. For the colour version, please refer to the plate section.)

tranexamic acid (TXA). Several risk factors have been directly associated with the presence of postoperative seizures. Open-chamber procedures, including valve and aortic repairs and cardiac transplants, have a higher incidence of complications than does coronary artery bypass graft surgery. The combination of TXA administration, especially high doses (>80 mg/kg) and open-chamber surgery has been confirmed in several studies as an important perioperative factor. Higher preoperative creatinine (>120 μmol/l), thoracic aortic surgery and early seizures onset (<4 hours) have also been found to increase risk of recurrent seizures (RS). Despite longer ICU stay and duration of mechanical ventilation, the presence of RS is not associated with significantly increased long-term morbidity or mortality.

Postcardiac Arrest

Clinical seizures occur in up to 40% of patients following cardiac arrest, mostly in the first 3 to 5 days. Seizures most commonly present as diffuse or multifocal myoclonus or focal and generalised tonic-clonic seizures, and contribute to decreased level of consciousness; they have important implications for prognosis.

Non-convulsive seizures may occur and often present as NCSE.

NCSE after cardiac arrest is very difficult to treat, and it is not clear if treatment improves neurological outcome or mortality. However, it is common: post-arrest patients treated with therapeutic hypothermia and receiving routine EEG or cEEG monitoring have a prevalence of NCSE/SE of around 30%. Clinical seizures typically begin within the first 2 days following cardiac arrest but it is not uncommon to see earlier electrographic seizures on the EEG. Several studies have shown that initial electrographic seizures are typically not associated with any clinical correlate of myoclonus or other motor seizure types by day 2 to 3.

Myoclonus can also occur in patients with hypoxic brain injury and may be either acute or chronic. Acute post-hypoxic myoclonic status epilepticus (MSE) occurs soon after a hypoxic insult and is a clinical diagnosis consisting of unrelenting diffuse myoclonus involving the face, limbs and torso that is often precipitated by stimulation. It is strongly associated with poor outcome if onset is during the first 24 hours postarrest, and this association remains true with therapeutic hypothermia, although the onset may be delayed until 3 to 5 days after cardiac arrest. It is important to appreciate that although rare (less than 5%) there have been reports of survivors of MSE with good cognitive outcome. Most of these patients were treated with at least three to four antiepileptic drugs (including high dose anaesthetics), had preserved brainstem reflexes, intact cortical somatosensory evoked potential responses and reactive EEG backgrounds.

Subcortical structures are involved in MSE and therefore the EEG does not show the same electrographic features. Instead the EEG may show generalised periodic discharges (GPDs) and/or a burst suppression pattern. A brainstem origin of postanoxic myoclonus may be suspected when there is sequential activation of muscles innervated by cranial nerves (reticular reflex myoclonus) and characterised by non-specific EEG changes (non-epileptiform patterns such as diffuse alpha activity). By contrast, cortical action-reflex myoclonus instead presents with epileptiform discharges and/or polyspikes and typically (but not necessarily) affects a few muscles in a localised distribution.

MSE may be confused with chronic post-hypoxic myoclonus (Lance–Adams Syndrome, LAS). LAS is a distinct entity that may also appear after a period of cerebral hypoxia in patients with a more prolonged coma or period of sedation. In contrast to MSE, LAS develops later, days or weeks after the initial hypoxic event, and does not respond to anticonvulsant treatment. Crucially, however, such patients regain consciousness, but may exhibit muscle jerks affecting face, trunk or limbs often provoked by sensory stimuli and strikingly elicited by the willed voluntary action. LAS is rare, but its differentiation from MSE is important to avoid incorrect prognostication and for the institution of timely rehabilitation.

General Intensive Care Considerations

In the cardiac ICU, anoxic brain injury is a common cause of severe encephalopathy as well as seizures, and ischaemic or haemorrhagic stroke must be suspected in patients who had cardiac surgery and develop postoperative seizures or SE. However, there are many possible causes for seizures in the critically ill and a single cause may often never be identified.

Sepsis is the most frequent cause of altered mental status in the general ICU as sepsis related encephalopathy has been associated with neuronal damage, mitochondrial and endothelial injury, and disturbances in neurotransmission. Metabolic alterations due to hepatic and/or renal dysfunction can lead to a background of encephalopathy.

Other primary systemic diseases can present as altered mental status and are associated with seizures (such as posterior-reversible leukoencephalopathy secondary to malignant hypertension, eclampsia, metabolic and electrolyte disturbances, embolic cerebral infarcts or mycotic aneurysms from endocarditis, central nervous system vasculitis from an underlying autoimmune disease such as polyarteritis nodosa, systemic lupus erythematosus, and Sjøgren's syndrome, paraneoplastic syndromes and limbic encephalitis).

Transplant patients in the postsurgical ICU are another population at risk for altered mental status and seizures. Seizures in these patients are often multifactorial with causes including severe metabolic derangements, toxicity from immunosuppressive therapy, and other postoperative complications. Central nervous system infections are an important cause of seizures, and this is of particular significance in patients who are immunosuppressed.

Management of Seizures

SE is an emergency and must be treated aggressively and early as the longer an episode of SE persists, the more refractory the patient will become to treatment. Also, clinically evident seizures should be treated immediately without waiting for the EEG but cEEG should ideally be started if a patient requires continuous neuromuscular blockade after initial treatment with antiepileptic drugs (AEDs).

It is important to assess and manage the patient's airway because apnoea or airway soiling can occur with generalised seizures and intubation may be required. The use of short-acting paralytics is preferable for intubation so that on-going seizure activity will not be masked. Autonomic instability may accompany seizures and cardiovascular support may be required.

Once SE has become established, rapid administration of intravenous therapy is required to control seizures. Whilst any benzodiazepine may be effective, lorazepam is the drug of choice as it has a long redistribution half-life (3–10 hours) reducing the likelihood of rebound seizures. If the first bolus (usually 2–4 mg in adults) fails, then a second bolus can be given followed by a loading dose of phenytoin (20 mg/kg infused at a maximum rate of 50 mg/minute).

A significant minority of patients with SE may be refractory to adequate doses of two AEDs. If SE has not responded to this first line treatment and lasts 60–90 minutes, patients will risk physiological compromise, neuronal damage and increasing drug resistance. The patient should be anaesthetised and transferred to the ICU to stop seizure activity. Propofol is likely to be the most familiar agent and is an effective anticonvulsant, although midazolam may be employed. More rarely barbiturates such as thiopentone may be required but specialist advice should be sought.

Laboratory tests to pursue include the following: blood glucose, full blood count, metabolic profile, liver function test, magnesium, phosphate, urine toxicology, serum ethanol levels, troponin, creatine kinase (CK), urinalysis, urine and blood cultures, and AEDs levels. If vitamin B1 deficiency is suspected (history of dietary insufficiency/inadequacy), intravenous thiamine should be administered before giving glucose to avoid precipitation of Wernicke's encephalopathy. Acid-base alterations and hyperthermia are common during SE and should be treated as soon as possible. A degree of rhabdomyolysis is common and can lead to acute kidney injury or even renal failure. Depending on CK levels, urine output should be maintained and alkalinisation with intravenous sodium bicarbonate considered. If CK is severely elevated, then renal replacement should be commenced from the outset to remove circulating myoglobin, although this is rare in the context of seizures alone.

A CT head scan must be performed once the patient is stabilised and clinically apparent seizures have stopped. If the aetiology is unknown and the CT head scan is negative, an MRI head scan should be performed. In patients with SE of unknown origin, a lumbar puncture is indicated and empirical cover with CNS-penetrating antibiotics and antivirals should be considered while CSF analysis, microscopy, culture and PCR studies are being obtained. This is particularly important in febrile or immunocompromised patients.

Phenytoin has gained widespread acceptance as a first line antiepileptic drug (AED) due to its availability, intravenous formulation, effectiveness and familiarity. However, its use in the cardiac intensive care unit must be carefully considered. In patients with postcardiac arrest SE and after cardiac surgery, special attention should be given to the risk of cardiac dysrhythmia (bradycardia occasionally progressing to heart block) or hypotension in this very susceptible population. In addition, phenytoin and warfarin have complex and poorly understood interactions that vary with cytochrome p450 genetic polymorphisms, which may limit its use in patients requiring anticoagulation.

Phenytoin has a long half-life and dosing must be carefully considered. It is also strongly protein bound and levels should be checked regularly and be adjusted for serum albumin levels to avoid inadvertent overdose:

$$[\text{Corrected phenytoin}] = [\text{Measured phenytoin}] / (0.29 \times \text{Albumin} + 0.1).$$

For CrCl <10 ml/minute or in renal replacement therapy use:

$$[\text{Corrected phenytoin}] = [\text{Measured phenytoin}] / (0.1 \times \text{Albumin} + 0.1).$$

Valproate is an alternative to phenytoin. It is not associated with significant cardiac side effects, can be loaded quickly intravenously (30 to 60 mg/kg infused over 30 to 60 minutes followed by maintenance 15 to 20 mg/kg in divided doses) and is very well tolerated. It is hepatically metabolised but is safe even in patients with mild to moderate liver dysfunction. Valproate has been demonstrated to be at least as effective as phenytoin in treating SE. A rare side effect that must be suspected in prolonged recovery after seizures in patients loaded with valproate is hyperammonaemia, an idiosyncratic metabolic response.

Another option that is gaining popularity in all ICU settings is levetiracetam, due to its minimal drug–drug interactions and unchanged excretion such that hepatic disease does not preclude its use. The dose should be adjusted in renal failure to allow for decreased clearance. A starting dose of 500 mg twice a day is thought to achieve therapeutic levels in most patients, although this may rapidly be increased over a few days to 1500 mg twice daily if required. Valproate, benzodiazepines and levetiracetam have shown some efficacy in reducing postanoxic myoclonus.

In the rare situations where moderate or high doses of barbiturates have been used, any neurological prognostication should be delayed because of their prolonged sedative effect. A randomised trial of refractory SE found a median duration of intubation of 14 days in survivors in the thiopental or pentobarbital infusion arm, versus 4 days for survivors in the propofol arm with no differences in mortality. Laboratory barbiturate assay is possible but not locally available in most hospitals.

Once the patient has been sedated, EEG (ideally cEEG) is helpful in establishing on-going AED effectiveness, whether a second AED is needed and what maintenance therapy will be required after sedation withdrawal. Once all seizure activity has stopped for more than 24 hours, and provided there are adequate blood levels of AEDs, then the anaesthetic can be slowly weaned. Should SE recur, other drugs may be tried, but good clinical trials are lacking to date.

Seizures versus Epileptiform Activity: To Treat or Not To Treat?

In addition to definitive seizure activity, the EEG may also reveal abnormal epilepsy-like activity. Although strictly speaking such epileptiform discharges are not seizures, they may be important as their presence is highly associated with both convulsive and non-convulsive seizures. Periodic discharges (PDs) are stereotyped repetitive discharges with diverse electrographic morphology that occur at regular intervals and may be localised to one hemisphere (lateralised PDs, LPDs) (Figure 33.2) or bilateral (bilateral independent PDs, BIPDs and generalised PDs, GPDs).

The clinical significance and management of epileptiform activity is controversial, especially in comatose patients. In the general ICU more than 20% of patients are estimated to suffer electrographic seizures or PDs. The presence of PDs is associated with a higher incidence of death or severe disability at hospital discharge; however, the clinical significance of PDs and their association with underlying structural injury are still controversial. Whether epileptiform activity is a true interictal pattern or instead simply represents a predisposition to seizures is unclear. Evidence for improvement in outcome from treatment with AEDs is lacking. Nevertheless these patterns are pathological: the clinical significance and management of such epileptiform findings should therefore be considered on a case-by-case basis.

Learning Points

- Seizures are common in both the general ICU and cardiac ICU in particular. Seizures are associated with poorer outcomes.
- Seizures are an important reversible cause of unexplained unconsciousness.

- Many seizures in the critically ill are non-convulsive and therefore may go unrecognised.
- Electroencephalography is required for the diagnosis of seizures and a range of seizure-like pathologies.
- EEG equipment is complex to set up and interpretation requires specialist expertise.

Further Reading

Chen JW, Wasterlain CG. Status epilepticus: pathophysiology and management in adults. *Lancet Neurology*. 2006; 5: 246–256.

Claassen J, Mayer SA, Kowalski RG, Emerson RG, Hirsch LJ. Detection of electrographic seizures with continuous EEG monitoring in critically ill patients. *Neurology*. 2004; 62: 1743–1748.

Fugate JE, Wijdicks EF, Mandrekar J, et al. Predictors of neurologic outcome in hypothermia after cardiac arrest. *Annals of Neurology*. 2010; 68: 907–914.

Herman ST, Abend NS, Bleck TP, et al. Consensus statement on continuous EEG in critically ill adults and children, part II: personnel, technical specifications, and clinical practice. *Journal of Clinical Neurophysiology*. 2015; 32: 96–108.

Hosokawa K, Gaspard N, Su F, et al. Clinical neurophysiological assessment of sepsis-associated brain dysfunction: a systematic review. *Critical Care*. 2014; 18: 674.

Hunter GR, Young GB. Seizures after cardiac surgery. *Journal of Cardiothoracic and Vascular Anesthesia*. 2011; 25: 299–305.

Kalavrouziotis D, Voisine P, Mohammadi S, Dionne S, Dagenais F. High-dose tranexamic acid is an independent predictor of early seizure after cardiopulmonary bypass. *Annals of Thoracic Surgery*. 2012; 93: 148–154.

Oddo M, Carrera E, Claassen J, Mayer SA, Hirsch LJ. Continuous electroencephalography in the medical intensive care unit. *Critical Care Medicine*. 2009; 37: 2051–2056.

Wijdicks EF, Hijdra A, Young GB, Bassetti CL, Wiebe S, Quality Standards Subcommittee of the American Academy of Neurology. Practice parameter: prediction of outcome in comatose survivors after cardiopulmonary resuscitation (an evidence-based review): report of the Quality Standards Subcommittee of the American Academy of Neurology. *Neurology*. 2006; 67: 203–210.

MCQs

1. **Any seizure lasting longer than what period of time is defined as status epilepticus?**
   (a) 1 minute
   (b) 5 minutes
   (c) 30 minutes
   (d) 60 minutes

2. **When we are awake and very alert, the EEG normally shows:**
   (a) Beta waves (13–30 Hz)
   (b) Theta waves (5–7 Hz)
   (c) Alpha waves (8–12 Hz)
   (d) Delta waves (1–4 Hz)

3. **Which one of the following cardiac surgery risk factors would be more likely to be present in patients with postoperative seizures?**
   (a) High doses of tranexamic acid
   (b) Open-chamber procedures
   (c) Stroke
   (d) All of the above

4. **Which one of the following regarding neurological outcome after cardiac arrest is true?**
   (a) The Lance–Adams syndrome is associated with a good neurological outcome
   (b) It can be predicted at 24 hours in patients who have undergone therapeutic hypothermia
   (c) Targeted-temperature management to 36 °C is not associated with better neurological outcome
   (d) EEG/cEEG should be recorded only in patients with clinical signs of seizures/SE

5. **Which of the following is the drug of first choice in a patient with generalised convulsive status epilepticus?**
   (a) Propofol
   (b) Phenytoin
   (c) Pentobarbital
   (d) Lorazepam

Exercise answers are available on p.469. Alternatively, take the test online at www.cambridge.org/CardiothoracicMCQ

The Acute Abdomen in the Cardiac Intensive Care Unit

Simon JA Buczacki and Justin Davies

Introduction

Abdominal complications following cardiothoracic surgery are infrequent (0.3–5.5%) but carry a significant mortality rate of around 30% (14–63%). This figure is far greater than is seen with the same pathologies in the general population, suggesting the physiological changes imparted by cardiothoracic surgery have a major and deleterious result in the body's ability to respond to abdominal pathology. Many of the abdominal complications discussed, such as mesenteric ischaemia, can have subtle initial presentations where early intervention can have the most benefit to prevent abdominal catastrophe. These findings suggest there should be a high index of suspicion for abdominal pathology in the postoperative cardiothoracic patient who is failing to progress in the intensive care environment.

Risk Factors and Prediction

Large retrospective and prospective studies have identified several risk factors for the development of abdominal pathology after cardiothoracic surgery:

- Old age (>70 years)
- Low cardiac output (secondary to AF or congestive cardiac failure)
- Peripheral vascular disease
- Reoperation secondary to haemorrhage
- Renal failure (chronic and acute)
- Prolonged cardiopulmonary bypass (CPB) time (>150 minutes)
- Use of an intra-aortic balloon pump
- Preoperative inotropic support
- Active smoker
- Chronic obstructive pulmonary disease
- Prolonged ventilation
- Valve surgery
- Sepsis
- Deep sternal infection
- Liver failure
- Myocardial infarction.

Although extended CPB times are associated with elevated risk, the issue of whether off-pump CABG (OPCABG) is protective has been extensively debated in the literature. A study reported in 2003 by Raja et al. suggested that OPCABG decreased the incidence of gastrointestinal complications from 7.3% to 0.6%. These results, however, have failed to be replicated by other groups; indeed it has further been shown that during OPCABG when accessing difficult to reach coronaries, the superior mesenteric artery blood supply is disturbed. General consensus currently is that OPCABG is not protective but the question remains to be definitively answered.

Although not designed specifically for this purpose, EuroSCORE has been used to predict the development of gastrointestinal complications. An alternative scoring model termed the gastrointestinal complication score (GICS) has been developed with the aim to more accurately predict the development of these pathologies. Using prospective collection of data from over 5500 patients, the authors identify that those with a GICS of ≥15 have a probability of developing GI complications of >20% whereas a score of ≤5 has a probability of <0.4%. The authors identify several independent predictors of these complications, which are weighted accordingly (Table 34.1).

The GICS has been tested on a validation set of over 1000 patients and is reported to have a sensitivity of 56% and a specificity of 88% for a GICS of 5; and a sensitivity of 13% with a specificity of 99.8% when the score is ≥15. GICS had a larger area under the curve than EuroSCORE when receiver operating characteristic (ROC) curve analysis was performed, although of note this only reached statistical significance in the developmental data set. Overall, GICS appears to provide a useful adjunctive tool to help identify patients at risk of postoperative gastrointestinal complications. Although GICS is useful in predicting which patients may develop abdominal complications, the nature of the pathologies is such that prophylactic measures introduced in those with high scores are unlikely to be of benefit.

Incidence of Abdominal Complications

Abdominal complications after cardiac surgery are not common, although the associated risk of mortality is great (Table 34.2). In addition to the postoperative pathologies described below, it is important not to forget that common causes of the acute abdomen in the general population can also, coincidentally, occur in the patient after cardiac surgery. These can include adhesive small bowel obstruction, incarcerated/strangulated herniae, appendicitis or pyelonephritis to name but a few.

Diagnosis and Management of the Common Intra-abdominal Complications

Gastrointestinal Haemorrhage

The vast majority of postoperative gastrointestinal bleeds are from the upper gut. Patients in the cardiothoracic ICU are more susceptible due to the common use of antiplatelet agents and also instrumentation of the upper GI tract with transoesphageal echo (TOE). The patient with an upper GI bleed may present with frank haematemesis, cardiogenic shock or melaena. It is important not to forget that a significant upper GI bleed can present solely with fresh blood per rectum, thereby mimicking a lower GI bleed. Upper GI bleeds can cause elevations in serum urea levels as well as the more characteristic drop in haemoglobin. Abdominal signs are often lacking and tenderness is normally absent. After resuscitation and correction of any clotting abnormalities, the first line investigation in any significant GI bleed is an upper GI endoscopy to exclude a bleeding peptic ulcer or alternative upper GI pathologies such as oesophageal varices. Should a peptic ulcer be identified, dual-modality therapy is recommended with the options including adrenalin injection, clips or diathermy. High dose proton pump inhibitor therapy should be commenced and *Helicobacter pylori* eradication therapy started if biopsy (CLO test) results confirm infection. Should the patient suffer a rebleed after primary endoscopy, the options are either repeat endoscopy, interventional radiology (IR) with possible embolisation of the bleeding vessel (usually the gastroduodenal artery) or if these fail, surgery. Surgery involves an upper midline laparotomy and underrunning of the bleeding vessel following enterotomy. Alternative diagnoses such as bleeding oesophageal varices can be managed endoscopically with the application of ligation rubber bands in conjunction with medical control of portal venous hypertension.

Significant lower GI bleeds which fail to stop early with resuscitation and correction of clotting abnormalities can be extremely difficult to manage.

The use of adjunctive medical therapies can be helpful in these situations, in particular intravenous tranexamic acid can, on occasion, slow down or

Table 34.1 Gastrointestinal complication score (GICS)

Postoperative vascular complication	9.5
Preoperative inotropic support	4.0
Postoperative heart failure	3.5
Reoperation for haemorrhage	3.5
Age >80 years	2.5
Current smoker	2.5
Cardiopulmonary bypass >150 minutes	2.5
Postoperative atrial fibrillation	2.5
NYHA class III–IV	2.0

Table 34.2 Approximate incidence and mortality rates of common postoperative abdominal complications (data from Rodriguez et al., 2010)

	Incidence	Mortality
Gastrointestinal bleed (upper GI (90%) lower GI (10%))	0.39	19
Ischaemic bowel	0.16	50
Pancreatitis	0.13	20
Acute cholecystitis	0.11	27
Perforated peptic ulcer	0.07	36
Pseudo-obstruction	0.06	50 (with perforation)
Diverticulitis	0.03	21

even stop significant colonic bleeds. It is imperative in situations of massive rectal bleeds to first exclude an upper GI bleed by endoscopy as well as bleeding haemorrhoids by using bedside proctoscopy. Should these tests fail to identify a source for the bleed and if the patient is generally haemodynamically stable, then a CT angiogram should be obtained. In order for this investigation to successfully identify a bleeding point, the patient needs to be bleeding at a rate of >0.5 ml/minute. However, if a location is identified this facilitates the possibility of an IR approach using conventional angiography in conjunction with embolisation. In the absence of IR, CT angiogram can still be of help as it can direct targeted therapeutic colonoscopy or surgical resection. If the bleeding patient is more unstable, or if CT angiogram fails to identify a bleeding location, the next option is therapeutic colonoscopy which can be performed in the operating theatre. Careful wash-out and mucosal inspection can permit diagnosis and therapeutic intervention, with the use of clips and/or adrenaline injection to achieve haemostasis. In the case of a patient continuing to bleed profusely and no active bleeding site identified, the endoscopy can be augmented by a laparotomy to aid wash-out of the colon through the appendix, and should the colon be cleared as a source of bleeding, sequential enterotomy and small bowel endoscopy to identify the site can then be undertaken. However, undertaking a laparotomy when the site of bleeding is not known in advance should be avoided whenever possible.

Mesenteric Ischaemia

Postoperative mesenteric ischaemia carries a very high mortality rate. Two forms of ischaemia are described: occlusive and non-occlusive. Occlusive disease occurs as a result of migration of emboli or the development of de novo thrombus. Non-occlusive disease is more common in this patient group and develops secondary to hypoperfusion from low cardiac output or the use of vasoconstrictors. Occlusive ischaemia tends to follow a very rapid course with the development of acidosis and ultimately intestinal infarction. Non-occlusive disease generally follows a slower clinical trajectory and in the intubated and sedated patient can be problematic to diagnose. In the awake patient, pain, nausea/vomiting and bloody diarrhoea can be present with the pain classically being 'out of proportion' to the abdominal signs, which commonly only occur late. However, in the sedated patient the suggestion of non-occlusive ischaemia can be subtle, varying from increasing nasogastric outputs, diarrhoea ± blood or a slowly rising unexplained metabolic acidosis in combination with raised serum lactate. In the stable patient, the investigation of choice if mesenteric ischaemia is suspected is a contrast enhanced CT scan. Endoscopy (both upper and lower) can also be performed if CT is equivocal. Ultimately, however, laparotomy is not uncommonly used as a diagnostic tool in sick patients, and should be considered in a patient where there is a high risk of clinical suspicion for mesenteric ischaemia even if the CT scan is non-diagnostic.

In non-occlusive mesenteric ischaemia, priority should be given to resuscitation and improvement of cardiac output once the diagnosis is made or suspected. If the clinical picture progresses and the patient deteriorates then laparotomy may be the only option for survival.

In both occlusive and non-occlusive mesenteric ischaemia it is not uncommon to find the entire intestine may be non-viable. Depending on the amount of intestine and other associated viscera that have infarcted, the surgical options are either resection with stoma formation accepting the high likelihood of lifelong parenteral nutrition dependency or 'open-and-shut' where the degree of ischaemia is extensive and not compatible with ongoing life.

Hepatobiliary (HPB) Complications

Pancreatitis

As with all the other pathologies here described, the mortality rate from pancreatitis in this patient cohort (20%) exceeds that of pancreatitis in the general population (5%). However, the management of the condition follows the same principles. As with mesenteric ischaemia, the diagnosis of pancreatitis can be difficult as the symptoms and signs can be impossible to elicit in the sedated patient. The aetiology of pancreatitis here is more commonly secondary to reduced perfusion although the possibility of 'traditional' gallstone pancreatitis should not be dismissed.

An elevated serum amylase level is reportedly present in 30–40% of all patients following cardiac surgery, although only 1–3% of these will have pancreatitis. Elevated serum lipase levels can be used to aid the diagnosis but do not appear to confer any additional sensitivity over and above amylase per se. It has been suggested, however, that the combination of an elevated amylase *and* lipase level can imply subclinical pancreatitis. Contrast enhanced CT scanning can be used to confirm the diagnosis, and the management for the first couple of weeks is invariably organ supportive. Parenteral or nasojejunal nutrition should be commenced if nasogastric (NG) aspirates are high, although NG feeding itself is not contraindicated in this group. There is no evidence for the use of prophylactic antibiotics and these should be reserved for cases of infected necrosis where sensitivities can be obtained by radiologically guided percutaneous aspiration. Rarely, in cases of advanced necrotising pancreatitis, surgical necrosectomy is required which should ideally be performed via a minimally invasive approach, or via an open transabdominal or retroperitoneal approach if not. Attention should be drawn during the course of pancreatitis to development of acute haemodynamic instability as this can suggest a ruptured splenic artery aneurysm secondary to the local inflammatory process. A specialist HPB opinion should always be sought in cases of acute pancreatitis in this patient group.

Acalculous Cholecystitis

In the general population acalculous cholecystitis is relatively rare, presenting in the sick and diabetics. In patients following cardiac surgery it occurs at least as frequently as calculous cholecystitis. The aetiology of acalculous cholecystitis in this group is not entirely clear but associations have been drawn with reduced gallbladder contraction and ischaemia. The disease is suggested by intra-abdominal sepsis in the presence of abnormal liver function tests as well as right upper quadrant pain in the awake patient. Diagnosis is confirmed by ultrasound or CT scanning. Aggressive and early treatment is essential to prevent deterioration and should consist of resuscitation and broad spectrum antibiotics. The risk of gangrene and subsequent perforation is far higher in patients with acalculous compared to classical calculous cholecystitis and for those that fail to improve rapidly early surgical intervention is recommended, with cholecystectomy for those fit enough and percutaneous cholecystostomy for those more acutely unwell.

Pseudo-obstruction

Pseudo-obstruction or Ogilvie's syndrome is not common after cardiac surgery but is an important condition to diagnose as failure to treat this appropriately can lead to haemodynamic compromise due to an abdominal compartment syndrome and colonic perforation, which carries a 50% mortality rate. It is defined as massive acute colonic dilatation as a result of an imbalance in the autonomic supply to the colon rather than a true mechanical blockage. The diagnosis is suggested upon the presence of increasing abdominal girth with a tense, tympanic abdomen together with the inability to pass faeces or flatus. Diagnostic confirmation can be made with an abdominal radiograph; however, a CT scan provides greater information and rules out the small possibility of a true mechanical blockage being present (e.g. sigmoid or caecal volvulus). Pseudo-obstruction is more likely to occur in patients with electrolyte imbalances, in particular potassium and magnesium. Indeed sometimes the condition can be adequately treated with restoration of homeostatic levels of these cations alone. Should colonic diameter exceed 10 cm or if the patient (if awake) complains of right iliac fossa tenderness, then urgent intervention is required as the possibility of imminent perforation exists. Generally, endoscopic decompression with a colonoscope can relieve the impending perforation and on occasion a flatus tube is left in situ to aid the ongoing decompression. In the general population the parasympathomimetic neostigmine has been used in refractory cases of pseudo-obstruction; however, the cardiac risk profile of this drug suggests its use may be limited in patients following cardiac surgery. Surgical intervention is only required in cases of perforation where colonic resection, abdominal wash-out and stoma formation are generally required. A drainage caecostomy tube, which can be placed radiologically, is only used in very rare cases of repeated caecal dilatation in a patient where laparotomy is not possible or safe.

Solid Viscus Perforation

Gastro-oesophageal perforation is a recognised complication of TOE. Presentation is often insidious, diagnosis delayed and outcomes poor. Detection requires a high index of suspicion particularly when there has been difficulty in passing the probe or blood noted on removal, and in those with known gastro-oesophageal pathology, small stature, advancing age, chronic steroid use or undetermined source of sepsis. Oesophageal perforation may also occur following radiofrequency ablation for atrial fibrillation, and in this instance there may be a coexisting atrial-oesophageal fistula. Once suspected, the patient should be made nil by mouth, commenced immediately on broad spectrum antimicrobials, and should undergo prompt investigation with fluoroscopy or CT. Treatment options include medical, endoscopic and surgical approaches; early involvement of upper GI specialists is essential but despite this mortality is high.

Perforated peptic ulcers have become far less common since the widespread use of prophylactic proton pump inhibitors. Nevertheless, the condition does still occur and the diagnosis should be entertained in the presence of an acute episode of intra-abdominal sepsis accompanied by pain in the awake patient. The diagnosis can be made by either an erect chest radiograph or a CT scan, with CT scan having the greatest sensitivity. Even with CT scanning it can be difficult to locate the anatomical source for the free air seen radiologically. Increasingly, in the elderly and unfit, these perforations can be managed conservatively as the omentum will often adhere and seal the perforation without intervention. The decision on non-operative versus operative management should only be made in conjunction with a senior and experienced general surgeon. Operative options vary from simple omental patching to, in advanced cases, partial gastrectomy. In virtually all cases, managed either conservatively or operatively, nasogastric drainage, parenteral nutrition and broad spectrum antibiotics (including *H. pylori* eradication) are essential. If there is any septic deterioration following conservative or operative management, then concern should exist that the repair/patch has broken down or an intra-abdominal collection has developed. Repeat CT scanning is essential in this situation to define the problem, and allow potential radiological drainage of any collection

Diverticulitis

Diverticular disease is very common in the elderly – it is reported that over 60% of patients >70 years of age have diverticulosis. Around 10–25% of those with diverticular disease will, at some stage, suffer an episode of diverticulitis. Whilst the majority of cases of diverticular disease in the Western population occur in the sigmoid colon, pan-colonic diverticular disease can also present. The phenomenon of 'right-sided diverticular disease' where multiple diverticula are seen in the caecum and ascending colon, is more common in an Asian population. Diverticulitis is a rare intra-abdominal complication following cardiac surgery but again has a mortality rate that exceeds that seen in the general population. The condition is suggested by the presence of intra-abdominal sepsis and lower abdominal pain which, whilst commonly is located in the lower left quadrant, can also be felt in the suprapubic region or lower right quadrant (as a result of the sigmoid colon sometimes having a long mesentery). Diagnosis is made by contrast enhanced CT scanning. The treatment in uncomplicated cases (non-perforated) is broad spectrum antibiotics and clinical observation. Patients with pericolic collections or abscesses can be treated with radiological drainage in addition to antibiotics. However, for those with generalised peritonitis or a free perforation radiologically, surgical intervention is required. Historically, this would involve a Hartmann's procedure consisting of sigmoid colectomy with an end colostomy. Contemporary approaches, whilst still mandating the use of Hartmann's procedure for those cases of generalised faecal peritonitis, also now include primary anastomosis ± defunctioning stoma or laparoscopic wash-out and drain insertion for less advanced cases. Any septic deterioration in a patient managed conservatively or otherwise should suggest an intra-abdominal collection which can be diagnosed with a CT scan and managed with antibiotics ± radiological drainage for those >2 cm in size.

Conclusion

Although not common, intra-abdominal complications occur at an elevated frequency in patients following cardiac surgery and carry a mortality rate out of keeping with the pathological process. The diagnosis of these conditions is made ever the more complex as they commonly occur in the early postoperative course where clinical signs are unreliable due to anaesthesia/sedation. Any suggestion of the development of an acute abdomen should immediately warrant early involvement of an experienced general surgeon to guide appropriate investigations and management. Delayed diagnosis should be avoided at all costs as mortality and morbidity rates are particularly high in this unique population group.

Learning Points

- Intra-abdominal complications are uncommon post cardiac surgery but carry a very high mortality rate.

- Many gastrointestinal complications are difficult to diagnose in the critical care environment and may present subtly.
- The GICS (gastrointestinal complication score) is a useful predictive tool to identify at risk patients.
- Failure to progress in high risk patients should raise the possibility of a significant intra-abdominal pathological process.
- Early involvement of an experienced general surgeon is essential to prevent a poor outcome.

Further Reading

Anastassiades CP, Baron TH, Wong Kee Song LM. Endoscopic clipping for the management of gastrointestinal bleeding. *Nature Clinical Practice Gastroenterology & Hepatology*. 2008; 5: 559–568.

Andersson B, Andersson R, Brandt J, et al. Gastrointestinal complications after cardiac surgery – improved risk stratification using a new scoring model. *Interactive Cardiovascular and Thoracic Surgery*. 2010; 10: 366–370.

British Society of Gastroenterology Endoscopy Committee. Non-variceal upper gastrointestinal haemorrhage: guidelines. *Gut*. 2002; 51(Suppl 4): 1–6.

D'Ancona G, Baillot R, Poirier B, et al. Determinants of gastrointestinal complications in cardiac surgery. *Texas Heart Institute Journal*. 2003; 30: 280–285.

Filsoufi F, Rahmanian PB, Castillo JG, et al. Predictors and outcome of gastrointestinal complications in patients undergoing cardiac surgery. *Annals of Surgery*. 2007; 246: 323–329.

Fiore G, Brienza N, Cicala P, et al. Superior mesenteric artery blood flow modifications during off-pump coronary surgery. *Annals of Thoracic Surgery*. 2006; 82: 62–67.

Musleh GS, Patel NC, Grayson AD, et al. Off-pump coronary artery bypass surgery does not reduce gastrointestinal complications. *European Journal of Cardio-Thoracic Surgery*. 2003; 23: 170–174.

Nashef SA, Roques F, Michel P, et al. European system for cardiac operative risk evaluation (EuroSCORE). *European Journal of Cardio-Thoracic Surgery*. 1999; 16: 9–13.

Passage J, Joshi P, Mullany DV. Acute cholecystitis complicating cardiac surgery: case series involving more than 16,000 patients. *Annals of Thoracic Surgery*. 2007; 83: 1096–1101.

Pfutzer RH, Kruis W. Management of diverticular disease. *Nature Reviews Gastroenterology & Hepatology*. 2015; 12: 629–638.

Rattner DW, Gu ZY, Vlahakes GJ, Warshaw AL. Hyperamylasemia after cardiac surgery. Incidence, significance, and management. *Annals of Surgery*. 1989; 209: 279–283.

Rodriguez R, Robich MP, Plate JF, Trooskin SZ, Sellke FW. Gastrointestinal complications following cardiac surgery: a comprehensive review. *Journal of Cardiac Surgery*. 2010; 25: 188–197.

Sessions SC, Scoma RS, Sheikh FA, McGeehin WH, Smink (Jr) RD. Acute acalculous cholecystitis following open heart surgery. *American Surgeon*. 1993; 59: 74–77.

Toumpoulis IK, Anagnostopoulos CE, DeRose JJ, Swistel DG. Does EuroSCORE predict length of stay and specific postoperative complications after coronary artery bypass grafting? *International Journal of Cardiology*. 2005; 105: 19–25.

UK Working Party on Acute Pancreatitis. UK guidelines for the management of acute pancreatitis. *Gut*. 2005; 54(Suppl 3): 1–9.

Vennix S, Musters GD, Mulder IM, et al. Laparoscopic peritoneal lavage or sigmoidectomy for perforated diverticulitis with purulent peritonitis: a multicentre, parallel-group, randomised, open-label trial. *Lancet*. 2015; 386: 1269–1277.

Zacharias A, Schwann TA, Parenteau GL, et al. Predictors of gastrointestinal complications in cardiac surgery. *Texas Heart Institute Journal*. 2000; 27: 93–99.

MCQs

1. **What is the commonest form of postoperative gastrointestinal complication?**

   (a) Diverticulitis

   (b) Mesenteric ischaemia

   (c) Perforated peptic ulcer

   (d) Pancreatitis

   (e) Gastrointestinal haemorrhage

2. **How quickly does a patient have to be bleeding in order for a CT angiogram to identify a bleeding location?**
   (a) ≥0.1 ml/minute
   (b) ≥0.3 ml/minute
   (c) ≥0.5 ml/minute
   (d) ≥1 ml/minute
   (e) ≥5 ml/minute
3. **What is the most appropriate first line test in a patient suffering a massive rectal bleed?**
   (a) CT angiogram
   (b) Oesphogo-gastro-duodenoscopy (OGD)
   (c) Colonoscopy
   (d) Red cell scan
   (e) MRI
4. **Which electrolyte is most important in the pathogenesis of colonic pseudo-obstruction?**
   (a) Calcium
   (b) Sodium
   (c) Potassium
   (d) Phosphate
   (e) Chloride
5. **In non-occlusive mesenteric ischaemia what is the most appropriate first line management?**
   (a) Laparotomy
   (b) Angiogram and embolisation
   (c) Resuscitation and restoration of cardiac output
   (d) Tranexamic acid
   (e) Broad spectrum antibiotics

Exercise answers are available on p.469. Alternatively, take the test online at www.cambridge.org/CardiothoracicMCQ

Chapter 35

Cardiothoracic Trauma

Alia Noorani and Ravi J De Silva

Background

Trauma accounts for up to 720,000 annual admissions, and over 6 million attendances to the emergency department in the UK. Thoracic injuries directly account for 20–25% of deaths due to trauma and contribute to 25–50% of the remaining deaths. Figures from the USA suggest that there are over 17,000 deaths per year, directly attributable to chest trauma.

Unsurprisingly, there has been a steady increase in the number of penetrating injuries presenting to hospitals. Concurrently, however, there have also been significant improvements in pre-hospital and perioperative care facilities, meaning that there are now more opportunities to save patients who, previously, would have been declared unsalvageable.

The earliest written description of thoracic injuries dates back to the Edwin Smith Surgical Papyrus in 3000 BCE. Later, Galen reported attempts to treat gladiators with chest injuries and Labeza in 1635 reported surgical removal of an arrowhead from the chest wall of a Native American. In 1814 Napoleon's military surgeon reported various injuries to the subclavian vessels. Until the late nineteenth century most agreed with the sayings of Boerhaave that 'all penetrating cardiac trauma is fatal', until the German physician Rehn in 1896 performed the first successful cardiorrhaphy for a right ventricular injury sustained during a fencing match.

Mechanisms of Cardiothoracic Trauma

Cardiothoracic trauma can be broadly divided into penetrating or blunt trauma (Table 35.1). Blunt trauma encompasses crush injuries, acceleration and deceleration, blast injuries and direct blunt trauma. Penetrating injuries include gunshot wounds, stabbing and shrapnel injuries (Figures 35.1–35.3). Only 10–15% of patients with blunt trauma and 15–30% of those with penetrating trauma require surgery.

Clinical Assessment and Resuscitation

As is usual management for any trauma patient, the ABC (airway, breathing, circulation) are established, although modification of the ABC may be required in order to diagnose the extent of the injury and resuscitate the patient simultaneously.

Any patient with a compromised airway should undergo endotracheal intubation; this may prove challenging, particularly in those with suspected cervical spine injury, as their neck must be immobilised. Immediate chest decompression for a tension pneumothorax is indicated, without requiring a chest radiograph, and a sucking chest wound requires cover to allow adequate ventilation. Presence of a haemothorax requires chest drainage. Control of ongoing haemorrhage and volume resuscitation are essential to maintain an adequate circulation.

On examination of the patient, it is essential to note the exact location of the injury and, in the case of a missile injury, the entry and exit points.

An entry wound below the nipples and inferior to the scapula should be considered to be a trajectory for an injury breaching the abdominal cavity. Gunshot wounds can penetrate any region of the body and in the absence of an exit point with a definitive entry point, a retained projectile has to be considered. Besides causing direct injury, this could also have the potential to embolise within the vasculature. Cardiac injury should be considered if entry points are present anywhere between the two midclavicular lines. The commonest chambers to be injured are the right ventricle and the left ventricle.

Imaging

A chest radiograph may confirm the presence of a haemothorax or pneumothorax or a chest wall injury such as fractured ribs and flail chest as well as diaphragmatic injuries. Echocardiography can provide a

Table 35.1 Types of cardiothoracic trauma and subsequent effects

Penetrating	Laceration of heart, great vessels, intercostal vessels, lung parenchyma, airways, oesophagus, diaphragm
Blunt	Cardiac/pulmonary contusion Rib fractures with or without flail segments, thoracic spine fractures
Crush	Ruptured bronchus, ruptured oesophagus, cardiac and pulmonary contusion
Deceleration	Aortic disruption, major airway injury, diaphragmatic rupture
Blast	Disruption of any intrathoracic organ

quick means to assess for the presence of pericardial fluid; however this is an operator dependent imaging modality and clinical signs should override an apparently negative scan. CT scanning provides definitive and rapid imaging for more subtle injuries that cannot be diagnosed by clinical examination or simpler modalities alone. The clinical stability of the critically injured patient is paramount and no imaging should take priority over management.

Specific Injuries

Chest Wall

The function of the chest wall is twofold: firstly to to provide structural and functional assistance with respiration and secondly to provide a rigid structure comprising muscles and bony skeleton to protect the intrathoracic and upper abdominal organs from external forces.

In general, the majority of injuries to the chest wall can be managed conservatively, with effective pain control, pulmonary physiotherapy and early mobilisation. Specific patterns of injuries and the age of the patient are important factors to consider, and may require specialist care. For example, multiple rib fractures in the elderly may require early fixation to aid with respiratory mechanics and avoid prolonged ventilator assistance. Early epidural analgesia should be considered in those with multiple rib fractures and certain trauma guidelines suggest that thoracic epidurals should be used in patients over the age of 65 years with four or more rib fractures

Injuries to the first and second ribs indicate a high velocity injury with significant impact force, and other associated injuries must be sought and treated.

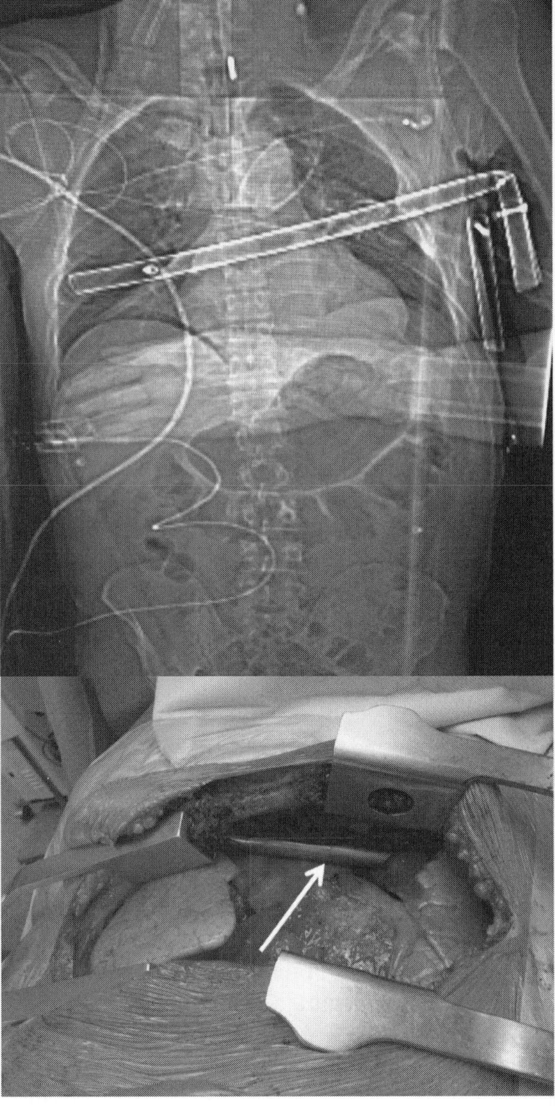

Figure 35.1 Penetrating trauma. This 42 year old man was impaled by a camping chair when he fell 15 feet off his roof into the garden. The steel chair leg was seen to be sitting anterior to the heart and had caused only minor injury to the left lower lobe. Note that the bent leg of the chair can be seen outside the chest wall. The arrow is pointing to the leg of the chair in the coloured photograph.

Surgical management of flail chest segments (defined as at least two fractures per rib in two or more ribs, which are therefore unable to contribute to lung expansion) have been shown to have benefits, such as reduced duration of mechanical ventilation and ICU stay, as well as lower odds of pneumonia or death.

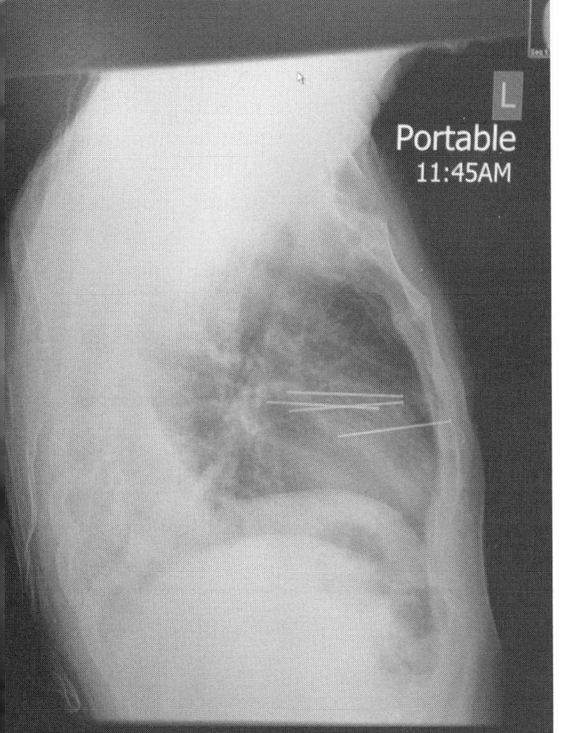

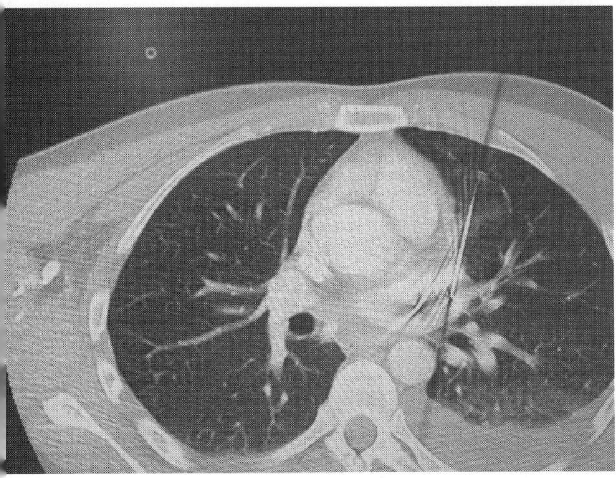

Figure 35.2 Penetrating trauma. This 45 year old patient had a nail gun fired accidentally into his chest. The CT scan demonstrates penetration of the left atrium and a left haemothorax.

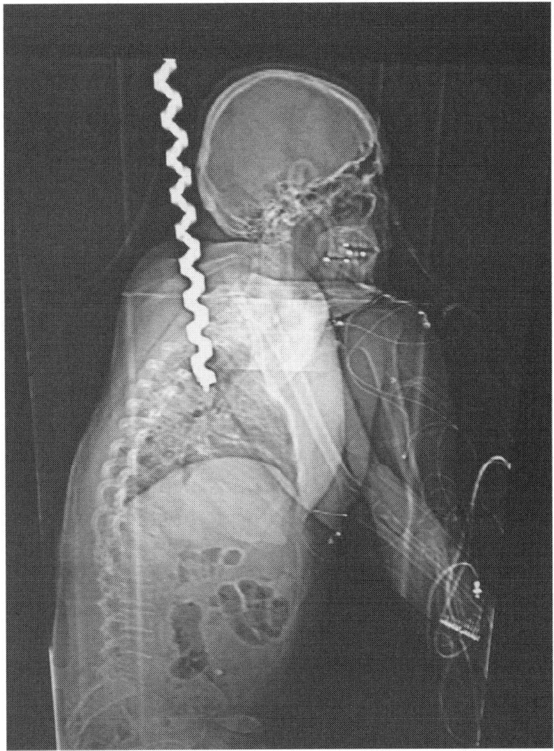

Figure 35.3 Penetrating trauma. This 28 year old patient was impaled by an industrial drill bit whilst working on a construction site.

Table 35.2 Indications for immediate thoracotomy

Immediate drainage of over 1500 ml of blood on chest drain insertion
Ongoing bleeding at a rate of 200 ml/hr
Massive air leak
Persistent haemothorax despite adequate chest drainage

Lung Injuries

Blunt trauma can lead to significant pulmonary contusions, air leaks and haemothorax. Penetrating trauma leads to contusions from direct trauma as well as the dissipation of kinetic energy. In general, the management for pulmonary contusions is chest tube insertion, which itself although a commonly performed procedure, is not without complications and should be undertaken by individuals with adequate training and experience.

Lung lacerations can be minor, or major, resulting in bisection of a lobe, although even if a thoracotomy is required, the majority of injuries can be managed by simple stapling or over sewing. Major injuries requiring a pneumonectomy are rare (less than 3%).

Tracheobronchial Injuries

These injuries can frequently be immediately fatal due to loss of the airway. Autopsy reports indicate that over

3% of all trauma deaths have associated tracheobronchial injuries. For those patients surviving to make it to the hospital, early suspicion and recognition of signs is key. These injuries can present with subcutaneous emphysema, pneumothorax, massive air leak once a chest tube is in situ and haemoptysis. Urgent management of the unstable patient requires immediate securing of the airway followed by diagnostic flexible bronchoscopy. Surgical repair is the treatment of choice for major lacerations, and the technique of repair should be tension free to allow for optimal healing.

Cardiac Injuries

Blunt cardiac injury occurs due to an anterior force compressing the chest. The most common mechanism is compression of the heart between the sternum and the thoracic spine, although deceleration causes injury when the heart strikes the sternum freely. Cardiac contusions can lead to dysrhythmias, valvular disruptions, myocardial infarction, myocardial rupture and tamponade. Clinical evaluation includes an ECG and an echocardiogram. Common ECG findings are a sinus tachycardia or atrial fibrillation. Echocardiography can help rule out valvular insufficiency or tamponade.

Penetrating cardiac injuries are a highly lethal entity but urgent diagnosis and appropriate treatment can save patients. As a general rule, any wounds in the 'cardiac box' area bounded by the midclavicular lines laterally, the clavicles superiorly and the costal margins inferiorly should raise the suspicion of cardiac injury. Stab wounds fare better than gunshot wounds and outcomes for single chamber injuries are better than when two or more chambers are affected. Although the clinical signs of tamponade (Beck's triad) are present in 30% of cases, they are easily missed in a busy emergency department setting.

Immediate surgical intervention is recommended for penetrating injuries to the anterior chest in a clinically unstable patient who cannot wait for diagnostic imaging. Occasionally an emergency room thoracotomy may have to be undertaken to salvage a dying patient. The American College of Surgeons guidelines on emergency department thoracotomy include the following:

- Precordial wound in a patient with an out of hospital cardiac arrest.
- A trauma patient with cardiac arrest after arrival into the emergency department.
- Penetrating cardiac injuries with a short transport time and with witnessed physiological signs of life such as a pupillary response, spontaneous ventilation, measurable blood pressure and a palpable carotid pulse, extremity movement and electrical cardiac activity.

Victims of penetrating trauma usually fare better than those of blunt trauma, and of the victims of penetrating trauma, those with stab wounds fare better than those with gunshot wounds. A generous anterior thoracotomy or bilateral anterior thoracotomies (clam shell) should be performed. Once the chest is entered, evidence of tamponade is sought and relieved, if present. Immediate indications for a thoracotomy in a case of penetrating injury with cardiac arrest are shown in Table 35.2.

Aortic and Other Great Vessel Injury

Up to 15% of all deaths due to road traffic accidents are due to injury to the thoracic aorta. Many of these deaths are as a result of complete aortic transection.

The majority of thoracic great vessel injuries occur due to penetrating thoracic trauma and about 20% of patients subjected to blunt aortic injury survive long enough to reach hospital, and of these the injuries are usually to the descending aorta. Blunt aortic injury is second to blunt head injury as the leading cause of death due to road traffic accidents.

The descending aorta is a relatively fixed structure compared to the mobile aortic arch. The majority of aortic injuries therefore affect the junction of the arch and descending aorta at the site of the ligamentum arteriosum (isthmus). Endovascular management of these is now routine in specialist hands, and this approach is supported by meta-analysis data.

Traumatic transection or dissection in the ascending aorta will require open surgical intervention although these patients frequently do not make it to the hospital alive.

In the case of a clinically stable patient, further diagnostic imaging can be carried out to guide definitive treatment. A chest X-ray is a useful screening tool and the presence of a left sided pleural effusion, widened mediastinum or tracheal deviation may provide clues, although a CT scan would confirm these findings and indicate the precise location of the injury.

Oesophageal Injuries

The oesophagus is infrequently involved in blunt or penetrating trauma due, in part, to its protected location. Additionally, injuries affecting the oesophagus are frequently associated with other severe injuries (great vessels), which are often fatal even before the patient presents to hospital. The presence of a major oesophageal injury, however, can have seriously detrimental effects on the patient, leading to mediastinitis, multiorgan failure and death. The stable patient can undergo additional investigations including a CT scan and fluoroscopy. Endoscopy should be undertaken in those with unclear imaging results.

The clinical management of these patients includes haemodynamic stability followed usually by surgical repair. Injuries diagnosed early can be treated with primary repair, whereas those over 12 hours old are best managed by multiple chest drain insertion.

Diaphragmatic Injury

In general, blunt thoracoabdominal trauma leads to larger defects in the acute setting and the defect from a penetrating injury may be quite small to begin with but enlarges over time due to a pressure gradient between the abdominal and chest cavities. Visceral herniation and subsequent ischaemia due to strangulation is a serious complication of left sided trauma and requires urgent repair. Right sided injuries are thought to be less dire as the liver acts as a barrier for herniation of bowel.

Further Reading

Altinok T, Can A. Management of tracheobronchial injuries. *Eurasian Journal of Medicine*. 2014; 46: 209–215.

Bertelsen S, Howitz P. Injuries of the trachea and bronchi. *Thorax*. 1972; 27: 188–194.

Karmy-Jones R, Wood DE. Traumatic injury to the trachea and bronchus. *Thoracic Surgery Clinics*. 2007; 17: 35–46.

Pang D, Hildebrand D, Bachoo P. Thoracic endovascular repair (TEVAR) versus open surgery for blunt traumatic thoracic aortic injury. *Cochrane Database of Systematic Reviews*. 2015; 9: CD006642.

Simon BJ, Cushman J, Barraco R, et al. Pain management guidelines for blunt thoracic trauma. *Journal of Trauma*. 2005; 59: 1256–1267.

Slobogean GP, MacPherson CA, Sun T, Pelletier M-E, Hameed SM. Surgical fixation vs nonoperative management of flail chest: a meta-analysis. *Journal of the American College of Surgeons*. 2013; 216: 302–311.

Working Group, Ad Hoc Subcommittee on Outcomes, American College of Surgeons, Committee on Trauma. Practice management guidelines for emergency department thoracotomy. *Journal of the American College of Surgeons*. 2001; 193: 303–309.

MCQs

1. **The management of the trauma patient begins with assessment of the:**
   (a) Airway and cervical spine
   (b) Breathing
   (c) Circulation
   (d) Fractures
   (e) Head injuries

2. **The commonest cardiac chamber to be injured by penetrating trauma is the:**
   (a) Left atrium
   (b) Right atrium
   (c) Left ventricle
   (d) Right ventricle

3. **Diaphragmatic injuries:**
   (a) Are often left sided
   (b) May result in herniation of abdominal contents into the thorax
   (c) May present with acute respiratory distress
   (d) Often require repair via laparotomy
   (e) All of the above

4. **The second leading cause of death from blunt trauma after head injury is:**
   (a) Oesophageal perforation
   (b) Aortic injury
   (c) Cardiac arrthymias

(d) Rib fractures

(e) Pelvic fractures

5. **Indications for immediate thoracotomy in the trauma setting include:**

   (a) Immediate drainage of over 1500 ml of blood on chest drain insertion following penetrating injury that has resulted in cardiac arrest

   (b) Tension pneumothorax

   (c) Hypotension with systolic blood pressure of 120 mmHg

   (d) Flail chest

   (e) Blast injuries

Exercise answers are available on p.469. Alternatively, take the test online at www.cambridge.org/CardiothoracicMCQ

Chapter 36

The Bleeding Cardiac Surgical Patient

Jerrold H Levy, Kamrouz Ghadimi and Ian J Welsby

Introduction

Bleeding is the commonest complication following cardiac surgery. The amount of blood loss is used to stratify patients in groups and judge their need for return to theatre, risks of postoperative complications, and need for transfusion of blood products. However, what is important for each individual patient is their demographic parameters, premorbid state, type of surgery and the risks of undertaking repeat operation.

Some patients suffer massive blood loss and surgical control may not be possible. These patients may need to be transferred to the intensive care unit with their chest open and packed with swabs. During the time spent in intensive care, the coagulation abnormalities can be largely corrected, providing better opportunities for haemostasis when returning to theatre.

An important feature of the bleeding patients in intensive care is the haemodynamic manifestation. This presents two types of problems: exsanguination and compression of structures by a clot. The intravascular blood volume lost needs merely to be replaced. However, the correct formula for which product and how much is difficult to determine for each patient. Laboratory blood tests and algorithms for how this should be done are described below. It is also important to remember that sometimes the bleeding is so fast that mechanical infuser devices and cell savers are needed. The second haemodynamic problem, compression of structures by a clot, is more challenging. A small amount of clot or fluid may be present in all cardiac surgical patients. When the amount of clot or fluid impedes filling of chambers or vessels, or causes a compression effect (tamponade, Figure 36.1), it has to be evacuated. Clinical examination, vital signs monitoring and echocardiography are used to guide decision making in these circumstances.

The bleeding patient in cardiac intensive care is also resource consuming. The patient often requires more than one nurse to help with blood sampling, requesting products, administering volume, operating cell savers, controlling temperature and frequent observations. The medical staff are often by this particular patient's bedside. When numerous discussions on how this patient is best managed are added, the effort consumption detracts resources from other patients in the unit at the same time. Ironically, the bleeding patient is not only in a perilous state themselves, but also exposes other patients to detriment. Therefore careful early assessment and early management are essential for successful outcome.

The Bleeding Patient

Following cardiac surgery, bleeding is one of the major expected associated problems. Therapeutic approaches include both prevention and treatment, and provide a unique opportunity to use prophylactic therapies including antifibrinolytics. In the bleeding patient, standard therapeutic approaches include blood product administration, multiple concomitant pharmacological agents, and the increasing use of both purified and recombinant haemostatic factors. It has been suggested that approximately 5–7% of patients bleed greater than 2 l of what may be reflected by chest tube drainage within the first postoperative 24 hours. When bleeding occurs, about 5% of patients require surgical re-exploration for bleeding. When cardiac surgical patients develop bleeding, this will increase the length of stay and is associated with a higher mortality.

Multiple factors contribute to the complex causes of bleeding in cardiac surgical patients. This includes surgical site bleeding, the effects of anticoagulants, including heparin, on platelet activation, contact activation, fibrinolytic and inflammatory pathway

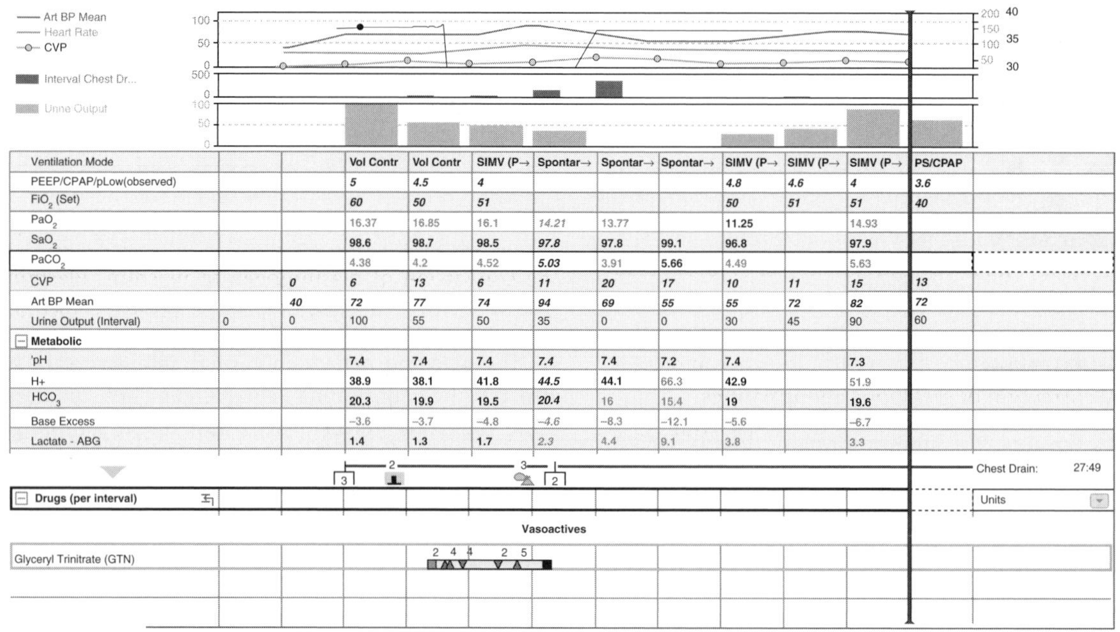

Ventilation Mode			Vol Contr	Vol Contr	SIMV (P→	Spontar→	Spontar→	Spontar→	SIMV (P→	SIMV (P→	SIMV (P→	PS/CPAP
PEEP/CPAP/pLow(observed)			5	4.5	4				4.8	4.6	4	3.6
FiO_2 (Set)			60	50	51				50	51	51	40
PaO_2			16.37	16.85	16.1	14.21	13.77		11.25		14.93	
SaO_2			98.6	98.7	98.5	97.8	97.8	99.1	96.8		97.9	
$PaCO_2$			4.38	4.2	4.52	5.03	3.91	5.66	4.49		5.63	
CVP		0	6	13	6	11	20	17	10	11	15	13
Art BP Mean		40	72	77	74	94	69	55	55	72	82	72
Urine Output (Interval)	0	0	100	55	50	35	0	0	30	45	90	60
Metabolic												
'pH			7.4	7.4	7.4	7.4	7.4	7.2	7.4		7.3	
H+			38.9	38.1	41.8	44.5	44.1	66.3	42.9		51.9	
HCO_3			20.3	19.9	19.5	20.4	16	15.4	19		19.6	
Base Excess			–3.6	–3.7	–4.8	–4.6	–8.3	–12.1	–5.6		–6.7	
Lactate - ABG			1.4	1.3	1.7	2.3	4.4	9.1	3.8		3.3	

Figure 36.1 Clinical Information System (CIS) illustration of reducing urine output, followed by reduction in blood pressure and increase in CVP and blood loss. (A black and white version of this figure will appear in some formats. For the colour version, please refer to the plate section.)

activation, dilutional changes, hypothermia, and other factors. Patients often are also on routine anticoagulants and antiplatelet agents that include oral anticoagulants (warfarin, dabigatran, rivaroxaban, apixaban, edoxaban) and platelet inhibitors (P2Y12 receptor inhibitors – clopidogrel, prasugrel or ticagrelor). Thus, bleeding and coagulopathy following cardiac surgery are due to multiple factors that can be highly problematic after cardiopulmonary bypass.

Transfusion Algorithms and Bleeding

Developing a specific therapeutic plan, especially with the use of transfusion algorithms, has been shown to consistently reduce allogeneic blood administration. It is important to realise that any laboratory testing that prevents empirical blood product administration is important as part of a multimodal approach to blood conservation and reduction of allogeneic blood product use. Transfusion algorithms generally recommend the following: administration of fresh frozen plasma (FFP) when bleeding is accompanied by a PT or a PTT > 1.5 times normal value, platelet transfusions for thrombocytopenia with a platelet count <50,000–100,000, or cryoprecipitate or fibrinogen concentrates when fibrinogen levels are <200 mg/ dl (2 g/l). As will be discussed later, the critical role for fibrinogen levels continues to evolve, with most data suggesting the importance of normalising fibrinogen in a bleeding patient. With critical bleeds, and longer turnover time in standard laboratory testing, point-of-care testing including rotational thromboelastometry (ROTEM©, Tem International, Munich, Germany), thromboelastography (TEG©, Haemonetics, Inc., Braintree, MA USA) and/or platelet function testing, is important. In the actively bleeding patient, testing for platelet dysfunction is unreliable as most tests need a relatively normal platelet count and most of the platelet function testing may not work following dilutional changes and activation after cardiopulmonary bypass.

Allogeneic Blood Product Administration

In the haemorrhagic patient, and from lessons learned in traumatic coagulopathy, the use of crystalloid and/or colloid administration may be helpful as first line therapy. With massive haemorrhage or uncontrollable bleeding, however, these compounds do not provide appropriate platelets or coagulation factors. The use of massive transfusion protocols, derived from lessons learned in traumatic coagulopathy, should be considered and implemented during uncontrollable bleeding in cardiac surgical patients. This routinely includes, in addition to red blood cells, FFP, platelets and cryoprecipitate (or fibrinogen concentrates). In European countries, factor concentrates (e.g., fibrinogen and prothrombin complex concentrates) are increasingly used to restore circulating levels of critical factors for haemostasis, and have been the subject of recent studies. In addition, in the patient with massive haemorrhage, hypothermia and acidosis frequently occur, requiring maintenance of normothermia and additional correction of metabolic abnormalities.

Of all the blood product administration used clinically, data elucidating when platelet transfusion should be administered are not clear. This is in part due to the problem of measuring platelet function after cardiopulmonary bypass. In the bleeding patient, because of dilutional thrombocytopenia and acquired platelet dysfunction, platelets are often transfused, but again monitoring platelet dysfunction is problematic in this setting. This is further complicated by extensive use of antiplatelet medications as outlined above. Whole blood clotting tests, including ROTEM© and TEG©, have been used as a monitor of platelet–fibrinogen interaction based on maximal clot firmness or clot strength. With that said, these values are indirect correlates and are highly affected by fibrinogen levels. Most of the data on platelet administration are from oncology patients and we still do not know the critical platelet mass for surgical patients. Thrombocytopenia may not always correlate with abnormal bleeding.

In the patient with ongoing haemorrhage, a massive transfusion coagulopathy can develop, which is defined as 10 or more units of packed red blood cells (PRBCs) transfused in a 24 hour period, although most of this literature is from trauma patients and retrospective evaluations. Laboratory testing often lags behind blood product administration during these scenarios. As a result, transfusion protocols have been developed using fixed doses of FFP, PRBCs and platelets that are administered as a fixed 1:1:1 ratio. In cardiac surgical patients, there are few data to determine whether these therapeutic approaches improve bleeding outcomes although it may be logical to adopt massive transfusion protocols. In trauma and battlefield patients, however, fixed ratios have become the mainstay of therapy although much of these data are from retrospective analyses of large databases.

Details of the variety of blood products are discussed in Chapter 13.

Fibrinolysis and Cardiac Surgery

Activation of the fibrinolytic system is an important mechanism of vascular homeostasis. Mechanistically, plasmin generation is the enzymatic serine protease responsible for fibrinolysis and is formed following the conversion of plasminogen to plasmin. Plasmin is an enzyme that cleaves multiple proteins, including fibrin but also fibrinogen. Following cardiopulmonary bypass and/or tissue injury that occurs with surgery or trauma, fibrinolysis is activated and represents an important cause of coagulopathy. In trauma, orthopaedic surgery, and most importantly cardiac surgery, multiple studies report the role of antifibrinolytic agent administration in order to decrease bleeding and the need for allogeneic transfusions. These synthetic antifibrinolytic agents include the lysine analogues, epsilon aminocaproic acid (EACA) and tranexamic acid (TXA) that interfere with the binding of plasminogen to fibrin, necessary for activating plasmin. Aprotinin, a broad spectrum protease inhibitor, is a direct plasmin inhibitor. The specific antifibrinolytic agents will be considered as follows.

Lysine Analogues

The two antifibrinolytic agents administered clinically include EACA and TXA. As previously mentioned, EACA and TXA competitively inhibit plasminogen conversion to the active enzymatic agent plasmin. TXA can also inhibit plasmin but at higher plasma levels. Most of the studies and efficacy data with the lysine analogues are reported with TXA, but EACA continues to be extensively utilised in the USA. EACA does not consistently reduce transfusion requirements or surgical re-exploration, but it is inexpensive and tends to be frequently substituted for TXA in the USA. Although multiple studies, primarily meta-analyses of randomised controlled trials, have reported a decrease in bleeding in cardiac surgical patients, there are limited safety data about the use of antifibrinolytic agents. Most dosing studies include EACA at ~20 to 30 g per case, or TXA at doses that range from 2 to 25 g, although most TXA dosing regimens involve 2 to 8 g dosing.

One issue with TXA is the potential increased risk of seizures. The incidence of postoperative convulsive seizures in a German hospital increased from 1.3% to

3.8% after cardiac surgery, a finding that was noted to be temporally associated with high-dose TXA. They noted 24 patients who developed seizures postoperatively and had received high doses of TXA that ranged from 61 to 259 mg/kg. The mean age of the patients was ~70 years, and 21/24 had undergone valve surgery/open chamber procedures. Although the underlying mechanisms are not fully elucidated, TXA enhances neuronal excitation by antagonising inhibitory gamma-aminobutyric acid (GABA) neurotransmission. Lecker showed that TXA inhibits neural glycine receptors, while inhibition of the inhibiting neurotransmitter glycine is an established cause of seizures. Viewing the similarities in the chemical structure of TXA, GABA and glycine, it is conceivable that an interaction of TXA with the receptors of both inhibitory neurotransmitters contributes to the increase in clinical seizures observed when TXA is given. However, in view of the chemical structure of EACA and its close similarity to GABA and glycine as well, it is noteworthy that it has not been reported to produce neurological side effects.

Aprotinin

This is a bovine serin protease inhibitor, which inhibits complement and contact factor activation via kallikrein and plasmin activation. The half-life is 5–10 hours. In 2008 Managno reported increased incidence of renal failure, myocardial infarction and heart failure in recipients. This led to the BART trial in 2008, resulting in revoking of the drug license when an excess mortality was found, despite beneficial effects on blood loss and transfusion. These findings have been disputed and aprotinin is available on a named patient basis for low risk cases. Aprotinin affects celite based tests such as some aPTT reagents and can suggest profound coagulopathy when in actual fact the patient has no excessive bleeding. Heparin monitoring is also affected.

Other Pharmacological Adjuncts to Bleeding

Protamine

Protamine is a highly basic polypeptide with molecular weight around 5000 Da that contains ~70% arginine residues. Protamine is isolated from salmon sperm, and exists in nature as a histone, a basic nuclear protein that binds to DNA to provide structural integrity in the nucleus. Currently, it is the only reversal agent for unfractionated heparin. This basic protein inactivates the acidic heparin molecule via a simple acid–base interaction. Interestingly, protamine does not reverse low molecular weight heparin. Following cardiac surgery, patients are routinely overdosed with protamine for heparin reversal because most fixed dose regimens for reversal involve protamine administration based on initial or total heparin dose, and do not account for the pharmacokinetics and/or relatively short half-life of approximately 1 hour. Excess protamine should be avoided when reversing heparin as it potentially contributes to coagulopathy. Protamine is an inhibitor of serine proteases involved in clot formation as well as platelets.

Studies suggest that maintaining 'adequate' heparin levels during cardiopulmonary bypass and reversal doses of protamine based on the circulating heparin levels significantly reduce postoperative bleeding and the need for transfusions. Part of this efficacy may be related to the effects of excess protamine on coagulation factors and platelets. Protamine has been shown to prolong the activated clotting time and cause platelet dysfunction. When protamine is administered using specific assays that determine the circulating heparin levels, and based on the exact amount of protamine needed, more complete reversal occurs with the lowest activated clotting time (ACT) values. Additional studies have also reported that lower protamine doses reduce bleeding and transfusion requirements.

Other important causes of bleeding after protamine reversal include heparin rebound. This usually occurs approximately 2–3 hours after the initial protamine dose, typically after the patient has been transferred to the intensive care unit. Heparin levels during this rebound time period usually range from 0.1 to 0.3 IU/ml. Protamine doses of 5–15 mg at the time of rebound may be effective at reversing heparin rebound, rather than the 50 mg dose normally contained in the small ampoule which is commonly administered. Studies have evaluated the ROTEM© assay for determining the need for additional protamine administration and note that most patients may not need additional protamine within 30 minutes of initial administration. Moreover, the ACT is not a sensitive indicator of low heparin concentrations and is impacted by platelet counts and fibrinogen levels.

Desmopressin

Desmopressin (DDAVP) is the V2 analogue of arginine vasopressin used to treat diabetes insipidus but also stimulates the release of von Willebrand factor (vWF) multimers from vascular endothelium. vWF is a critical protein that facilitates platelet adherence to damaged vascular subendothelium by acting as a protein bridge between platelet glycoprotein Ib receptors and subendothelial vascular basement membrane proteins. DDAVP will decrease bleeding times with mild forms of both haemophilia A or von Willebrand disease. Beyond these indications and despite widespread perioperative use, efficacy is limited. Surgical patients who potentially benefit from use of DDAVP are not well established, despite its frequent administration. DDAVP is administered intravenously at doses of 0.3 μg/kg, and should be infused over 15–30 minutes to avoid aberrancies in blood pressure or cardiac chronotropy. Most studies have not demonstrated efficacy or usefulness in cardiac surgical patients. Mannucci reported that, despite 18 trials of desmopressin in 1295 patients undergoing cardiac surgery, there was only a minimal reduction of perioperative blood loss (median decrease, 115 ml). Furthermore, vasopressin is often administered to cardiac surgical patients, which also has V2- and V1-receptor mediated effects, and the additional benefit of administering DDAVP in these patients is not clear.

Recombinant Activated Factor VIIa (rF VIIa)

Recombinant FVIIa is approved for treatment of bleeding episodes and perioperative management in adults and children with haemophilia A or B with inhibitors, congenital factor VII deficiency, and Glanzmann's thrombasthenia with refractoriness to platelet transfusions, with or without antibodies to platelets; and for treatment of bleeding episodes and perioperative management in adults with acquired haemophilia. However, it is also used off-label as a prohaemostatic agent for life threatening haemorrhage. rFVIIa produces a prohaemostatic effect to mechanisms thought to be related to binding with tissue factor (TF) expressed at the site of vascular injury to locally produce thrombin and amplify haemostatic activation. The active form of FVII (FVIIa) accounts for ~1% of circulating FVII, and has no effect until bound with TF. The therapeutic dose of rFVIIa in non-haemophilia patients has not been established. However, guidelines for off-label use are reported by Goodnough and Despotis for life threatening haemorrhage. Controlled clinical trials report the incidence of thrombotic complications among patients who received rFVIIa to be relatively low and similar to that among patients who received placebo. However, most case reports giving rFVIIa as rescue therapy include patients who have impaired coagulation, have received multiple transfusions and are at a high risk for adverse events. The complex role that transfusion therapy has in producing adverse outcomes is increasingly being noted in the literature. In a large and comprehensive cohort of persons in placebo-controlled trials of rFVIIa, treatment with high doses of rFVIIa on an off-label basis significantly increased the risk of arterial, but not venous, thromboembolic events, especially among the elderly.

In the most recent cardiac surgical study, patients bleeding postoperatively >200 ml/hour were randomised to placebo ($n = 68$), 40 μg/kg rFVIIa ($n = 35$) or 80 μg/kg rFVIIa ($n = 69$). The primary end points were the number of patients suffering critical serious adverse events. Secondary end points included rates of reoperation, blood loss and transfusions. Although more adverse events occurred in the rFVIIa groups, they did not reach statistical significance (placebo, 7%; 40 μg/kg, 14%; $P = 0.25$; 80 μg/kg, 12%; $P = 0.43$). However, after randomisation, significantly fewer patients in the rFVIIa group underwent a reoperation because of bleeding ($P = 0.03$) or needed allogeneic transfusions ($P = 0.01$).

Summary

The potential for haemorrhage in cardiac surgical patients represents an ongoing concern for management. Anticoagulation monitoring using point-of-care testing, optimal use of transfusional therapies and adjunct administration of antifibrinolytics, as well as purified and recombinant therapies, provide clinicians with the ability to administer key coagulation proteins to treat haemorrhage. Although factor concentrates represent an important potential therapeutic approach to coagulopathy, other considerations should include treating hypofibrinogenaemia, thrombocytopenia and platelet disorders, or repairing surgical sources of bleeding. The integration of optimal use of pharmacological, transfusional and factor concentrates into a comprehensive perioperative coagulation treatment algorithm for bleeding is an important therapeutic approach for managing bleeding in cardiac surgical patients.

Learning Points

- Bleeding after cardiac surgery is multifactorial.

- Antifibrinolytic agents are an important part of management.
- Transfusion algorithms are important for reducing blood product administration and bleeding.
- Fibrinogen is a critical component to target in the bleeding patient.
- Factor concentrates are increasingly used as therapies in managing bleeding.

Further Reading

Despotis GJ, Grishaber JE, Goodnough LT. The effect of an intraoperative treatment algorithm on physicians' transfusion practice in cardiac surgery. *Transfusion*. 1994; 34: 290–296.

Gill R, Herbertson M, Vuylsteke A, et al. Safety and efficacy of recombinant activated factor VII: a randomized placebo-controlled trial in the setting of bleeding after cardiac surgery. *Circulation*. 2009; 120: 21–27.

Hein OV, Birnbaum J, Wernecke KD, et al. Three-year survival after four major post-cardiac operative complications. *Critical Care Medicine*. 2006; 34: 2729–2737.

Koster A, Faraoni D, Levy JH. Antifibrinolytic therapy for cardiac surgery: an update. *Anesthesiology*. 2015; 123: 214–221.

Levi M, Cromheecke ME, de Jonge E, et al. Pharmacological strategies to decrease excessive blood loss in cardiac surgery: a meta-analysis of clinically relevant endpoints. *Lancet*. 1999; 354: 1940–1947.

Mannucci PM, Levi M. Prevention and treatment of major blood loss. *New England Journal of Medicine*. 2007; 356: 2301–2311.

Sniecinski RM, Chandler WL. Activation of the hemostatic system during cardiopulmonary bypass. *Anesthesia & Analgesia*. 2011; 113: 1319–1333.

Steiner ME, Despotis GJ. Transfusion algorithms and how they apply to blood conservation: the high-risk cardiac surgical patient. *Hematology/Oncology Clinics of North America*. 2007; 21: 177–184.

Whitlock R, Crowther MA, Ng HJ. Bleeding in cardiac surgery: its prevention and treatment – an evidence-based review. *Critical Care Clinics*. 2005; 21: 589–610.

MCQs

True or False

1. **Multiple factors contribute to bleeding in cardiac surgical patients, including:**
   (a) Effects of antithrombolytics
   (b) Hyperthermia
   (c) Contact activation
   (d) Inhibition of fibrinolytic pathway
   (e) Dilutional changes
2. **In the bleeding patient, therapeutic approaches include administration of:**
   (a) Altepase
   (b) Protamine
   (c) DDAVP
   (d) Apixaban
   (e) Prothrombin complex concentrate
3. **Tranexamic acid:**
   (a) Activates conversion of plasminogen to plasmin
   (b) Is typically given in doses of greater than 200 g
   (c) Is associated with a decrease in bleeding
   (d) Promotes fibrinolysis
   (e) Is associated with occurrence of seizures
4. **Protamine:**
   (a) Is an acidic polypeptide
   (b) Has a molecular weight around 5000 Da
   (c) Is isolated from salmon sperm
   (d) Can cause coagulopathy
   (e) Is an effective reversal agent for low molecular weight heparin
5. **Desmopressin (DDAVP) is:**
   (a) An analogue of arginine vasopressin
   (b) Inhibits V2 receptors
   (c) Stimulates the release of von Willebrand factor (vWF)
   (d) Is administered subcutaneously at doses of 0.3 μg/kg

Exercise answers are available on p.469. Alternatively, take the test online at www.cambridge.org/CardiothoracicMCQ

Chapter 37

Management after Coronary Artery Bypass Grafting Surgery

Sam Nashef and Paolo Bosco

Professor Kolesov performed the first beating-heart left internal mammary artery to left anterior descending coronary artery bypass graft in February 1964 in Leningrad, Russia, whilst Dr Favaloro performed the first saphenous vein coronary artery bypass graft (CABG) surgery in May 1967 at the Cleveland Clinic in the USA. Until then, treating angina using surgery, and the feasibility of operating on the delicate and small coronary arteries had been unimaginable. Fifty years later, several million CABG operations have been performed worldwide and it remains the most common operation performed by cardiac surgeons with excellent outcome and very low mortality.

Patient Population

Isolated CABG operations represent about 50–60% of the cardiac surgery workload in the UK. As percutaneous coronary intervention is now often offered early in the course of ischaemic heart disease, patients presenting for CABG are now older and sicker and this trend is set to continue. In addition, people live longer due to advances in treatment of chronic diseases, including hypertension, elevated lipids, diabetes and others. Despite this, mortality from CABG is at an all-time low of between 1 and 2% due to better perioperative management. A low-risk patient with a competently executed CABG operation should have a smooth and uneventful recovery, an ITU stay shorter than 24 hours and an overall hospital stay of around 5 days. In a high-risk patient, however, with multiple risk factors and comorbidities, or after a suboptimally performed CABG operation, the procedure may be followed by complications and longer postoperative hospitalisation.

The limited functional reserve of elderly patients, the presence of chronic kidney disease, peripheral vascular disease, COPD, diabetes and impaired cardiac function are but a few of the challenges which may be faced in the management of this high-risk population.

Haemodynamic Management

In the majority of low-risk patients, there is no need for cardiovascular support and an adequate cardiac output can be obtained just with fluid management and rate control by means of temporary pacing wires.

$CO = HR \times SV.$

The stroke volume, SV, is determined by preload, contractility and afterload.

If contractility and afterload are within the normal range, it is obvious that cardiac output can be optimised with fluids (preload) or by simply increasing the heart rate with temporary cardiac pacing. Determination of the optimal filling pressure is often empirical and can be estimated with the use of a fluid challenge and observing the haemodynamic response (see Chapter 14).

If adequate perfusion pressure cannot be maintained with these simple, first line measures, contractility and afterload may need to be addressed pharmacologically. Before making the diagnosis of impaired contractile cardiac function, it is important to exclude tamponade (see Chapter 3). Impaired contractility can be improved with either pharmacological or mechanical means. Dopamine and catecholamines are often the first choice but phosphodiesterase inhibitors may be beneficial in right ventricular dysfunction and elevated pulmonary vascular resistance (see Chapter 15).

The most commonly used mechanical support device is the intra-aortic balloon pump (IABP) (see Chapter 21) which, by simultaneously decreasing myocardial workload and improving coronary perfusion, can immediately alleviate myocardial ischaemia and improve poor cardiac function. The routine use of IABP in routine CABG is not necessary, but in selected high-risk patients there is a significant advantage in survival provided by this device. This was supported by several randomised trials and a recent meta-analysis.

The use of inotropic drugs, vasoconstrictors and mechanical support in the postoperative management of the CABG patient can be guided by clinical assessment. Features of low cardiac output include hypotension, poor peripheral perfusion, falling urine output despite adequate preload and metabolic evidence of impaired perfusion, such as acidosis. In a CABG patient with low blood pressure and inadequate perfusion, it can sometimes be difficult to differentiate between inadequate filling (preload), poor cardiac function (contractility) or low systemic vascular resistance (afterload). The cause may also be multifactorial. If there is doubt in interpreting clinical and simple haemodynamic findings, more invasive haemodynamic monitoring using transoesophageal echocardiography or a pulmonary artery catheter will directly provide information on the cardiac output and on the state of preload and afterload of both the pulmonary and systemic circulations, thus helping tailor the therapy to the haemodynamic needs of the patient. Routine use of a pulmonary artery catheter is controversial and is not supported by clear evidence. Nevertheless, it may play a role in high-risk patients, but the risk of adverse events and the costs associated with it suggest that its use be restricted to those patients in whom the aetiology of the haemodynamic instability cannot be identified by more simple methods and those who require multiple vasoactive agents and their fine titration.

Myocardial Infarction

Myocardial ischaemic event presenting soon after CABG surgery is a rare but troublesome finding that can be difficult to diagnose and to treat. Many factors can contribute to myocardial injury during a CABG operation, including surgical trauma due to manipulation and suturing, less than ideal myocardial protection, incomplete revascularisation, acute graft thrombosis and iatrogenic injury to the native vessels. Because of these confounding factors, the diagnosis of MI following CABG is not straightforward and uncertainties remain around the correct threshold for biomarker elevation and the need for associated criteria. According to the 2012 third universal definition of myocardial infarction after CABG, at least two of the following criteria should be present for diagnosis: cardiac biomarkers (with troponins preferred) rise >10 times 99% upper reference limit from a normal preoperative level; and new pathological Q-waves or new left bundle branch block (LBBB) or imaging or angiographic evidence of new occlusion of native vessels or grafts, new regional wall motion abnormality, or loss of viable myocardium. In daily clinical practice in many centres, cardiac biomarkers are not routinely measured after CABG surgery. Therefore, in the immediate postoperative period, when the patient is fully sedated and intubated, the first sign of possible ongoing myocardial ischaemia or infarction may be unexpected haemodynamic or rhythm instability. This finding should lead to a thorough assessment of the patient, which includes ECG for new abnormalities, echocardiogram for new regional wall motion abnormalities and cardiac biomarkers. If it is then believed that myocardial ischaemia is a genuine possibility, a low threshold for emergency angiography should be adopted. If a technical problem such as acute graft or native vessel occlusion is demonstrated, surgical revision and emergency re-grafting of the affected territory should be considered as it may save both myocardium and life. Additional treatment options include an intra-aortic balloon pump, GTN infusion, antiplatelet agents and beta-blockers.

Acute Kidney Injury

Acute kidney injury (AKI) is a common postoperative complication of cardiac surgery and is associated with an increased risk of morbidity, mortality and length of stay

Between 5% and 30% of patients undergoing CABG may suffer this complication in the postoperative period. The use of serum creatinine rather than urine output as main criterion for the diagnosis of postoperative AKI is appropriate in the cardiac surgery population, since manipulation of the urine output with diuretics makes this a less reliable indicator of AKI. A limitation of defining AKI based on serum creatinine measurements is the delay in detecting the onset of injury. Optimisation of renal perfusion, avoidance of hypovolaemia and avoidance of nephrotoxins are the only options to prevent or mitigate the effects of postoperative AKI. Pharmacological interventions have been attempted with inconsistent results, and there are no drugs that have demonstrated a definitive renal protection.

The widely used drug furosemide was found not to be protective and to be potentially harmful, as the incidence of AKI was twice that of the dopamine or placebo group in a double-blind randomised controlled trial. Similar negative results have been seen in other studies.

Other Postoperative Complications

Arrhythmia: Postoperative arrhythmia is common in cardiac surgical patients. The commonest observed arrhythmia is atrial fibrillation. The precise reasons for developing arrhythmias are not always clear, but overall the prognosis is good as frequently these recover and sinus rhythm is restored. It is important to exclude poor right ventricular perfusion as a cause of malignant ventricular arrhythmias. Occlusion of right coronary graft needs be ruled out in such cases. The treatment of postoperative arrhythmia is no different from the treatment for other patients in the ICU, and is described in Chapter 10.

Heart block: Temporary heart block is not a prominent feature of the CABG patients, but can occur. It normally resolves in the first few days, but sometimes needs implantation of a pacemaker system.

Postoperative bleeding: Patients undergoing coronary surgery often receive antiplatelet medication, which may have long lasting effects, and hence they are at a higher risk of coagulopathy. Thus postoperative bleeding can be a problem. The management of this problem is discussed in detail in Chapter 36.

Haemothorax: CABG patients are at a higher risk than other cardiac patients of bleeding in the left hemithorax when the left internal mammary artery has been used. The ICU team needs to be vigilant for this complication if haemodynamic instability is a problem or if there is a massive blood loss postoperatively.

Prevention of Early and Late Graft Occlusion

Several randomised controlled studies, including a meta-analysis, have shown a clear benefit of early administration of aspirin in the prevention of early and late vein graft occlusion. This beneficial effect of early aspirin declines after 24 hours and disappears after 48 hours. In the appropriate clinical settings, early administration of postoperative aspirin following CABG is not associated with increased blood loss or transfusion requirement. The advantages of early aspirin administration include a reduction in mortality, myocardial infarction, stroke, renal failure and bowel ischaemia. The antithrombotic effect of aspirin is greatly potentiated when used in combination with clopidogrel. The use of dual antiplatelet therapy following CABG is still controversial and a clear benefit in vein graft patency has not been clearly demonstrated. In conclusion, the use of aspirin within 6 hours following CABG is strongly recommended and supported by clinical evidence.

Learning Points

- CABG is the most common operation performed by cardiac surgeons, with an overall mortality between 1 and 2%.
- The risk profile of the patient population is changing, multiple comorbidities and advanced age are now common features of the patient referred for CABG.
- Fluid challenges and different pacing strategies can significantly increase the cardiac output.
- Haemodynamic instability in the early postoperative period may represent the first sign of ongoing myocardial ischaemia.
- In the appropriate clinical setting, the use of aspirin within 6 hours following CABG is strongly recommended.

Further Reading

Chaikhouni A. The magnificient century of cardiothoracic surgery. *Heart Views*. 2010; 11(1): 31–37.

Dunning J, Versteegh M, Fabbri A, et al. Guideline on antiplatelet and anticoagulation management in cardiac surgery. *European Journal of Cardio-Thoracic Surgery*. 2008; 34: 73–92.

Gukop P, Gutman N, Bilkhu R, et al. Who might benefit from early aspirin after coronary artery surgery? *Interactive Cardiovascular and Thoracic Surgery*. 2014; 19: 505–511.

Lassnigg A, Donner E, Grubhofer G, et al. Lack of renoprotective effects of dopamine and furosemide during cardiac surgery. *Journal of the American Society of Nephrology*. 2000; 11: 97–104.

Lombardi R, Ferreiro A, Servetto C. Renal function after cardiac surgery: adverse effect of furosemide. *Renal Failure*. 2003; 25: 775–786.

Mangano DT. Multicenter study of Perioperative Ischemia Research Group. Aspirin and mortality from coronary bypass surgery. *New England Journal of Medicine*. 2002; 347: 1309–1317.

Mehta RL, Kellum JA, Shah SV, et al. Acute Kidney Injury Network: report of an initiative to improve outcomes in acute kidney injury. *Critical Care*. 2007; 11(2): R31.

Sandham JD, Hull RD, Brant RF, et al. A randomized, controlled trial of the use of pulmonary-artery catheters in high-risk surgical patients. *New England Journal of Medicine*. 2003; 348: 5–14.

Thygesen K, Alpert JS, Jaffe AS, et al. Writing Group on behalf of the Joint ESC/ACCF/AHA/WHF Task Force for the Universal Definition of Myocardial Infarction. Third universal definition of myocardial infarction. *European Heart Journal*. 2012; 33: 2551–2567.

Zangrillo A, Pappalardo F, Dossi, et al. Preoperative intra-aortic balloon pump to reduce mortality in coronary artery bypass graft: a meta-analysis of randomized controlled trials. *Critical Care*. 2015; 19: 10.

MCQs

1. **One hour following a routine CABG operation the mean pressure of your patient is dropping below 60 mmHg. Looking at the monitor you notice a sinus rhythm of 50 bpm and a CVP of 12. The patient is not bleeding, there is no suspicion of tamponade and urine output is adequate. You want to increase the cardiac output in order to prevent obvious complication due to hypoperfusion. What is your strategy?**
   (a) Insert an intra-aortic balloon
   (b) Start noradrenaline
   (c) Pace the atrium at 90 bpm
   (d) Start adrenaline
   (e) Pace the ventricle at 90 bpm

2. **Your patient has just arrived in the unit. Mr Cabbage has just received a total arterial revascularisation by a very experienced surgeon. When the nurses looking after him roll him slightly in order to insert the sliding sheet and reposition him in the bed, you notice a sudden drop of the blood pressure. The monitor shows a BP of 50/30 a heart rate of 100 and a CVP of 4. What is your first action?**
   (a) Give a rapid bolus of fluid
   (b) Pace the heart at 120 bpm
   (c) Call the cardiac arrest team
   (d) Give a bolus of metaraminol
   (e) Call the surgeon

3. **Mr Bacon is a 66 year old man with diffuse coronary disease. His LIMA was not used since the flow was considered poor, and he received a triple vein graft. The surgeon is not too happy about him since the conduits and the targets were poor. The patient shows some haemodynamic instability with a blood pressure of 80 over 55, CVP of 16 and a heart rate of 100 bpm. The urine output is low and peripheral perfusion is poor. What is your first action?**
   (a) Start adrenaline
   (b) Give fluids
   (c) Request ECG and echocardiogram
   (d) Insert an intra-aortic balloon
   (e) Start GTN infusion

4. **Mr Stone underwent a CABG operation in the morning. Now it is 2 pm and the nurse calls you for poor urine output since his arrival in the unit. Blood pressure is 130/70, heart rate 80, CVP 10. Haemoglobin is 95, base excess is −2 and lactate 2.5. On examination you notice cold peripheries, but Mr Stone is otherwise unremarkable. What is your approach?**
   (a) Start noradrenaline
   (b) Start GTN
   (c) Start a furosemide infusion
   (d) Give a fluid challenge
   (e) Wait and see

5. **You are asked to prescribe the standard medication to be administered in the first 24 hours following a routine CABG operation for Mrs Dark. Which of the following should be included in the list?**
   (a) Sildenafil
   (b) Warfarin
   (c) Vasopressin
   (d) Aspirin
   (e) Lorazepam

Exercise answers are available on p.469. Alternatively, take the test online at www.cambridge.org/CardiothoracicMCQ

Chapter 38

Intensive Care Unit Management Following Valve Surgery

Yasir Abu-Omar and Shakil Farid

The post cardiac valve surgical patients follow the same general management principles as any other cardiac surgical patients. Adequate basic requirements such as oxygenation, ventilation management, optimal heart rate and cardiac output, coagulation management and early detection and management of pericardial tamponade, as well as pain management, are not different. However, patients undergoing valve surgery tend to have higher risks of morbidity and mortality. They may require more invasive monitoring, including with a pulmonary artery catheter, and infusion of vasoactive medication. Early re-evaluation of post-intervention valvular function by echocardiography is frequently needed. Electrophysiological interventions and pacing techniques are needed more often than for uncomplicated coronary artery bypass graft surgery patients. Sometimes, patients at a particularly high risk need preoperative ICU admission for preoptimisation. In this chapter we will discuss the salient features and basic principles of preoperative and postoperative heart valve pathology challenges and management in the cardiac surgical ICU.

Aortic Valve Surgery

Aortic valve replacement is generally indicated in patients with symptomatic severe aortic stenosis and/or regurgitation.

Options for aortic valve replacement include stented and stentless xenograft tissue valves, mechanical valves, homografts and, less commonly, pulmonary autografts.

Anatomical Considerations

The commonest cause for aortic stenosis in elderly patients is degenerative calcific disease, while in younger patients the commonest aetiology is congenital bicuspid aortic valve.

Several important structures that are in close proximity to the aortic valve may be damaged at the time of surgery. These include the bundle of His, the anterior leaflet of the mitral valve and the ostial origin of the coronary arteries. The bundle of His runs beneath the commissure between right coronary and non-coronary cusps. A deep suture placed in this region may result in injury with resultant complete heart block. The anterior leaflet of the mitral valve is separated from the aortic annulus by the aortomitral curtain in the region of the non-coronary cusp and left coronary cusps. Iatrogenic damage to the anterior leaflet of the mitral valve may result in mitral regurgitation. Lastly, due to the close proximity of the coronary ostia to the aortic annulus, there is a risk of coronary ostial blockade or compromise and ensuing ischaemia. Accurate suture placement and carefully securing the prosthesis in place should reduce the risks of paravalvular leak.

Intraoperative transoesophageal echocardiogram is essential in all cases of valvular surgery, allowing for early detection and immediate correction of complications.

Physiological Considerations

In aortic stenosis, there is pressure overload of the left ventricle that results in concentric hypertrophy and diastolic dysfunction. The stiff non-compliant ventricle is dependent on adequate preload and atrial contraction – the latter may contribute up to 30% of left ventricular filling.

In chronic aortic regurgitation there is a volume as well as pressure load to the left ventricle, resulting in dilatation and hypertrophy. In the acute setting of aortic regurgitation, such as in cases of aortic regurgitation secondary to infective endocarditis or aortic dissection, the left ventricle may be normal in size. These patients often display marked haemodynamic compromise with a small ventricle that has not adapted to the large regurgitant volume during diastole.

Common ICU Problems

Aortic Stenosis

Arrhythmia: Atrial arrhythmia must be immediately treated with antiarrhythmic medications as the atrial contraction contributes up to 30% of the ventricular filling. The threshold for synchronised cardioversion to maintain atrioventricular synchrony should be low, especially in patients with haemodynamic compromise.

Bradycardia: Postoperative bradycardia is treated with atrioventricular sequential pacing in order to maximise the cardiac output. Transient or permanent complete heart block may occur following aortic valve surgery due to oedema, haemorrhage, debridement or damage to the atrioventricular bundle. If complete heart block persists for more than 4–5 days then due consideration should be given to the placement of a permanent pacemaker.

Hypotension: Adequate preload is essential for patients with aortic valve disease due to accompanying diastolic dysfunction. Hypotension and hypovolaemia must be avoided as they could lead to a vicious cycle of coronary hypoperfusion, reduced cardiac output and worsening hypotension.

Hypertension: Hypertension tends to develop a few hours following surgery secondary to the relief of left ventricular outflow tract obstruction, often in the setting of left ventricular hypertrophy. Severe hypertension should be aggressively treated in order to protect the surgical aortic suture lines and reduce myocardial oxygen demand.

Stroke: Stroke may be caused by emboli in the presence of atheromatous aortic disease, particularly in elderly patients and/or those with known history of cerebrovascular disease. Cerebral hypoperfusion may also lead to cerebral ischaemic injury with or without concomittent embolism in light of the high prevalence of large and small vessel cerebral vascular disease.

TAVI Patients in ICU: Novel technology of minimally invasive treatment for aortic valve stenosis by percutaneous valve implantation has allowed for patients with greater comorbidities and hence high surgical risk to be treated. These patients do not normally need ICU post-surgical admission. However, in case of complications intraoperatively and postoperatively, these patients can need intensive care. Common reasons for ICU admissions are haemodynamic instability (bradycardia, arrhythmia, hypotension, hypertension), pulmonary oedema, renal failure and stroke. The support for these patients follows the same principles as for surgical aortic valve patients.

Aortic Regurgitation

Hypovolaemia: In the setting of diastolic dysfunction that accompanies ventricular hypertrophy, large fluid challenges often result in minimal change in filling pressures. Adequate preload is important in these patients for maintenance of an adequate cardiac output.

Hypotension: Hypotension is not uncommon following aortic valve replacement for regurgitation. The reasons can be multifactorial, and include post cardiopulmonary bypass vasodilatation, low cardiac output due to reduced contractility, pericardial collection or reduced preload. Post cardiopulmonary bypass vasodilatation is not uncommon and is readily treated with vasopressor medication. However, it is important to establish that this is the reason for hypotension, and not reduced cardiac output or pericardial collection. Therefore, use of ultrasound imaging to rule out a pericardial collection and cardiac output measurement is advisable.

Bradycardia and **complete heart block** should be treated in a similar fashion as for aortic stenosis (see above).

Mitral Valve Surgery

Mitral valve surgery is generally indicated in patients with severe mitral stenosis not amenable to percutaneous mitral balloon valvuloplasty and those with severe symptomatic mitral regurgitation.

Mitral valvular pathology may arise due to dysfunction of the mitral annulus, leaflets, subvalvular apparatus as a result of ventricular dysfunction or a combination of some or all of these components.

Anatomical Considerations

Rheumatic heart disease is the commonest cause of mitral stenosis, whereas degenerative disease is the commonest cause of mitral regurgitation. Other causes of mitral regurgitation include ischaemic heart disease, rheumatic disease and endocarditis.

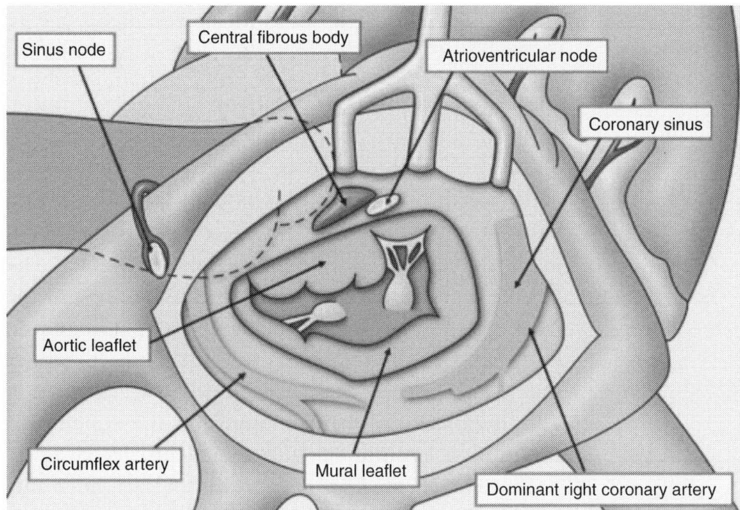

Figure 38.1 Mitral valve and its relation to various structures. (A black and white version of this figure will appear in some formats. For the colour version, please refer to the plate section.)

The mitral valve is a complex structure that has an important role in the left ventricular geometry and function. The subvalvular apparatus, which includes the chordae tendinea and papillary muscles, plays an important role in maintaining the integrity of the mitral valve as well as the function of the left ventricle. The anterior and posterior leaflets of the mitral valve are arbitrarily divided into A1, A2, A3 and P1, P2, P3 regions, respectively. The circumflex artery runs in the atrioventricular groove near the posteromedial commissure and in close proximity to the medial half of the posterior leaflet of the mitral valve. Injury or compression to the circumflex artery results in inferobasal and lateral wall ischaemia (Figure 38.1).

The coronary sinus is close to the anterolateral commissure and adjoining part of the posterior leaflet, while part of the anterior leaflet is close to the non-coronary cusp of the aortic valve. Care must be taken when annular sutures are placed in these regions.

Mitral annular calcification causes difficulties and challenges during mitral valve surgery. Overenthusiastic decalcification of the mitral annulus may result in atrioventricular disruption, which is associated with high mortality and morbidity. Excessive removal of the subvalvular apparatus may result in left ventricular rupture.

Physiological Considerations

Mitral stenosis is generally associated with a small left ventricular cavity size. Advanced cases may be complicated by pulmonary hypertension (which may be reversible or irreversible) and occasionally right heart dysfunction. Affected patients are prone to low cardiac output postoperatively as a result of low end-diastolic and end-systolic volumes. The onset of congestive heart failure may coincide with the development of atrial fibrillation. Postoperatively, stroke volume is largely dependent on the maintenance of adequate ventricular preload. The pathology of degenerative disease of the mitral valve causing mitral regurgitation ranges from fibroelastic deficiency to Barlow's disease. Barlow's disease is characterised by pronounced annular dilatation, bileaflet prolapse and the presence of thick, spongy leaflets due to excessive myxomatous tissue proliferation. It may also be associated with annular calcification. Fibroelastic deficiency is found in older patients whereas Barlow valve with congenitally excessive valve tissue is seen in younger patients.

There may be prolongation or rupture of the chordae giving rise to a flail or prolapsing leaflet. Chronic mitral regurgitation causes volume overload of the left ventricle that leads to ventricular and atrial dilatation. Mitral regurgitation leads to increased ventricular preload as the regurgitate volume generated during systole returns to the ventricle during diastole. There is also reduced ventricular stress along with reduced afterload due to offloading of the ventricle. As the ventricle accommodates to the excess volume by dilatation, there is minimal elevation of the pulmonary vascular resistance initially. Increased pulmonary vascular resistance occurs due to chronic volume overload, ultimately leading to left ventricular failure.

Acute ischaemic mitral regurgitation is most often due to annular dilation and malfunction of coaptation due to ventricular remodelling. However, it can also be due to ruptured chordae or head of the papillary muscle following myocardial infarction. The posteromedial papillary muscle is most commonly involved as it is only supplied by the posterior descending branch of the right coronary artery (or the circumflex artery in the case of a left dominant coronary circulation). The heart has little time to adapt to the regurgitant mitral valve, which results in rapid rise of pulmonary pressure, pulmonary oedema and development of cardiogenic shock. This is associated with high mortality.

Chronic ischaemic mitral regurgitation is generally a disease of the ventricle. Features include annular dilatation and tethering of the papillary muscle and posterior leaflet due to ventricular remodelling following ischaemia.

Common ICU Problems

Ventilatory failure: This can occur in patients with long standing mitral stenosis who have pulmonary hypertension. It is important to avoid hypoxia and hypercarbia in the early postoperative period. Therefore management of pulmonary congestion by reducing preload (diuresis, haemofiltration, vasodilatation), pulmonary vasodilatation and mechanical ventilator support is important. Where prolonged mechanical ventilation of the lungs is needed, the team need to judge the risks of ventilator associated pneumonia and other complications of mechanical ventilation versus earlier extubation.

Right ventricular dysfunction: Following surgery for mitral stenosis, right ventricular dysfunction normally improves over time. However, right ventricular dysfunction can be problematic. A pathophysiological approach to treatment is advisable. Optimising preload, and maintaining adequate contractility, along with reduction in right ventricular afterload where possible, are the usual strategies. Medical treatment with phosphodiesterase inhibitors, intra-aortic balloon counterpulsation and right ventricular extracorporeal support (temporary right ventricular assist device, Impella) may be needed.

Left ventricular dysfunction: Correction of valvular regurgitation often unmasks left ventricular dysfunction and may require treatment with appropriate inotropes.

Atrial fibrillation: Many patients undergoing mitral valve surgery have pre-existing paroxysmal or chronic atrial fibrillation. The Maze procedure or pulmonary vein isolation may be used as an adjunct to mitral valve surgery in these patients. A left atrial diameter of less than 5 cm and duration of atrial fibrillation of less than 5 years is associated with greater success of the Maze procedure. The left atrial appendage may also be excised or obliterated in these patients to reduce the risk of stroke due to chronic atrial fibrillation and embolisation of thrombus from the appendage. In addition, around 30–40% of patients develop new onset of atrial fibrillation following mitral valve surgery needing electrical or chemical cardioversion with amiodarone therapy.

Tricuspid Valve

Tricuspid valve surgery is commonly indicated for moderate–severe functional tricuspid regurgitation due to left sided valvular heart disease or less commonly pulmonary vascular disease. Tricuspid valve surgery is also indicated for right heart failure refractory to medical therapy or progressive dilatation of the right ventricle. Severe tricuspid regurgitation is not a benign process because of its effects on systemic venous congestion, atrial rhythm and right ventricular function.

The tricuspid valve has three leaflets: septal, anterior and posterior. The septal leaflet abuts the fibrous skeleton of the heart, as a result of which it cannot dilate.

The anterior leaflet is the largest of all the leaflets. The tricuspid valve has papillary muscle and chordal attachments to the ventricular septum, unlike the mitral valve. The atrioventricular node lies just posterior to the commissure between the anterior and septal leaflets. Deeply placed sutures in the medial half of the septal leaflet may result in atrioventricular block. The right coronary artery lies in close proximity to the posterior leaflet. A deep suture placed in this region may result in injury to the coronary artery or kinking of the artery.

Most cases of tricuspid valve dysfunction are caused by failure of the coaptation of the leaflets due to annular dilatation. Tricuspid valve replacement is only rarely indicated, as an annuloplasty ring is adequate to correct functional tricuspid insufficiency in most cases.

Valve Implant Considerations

Choice of Prosthesis

According to the American Heart Association Guidelines 2014, bioprostheses are recommended for patients over the age of 70 years while mechanical prostheses are recommended below 60 years of age provided there are no contraindications to anticoagulation. Between 60 and 70 years either prosthesis is reasonable. Patient choice is essential in the decision making process.

Postoperative Anticoagulation

Prosthetic heart valves are susceptible to thrombosis. For patients with mechanical mitral valves and those with associated risk factors (i.e. atrial fibrillation, previous thromboembolism and hypercoagulable condition) receiving mechanical aortic valves, aspirin (75—100 mg once daily) as well as warfarin (with a target INR of 3) should be commenced in the early postoperative period and continued in the long term. Bridging anticoagulation with unfractionated heparin should be considered if warfarin therapy is interrupted for any future cardiac or non-cardiac procedures.

For mechanical aortic valves without risk factors, warfarin therapy with a lower target INR (2.5) and long-term aspirin (75—100 mg once daily) should be used.

Aspirin (75—100 mg once daily) and warfarin therapy (target INR 2.5) is recommended for the first 3 months following mitral valve repair or replacement with bioprostheses.

Special Considerations

Mitral valve

Repair of the mitral valve is preferable to replacement. If replacement is carried out, the subvalvular apparatus (papillary muscle and chordae) should be preserved in order to maintain left ventricular function. Mitral repair is associated with better short-term and long-term survival and less incidence of thromboembolism when compared to replacement.

Systolic anterior motion

Mitral valve repair is occasionally complicated by systolic anterior motion (SAM). SAM has long been recognised as a risk factor for left ventricular outflow tract obstruction and residual mitral regurgitation following mitral valve surgery. SAM results from the 'Venturi effect' pulling the mitral valve leaflets into the left ventricular outflow tract (LVOT). This may result in obstruction of the LVOT along with severe mitral regurgitation due to displacement of the anterior leaflet.

Intraoperative echocardiogram is essential to identify the risk of SAM and detection should this occur.

Predisposing factors for systolic anterior motion include the following:

1. Narrow aortomitral angle (<120° pre repair).
2. Distance of the ventricular septum to coaptation point of the mitral leaflet <2.5 cm.
3. Posterior leaflet height >1.5 cm.
4. Basal septal diameter >1.5 cm.

When identified intraoperatively, initial measures include maintenance of adequate preload and reduction of tachycardia. If these conservative measures fail then insertion of a larger annuloplasty ring or a sliding annuloplasty should be performed in order to reduce the height of the posterior leaflet.

Postoperative management for prevention of systolic anterior motion includes the following:

1. Maintenance of adequate preload.
2. Increase afterload by using alpha agonists.
3. Reduce tachycardia by using beta adrenoreceptor blockers.
4. Avoidance of inotropic agents.

Combined valvular pathologies

Different valvular pathologies can occur in combination. The combination of aortic regurgitation along with mitral regurgitation carries high perioperative morbidity and carries the worst prognosis if left untreated. The combination of these two pathologies causes left ventricular enlargement, increasing volume overload and ultimately ventricular failure.

Key Points

- Following valve procedures, maintenance of sinus rhythm is beneficial in order to optimise cardiac output, as is careful optimisation of ventricular filling pressures.
- Valve procedures can be complicated by heart block due to haemorrhage, oedema, suturing

or aggressive debridement near the conductive tissue.

- Degenerative disease is the commonest cause of mitral regurgitation. Localised ventricular infarct along with asymmetric ventricular remodelling affecting the posterolateral ventricular wall causes ischaemic mitral regurgitation. Functional mitral regurgitation is caused by a severely impaired and dilated left ventricle.
- Although mitral and aortic valve diseases are the commonest indications for heart valve surgery, the tricuspid valve can be a potential source of considerable morbidity and mortality. Tricuspid valve disease commonly occurs secondary to left heart disease or pulmonary vascular disease.
- The type of valve prosthesis used is dependent on the patient age, valve preference, comorbidities, valvular pathology and the contraindications to the use of anticoagulants.

Further Reading

Bojar RM. *Manual of Perioperative Care in Adult Cardiac Surgery*, 5th edition. Oxford: Wiley-Blackwell, 2011.

Loulmet DF, Yaffee DW, Ursomanno PA, et al. Systolic anterior motion of the mitral valve: a 30-year perspective. *Journal of Thoracic and Cardiovascular Surgery*. 2014; 148: 2787–2793.

Mackay JH, Arrowsmith JE (Eds). *Core Topics in Cardiac Anesthesia*, 2nd edition. Cambridge: Cambridge University Press, 2012.

Nishimura RA, Otto CM, Bonow RO, et al. 2014 AHA/ACC guideline for the management of patients with valvular heart disease: a report of the American College of Cardiology/American Heart Association Task Force on Practice Guidelines. *Journal of Thoracic and Cardiovascular Surgery*. 2014; 148: e1–e132.

Varghese R, Itagaki S, Anyanwu AC, et al. Predicting systolic anterior motion after mitral valve reconstruction: using intraoperative transoesophageal echocardiography to identify those at greatest risk. *European Journal of Cardio-Thoracic Surgery*. 2014; 45: 132–138.

MCQs

1. **A 28 year old female needs an aortic valve replacement for severe symptomatic aortic stenosis. She wants to complete her family within the next few years. What are the options for management?**

   (a) Mechanical prosthesis

   (b) Bioprosthesis

   (c) Ross procedure

   (d) (b) or (c)

   (e) Medical treatment until she completes her family.

2. **An 80 year old female underwent mitral valve repair for severe mitral regurgitation. After coming off bypass her parameters were as follows: mean arterial pressure 45 mmHg, heart rate 95 beats/minute, central venous pressure 10 mmHg. TOE revealed systolic anterior motion of the mitral valve. What should be the next appropriate step?**

   (a) Increase the heart rate to 110 beats/minute

   (b) Start inotrope

   (c) Fluid bolus

   (d) Start noradrenaline

   (e) Observe

3. **After coming off bypass following aortic valve replacement for severe aortic stenosis, the patient has a mean arterial pressure of 50 mmHg, heart rate of 45 beats/minute and a central venous pressure of 12 mmHg. Atrial and ventricular wires had been inserted before coming off bypass. In order to increase the heart rate what is the best pacemaker mode that should be selected in order to optimise cardiac output?**

   (a) VVI

   (b) AOO

   (c) DOO

   (d) DDD

   (e) VOO

4. **What is the commonest cause of mitral stenosis?**

   (a) Degenerative

   (b) Rheumatic

   (c) Endocarditis

   (d) Congenital heart disease

   (e) Carcinoid

5. **After coming off bypass following mitral valve replacement there are ST depressions in leads I, II, V5, V6 and regional wall motion abnormalities in the lateral wall on TOE. What is the possible cause of the wall motion abnormalities?**

   (a) Injury to the right coronary artery

   (b) Injury to the circumflex coronary artery

   (c) Injury to the left anterior descending artery

   (d) Air embolism of the coronary arteries

   (e) Inadequate cardioprotection

Exercise answers are available on p.469. Alternatively, take the test online at www.cambridge.org/CardiothoracicMCQ

Chapter 39

Pulmonary Endarterectomy Patients in Cardiothoracic Critical Care

Choo Yen Ng

Introduction

Chronic thromboembolic pulmonary hypertension (CTEPH) arises from total or partial occlusion of the pulmonary vascular bed from non-resolving thromboemboli. Although pulmonary embolism (PE) is one of the more common cardiovascular diseases, CTEPH remains an under-diagnosed condition. CTEPH is defined as precapillary pulmonary hypertension with mean pulmonary artery pressure (mPAP) of more than 25 mmHg, pulmonary capillary wedge pressure (PCWP) of less than 15 mmHg and pulmonary vascular resistance (PVR) of more than 2 Wood units.

CTEPH is a relatively rare but important sequela of deep venous thrombosis (DVT) and PE, where in up to 4% of patients, the acute embolic material fails to resolve. Given that DVT and PE is as common as 1/1000 population per year, the annual incidence of CTEPH may be of the order of 8–40 cases/million population. However, because some patients diagnosed with chronic thromboembolic disease have no preceding history of acute embolism, the true incidence of this disorder could be much higher.

The majority of DVT and acute PE are managed medically with anticoagulation. Cardiothoracic surgeons rarely become involved in management of acute PE, unless it is in a hospitalised patient who survives a massive embolism that causes life-threatening acute right heart failure and shock. Conversely, the majority of CTEPH cases are amenable to surgical treatment by pulmonary endarterectomy (PEA). PEA is the definitive, and in most cases the curative, treatment for CTEPH. The objective of the surgery is the normalisation of pulmonary artery pressure with resultant significant symptomatic and prognostic benefit. Medical management is only palliative, and lung transplantation has an inferior outcome compared with PEA and is only relevant for very selected patients with distal disease and extreme pulmonary hypertension (PH).

Pathophysiology

It is uncertain why some patients have unresolved emboli, but a variety of factors play a role, alone or in combination. Initially, thrombus resolution probably results from a combination of thrombus fragmentation and endogenous fibrinolysis. In the majority of patients this leads to complete clot resolution. Further resolution relies on clot organisation and neovascularisation, during which the obstructed vessel becomes recanalised and vessel patency is partially restored.

After the clot becomes wedged in the pulmonary artery, one of two processes occurs:

1. The organisation of the clot proceeds to canalisation, producing multiple small endothelialised channels separated by fibrous septa (i.e. bands and webs).
2. Complete fibrous organisation of the fibrin clot without canalisation may result, leading to a solid mass of dense fibrous connective tissue totally obstructing the arterial lumen.

The generation of PH in CTEPH is not just the result of simple obstruction of the pulmonary arterial bed; indeed, there is little rise in pulmonary artery pressure following a pneumonectomy. The increased pressure as a result of redirected pulmonary blood flow in the unobstructed pulmonary vascular bed can create an arteriopathy in the small precapillary blood vessels similar to that seen in idiopathic pulmonary arterial hypertension. Hence, the pathogenesis of chronic thromboembolic occlusion in CTEPH with resultant raised PVR is thought to be secondary to obstruction by thromboemboli and remodelling of the previously normal pulmonary vascular bed.

Clinical Presentation and Diagnosis

Clinical Presentation

There are no symptoms specific for chronic thromboembolism. The most common symptom associated with thromboembolic pulmonary hypertension, as with all other causes of pulmonary hypertension, is exertional dyspnoea. This dyspnoea is out of proportion to any abnormalities found on clinical examination. Syncope, or presyncope, is another common symptom in severe pulmonary hypertension.

The physical signs of pulmonary hypertension are the same no matter what the underlying pathophysiology. Initially the jugular venous pulse is characterised by a large 'A' wave. As the right heart fails, the 'V' wave becomes predominant. The right ventricle is usually palpable near the lower left sternal border. The second heart sound is often narrowly split and varies normally with respiration. In the later stages of the disease, signs of right heart failure predominate with oedema and ascites. Tricuspid regurgitation can be severe, with a pansystolic murmur and an enlarged pulsatile liver.

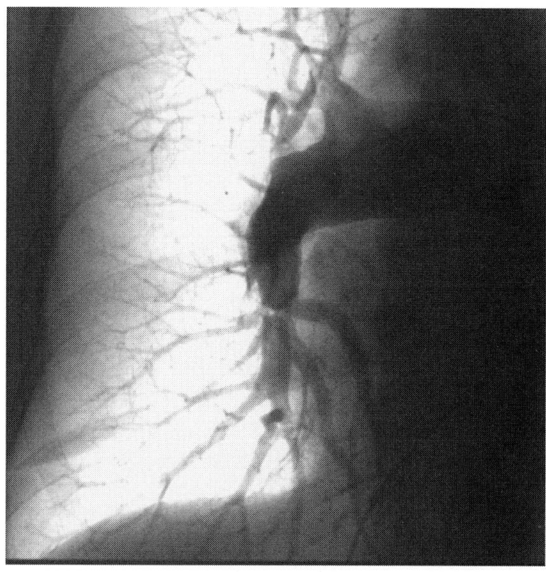

Figure 39.1 Right pulmonary angiography of a patient with CTEPH demonstrating a web in the trifurcation of the lower lobe vessels with complete occlusion of two segments of the lower lobe and both segments of the middle lobe.

Diagnosis

High index of suspicion and awareness of the disease is crucial. The chest radiograph may be entirely normal. Pulmonary function tests reveal minimal changes in lung volume and ventilation. Diffusion capacity is often reduced and may be the only abnormality on pulmonary function testing. Most patients are hypoxic. Dead space ventilation is increased.

The ventilation-perfusion lung scan is the essential test for establishing the diagnosis. An entirely normal lung scan excludes the diagnosis of both acute and chronic thromboembolism.

Transthoracic echocardiogram (TTE) is usually the test that gives the first indication of the presence of PH. Systolic pulmonary artery pressure is significantly raised. Features that may be seen on TTE depend on the chronicity and degree of right ventricular failure; raised right ventricular dimension, impaired right ventricular function and right ventricular hypertrophy.

Currently, pulmonary angiography is said to be the gold standard imaging test for evaluation of operability in CTEPH, but experience is essential for the proper interpretation of pulmonary angiograms. Organised thrombi appear as filling defects, webs or bands, or as completely thrombosed vessels 'missing' (Figure 39.1). Distal vessels demonstrate the rapid tapering and pruning characteristic of pulmonary hypertension. Other modalities of imaging, including multislice CT pulmonary angiogram and magnetic resonance angiography, are gaining acceptance and are now favoured over conventional angiography in some centres.

Right heart catheterisation is crucial for the diagnosis of pulmonary hypertension, defined as a mPAP >25 mmHg at rest. Right atrial pressure, right ventricular end-diastolic pressure, pulmonary artery pressure and mixed venous O_2 saturation are measured directly. Cardiac output and PVR can then be calculated. Coronary angiography and other cardiac investigations are recommended for patients over 40–45 years being considered for surgery.

Management – Medical Treatment

The main treatment of CTEPH is surgical and all patients with suspected CTEPH should be referred to an experienced unit able to perform PEA. Untreated, the prognosis of CTEPH is very poor with severe debilitation and premature death from right heart failure. In historical case series, the mean survival is 6.8 years, and when the mPAP of patients with thromboembolic disease reaches 50 mmHg or more, the 3-year mortality is about 90%.

Chronic anticoagulation represents the mainstay of the medical regimen. Anticoagulation is primarily used to prevent future embolic episodes, but it also serves to limit the development of thrombus in regions of low flow within the pulmonary vasculature. Historically, inferior vena caval filters were used routinely to prevent recurrent embolisation but this is now not recommended, as there are few data to support this indication.

Data from clinical drug trials in CTEPH are limited. Specific disease targeted drug therapy is therefore not licensed for CTEPH patients, but drugs used for the treatment of idiopathic pulmonary arterial hypertension such as Bosentan and Sildenafil are sometimes used and may provide symptomatic improvement in some patients.

Pulmonary Endarterectomy

Operative Principles

The basis of the operation is the removal of the obstruction of the pulmonary vascular bed by endarterectomy within the superficial media of the arterial wall. Therefore, the reduction in the PVR after pulmonary endarterectomy is dependent on the burden of 'clearable' disease as defined on preoperative imaging. The correlation between the degree of 'clearable' disease in imaging studies and PVR is the main determinant of operability. The absolute preoperative and resultant postoperative PVR are also the main factors that determine outcome after endarterectomy. Mortality following endarterectomy may be five- to ten-fold higher in patients with a preoperative PVR > 1200 dyne s/cm^5. Similarly, a postoperative residual PVR of > 500 dyne s/cm^5 is a risk factor for in-hospital mortality.

Although preoperative imaging helps to determine operability, the true extent of the disease can only be determined intraoperatively and has been classified in four types:

Type 1: Central disease where major vessel clots (fresh and/or mature) are present.

Type 2: Lobar and segmental disease where thickened intima is present with webs in the lobar and segmental branches.

Type 3: Subsegmental disease where the disease begins distally at the subsegmental branches.

Type 4: Distal disease where small vessel disease is present and represents inoperable disease.

Surgery is more successful in patients with types 1 and 2 disease, with a greater reduction in PVR and lowest mortality. Surgery in patients with the more distal type 3 disease is more challenging with a smaller reduction in PVR and higher risk. Patients with predominant type 4 disease are considered 'non-operable' or to have 'non-surgical' disease.

Patient Selection

Main indications for surgery are symptoms and prognosis. A patient with CTEPH, in WHO Class II–IV with significant pulmonary hypertension (mPAP more than 25 mmHg), stands to benefit from PEA.

This must be weighed against the amount of 'clearable' disease based on imaging and correlated to the pulmonary vascular resistance measured preoperatively.

Other patient comorbidities that will be significant in a prolonged cardiopulmonary bypass time such as age, known cerebrovascular condition, renal impairment and intrinsic lung parenchymal disease should also be considered.

Surgical Techniques

The approach is via a median sternotomy with cardiopulmonary bypass (CPB). The patient is cooled systemically to 20 °C and right and left pulmonary arteriotomies are performed within the pericardium. Adequate visualisation for distal dissection necessitates reduction in bronchial arterial collateral return to the pulmonary arteries. This is achieved by periods of complete deep hypothermic circulatory arrest for up to 20 minutes at a time with an intervening period of 10 minutes of re-perfusion on CPB. A cast of the inner layer of the pulmonary arterial tree is then dissected free (Figure 39.2).

After completion of the endarterectomies, the patient is rewarmed slowly on full CPB. The procedure time is long because of the time necessary to cool and warm on bypass.

The aim is to achieve an immediate fall in mean PA pressure by approximately 50%, and reduction in PVR to approximately one third of the preoperative level in the majority of patients.

Critical Care Management

General Principles

Most of the general principles of postoperative cardiac surgical care apply, but these principles centre around

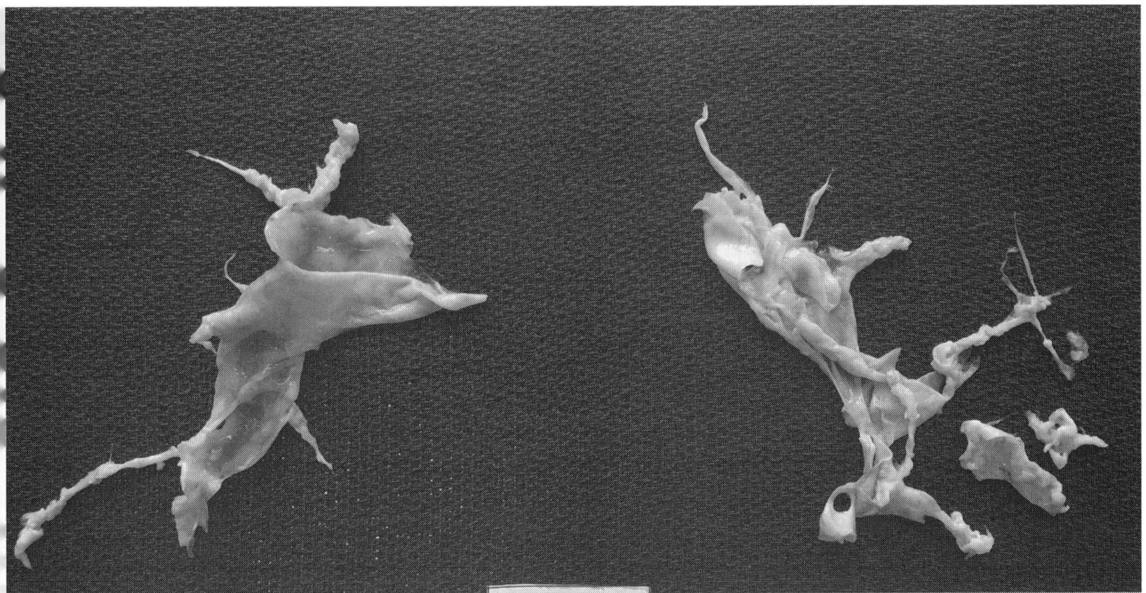

Figure 39.2 Endarterectomy casts from both pulmonary arteries of the same patient in Figure 39.1, demonstrating long tapering 'tails' which is a hallmark of good clearance. (A black and white version of this figure will appear in some formats. For the colour version, please refer to the plate section.)

the management of the left ventricle. The management of patients following PEA involves these two principles:

- Careful management of the right ventricle;
- Minimising the pulmonary vascular resistance.

Most patients with CTEPH have a normal functioning left ventricle in the absence of coronary atherosclerosis and 'left-sided' heart valvular disease. Therefore left ventricular cardiac output and ultimately end-organ perfusion is usually dependent on the contractile reserve of the right ventricle and pulmonary vascular resistance in the post-PEA patients.

The contractile reserve of the right ventricle in the post-PEA patients depends on the following:

- The varying degree of right ventricular impairment secondary to CTEPH in the preoperative period;
- The post-PEA pulmonary vascular resistance that is dependent on the amount of disease cleared during PEA with resultant fall in pulmonary artery pressure. High PVR in the postoperative period can be due to technical failure to clear 'surgical' disease and/or presence of type 4 distal disease (inoperable):
- Prolonged cardiopulmonary bypass, prolonged myocardial ischaemic time and inadequate right ventricular myocardial protection during PEA which impacts on right ventricular performance upon weaning from cardiopulmonary bypass.

Pulmonary vascular resistance in the post-PEA patient can be affected by the following:

- Right ventricular function, hence inexplicably linked;
- Hypoxia secondary to poor perfusion matching, intrinsic lung parenchymal disease, fluid overload, lung sepsis and mechanical complications such as pneumothorax;
- Vasoconstrictor agents such as noradrenaline;
- High peak airway pressures.

Considering the above factors when receiving a patient onto the Critical Care Area (CCA) following PEA surgery will help plan for potential problems that may be encountered during the postoperative period.

Monitoring

Patients returning from the operating room following PEA surgery should have the following monitoring:

- 3 lead ECG monitoring;
- Pulse oximetry;
- Invasive radial and femoral arterial pressure;
- Invasive central venous pressure;
- Invasive pulmonary artery pressure;

- Peripheral oxygen saturation and respiratory rate;
- Blood temperature and end-tidal CO_2 measurement.

The femoral arterial line, which is placed after induction, is used in preference to the radial line due to damping associated with cooling and rewarming during surgery. It is used for the first 12 hours in CCA before being removed and arterial monitoring reverts back to the radial line.

The balloon at the tip of the pulmonary artery catheter is disabled and never inflated. Pulmonary artery wedge pressure is taken as a default at 10 mmHg to allow comparison of pulmonary vascular resistance over time. Cardiac output and other haemodynamic measurements are taken at 4 hourly intervals during the first 24 hours. The pulmonary arterial catheter is usually removed 24 hours after the patient is extubated, and providing there are no concerns regarding residual pulmonary hypertension.

Ventilation

Patients are connected to the ventilator in the operating room before weaning of cardiopulmonary bypass. The patient is then transferred to the CCA with the same ventilator to ensure a continuous level of positive end-expiratory pressure (PEEP).

A chest radiograph is usually obtained within an hour of arrival in the CCA, to exclude the presence of pneumothorax and early signs of reperfusion lung injury (see below).

The patient is nursed in a slight upright position of at least 30° to reduce the preload on the right ventricle.

Recommended ventilator settings on arrival to the CCA are as follows:

- SIMV or SIMV PRVC mode;
- Fraction inspired oxygen percentage (FiO_2) of 80%;
- Tidal volume set at 10 ml/kg;
- Respiratory rate at 16/minute;
- PEEP of 6 cmH_2O;
- Pressure support of 12 cmH_2O above PEEP level.

An aggressive ventilator weaning protocol is adopted with the aim of facilitating extubation by the first postoperative day. The FiO_2 is decreased by 10% every second hour, as long as the PaO_2 is above 12 kPa (or every hour if PaO_2 is above 25 kPa). Once FiO_2 of 40% is reached, the PEEP is decreased at a rate of 1 cmH_2O every hour down to a minimum of 2 cmH_2O. Peak airway pressure should be less than 30 cmH_2O.

Most patients who have had a good surgical clearance during PEA surgery with resultant mPAP of less than 25 mmHg and a low PVR, who are haemodynamically stable with satisfactory acid–base balance, should achieve these ventilator targets by the first postoperative day. The sedation is then turned off and the patient is allowed to wake up and is extubated.

In some cases, it may be necessary to extubate the patient onto a continuous positive airway pressure (CPAP) mask, especially when the PaO_2 is borderline low or the patient is cerebrally agitated or obtunded, to avoid hypoxia and maintain normocapnoea.

Drugs and Antibiotic Prophylaxis

The specific aim is to achieve a negative daily fluid balance and support the right ventricle. Mannitol (12.5 g, 6 hourly for 6 doses) and furosemide (40 mg, 6 hourly for 6 doses then decrease to 8 hourly on day 2 and 12 hourly on day 3) are used to keep these patients 'dry'. At Papworth Hospital NHS Foundation Trust, the standard inotropic support following PEA surgery is dopamine at 3–5 μg/kg/min until the patients are discharged to the ward.

Rarely, the patients develop systemic hypertension during the first 24 hours due to a systemic vascular resistance that remains high and this is associated with low or borderline low cardiac indices. Most patients can tolerate this and do not require intervention unless the low cardiac output impacts on end-organ perfusion such as renal function. Phosphodiesterase inhibitor such as Enoximone is sometimes used in this situation.

In situations where residual pulmonary hypertension remains post PEA surgery, preoperative drugs such as Bosentan and Sildenafil may be continued in the postoperative period. In cases where residual pulmonary hypertension is significant post PEA with concomitant right ventricular impairment or failure, ilioprost (nebulised) is frequently used as an adjunct (see residual PH and right ventricular failure below).

The prophylactic antibiotic of choice is Tazocin, which is a combination antibiotic containing extended-spectrum penicillin antibiotic piperacillin and β-lactamase inhibitor tazobactam. The combination has activity against many Gram-positive and Gram-negative pathogens and *Pseudomonas aeruginosa*. This covers both the sternotomy wound and the potential pathogens that the lung may be exposed to. In patients who have penicillin allergy, vancomycin and aztreonam are used instead.

Fluid Balance and Renal Support

The patient's haematocrit is maintained above 30% (haemoglobin above 100 g/l) and human albumin solution (4%) is the colloid of choice. Crystalloid is avoided at all times.

In patients who develop acute or acute-on-chronic kidney injury secondary to the effects of prolonged cardiopulmonary bypass and surgery, maintaining aggressive diuresis can be challenging. Furosemide may be switched to an infusion. Haemofiltration is often used to maintain acid–base balance and maintain negative balance, especially when the kidney injury impacts on ventilatory weaning and haemodynamic stability.

Haematology and Anticoagulation

Dilutional and consumptive coagulopathy is not uncommon after a prolonged cardiopulmonary bypass with low platelet counts and clotting factors. Unless there is significant bleeding, transfusion of blood products such as pooled platelets, fresh frozen plasma and cryoprecipitate are to be avoided in the first 24–48 hours. Infusion of these products into a pulmonary vasculature that is denuded of its intimal layer can result in release of cytokines and formation of microemboli, which result in a rise of the mPAP and PVR.

Enoxaparin 40 mg once daily is usually started on the evening of the first postoperative day. If the patient is extubated, warfarin is commenced on the second postoperative day. If warfarin cannot be instituted, heparin infusion is commenced. This is an important part of PEA management as anticoagulation with warfarin or another novel direct Xa inhibitor like Rivaroxaban is the mainstay of CTEPH prevention post PEA surgery.

Cerebrovascular

Prolonged cardiopulmonary bypass and periods of deep hypothermic circulatory arrest may impact on the neurological function especially in the elderly. In addition, elderly patients on long term warfarin have a very small but significant prevalence of chronic subdural haematomas. Combined with a coagulopathy in the immediate postoperative period, all these can contribute to cerebral agitation or obtunded neurological state when sedation is switched off. In addition, tranexamic acid infusion (started during surgery to prevent fibrinolysis) may give rise to small incidences of epileptic fits.

Therefore, the threshold to perform CT brain scans in these patients who do not wake up appropriately should be low to avoid missing treatable causes of an altered neurological state. Otherwise, if the CT scans are inconclusive, the treatment is largely supportive and patients usually recover with conservative management.

Specific Complications

Reperfusion Lung Injury

Reperfusion injury is defined as new radiological opacity in the lungs within 72 hours of pulmonary endarterectomy with associated hypoxia. The clinical manifestation is that of focal or diffuse pulmonary oedema. The radiological opacity can be segmental or unilateral and is thought to reflect the segmental area where surgical clearance was most effective with resultant sudden increase in perfusion.

Reperfusion injury that directly adversely impacts the clinical course of the patient occurs in approximately 10% of patients. In its most dramatic form, it occurs soon after operation (within a few hours) and is associated with profound desaturation with rapidly worsening PaO_2:FiO_2 ratio.

Early measures should be taken to minimise the development of pulmonary oedema with diuresis, maintenance of the haematocrit levels, and the early use of peak end-expiratory pressure. Once the capillary leak has been established, treatment is supportive because reperfusion pulmonary oedema will eventually resolve if satisfactory haemodynamics and oxygenation can be maintained. Venovenous extracorporeal membrane oxygenation (ECMO) is sometimes necessary to provide temporary support when failure of adequate oxygenation impacts significantly on end-organ functions.

Residual Pulmonary Hypertension and Right Ventricular Failure

The decrease in PVR level usually results in an immediate and sustained restoration of pulmonary artery pressure to normal levels. Therefore right ventricular function improves and cardiac output is often increased. In patients with residual PH, the postoperative course can be difficult and the risk of death is increased. The general principles outlined above explain the link between PVR and right ventricular performance and the various factors that can affect the relationship with often deleterious consequences.

Pulmonary vasodilators (iloprost) and inotropic support (enoximone and judicious use of vasoconstrictor) are used in an attempt to improve right ventricular performance and reduce PVR. If the surgical clearance has been adequate and it is thought there may be some reversibility (myocardial recovery following surgery and recovery from superimposed lung sepsis), venoarterial ECMO may allow time for recovery.

We have used ECMO to support patients with severe reperfusion lung injury and residual PH post PEA. Up to 2016, 33 patients have been supported with successful weaning in 70% and long-term survival in approximately 50%. The period of ECMO support has ranged from 48 to 1480 hours.

Pulmonary Haemorrhage

This is a rare, dramatic and often fatal complication of PEA that happens in the operating room around the time of cardiopulmonary bypass wean. The clinical manifestation is profound haemorrhage into the bronchial airways resulting in severe hypoxia. It results from perforation of the pulmonary arterial wall during dissection of the endarterectomy cast.

Single lung ventilation with isolation of the offending side is usually futile and the only option is conversion from cardiopulmonary bypass to central venoarterial ECMO and reversal of systemic heparinisation. If central venoarterial ECMO results in a viable patient, the patient is brought back to the CCA and maintained on ECMO until haemorrhage into the airway has stopped. Bronchial toilet is then performed to clear the airway before any attempts to wean from ECMO. Mortality from this complication is nearly 100%.

Outcomes

Since the year 2000, Papworth Hospital has been the sole commissioned centre for pulmonary endarterectomy in the UK and we have seen a steady increase in the number of operations and improvement in results over the last 10 years (Figure 39.3).

Over 1350 patients have now been operated on at Papworth and the current in-hospital mortality is 3–4%. In a recent cohort, the median age was 60 years (range 15–84) with concomitant surgery being carried out in 10% of the cases.

All PEA patients in the UK are reviewed at 3 months and 1 year after endarterectomy. In a recent review of 230 patients, we demonstrated a significant improvement in NYHA class following surgery (Figure 39.4). Five-year survival is nearly 90% even in patients over 70 years of age.

Learning Points

CTEPH is one of the most prevalent and increasingly recognised forms of pulmonary hypertension (PH) and should be considered in all cases with unexplained PH.

- Patients with CTEPH should receive lifelong anticoagulation and be considered for treatment with pulmonary endarterectomy.
- Pulmonary endarterectomy is the treatment of choice in selected cases and may be curative with normalisation of pulmonary artery pressures and significant symptomatic and prognostic benefit.
- Critical care management of patients following pulmonary endarterectomy involves careful management of the right ventricle and minimising pulmonary vascular resistance.
- Reperfusion injury and residual pulmonary hypertension with or without right ventricular failure are treatable in the most severe form with venovenous or venoarterial extracorporeal membrane oxygenation (ECMO).

Further Reading

Madani M, Auger WR, Pretorius V, et al. Pulmonary endarterectomy: recent changes in a single institution's experience of more than 2,700 patients. *Annals of Thoracic Surgery*. 2012; 94: 97–103.

Mayer E, Jenkins DP, Lindner J, et al. Surgical management and outcome of patients with chronic thromboembolic pulmonary hypertension: results from an international prospective registry. *Journal of Thoracic and Cardiovascular Surgery*. 2011; 141: 702–710.

NHS Information Centre for Health and Social Care. National Audit of Pulmonary Hypertension, 2nd annual report, 2011. Available at: www.ic.nhs.uk

Simonneau G, Robbins IM, Beghetti M, et al. Updated clinical classification of pulmonary hypertension. *Journal of the American College of Cardiology*. 2009; 54(Suppl): S43–S54.

Thistlethwaite PA, Makato M, Madani MM, et al. Operative classification of thromboembolic disease determines outcome after pulmonary endarterectomy. *Journal of Thoracic and Cardiovascular Surgery*. 2002; 124: 1203–1211.

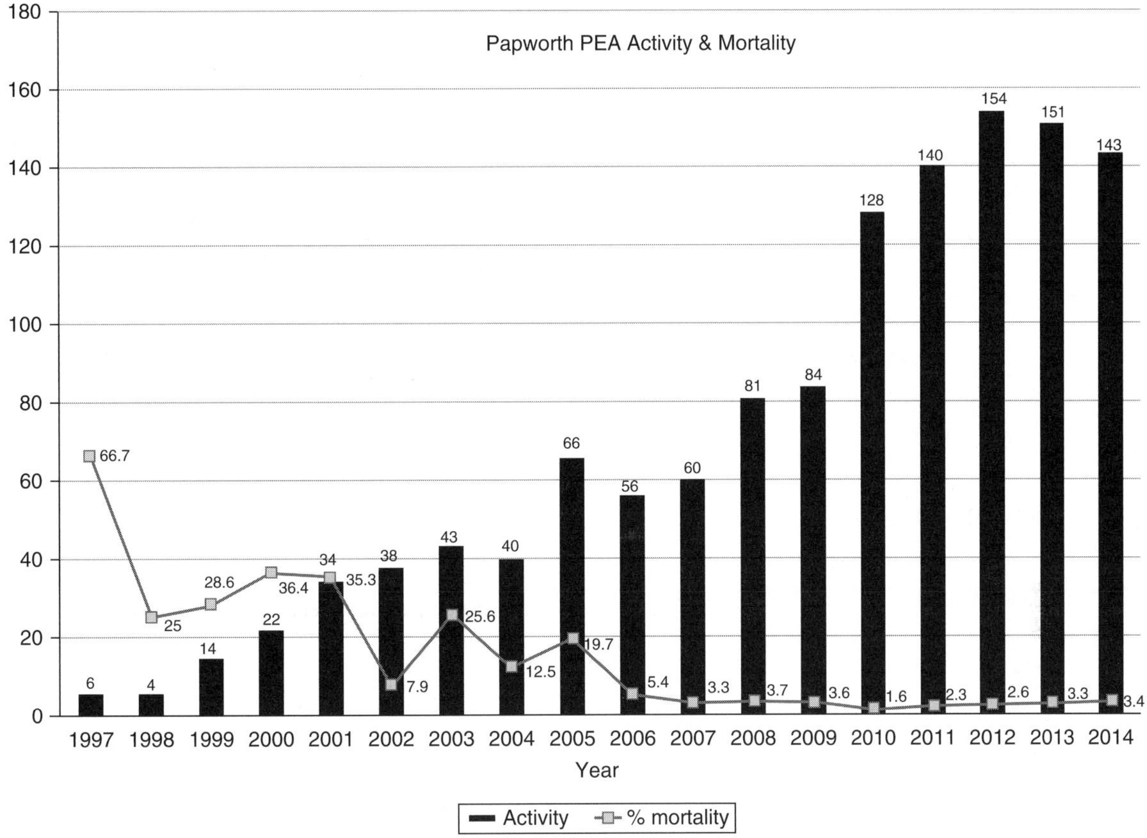

Papworth PEA Activity & Mortality

180
160
140
120
100
80
60
40
20
0

Year	Activity	% mortality
1997	6	66.7
1998	4	25
1999	14	28.6
2000	22	36.4
2001	34	35.3
2002	38	7.9
2003	43	25.6
2004	40	12.5
2005	66	19.7
2006	56	5.4
2007	60	3.3
2008	81	3.7
2009	84	3.6
2010	128	1.6
2011	140	2.3
2012	154	2.6
2013	151	3.3
2014	143	3.4

Year

Activity % mortality

Figure 39.3 Number of PEA operations in the UK.

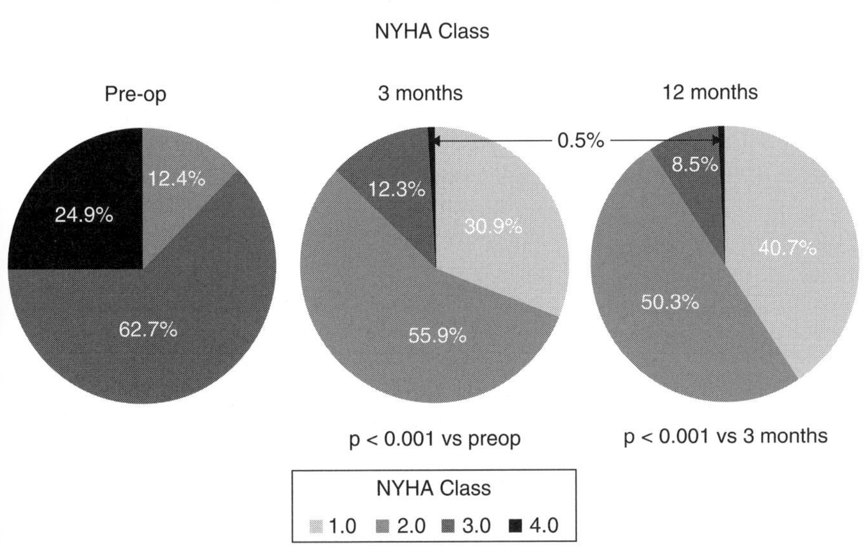

Figure 39.4 NYHA class: preoperative, at 3 months and 12 months follow-up.

MCQs

1. **Chronic thromboembolic pulmonary hypertension (CTEPH) is a precapillary pulmonary hypertension that can be defined by one of these criteria:**
   (a) Pulmonary artery wedge pressure of more than 20 mmHg
   (b) Central venous pressure of less than 10 mmHg
   (c) Mean pulmonary artery pressure of more than 25 mmHg
   (d) Cardiac index of less than 2.0 l/min/m^2

2. **Which one of these symptoms is the most common in patients with CTEPH?**
   (a) Persistent cough
   (b) Exertional dyspnoea
   (c) Paroxysmal nocturnal dyspnoea
   (d) Exertional angina

3. **Pulmonary endarterectomy is the definitive treatment for one of the following:**
   (a) Idiopathic pulmonary hypertension
   (b) Pulmonary venous hypertension secondary to mitral valvular disease
   (c) Eisenmenger 's syndrome
   (d) Chronic thromboembolic pulmonary hypertension

4. **Management of post-PEA patients in cardiothoracic critical care revolves around one of these principles:**
   (a) Inotropic support for the left ventricle
   (b) Aggressive use of vasoconstrictors
   (c) Prolonged ventilation
   (d) Management of the right ventricle and pulmonary vascular resistance

5. **Which one of these complications is NOT seen in post-PEA patients?**
   (a) Left to right shunt
   (b) Reperfusion lung injury
   (c) Residual pulmonary hypertension
   (d) Massive lung haemorrhage

Exercise answers are available on p.469. Alternatively, take the test online at www.cambridge.org/CardiothoracicMCQ

Chapter 40

Heart Transplantation

Stephen J Pettit and Anna Kydd

Introduction

Heart transplantation remains the definitive treatment for advanced heart failure that is refractory to conventional medical and surgical therapy. Over 110,000 heart transplants have been performed worldwide. Survival is excellent with a median survival of 11 years for all patients and 13 years for patients that survive the first year. The majority of patients return to a normal quality of life. Heart transplantation is limited by supply of suitable donor hearts. For this reason, the waiting time for heart transplantation is long and many patients deteriorate while waiting. Selected patients receive mechanical circulatory support with implantable or paracorporeal ventricular assist devices as a bridge to heart transplantation. These patients pose a particular challenge when they come to heart transplantation, but their outcomes need not be adversely affected.

The time of greatest risk for mortality after heart transplantation is during the immediate postoperative period when patients are on the critical care unit. It is important that cardiac surgeons, cardiologists and intensive care doctors share an awareness of the goals of treatment and common problems in order to deliver excellent outcomes. Greater institutional experience is associated with a lower incidence of complications and higher survival after heart transplantation. This is vital for the success of a transplant programme because outcomes are closely scrutinised by regulatory bodies.

Preoperative Assessment

Patients are assessed by a multidisciplinary team before acceptance onto a waiting list for heart transplantation. Assessment serves several purposes. The team must determine whether the patient is expected to derive symptomatic and prognostic benefit from heart transplantation. The team must identify any contraindications to heart transplantation; common problems that may preclude heart transplantation are listed in Table 40.1. Finally, the team must enable the patient to make an informed decision about whether they wish to be placed on the waiting list for heart transplantation. Intensive care doctors are important members of the multidisciplinary team. Problems with airway management, vascular access, ventilatory support, nutritional support and psychological difficulties may be predictable in certain patients. Postoperative critical care planning should begin at the time of preoperative assessment.

Transfer from the Operating Room

It is important to understand any problems that were encountered in the operating room at the point of admission to the critical care unit. An early indication of allograft function will be given by visual inspection of the donor heart as cardiopulmonary bypass is weaned, the amount of cardiovascular support required, invasive haemodynamic data (cardiac index, pulmonary capillary wedge pressure and right atrial pressure) and blood tests including mixed venous oxygen saturation and serum lactate. In the most severe forms of primary graft dysfunction, patients may leave the operating room with venoarterial extracorporeal membrane oxygenation (VA ECMO) support. The team in the critical care unit should receive the patient and ensure that they are in a satisfactory haemodynamic state. Any immediate surgical problems should be identified before the operating room team stand down.

Postoperative Care

Excellent long-term outcomes after heart transplantation are dependent on excellent postoperative care in the critical care unit. Patients change rapidly in the immediate postoperative period. Close observation

Table 40.1 Common absolute and relative contraindications to heart transplantation

Absolute contraindications	Relative contraindications
Transpulmonary pressure gradient >15 mmHg	Advanced age
Pulmonary vascular resistance >5 Wood units	Body mass index >32 or <17.5
Irreversible renal dysfunction	Recent pulmonary embolism
Sepsis or active infection	Smoking, alcohol or substance misuse
Microvascular complications of diabetes	Severe mental health disorder
Malignancy within 5 years (except skin)	

Table 40.2 Principles of care after heart transplantation

Support allograft function
Allow recovery of end-organ function
Establish immunosuppression
Avoid infection

by all members of the multidisciplinary team is vital. Treatment will need to be continually adjusted on an individual patient basis. The basic principles of care are outlined in Table 40.2.

A series of investigations are routinely performed to assess allograft function and look for common problems. These include regular blood gas analysis, daily venous blood tests, an electrocardiogram, chest radiography and transthoracic echocardiography. Additional investigations such as cross-sectional imaging and therapeutic drug monitoring assays are arranged if needed. Surveillance endomyocardial biopsy is usually performed on a weekly basis during the first month after heart transplantation, but this is generally deferred until the patient is discharged from the intensive care unit unless there is specific concern about acute rejection. Common problems after heart transplantation are summarised in Table 40.3.

Airway and Ventilation

All patients will be sedated and mechanically ventilated via an endotracheal tube until they are ready for extubation. Many sedative drugs cause vasodilatation and drive use of potentially deleterious vasopressors.

Table 40.3 Common problems after heart transplantation

Right ventricular dysfunction
Acute kidney injury
Bleeding into pericardial or pleural space
Sinus node dysfunction or high grade AV block
Atrial arrhythmias
Systemic inflammatory response syndrome

Mechanical ventilation must be used with care. Excessive tidal volume and positive end-expiratory pressure (PEEP) should be avoided. Both increase right atrial pressure, worsen tricuspid regurgitation and increase right ventricular work by increasing pulmonary vascular resistance. Hypoxia should not be permitted because it will cause pulmonary vasoconstriction, increase pulmonary vascular resistance and increase right ventricular work. Inhaled therapies such as nitric oxide and iloprost may be used to reduce pulmonary vascular resistance in selected patients.

Cardiovascular

Sinus node dysfunction and atrioventricular (AV) block are common after heart transplantation. All patients should leave the operating room with temporary epicardial pacing wires. It is important to ensure that these are attached to a temporary pulse generator and that the pacing system is working correctly. Sinus tachycardia should be expected in the denervated heart. However, this is not always present in the immediate post transplant period. Demand pacing in a dual chamber mode (DDD) with a lower rate limit of 90–100 beats per minute is routine. A relatively high heart rate may improve cardiac output in a transplanted heart when the ability to augment stroke volume is limited. Pacing threshold, sensing and underlying rhythm should be assessed on a daily basis. Sinus rhythm and AV conduction typically return within 1 to 3 weeks of transplantation but around 10% of patients will require a permanent pacemaker.

All patients require continuous invasive monitoring of cardiovascular performance in the immediate postoperative period. This is most commonly achieved with a pulmonary artery catheter. It is helpful to establish desirable haemodynamic ranges; an example is provided in Table 40.4. Measurements outside the desirable range should prompt review and exclusion of a surgical problem such as haemopericardium or haemothorax. In the absence of a surgical problem, abnormal haemodynamics may represent a target for treatment. Abnormalities such as hypovolaemia may be easy to identify and treat. It is important to recognise that right ventricular dysfunction is common after heart transplantation and a leading cause of primary graft failure. Risk factors for right ventricular dysfunction include older donor age, longer ischaemic time, low donor height/weight relative to recipient and high pulmonary vascular resistance in recipient. Right ventricular dysfunction is normally identified by a low cardiac index and rising right atrial pressure. Treatment of right ventricular dysfunction is complex and the principles are outlined in Figure 40.1. It is vital that high right atrial pressure is not permitted because this will lead to right ventricular distension and a downward spiral of right heart failure.

Table 40.4 Desirable haemodynamic parameters after heart transplantation

Haemodynamic parameter	Desirable range
Mean arterial pressure	70–90 mmHg
Mean right atrial pressure	5–12 mmHg
Mean pulmonary capillary wedge pressure	5–12 mmHg
Cardiac index	>2
Mixed venous oxygen saturation	>70%

Use of inotropic or vasoactive medications in isolation or combination after heart transplantation is common but there is no good evidence base to support the superiority of any particular regime. Agents should be selected according to individual patient physiology and the desired effect. The expected effects in a typical patient are outlined in Table 40.5. In general, the dose of inotropic or vasoactive medications should be minimised and the medications should be progressively weaned as recovery of allograft and end-organ function is seen. Intra-aortic balloon pump (IABP) counterpulsation will increase coronary blood flow and reduce left atrial pressure, both of which may be helpful in right ventricular dysfunction.

Mechanical circulatory support may be required when inotropic, vasopressor/vasodilator and intra-aortic balloon pump support is insufficient to achieve desired haemodynamic parameters. Percutaneous devices to mechanically support the right ventricle are now available but have not been widely used after heart transplantation. VA ECMO is thought to be the best treatment for severe primary graft failure. Central cannulation may be preferable to peripheral cannulation to allow longer support duration, permit left ventricular venting and reduce the risk of peripheral vascular complications. Primary graft dysfunction may improve sufficiently for VA ECMO to be weaned in up to 90% of patients within 1 week. In the most severe cases, central VA ECMO may be used as a bridge to acute re-transplantation.

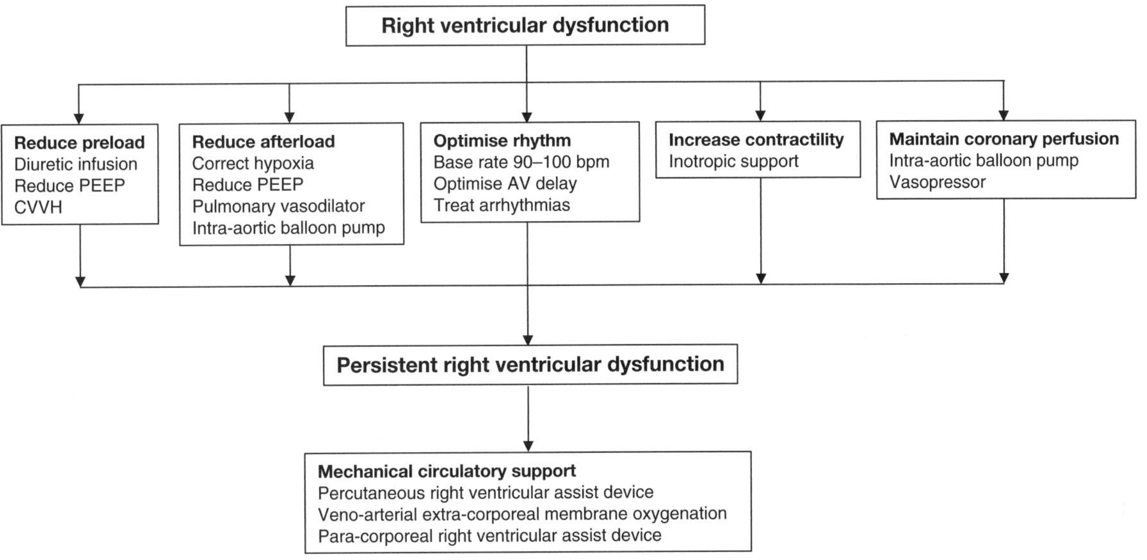

Figure 40.1 Treatment of right ventricular dysfunction. CVVH continuous venovenous haemofiltration.

Table 40.5 Expected effects of agents used for cardiovascular support after heart transplantation

Agent	Contractility	SVR	PVR
Adrenaline	Increased	Increased	Neutral
Noradrenaline	Increased	Increased	Increased
Dopamine	Increased	Increased	Neutral
Arginine vasopressin	Neutral	Increased	Increased
Type 2 PDEi	Increased	Decreased	Decreased
Hydralazine	Neutral	Decreased	Neutral

Renal

Most patients sustain acute kidney injury (AKI) at the time of transplantation and the risk is greater in patients with pre-existing renal dysfunction. It is imperative to avoid high right atrial pressure in order to avoid right ventricular distension and progressive right ventricular dysfunction. Patients require multiple intravenous medications in the immediate post-transplant period and a high urine output is essential to maintain fluid balance. Most patients are treated with loop diuretics to maintain neutral or negative fluid balance. Continuous venovenous haemofiltration (CVVH) may be required if patients have significant AKI and either important electrolyte disturbances, acidosis or a positive fluid balance and high right atrial pressure. One should aim to wean CVVH as soon as possible to avoid platelet consumption within the circuit and vascular access complications. Care must be taken to adjust doses of antimicrobial therapy in patients with postoperative renal dysfunction, and introduction of potentially nephrotoxic immunosuppressive medications may be delayed until recovery of renal function.

Immunosuppression

All recipients receive immunosuppression from the time of transplantation to reduce the risk of rejection. Hyperacute antibody-mediated rejection is rare in the modern era because of matching to avoid ABO or HLA incompatibility, but should be considered in the event of very early primary graft dysfunction. Acute cellular rejection remains a major problem and is challenging to diagnose due to lack of specific clinical features. In general, there should be a low threshold for treatment of suspected acute cellular rejection. Most centres use 10 mg/kg of intravenous methylprednisolone, administered on 3 consecutive days, for treatment of acute cellular rejection. Endomyocardial biopsy should ideally be performed before treatment, but treatment should not be delayed if it is not possible to perform endomyocardial biopsy in a timely fashion.

There is no consensus on the optimal regime for immunosuppression, and practice varies between transplant centres. Immunosuppression will also vary between patients for reasons including renal dysfunction and haematological abnormalities. Most patients are maintained on three immunosuppressive agents during the first year after transplantation and two immunosuppressive agents in the longer term.

Corticosteroids

All patients receive intravenous corticosteroids at the time of transplantation and these are continued until gastrointestinal absorption recovers. Steroids are started at high doses, equivalent to 1 mg/kg prednisolone per day, then slowly weaned to a maintenance dose, equivalent to 0.2 mg/kg prednisolone per day. Further reductions in corticosteroid dose and discontinuation are guided by surveillance endomyocardial biopsy.

Proliferation inhibitors

All patients receive a proliferation inhibitor at the time of transplantation and these are continued lifelong. The first choice agent is mycophenolate mofetil (MMF). A specific preparation is prescribed due to differences in bioavailability. Patients will receive intravenous MMF until gastrointestinal absorption recovers. Oral MMF should be taken with meals to reduce the incidence of gastrointestinal adverse effects. Azathioprine may be used if MMF is not tolerated. Leucopenia is a common adverse effect and the full blood count must be regularly measured. Proliferation inhibitors should be reduced or stopped if there is significant leucopenia, particularly in the context of infection.

Calcineurin inhibitors (CNI)

Most patients are treated with ciclosporin or tacrolimus after heart transplantation. Tacrolimus has a more favourable profile of adverse effects than ciclosporin, but there is no difference in survival. CNI may be started at the time of transplantation or delayed until recovery from AKI if an induction agent is used. Therapeutic drug monitoring is required to achieve a balance between efficacy and toxicity. The most common adverse effect of CNI is renal dysfunction, due to renal arteriolar vasoconstriction. Patients may receive sublingual tacrolimus or intravenous ciclosporin if they are unable to absorb medications from the gastrointestinal tract.

Mammalian target of rapamicin (mTOR) inhibitors

Sirolimus or everolimus may be used in place of CNI or proliferation inhibitors after heart transplantation. The major benefit over CNI is a lower incidence of renal dysfunction. However, mTOR inhibitors have a less favourable profile of adverse effects than CNI. Wound healing delay is a particular concern in the immediate post-transplant period.

Induction agents

Induction agents may be used at the time of heart transplantation. These are antibodies directed against components of the cell-mediated immune response. Anti-human thymocyte globulin (ATG) and anti-human lymphocyte globulin (ALG) are polyclonal antibodies. Muromonab is a monoclonal antibody directed against CD3, expressed on T lymphocytes. Basiliximab, daclizumab and inolimomab are monoclonal antibodies directed against the interleukin-2 receptor. Alemtuzumab is a monoclonal antibody directed against CD52, expressed on B and T lymphocytes, as well as macrophages, monocytes and natural killer cells. There is no evidence any induction agent improves survival but they may reduce the incidence of acute rejection and allow CNI to be withheld until resolution of AKI.

Antimicrobial Prophylaxis

Most centres administer prophylactic antibiotic therapy at the time of heart transplantation, based on local resistance patterns and recipient colonisation. In general, prophylactic antibiotics are stopped if donor culture results are negative. Co-trimoxazole is commonly used as prophylaxis against *Pneumocystis jirovecii* during the first year after heart transplantation. Prophylactic antiviral therapy may be used according to donor and recipient cytomegalovirus (CMV) status. Intravenous ganciclovir is started at the time of transplantation and switched to oral valganciclovir when possible. The optimal duration of CMV prophylaxis is uncertain. Many centres discontinue valganciclovir after 3 to 6 months depending on donor and recipient CMV status, then monitor for CMV reactivation or de novo CMV infection. Other antiviral agents may be used if there are specific concerns about infection such as hepatitis or human immunodeficiency virus (HIV) in either donor or recipient. Nystatin is used to prevent mucocutaneous *Candida* infection. Additional antifungal prophylaxis with an azole or an echinocandin may be used if there are specific risk factors for fungal infection in the recipient.

Other Issues

Many other issues must be addressed in the critical care unit that are not unique to heart transplantation. These include management and removal of pleural, mediastinal and pericardial drains. Feeding must be established as soon as possible and total parenteral nutrition may be required if the gastrointestinal tract cannot be accessed or is not functioning. Physiotherapy is an important part of the recovery process and should be commenced as soon as possible. Careful and close communication with the family is required. Psychological support is likely to be required for both patient and family, particularly if there are early problems with allograft function.

Discharge from the Critical Care Unit

Discharge from the critical care unit should occur when the patient has been successfully weaned from support and both allograft and end-organ function continue to recover. The receiving medical team need to know the date of transplantation, current cardiovascular function including any ongoing requirement for pacing, details of renal function including the need for postoperative CVVH, and details of current immunosuppression including any induction agents that have been administered.

Learning Points

- The period of highest risk for mortality occurs early after heart transplantation while patients are on the critical care unit.

- All patients will have a degree of right ventricular dysfunction after heart transplantation and require careful individualised cardiovascular support.
- High right atrial pressure must not be permitted because this will lead to right ventricular distension and a downward spiral of worsening right heart failure.
- Corticosteroids and proliferation inhibitors are started at the time of transplantation but introduction of calcineurin inhibitors may be delayed until renal recovery if an antibody is used for induction of immunosuppression.
- All patients require antimicrobial prophylaxis from the time of transplantation.

Further Reading

Banner NR, Bonser RS, Clark AL, et al. UK guidelines for referral and assessment of adults for heart transplantation. *Heart*. 2011; 97: 1520–1527.

Costanzo MR, Dipchand A, Starling R, et al. The International Society of Heart and Lung Transplantation guidelines for the care of heart transplant recipients. *Journal of Heart and Lung Transplantation*. 2010; 29: 914–956.

Dhital KK, Iyer A, Connellan M, et al. Adult heart transplantation with distant procurement and ex-vivo preservation of donor hearts after circulatory death: a case series. *Lancet*. 2015; 385: 2585–2591.

Grimm JC, Kilic A, Shah AS, et al. The influence of institutional volume on the incidence of complications and their effect on mortality after heart transplantation. *Journal of Heart and Lung Transplantation*. 2015; 34: 1390–1397.

Kobashigawa J, Zuckermann A, Macdonald P, et al. Report from a consensus conference on primary graft dysfunction after cardiac transplantation. *Journal of Heart and Lung Transplantation*. 2014; 33: 327–340.

Lahm T, McCaslin CA, Wozniak TC, et al. Medical and surgical treatment of acute right ventricular failure. *Journal of the American College of Cardiology*. 2010; 56: 1435–1446.

Lund LH, Edwards LB, Kucheryavaya AY, et al. The Registry of the International Society for Heart and Lung Transplantation: Thirty-second Official Adult Heart Transplantation Report-2015; Focus theme: early graft failure. *Journal of Heart and Lung Transplantation*. 2015; 34: 1244–1254.

Schulze PC, Jiang J, Yang J, et al. Preoperative assessment of high-risk candidates to predict survival after heart transplantation. *Circulation: Heart Failure*. 2013; 6: 527–534.

Singh TP, Milliren CE, Almond CS, et al. Survival benefit from transplantation in patients listed for heart transplantation in the United States. *Journal of the American College of Cardiology*. 2014; 63: 1169–1178.

Tallaj JA, Pamboukian SV, George JF, et al. Have risk factors for mortality after heart transplantation changed over time? Insights from 19 years of Cardiac Transplant Research Database study. *Journal of Heart and Lung Transplantation*. 2014; 33: 1304–1311.

MCQs

1. **Which of the following factors is not a contraindication to heart transplantation?**
   (a) Transpulmonary pressure gradient of 12 mmHg
   (b) Patient age 72 years
   (c) Complete resection of adenocarcinoma of colon 2 years ago
   (d) Pulmonary vascular resistance of 6.5 Wood units
   (e) Left lower lobe pneumonia
2. **Which of the following statements about RV dysfunction after heart transplantation is true?**
   (a) Shorter ischaemic time is a risk factor for development of RV dysfunction
   (b) Increasing pulmonary vascular resistance may be helpful in the treatment of RV dysfunction
   (c) High right atrial pressure may lead to worsening RV dysfunction
   (d) Venoarterial ECMO is not a treatment option for patients with severe RV dysfunction
   (e) Pacing should be minimised in patients with RV dysfunction by setting a lower rate limit of 50–60 bpm
3. **Regarding use of antibody induction agents in heart transplantation, which of the following is false?**
   (a) Antithymocyte globulin may be used for induction of immunosuppression

(b) Use of antibody induction agents may reduce the incidence of early rejection after heart transplantation

(c) Basiliximab may be used for induction of immunosuppression

(d) Use of antibody induction agents allows calcineurin inhibitor introduction to be delayed until recovery from acute kidney injury

(e) Use of antibody induction agents improves survival after heart transplantation

4. Regarding use of antimicrobial prophylaxis after heart transplantation, which of the following is false?

(a) Valganciclovir is used as prophylaxis against CMV infection for 3 to 6 months after heart transplantation

(b) Nystatin is used as prophylaxis against mucocutaneous *Candida* infection

(c) Co-trimoxazole is used as prophylaxis against *Pneumocystis jirovecii* infection

(d) Entecavir is used as prophylaxis in selected individuals at risk of hepatitis B infection

(e) Penicillin V is used as prophylaxis against encapsulated bacterial infection

5. Which of the following treatments is not used to decrease pulmonary vascular resistance after heart transplantation?

(a) Nebulised iloprost

(b) Intravenous noradrenaline

(c) Reduction of PEEP

(d) Inhaled nitric oxide

(e) Intravenous type II phosphodiesterase inhibitor

Exercise answers are available on p.469. Alternatively, take the test online at www.cambridge.org/CardiothoracicMCQ

Lung Transplantation

JS Parmar

Introduction

Lung transplantation is currently the most effective treatment in carefully selected patients with a variety of end-stage lung diseases. The major indications for lung transplantation are chronic obstructive pulmonary disease (COPD), cystic fibrosis (CF), pulmonary fibrosis (PF) and pulmonary hypertension (PH). Sadly there is a critical shortage of donor organs, which results in the need for careful selection of patients to maximise the benefit of a scarce resource. This careful selection includes an assessment of the patient's abilities to withstand the rigors of lung transplantation. This assessment has relied on clinical judgement of the patient's condition performed by the multidisciplinary team.

Although a successful therapy with both prognostic and quality of life benefit, it is not a risk free enterprise. Most large volume centres quote a 1-year survival of around 85% and 5-year survival of approximately 60% with a median survival of 6.8 years.

Lung transplant patients will routinely require support in the ICU in the immediate post transplant period but may also develop issues post transplant necessitating ICU admission. These two requirements are distinct clinical entities and are considered separately.

General ICU Issues

Lung transplant recipients are vulnerable to a number of specific issues related to their disease and treatment. However, if they become critically ill they are also vulnerable to the general range of problems that are seen in critically ill patients. These include problems with dysfunction of any of the major organ systems. Two that require specific mention are kidney and neuromuscular dysfunction. The entire transplant process places a huge strain on the renal system. Surgery, transfusion of blood products and the use of nephrotoxic drugs can all result in the loss of kidney function in the early postoperative period and this is associated with poorer outcomes.

Lung transplant patients are probably at higher risk of developing the ICU related neuromyopathy as a result of the requirement for high dose steroids as part of the immunosuppression protocol. This can have a significant impact on the process of rehabilitation, necessitating longer stays in the ICU. If severe, it can impact on the respiratory muscles and diaphragm, which can lead to poor airway clearance and the need for a tracheostomy.

Early Post Transplant

Primary Graft Dysfunction (PGD)

The transplant process from the declaration of death in the donor, to organ harvesting, cold storage and finally reperfusion in the recipient places a huge stress on the organ. All of these essential steps may create an inflammatory milieu that increases the possibility of alveolar oedema. The absence of lymphatic drainage in transplanted lungs, the primary mechanism for clearing excess alveolar fluid, means that the lung is exquisitely sensitive to these fluid shifts.

Primary graft dysfunction (PGD) is the syndrome complex that describes the early allograft dysfunction (<72 hours) and is the largest cause of early mortality. It is clinically manifest by progressive hypoxaemia associated with radiological infiltrates, and shares many similarities with acute respiratory distress syndrome (ARDS) in non-transplanted lungs. The syndrome is graded according to the International Heart and Lung consensus document (Table 41.1).

It is important to exclude other causes of early allograft dysfunction such as infection, volume overload, torsion of the lung or compromise of the pulmonary venous anastomosis, and acute rejection. In the majority of cases with grade 1 or 2 dysfunction, a relatively

Table 41.1 International Heart and Lung Transplantation consensus on primary graft dysfunction

Grade	PaO_2/FiO_2	Radiographic infiltrates consistent with pulmonary oedema
0	>300	Absent
1	>300	Present
2	200–300	Present
3	<200	Present

benign course is followed. However, the presence of persistent grade 3 PGD (>72 hours) is associated with a poor prognosis with estimates of 1-year survival varying from 30 to 60% and reduced long-term survival. A number of potential risk factors have been identified which include: recipients with PH, IPF, sarcoidosis or donors with obesity, older age, smoking, high alcohol intake, and possibly the use of cardiopulmonary bypass. Treatment of PGD is principally about careful fluid balance with supportive measures for oxygenation and haemodynamics. Aggressive diuresis and protective lung ventilation are the cornerstones of management for milder grades. For PGD grade 3, in addition to the above support, measures such as venovenous extracorporeal membrane oxygenation may be required (Figures 41.1 and 41.2). Some experimental approaches have included instillation of surfactant directly into the lung. Other potential treatments that are being explored include aspirin, statins, stem cells and aprotonin.

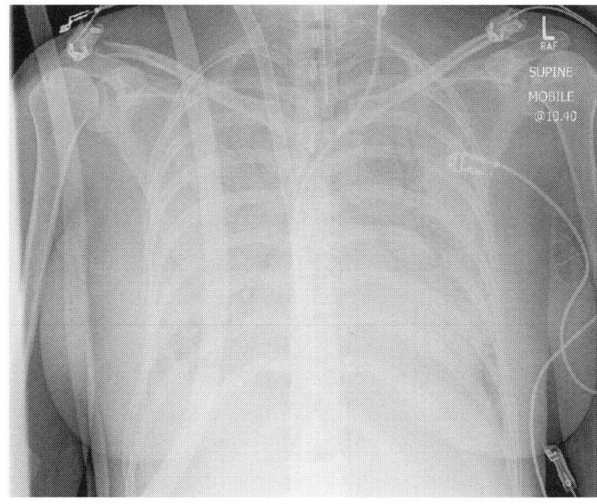

Figure 41.1 PGD grade 3 at 48 hours. The patient is very hypoxic despite being intubated and ventilated and is requiring ECMO support. The X-ray demonstrates extensive bilateral infiltrates.

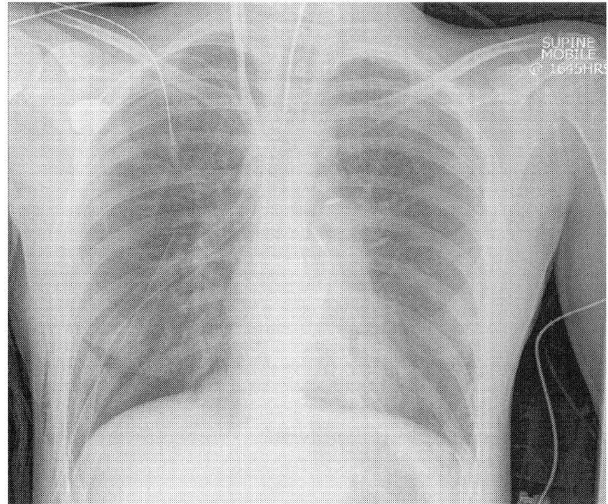

Figure 41.2 PGD grade 3 at 1 week. The patient remains intubated and ventilated but with clearance of the alveolar oedema and without ECMO support.

Infections

The second biggest cause of early mortality in lung transplant recipients in the ICU after PGD grade 3 is infection. The lung transplant recipient is particularly vulnerable to infection as the allograft is open to the atmosphere and a number of the usual defence mechanisms are compromised. Foremost of these are the impairment of mucociliary function, reduced cough, pain and compromise of the innate and adaptive immune responses by immunosuppression. In addition, the use of mechanical ventilation along with the multiple invasive catheters required to manage the patient are portals for entry for infection in an immunosuppressed patient. This vulnerability extends across the whole microbial constellation and means that susceptibility to bacterial, fungal and viral infections is increased. Whilst opportunistic infections with low virulence organisms such as *Pneumocystitis jirovecii* (PCP) can be problematic it should be remembered that the most common infections in this group are the same as for other critically ill patients. This high-risk profile is managed early post transplant with prophylaxis with broad spectrum antibiotics, oral and nebulised antifungals and target antiviral agents.

Bacterial Infections

Cultures are taken from the donor at the time of harvesting and the generic universal prophylactic antibiotic regime is adjusted if these are positive. Many recipients will have pre-existing respiratory infections that may have antibiotic resistances. This is particularly an issue in CF patients who are often colonised chronically with *Pseudomonas aeuroginosa,* which is present in the upper airways and often recolonises the new lungs. This is managed with a pre-existing agreed antibiotic protocol and usually consists of at least two anti-pseudomonal agents that are given for 2 weeks post transplantation.

Viral Infections

The desired T-cell inhibitory effects of the post-transplant immunosuppression increase the susceptibility to and reduce the recipient's capacity to deal with viral infections. Cytomegalovirus (CMV) is the commonest viral pathogen in lung transplant recipients and is associated with increased risk of chronic rejection in patients who develop CMV pneumonitis. The greatest risk is in CMV mismatched patients who are CMV naive and receive a positive organ. All CMV mismatched patients and positive patients receive prophylaxis with initially ganciclovir and subsequently valganciclovir.

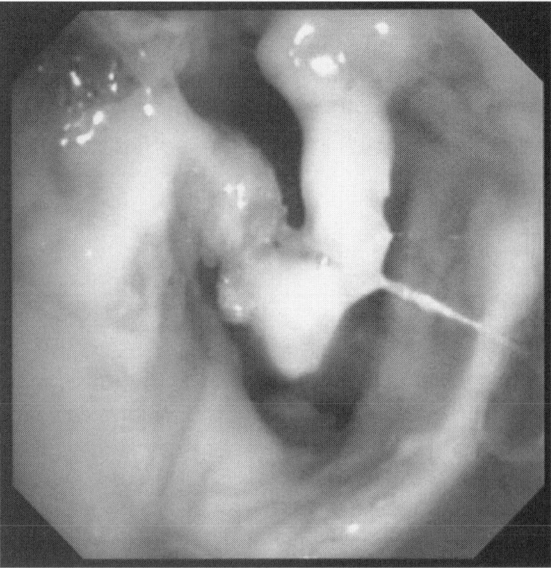

Figure 41.3 Bronchoscopic appearance of a right bronchial anastomosis, demonstrating a severely ischaemic airway with superadded *Aspergillus* infection. (A black and white version of this figure will appear in some formats. For the colour version, please refer to the plate section.)

Fungal Infections

Fungal infections cause significant morbidity and mortality in recipients post lung transplant. Lung transplants are particularly vulnerable to *Aspergillus fumigatus* infections of the airways. This can range from anastomotic infections that can result in airway complications to *Aspergillus* trachea-bronchitis (Figure 41.3). Fortunately, angioinvasive aspergillosis is a rare complication. To combat this potential complication, early post transplant most patients receive antifungal prophylaxis. Practices vary according to the risk profile of the centre. We employ both topical nebulised amphotericin and oral itraconazole until there is airway healing (Figure 41.4).

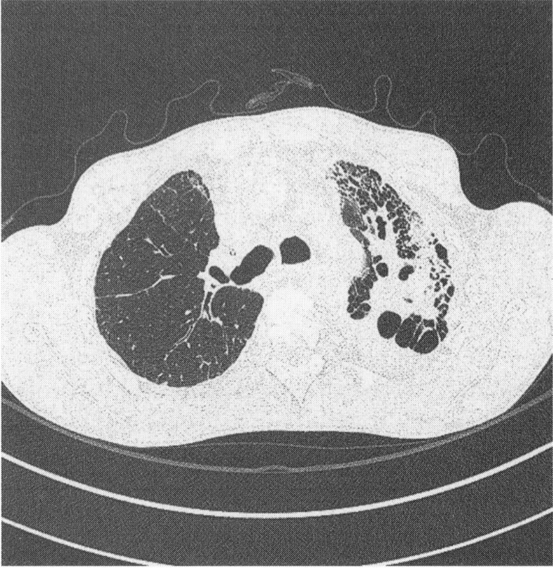

Figure 41.4 Extensive left sided *Aspergillus* bronchopneumonia complicating chronic rejection in a lung transplant recipient.

Disease Specific Issues

COPD

COPD remains the most common indication for lung transplantation in the UK. With the rapid developments occurring in all areas of medicine leading to increasingly complex and aged patients comes the potential for these patients to be more frail. Although not exclusively a feature of age, it is recognised that a significant proportion of elderly patients will have features of frailty and as such this is likely to be an increasingly relevant clinical concern. Increasing understanding of the impact of frailty on outcomes is emerging, suggesting that determination of frailty may help to guide the appropriateness of therapy in individuals. Currently frailty is not formally quantified in lung transplantation. A number of studies have highlighted its potential utility in determining outcomes in potential recipients. Early studies have suggested that patients with frailty syndrome are more likely to develop complications and be removed from the waiting list prior to transplantation.

Cystic Fibrosis

CF patients have markedly altered pharmacodynamics with rapid processing of a number of classes of medications. This is particularly evident in the early postoperative period when the requirements for analgesia may be very high. A delicate balance between comfort and respiratory depression may be difficult to achieve, often necessitating the need for either an epidural or patient controlled analgesia. The need for opiates can increase the inherent propensity for bowel blockages in some CF patients and can be a very difficult perioperative issue, which can have a major impact on their outcomes.

Idiopathic Pulmonary Fibrosis (IPF)

Patients with IPF have fibrosis of the lungs which results in shrinkage of the lung volumes and a consequence of this is a stiff and relatively poorly compliant chest. Post transplant these patients often have small stiff chests that require time to accommodate to the new lungs. This may require protracted ventilation and gentle weaning.

Pulmonary Hypertension (PH)

Patients with PH have the most difficult perioperative course with the worst 30-day survival. The presence of PH is an independent risk factor for PGD, in addition the preoperative anticoagulation and selective pulmonary vasodilators all add significantly to the bleeding risk. The right ventricle (RV) in these patients has accommodated to chronic strain and is used to high filling pressures. The principle of drying the lungs out and keeping the right sided filling low often means that the RV function is severely compromised and may need support with inotropes. These issues are the main reason for increased early mortality and morbidity. However, it is reassuring that once through this difficult period patients do have good median and long-term survival.

Drug Interactions

Immunosuppression targeted at T cells is the cornerstone of maintaining an allograft healthy in a recipient. Although there is a paucity of randomised controlled studies in lung transplantation to guide therapy, there is a wealth of clinical experience (over 30,000 transplants worldwide). Most transplant units use triple therapy consisting of steroids, a cell cycle inhibitor (mycophenolate or azathioprine) with a calcineurin inhibitor ((CNI) cyclosporin or tacrolimus). CNIs are highly dependent on normal renal function and processing by the cytochrome P450 system. Impairment in either of these systems can make adequately immunosuppressing a patient difficult, leading to either drug toxicities and infection from over immunosuppression or an increased risk of rejection from under immunosuppression. As a guiding principle, drugs which can have significant impact on the cytochrome P450 system, either by enzyme induction or inhibition, should only be started if absolutely necessary and with the appropriate dose adjustment for the immunosuppression (see Table 41.2).

Similarly, avoidance of medications that can adversely affect renal function is advisable (i.e. NSAIDs).

Table 41.2 Drug interactions

Interaction	Increased level of CNI	Decreased level of CNI	Increased nephrotoxicity	Increased hyperkalaemia
Drug	Amiodarone Clarithromycin Ciprofloxacin Diltiazem Erythromycin Fluconazole Itraconazole Voriconazole	Carbamazepine Phenytoin Rifampicin	Aminoglycosides Amphotericin Foscarnet NSAIDs	ACE inhibitor Amiloride Spironolactone

Bridging with ECMO

Patients who required respiratory support with mechanical ventilation whilst waiting for lung transplantation have historically had poor outcomes, and this has been regarded as a contraindication. The increasing experience and technical developments in the delivery of respiratory ECMO support (venovenous) has led to dramatic improvements in the utility of this treatment. A number of published case series have described the ability to bridge patients to successful lung transplantation. Transplants from ECMO are usually more complicated, have a poorer 1-year and 5-year survival, but do provide a possible intervention to extend the opportunity of transplant. In these patients, support with ECMO is time sensitive and this means that these patients require organs urgently. To support this, it is vital that organs are prioritised to these recipients.

Late Admissions to ICU (After 1 Year)

Most patients post lung transplantation enjoy good quality of life with little need for hospital inpatient care. Occasionally, they may require admission to ICU post transplant for allograft related issues. The two most common reasons are acute rejection and severe infections in the context of chronic lung allograft dysfunction (CLAD).

Acute rejection is most common in the first year post transplant. Approximately a third of patients have one episode in the first year. It usually presents with an increase in breathlessness associated with a decrease in exercise tolerance. These symptoms may be supported with a fall in lung function and non-specific infiltrates on X-ray. The gold standard for diagnosis is a transbronchial biopsy, which has a sensitivity and specificity of around 80%. Most patients will respond to enhanced immunosuppression with pulsed methylprednisolone; however, occasionally this may fail and these patients may require respiratory support to allow time for resolution of the rejection episode.

CLAD is sadly a progressive unresponsive disease which is the biggest cause of death in patients after 3 years post transplant. The disease is characterised by progressive scarring and obliteration of the airways. The pathology shows fibromyxoid scarring initially of the small airways. This results in a loss of respiratory function with increasing symptoms of breathlessness. In some patients with progressive allograft dysfunction, a significant infection may be the presenting or precipitating cause and support in this situation may be needed to allow adequate diagnosis. Often this may require ventilation to facilitate either bronchoscopy or CT scanning (Figure 41.5).

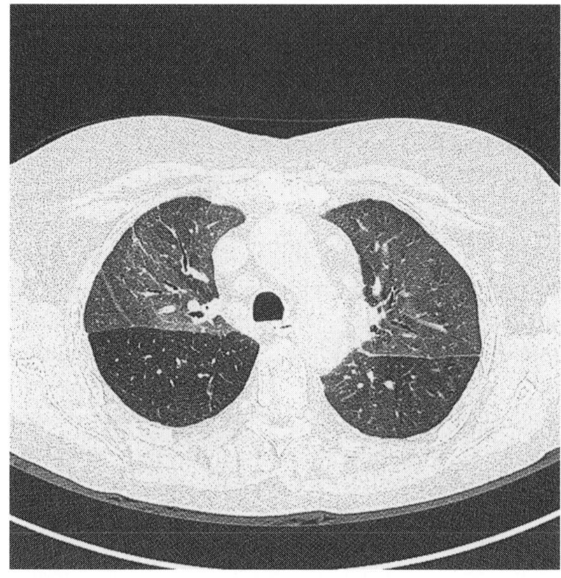

Figure 41.5 An unenhanced CT scan of a patient post lung transplantation. The CT scan demonstrates failure of the lung to empty as a result of gas trapping from airway obliteration.

Mobilisation

Lung transplant recipients are unique in that they need to start exercising the implanted organ immediately and expose it to air, which increases the risk of infections. Early mobilisation and physiotherapy can improve the physiological parameters of the new organ and avoid sputum retention and atelectasis. Additionally, many patients are relatively malnourished prior to surgery, and mobilisation and nutrition can help build their strength to improve mechanics of respiration.

Pain control after surgery is therefore important, and analgesia needs to be carefully balanced. Depending on the surgical approach, patient tailored analgesia should be used as soon as the sedation has been stopped. In general, patients undergoing sternotomy have relatively little pain and intravenous morphine or simple analgesics may be sufficient to facilitate physiotherapy and mobilisation. Anterior mini-thoracotomies are also relatively favourable with regard to pain control. However, posterior thoracotomies involving rib resections and extreme rib retraction, as well as clam-shell incisions, tend to be more painful. Many of these patients need regional anaesthesia in the form of nerve blocks or thoracic epidurals. In general pre-emptive epidurals are avoided for two reasons: not all patients need them; there is a risk of intraoperative need for extracorporeal support or cardiopulmonary bypass involving systemic anticoagulation, hence a high risk of epidural haematoma and paraplegia. If needed, epidurals are usually offered to selected patients postoperatively in the ICU.

Good analgesia facilitates early mobilisation and physiotherapy, as well as lowering the risk of nausea and gastrointestinal failure. The lower risk of gastrointestinal failure allows for early nutrition and recovery.

Conclusions

Lung transplant recipients are an extremely vulnerable cohort of patients, who require careful attention to detail to ensure that they gain the best outcome from their treatment. The combination of sick recipients with complex and involved surgery, immunosuppression and the heightened risk of infection adds complexity to their management.

Although transplantation is not a risk free enterprise and in lung transplantation the risks are high, it is also a highly rewarding endeavour offering the patients both prognostic benefit and improvement in quality of life.

Learning Points

- Lung transplantation is limited by shortage of donor organs. The hospital mortality is approximately 10%.
- Early complications such as rejection and infections can be successfully treated in most patients and require a multidisciplinary approach.
- Post-transplant infections are common and the microbiological history of both the donor and recipient is essential for their management.
- Numerous drug related complications are possible in the early postoperative period, and detailed knowledge of drug interactions is important.
- Avoidance of renal dysfunction is important in the early postoperative period as it can hinder mobilisation and healing.

Further Reading

Bulack BC, Hirji SA, Hartwig MG. Bridge to lung transplantation and rescue post-transplant: the expanding role of extracorporeal membrane oxygenation. *Journal of Thoracic Disease*. 2014; 6: 1070–1079.

Christie JD, Carby M, Bag R, et al. Report of the ISHLT Working Group on Primary Lung Graft Dysfunction part II: definition. A consensus statement of the International Society for Heart and Lung Transplantation. *Journal of Heart and Lung Transplantation*. 2005; 24: 1454–1459.

Christie JD, Edwards LB, Kucheryavaya AY, et al. International Society of Heart and Lung Transplantation. The Registry of the International Society for Heart and Lung Transplantation: 29th adult lung and heart-lung transplant report – 2012. *Journal of Heart and Lung Transplantation*. 2012; 31: 1073–1086.

Issa N, Kukla A, Ibrahim HN. Calcineurin inhibitor nephrotoxicity: a review and perspective of the evidence. *American Journal of Nephrology*. 2013; 37: 602–612.

Javidfar J, Bacchetta M. Bridge to lung transplantation with extracorporeal membrane oxygenation support. *Current Opinion in Organ Transplantation*. 2012; 17: 496–502.

Kotloff RM, Thabut G. Lung transplantation. *American Journal of Respiratory and Critical Care Medicine*. 2011; 184: 159–171.

Malagon I, Greenhalgh D. Extracorporeal membrane oxygenation as an alternative to ventilation. *Current Opinion in Anaesthesiology*. 2013; 26: 47–52.

Shah RJ, Diamond JM, Cantu E, et al. Objective estimates improve risk stratification for primary graft dysfunction after lung transplantation. *American Journal of Transplantation*. 2015; 15: 2188–2196.

Singer JP, Diamond JM, Gries CJ, et al. Frailty phenotypes, disability, and outcomes in adult candidates for lung transplantation. *American Journal of Respiratory and Critical Care Medicine*. 2015; 192: 1325–1334.

Weill D, Benden C, Corris PA, et al. A consensus document for the selection of lung transplant candidates: 2014 – an update from the Pulmonary Transplantation Council of the International Society for Heart and Lung Transplantation. *Journal of Heart and Lung Transplantation*. 2015; 34: 1–15.

MCQs

1. **What is the 30-day and 1-year survival post lung transplantation?**
   (a) 99% and 85%
   (b) 90% and 85%
   (c) 85% and 60%
   (d) 85% and 85%
   (e) 90% and 70%
2. **What is the leading cause of early mortality post lung transplantation?**
   (a) Infection
   (b) Primary graft dysfunction
   (c) Acute renal failure
   (d) Postoperative bleeding
   (e) Hepatic failure
3. **What factors make lung transplant patients particularly vulnerable to infection?**
   (a) Poor sterility in the intensive care unit
   (b) The graft is open to infection and has impaired immune defense
   (c) Physiotherapy
   (d) Antibiotic resistance
   (e) Multidisciplinary team management
4. **Which infections cause problems in lung transplant recipients?**
   (a) Bacterial
   (b) Viral
   (c) Fungal
   (d) Combined
   (e) All of the above
5. **Which of the immunosuppressant medications are particularly vulnerable to drug interactions?**
   (a) NSAIDs
   (b) Steroids
   (c) Calcineurin inhibitors
   (d) Potassium supplements
   (e) Anticonvulsants

Exercise answers are available on p.469. Alternatively, take the test online at www.cambridge.org/CardiothoracicMCQ

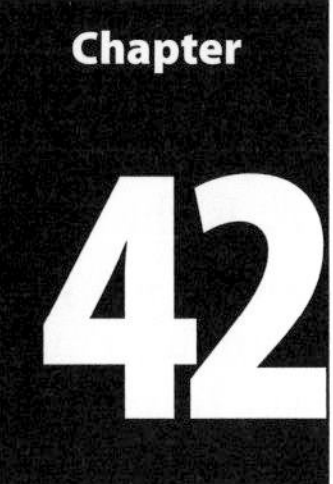

Aortic Surgical Patients in the Intensive Care Unit

Pedro Catarino and Swetha Iyer

Introduction

Aortic surgical patients in the ICU can be some of the most challenging patients. Further, these are the patients for whom good intensive care management can make a big difference to the outcome. Most of these patients are admitted to the ICU following an operation. Sometimes the patients may need to be admitted to the ICU for preoperative optimisation. Knowledge of the aortic disease pathology, the surgical interventions for it, and the expected ICU support is important for delivering optimal care for these complex patients.

Aortic Pathology and Treatment

There are three main conditions requiring aortic surgery.

Aortic Dissection/Acute Aortic Syndrome

Aortic dissection forms part of a group of interrelated pathologies where blood breaches the aortic lumen typically into the aortic media, to produce a so-called acute aortic syndrome. In aortic dissection there is an intimal tear. However, penetrating ulcer or rupture of vasa vasorum (intramural haematoma) causes similar presentation and imaging. The blood in the media may track proximally or distally, producing a dissection plane, which may rupture through the adventitia or back through the intima into the lumen again. The propagating dissection may also rupture into the pericardium, causing cardiac tamponade; it can disrupt the aortic valve, causing aortic regurgitation; or impinge on side branches of the aorta causing malperfusion syndromes (including cardiac ischaemia, stroke, intestinal or renal malperfusion and pulseless limbs).

Penetrating ulcer occurs in relation to atherosclerosis and has similar risk factors. Intramural haematoma and acute aortic dissection are typically associated with medial degeneration in the aorta. A number of conditions are known to predispose to these changes, including Marfan's syndrome, Loeys–Dietz syndrome, Ehlers–Danlos syndrome, Turner's syndrome and bicuspid aortic valve. Vasculitides such as giant cell arteritis and Takayasu's arteritis are also predisposing conditions. In all cases, hypertension is strongly implicated.

Presentation is most commonly with chest pain, described as severe and sharp and initially corresponding with the site of intimal tear then migrating according to the extent of dissection of the aorta. Syncope may occur, as may symptoms of malperfusion. There may be signs of haemodynamic upset or indeed hypertension, as well as aortic regurgitation, cardiac tamponade and reduced pulses. The most common differential diagnoses are myocardial infarction or pulmonary embolism. Diagnosis is urgent.

An anatomical classification (Figure 42.1) underpins clinical management. The Stanford classification divides acute aortic dissection according to whether or not the ascending aorta is involved, regardless of the site of intimal tear. In type A dissection, the ascending aorta is involved and emergency open surgery is indicated in a cardiothoracic centre. This is an emergency procedure with high (10–20%) operative mortality. The goal of surgery is to excise the intimal entry tear and direct blood down the true lumen by obliterating the false lumen proximally. Frequently, dissection extends down into the aortic root, causing prolapse of the aortic valve and regurgitation. Often reconstituting these layers with sutures and/or glue can resuspend the aortic valve and so it does not need to be replaced. If the root is already abnormal or irreparable, then a root replacement is required, with or without valve replacement depending on the condition of the aortic leaflets and the surgical expertise. Another principle of the surgery is that the aorta, which is left behind, should not have had a vascular clamp placed

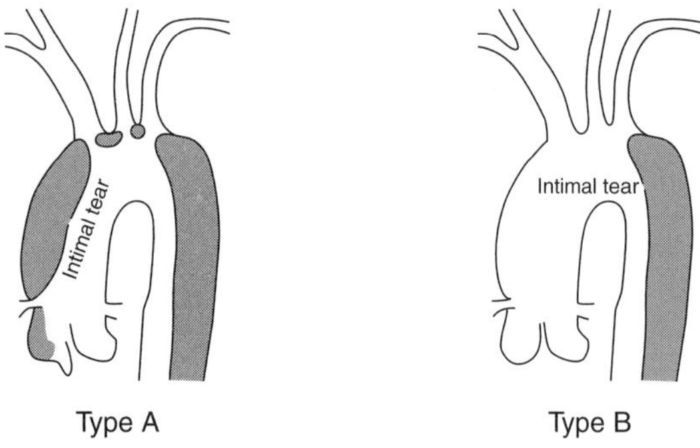

Figure 42.1 Classification of aortic dissection.

across it. This weakens the aorta, which is dissected and likely to be intrinsically abnormal. Therefore the distal repair is performed 'open', i.e. without a clamp, necessitating a period of circulatory arrest, which can be partial or total.

In type B dissection, the ascending aorta is not involved and surgery is usually not indicated for uncomplicated cases, which are typically managed by cardiologists in a CCU setting, with blood pressure control and serial imaging until symptoms settle and imaging is stable. Complicated cases involve malperfusion syndromes, ongoing pain or other suggestions of imminent rupture and then endovascular stenting is indicated in a vascular surgery unit.

Thoracic Aortic Aneurysm (TAA)

The thoracic aorta is never normal at 4 cm in diameter and this size serves as a pragmatic cut-off to diagnose TAA. Unlike abdominal aortic aneurysms, which are commonly the result of atherosclerosis, this is much less likely in TAA, although TAA shares a number of risk factors with atherosclerosis, including hypertension, smoking and chronic obstructive pulmonary disease. TAA is also predisposed by connective tissue defects due to a number of genetic syndromes or inflammatory disorders. There is an association with congenital bicuspid aortic valves, which affects 2% of the population. Atherosclerosis is more common in the descending thoracic aorta.

Since wall tension increases with greater diameter, TAA is an exponentially progressive condition with the result that the aorta is increasingly at risk of rupture or dissection. Patients occasionally present with symptoms such as change in voice (indicating recurrent laryngeal nerve palsy), chest pain or shortness of breath, and even dysphagia (mostly down to compression of surrounding structures). More typically, TAA is found incidentally on imaging for some other indication. Symptoms may be a reason for intervention, but more commonly size is the main factor driving intervention. In these cases, the predicted risk of rupture or dissection (per annum) must be balanced against the procedural risks (essentially one time) in the individual patient. Limited natural history studies have shown that the risk of an event increases significantly at 6 cm for the ascending and 7 cm for the descending aorta. In the absence of other factors therefore, a TAA of 5.5 cm in the ascending aorta and of 6.5 cm in the descending aorta would indicate intervention.

TAA is not a homogenous condition. The natural history varies according to the predisposing condition, and according to which segment of the thoracic aorta is affected. TAA is commonly associated with aortic valve disease, coronary artery disease and abdominal aortic aneurysm. Thoracoabdominal aortic aneurysms are a particular form, which include thoracic and abdominal components, typically in continuity. The management of TAA is influenced by anatomical factors, patient factors, pathological factors and institutional experience and is mostly decided by multidisciplinary teams.

The options for management include the following:

Open Surgery

This involves resection of the aneurysm and replacement of that segment with a polyester graft. Therefore that segment must be excluded from the circulation by vascular clamps or by arrest of circulation. For TAA of the ascending aorta, it is carried out through a median sternotomy with the patient on cardiopulmonary bypass. Adjunctive procedures on the heart are possible. It is also possible to deal with involvement of the arch and/or proximal descending aorta, but this requires advanced perfusion techniques such as deep hypothermic circulatory arrest or selective antegrade cerebral perfusion, and carries an additional risk of mortality, stroke, paraplegia and recurrent laryngeal nerve palsy. For TAA of the descending aorta, open surgery is carried out via lateral thoracotomy. There are a number of surgical techniques to augment the distal aortic perfusion to reduce the risk of paraplegia during clamping of the aorta, described below. Even with intercostal artery reimplantation, spinal cord ischaemia can occur, and adjuncts such as spinal cord drainage and motor evoked potentials may be used to mitigate this risk. Patients need to have a degree of physiological reserve to withstand this level of invasiveness and achieve suitable recovery times.

Endovascular Stent Graft (ESG)

This involves exclusion of the TAA. A guidewire is passed within the TAA, over which the ESG is passed from a peripheral artery, usually retrogradely. The ESG is positioned under X-ray guidance and deployed, resulting in exclusion of the aneurysm. A number of different devices are used, which are generally constructed of a polyester graft supported by nitinol or stainless steel Z, which self-expand when deployed. There are some anatomical requirements. First, the proximal and distal landing zones should be at least 2 cm in length to ensure an adequate fixation and seal. In addition, the access vessels should be sufficiently large to permit passage of the delivery system. There are ways of getting around both problems, such as performing extra-anatomical bypass or using branched or fenestrated stents to increase the potential landing zone, and using temporary surgical grafts to improve access to the aorta, but all these procedures add to the complexity of the intervention.

Medical Management

There is limited evidence to support cessation of smoking, blood pressure control and use of beta-blockers and losartan in reducing the rate of aneurysm expansion or events.

Other Issues

Anatomical factors refer to the exact site with respect to branches of the aorta and the extent of aorta involved. The site of the aneurysm determines the feasibility of both stent placement and/or clamp placement in open surgery without compromising important aortic branches. Patient factors include age and comorbidities, particularly respiratory and renal function. Pathological factors include whether there is a connective tissue defect, the presence of infection and whether the aneurysm is true or a chronic dissection.

Thoracic Aortic Injury/Aortic Transection

Blunt aortic injury is common in trauma from major decelerating forces, typically road traffic accidents, falls, or aeroplane crashes. The majority of patients die at the scene, but a significant proportion may reach hospital and may survive with timely diagnosis and treatment. Associated injuries are common and may complicate diagnosis and management.

Most injuries (80%) occur at the aortic isthmus just beyond the left subclavian artery. This is probably because this area is the transition between the mobile ascending arch and the immobile descending aorta. Other locations include the transverse arch, proximal ascending aorta and descending aorta just proximal to the diaphragm. Rupture of the intima and media occurs at the time of injury and exsanguination is prevented by the adventitia and surrounding tissues, but this remains at high risk without appropriate management.

There are no specific symptoms or signs. A chest radiograph may be suggestive, for example showing a widened mediastinum, but a normal physical examination does not exclude the condition. Chest CT is the investigation of choice.

The initial management is that of any trauma patient, applying ATLS guidelines, whilst making the diagnosis. If thoracic aortic injury is suspected then patients should be managed with a goal systolic blood pressure of approximately 100 mmHg and a pulse of <100. Repair of blunt thoracic aortic injury can be performed using open or endovascular techniques, with a growing preference for ESG.

Anaesthetic and Critical Care Management

Unstable Patients

Acute type A aortic dissection is a surgical emergency. There is a 1% per hour mortality in the first 48 hours, with 50% of untreated patients dead by 1 week. Transthoracic echo may show aortic regurgitation, pericardial effusion or even proximal dissection. However, CT imaging provides the most definitive and reliable information and is indicated immediately where there is clinical suspicion. Transoesophageal echo is best reserved for the anaesthetised patient to prevent hypertensive surges, which could lead to decompensation.

Acute rupture of TAA and aortic transection are also unstable conditions mandating emergency intervention, and anaesthetic management is similar.

Preoperative

Once the diagnosis is made, immediate transfer to a cardiothoracic centre is indicated. In the meantime, blood pressure control is paramount. Admission to an intensive care unit should be considered for close monitoring with insertion of an arterial line, wide-bore venous cannulae and urethral catheter. However, insertion of these lines should not delay transfer to theatre or an accepting hospital.

Medical therapy has the goal of reduction of systemic arterial pressure while at the same time blunting the force of contraction of the heart (*dP*/*dt*), and hence the shear forces in the aorta. Intravenous Labetalol is the agent of choice, having both alpha-blocking (blood pressure lowering) and beta-blocking (*dP*/*dt* lowering) effects. Infusions of 0.5–2 mg/minute should be administered, aiming for systolic BP 100–120 mmHg and heart rate of 60–70 beats/minute. Pain should be addressed with opiates as required. The patient should be monitored for evidence of malperfusion through ECG monitoring, recording neurological observations, attention to oliguria and abdominal pain, acid–base changes and limb pulses.

Intraoperative management

The transition period from preoperative to intraoperative is hazardous for these patients. The priority for the anaesthetist must be careful control of blood pressure and avoidance of worsening haemorrhage, which can result in either cardiac tamponade or exsanguination. The priority for the surgeon will be institution of cardiopulmonary bypass. The anaesthetist and surgeon must work together. If there is tamponade, then great care should be taken at the time of pericardial opening, since an acute rise in blood pressure may follow, producing exsanguination if bypass is not immediately available.

Numerous arterial cannulation strategies are feasible (Figure 42.2). The most common are right axillary artery or femoral artery or even carotid artery cannulation before sternotomy or direct aortic cannulation after sternotomy. Left ventricular apex and aortic cannulation after transection are also feasible. Almost invariably, the right atrium is cannulated for venous return, although in rare instances peripheral femoral venous cannulation may be preferred in order to commence bypass prior to chest opening.

Cardiopulmonary bypass is instituted and monitoring is observed to exclude induced malperfusion. The patient is systemically cooled, to 18–20 °C for total circulatory arrest, or 22–28 °C for partial arrest. For the latter, selective antegrade perfusion is continued, providing 10 ml/kg blood flow to the upper body via the right axillary artery (innominate artery clamped), or via separate catheters in the innominate artery itself and/or the left carotid artery. The aortic root can be operated on whilst the patient is cooling, or after the distal repair, whilst the patient is rewarming.

Intraoperative monitoring: Monitoring must cover the range of options for cannulation strategy since the surgeon's first choice may result in malperfusion, which only becomes evident once instituted, and therefore needs to be altered. Arterial monitoring proximal to the arch (right radial) and distal to the arch (left radial or femoral) is mandatory. It may be helpful to examine the CT to see whether the femoral arteries are included, to determine whether they are dissected or not. In the absence of CT guidance, the best pulse is usually chosen. Regardless of whether deep hypothermic circulatory arrest or selective antegrade cerebral perfusion is used, cerebral oximetry is required.

Stable Patients

The stable patients have time for careful discussion and planning between the surgeon, anaesthetist and perfusionist. The site of pathology determines the incision and options for perfusion.

Ascending Aorta

Surgery on the aortic root and/or ascending aorta, which does not involve the aortic arch, can be performed with a single arterial line, usual central venous catheter, and does not require any of the advanced adjuncts discussed below. Median sternotomy, or occasionally partial sternotomy is used; perfusion is mostly right atrial to ascending aortic bypass without significant systemic hypothermia, and with standard cardioplegic myocardial management.

Aortic Arch

The role of anaesthesia and intensive care in these patients is to:

- Facilitate surgery (positioning, perfusion and equipment);
- Ensure adequate organ protection/perfusion for the heart, brain, spine, kidneys;
- Prevent and allow aggressive management of coagulopathy;
- Minimise lung injury.

Since the supra-aortic vessels will be interrupted preparation for selective antegrade cerebral perfusion

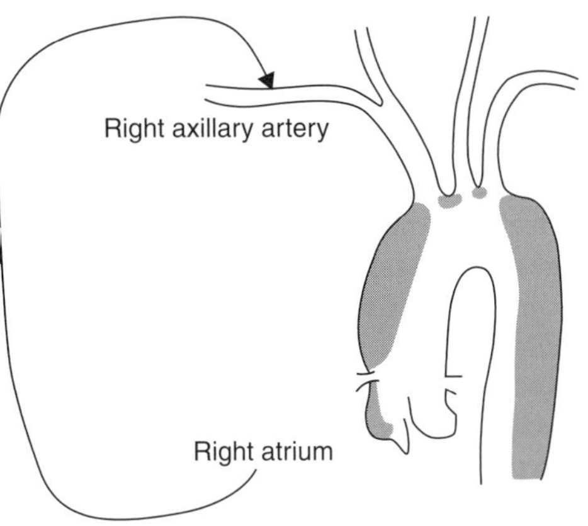

1. Full cardiopulmonary bypass, cool to 25°C

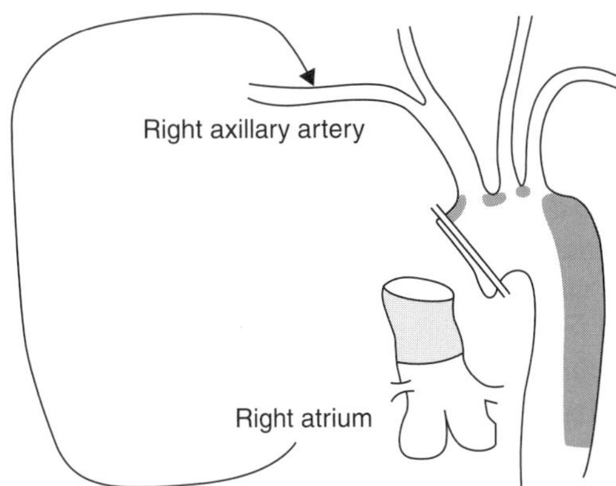

2. Clamp asc aorta, repair aortic valve, replace asc aorta

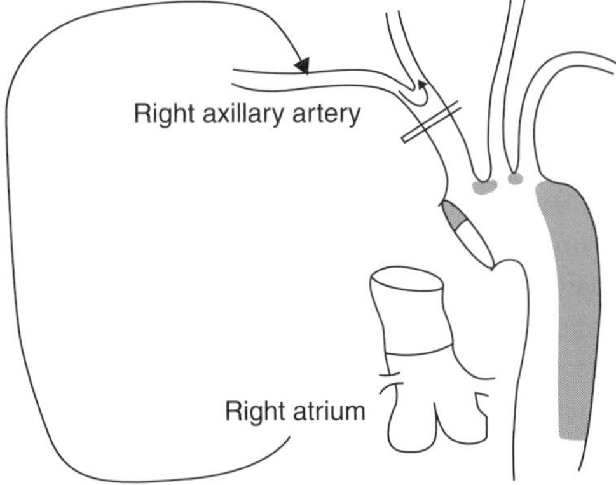

3. Circulatory arrest to body, clamp innominate art
Selective antegrade cerebral perfusion 10 ml/kg/min
Cut out clamp site asc aorta, reconstitute true lumen of arch

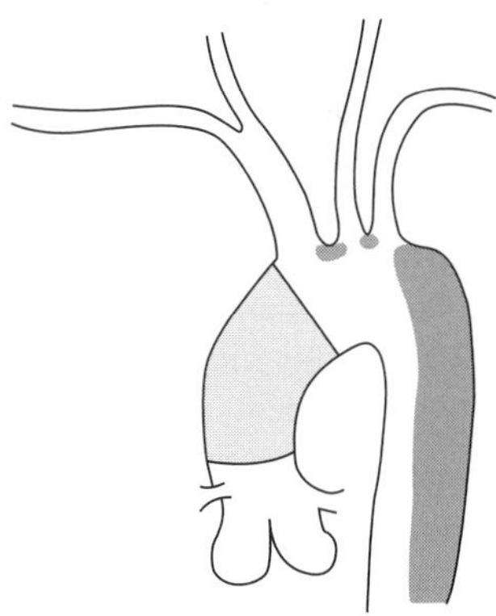

4. Distal anastomosis, rewarm, off bypass

Figure 42.2 Variety of cannulation techniques for aortic surgery.

(SACP) is preferred, i.e. right radial and post-arch (left radial or femoral) arterial lines, cerebral oximetry, and head cooling. Systemic hypothermia is invariably used, either 22–28 °C for SACP or 18–20 °C if total circulatory arrest is envisaged.

Bypass is typically right atrial to right axillary artery. A second arterial perfusion line is prepared which allows for either left carotid perfusion in the event that cerebral oximetry declines unacceptably, or for re-perfusion, once the arch graft is secured distally.

Frequently there are concomitant cardiac procedures requiring cardioplegia for myocardial management. However, if there are not, or not during the arch part of the surgery, it is common to perfuse the heart separately from the systemic circulation (i.e. clamp across the ascending aorta with perfusion line below this) with warm blood at 500–700 ml/min, which allows it to beat and avoids a prolonged ischaemic period. The ECG should be observed for adequacy of this perfusion.

Descending/Thoracoabdominal Aortic Operations

Operations on the descending thoracic aorta require left thoracotomy with the patient in a right lateral decubitus position. If the abdominal aorta is also operated on then an extensive thoracolaparotomy is performed, cutting across the left diaphragm and costal margin. Double lumen endotracheal tube is preferred. There are a number of options for perfusion, which is essential to maintain flow distal to any clamp below the aneurysm. Full cardiopulmonary bypass is one option, with femoral venous outflow (long cannula up to the right atrium) and femoral artery + axillary artery inflow, i.e. perfusing above and below the aneurysm. Partial cardiopulmonary bypass is an alternative, with left atrial outflow (cannulation of either pulmonary vein or left atrial appendage) and inflow to the femoral artery or distal descending aorta. Therefore the left heart is only partly drained, so that the heart ejects blood into the upper body including the coronaries, above any proximal clamp, and the bypass circuit pumps already oxygenated blood distal to any distal clamp. There is no oxygenator in the circuit, so less heparin is required, and the perfusion is normothermic so that the heart continues to beat normally. For both these forms of cardiopulmonary bypass, separate perfusion lines can be taken off the arterial line to continuously perfuse the coeliac axis, superior mesenteric artery and both renal arteries, in the case of thoracoabdominal procedures.

A final option for straightforward cases is a Gott shunt where the aortic arch is cannulated above the proximal clamp and the distal aorta cannulated below the distal clamp and these are connected with a short piece of heparin-coated tubing providing passive shunting to the distal aorta.

Right radial arterial lines for the upper body and femoral arterial lines for the lower body are essential. Spinal cord drain and motor evoked potentials are important adjuncts for addressing interruptions to spinal cord perfusion.

General ICU Goals for Management of Aortic Surgical Patients

Perioperative Coagulopathy Management

Persistent bleeding is common and it can lead to episodes of hypotension, which may increase the risk of spinal cord injury. Proactive coagulation management allows maintaining higher systemic perfusion pressure without excessive increment in the risk of bleeding. If coagulopathy is suspected or confirmed, conventional blood products should be used as per ICU protocols. If bleeding persists despite a first round of FFP, PLTs and cryoprecipitates/fibrinogen, a surgical review is required and the haematologist should be contacted.

Haemodynamics Goals

The majority of patients are likely to have normal ventricular function. Thus, hypotension is mainly associated with hypovolemia and vasodilation. Maintaining adequately high systemic arterial pressure and CVP is important.

If volume (i.e. cristaloids and blood products) does not achieve the above mentioned goals, then a rather early introduction of vasoconstrictors should be aimed for, to minimise the episodes of sustained hypotension.

Cardiac tamponade is less common in these patients. However, echocardiographic exam should be considered in patients with poor response to vasoconstrictors and volume administration.

Maintaining normothermia is important, unless the theatre team advise otherwise based on intraoperative events. Hyperthermia increases the risk of spinal injury and should be treated actively. Mild hypothermia (35.5–36.4 °C) can be accepted if the patient has good haemostasis.

Mechanical ventilation should be adjusted as per ICU protocol.

Spinal Cord Protection via CSF Drainage

Although the evidence behind this approach is not robust, many aortic centres use spinal catheters to drain SCF in an attempt to increase spinal perfusion pressure and reduce the risk of spinal cord damage. The spinal catheters are normally placed in the operating theatres; however, in rare cases when they are not used intraoperatively, and the patient wakes up paraplegic, a spinal catheter can be inserted in the ICU as a last attempt to reverse permanent paraplegia.

Spinal Cord Drainage

Paraplegia remains one of the most devastating complications of thoracic aortic surgery and is associated with a significant increase in both morbidity and mortality. One of these modalities that acts via optimising spinal cord blood flow is lumbar cerebrospinal fluid (CSF) drainage. The purpose of the drain is to allow control of the CSF pressure and help maintain blood flow up and down the anterior spinal artery. During the course of resecting a thoracoabdominal aneurysm, various vessels (intercostal arteries) that contribute to the anterior spinal artery are transected. Some of these

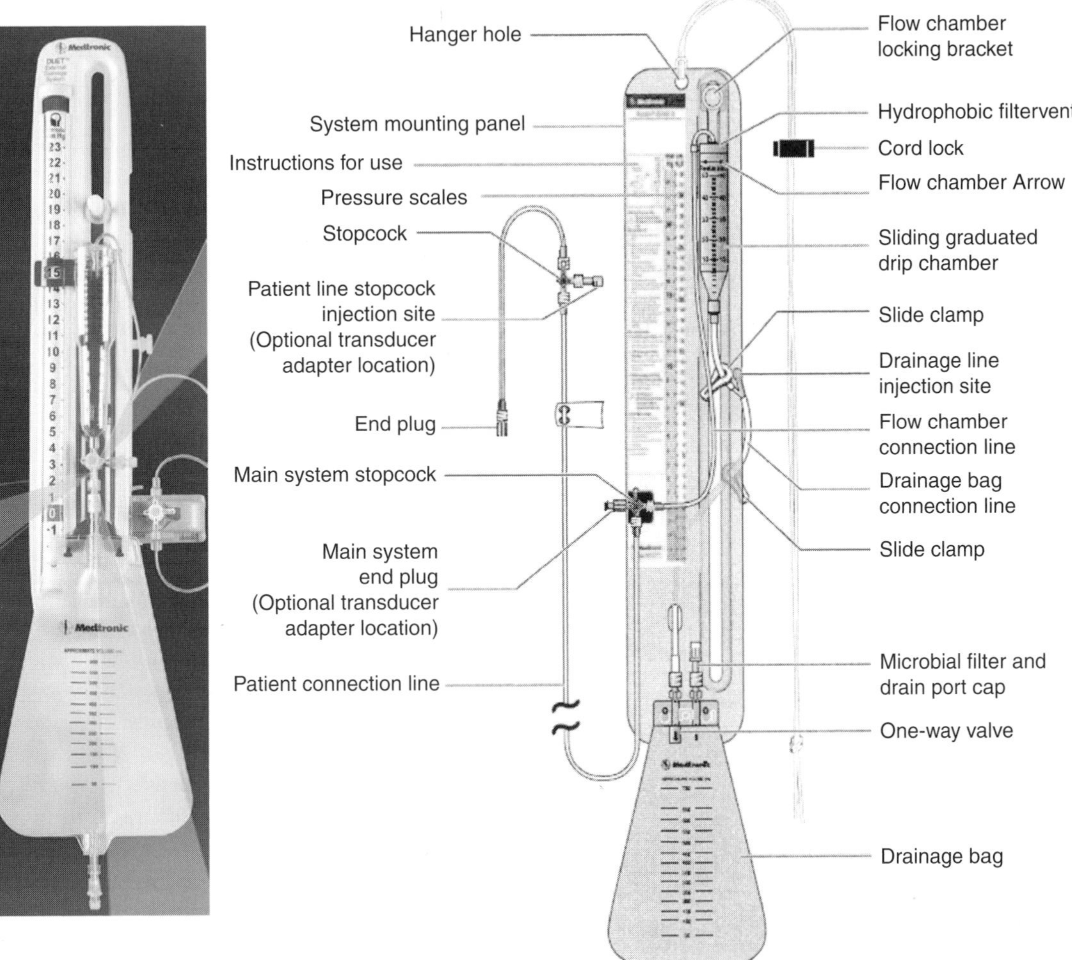

Figure 42.3 Spinal drain monitoring system.

vessels will be reattached to the graft that replaces the aorta, but it is not possible to do this with all of them.

The insertion of the spinal catheter should be carried out under strict and full aseptic conditions by the anaesthetist. The system (Figure 42.3) should be calibrated (zeroed) independently of all other pressure transducers. This should be performed at the level of the phlebostatic axis (location of right atrium) with the bed flat. The target CSF pressures are kept between 10 and 12 mmHg immediately following surgery and 12 and 15 mmHg once the patient is awake and moving.

Anaesthesia and ICU for ESG

Thoracic endovascular aortic repair (TEVAR) can be performed under general, regional or local anaesthesia. A key consideration is the ability to provide controlled hypotension at the time of stent deployment, and/or balloon inflation, minimising malposition, followed by relative hypertension once the stent is positioned. This can be achieved by administration of adenosine, which causes a transient heart block. The usual dose is 36 mg of adenosine (18 mg for subsequent episodes), which produces 4–6 seconds of cardiac asystole. Rapid pacing is another method to lower the cardiac output briefly. A temporary transvenous pacing electrode placed via the jugular vein before the procedure allows for rapid pacing at 160–180 beats/minute. After deployment, the rapid pacing is stopped, and the blood pressure is recovered. Hypertension once the stent is in place is aimed at enhancing spinal cord perfusion. Since a good number of intercostal arteries are covered by the stent, spinal cord drainage should also be considered prior to the procedure. This is indicated for extensive coverage, coverage without revascularisation of the left subclavian artery and previous abdominal aortic surgery.

Other Forms of Aortic Surgery

Coarctation or aberrant aortic vessels are also operated on and the same principles apply according to the anatomical site of the procedure. Typically these patients are younger and have better than average tissues and physiological reserve.

Learning Points

- Aortic surgery is complex, and it can be elective or emergency. In emergency operations, timing of diagnosis, transfer and treatment is crucial.
- Anaesthesia and intensive care can make a significant difference to patient outcome of aortic surgical patients.
- Spinal cord drain and motor evoked potentials are important adjuncts for addressing interruptions to spinal cord perfusion.
- The general ICU goals for management of aortic surgical patients are: coagulopathy management, blood pressure management and spinal cord protection.
- Bleeding following aortic surgery is common and it should be treated expectantly. Coagulopathy is common and should be treated promptly as delayed blood product administration leads to wasting of the already administered coagulation factors.

Further Reading

Erbel R, Aboyans V, Boileau C, et al. 2014 ESC Guidelines on the diagnosis and treatment of aortic diseases. *European Heart Journal.* 2014: 35: 2873–2926.

Fedorow CA, Moon MC, Mutch WA, Grocott HP. Lumbar cerebrospinal fluid drainage for thoracoabdominal aortic surgery: rationale and practical considerations for management. *Anesthesia & Analgesia.* 2010; 111: 46–58.

Foley LS, Yamanaka K, Reece TB. Arterial cannulation and cerebral perfusion strategies for aortic arch operations. *Seminars in Cardiothoracic and Vascular Anesthesia.* 2016; 20: 298–302.

Griepp RB, Griepp EB. Spinal cord protection in surgical and endovascular repair of thoracoabdominal aortic disease. *Journal of Thoracic and Cardiovascular Surgery.* 2015; 149: S86–S90.

Lee AW. Status of branched grafts for thoracic aortic arch endovascular repair. *Seminars in Vascular Surgery.* 2016; 29: 84–89.

Matsuda H. Treatment of uncomplicated type B aortic dissection. *General Thoracic and Cardiovascular Surgery.* 2017; 65: 74–79.

Wynn MM, Acher CW. A modern theory of spinal cord ischemia/injury in thoracoabdominal aortic surgery and its implications for prevention of paralysis. *Journal of Cardiothoracic and Vascular Anesthesia.* 2014; 28: 1088–1099.

MCQs

1. **The role of anaesthesia for aortic surgery is to:**
   (a) Facilitate surgery (positioning, perfusion and equipment)
   (b) Ensure adequate organ protection/perfusion for the heart, brain, spine, kidneys
   (c) Prevent and allow aggressive management of coagulopathy
   (d) Minimise lung injury
   (e) All of the above
2. **The risk of spinal cord injury during aortic surgery is highest in operations involving:**
   (a) Ascending aorta
   (b) Aortic root
   (c) Descending aorta
   (d) Aortic arch
   (e) Thoracoabdominal aorta
3. **Use of vasopressors in postoperative surgical patients:**
   (a) Is contraindicated as it reduces organ perfusion
   (b) Allows maintaining perfusion pressure
   (c) Should be initiated prior to fluid administration
   (d) Is more important than blood product administration
   (e) Should be used to provide supraphysiological perfusion pressure

4. **CSF drainage for spinal cord protection:**
   (a) Should be used in all cardiac surgical patients
   (b) Carries a risk of meningitis
   (c) Commonly produces dural puncture headache
   (d) Renders epidural analgesia contraindicated
   (e) Should only be done preoperatively

5. **Spinal cord damage following aortic surgery:**
   (a) Occurs only after open operations
   (b) Can be reliably prevented by CSF drainage
   (c) Can be prevented by intraoperative perfusion techniques
   (d) Is the most devastating complication of surgery
   (e) None of the above

Exercise answers are available on p.469. Alternatively, take the test online at www.cambridge.org/CardiothoracicMCQ

Thoracic Surgical Patients

J Irons and S Ghosh

Introduction

In the UK, 26,746 thoracic surgical procedures were recorded in the Society of Cardiothoracic Surgeons Thoracic Registry as having been performed in 2013–2014. Of these procedures, 6713 were primary lung cancer resections.

The association between lung cancer, smoking, emphysema and cardiovascular disease is widely accepted and thus thoracic surgical patients often have significant comorbid conditions. The preponderance of comorbid disease, together with the extent of surgery and the surgical approach, predispose to numerous potentially serious complications. Perioperative management of thoracic surgical patients should focus on the utilisation of techniques that promote early mobilisation and discharge. Key factors in achieving this aim are as follows:

- Optimisation of lung function preoperatively, for example by physiotherapy and treatment of infection or oedema/effusions
- Improving nutritional status preoperatively
- Limiting intraoperative lung injury, for example due to barotrauma or excessive fluid infusion
- Prompt return to spontaneous ventilation at the end of the procedure to reduce barotrauma, nosocomial infection and prolonged air leaks perpetuated by positive pressure ventilation
- Use of adjunctive intraoperative and postoperative analgesic techniques, for example central or peripheral nerve blocks, to ensure the patient is sufficiently pain free to cough and clear secretions.

Routine admission of patients to intensive care and high dependency units can lead to delay in patient mobilisation and recovery, increased nosocomial infections, bed occupancy issues and increased costs. The European Society of Thoracic Surgery (ESTS) states that low-risk patients should be admitted to a dedicated thoracic surgical ward and do not recommend the routine admission of high-risk patients to ICU. In the presence of an appropriate HDU, no thoracic surgical patient should be admitted to ICU electively; only those patients who require organ support as an emergency measure should be considered for ICU admission. Examples of valid indications for ICU admission in this group of patients include mechanical ventilation for acute respiratory support, haemofiltration for acutely deteriorating renal function or inotropes for acute cardiac failure.

Mortality

Mortality following lung resection has significantly improved over the years with improved diagnostic and treatment strategies. The overall mortality rate for lung resection in the UK in 2013–2014 was 1.7%. Pneumonectomy carried a higher mortality rate at 5.9% compared to open lobectomy at 2%, which in turn carried a higher mortality rate than VATS lobectomy at 0.7% and VATS wedge lung resections at 0.18%.

The most frequent cause of death is acute respiratory distress syndrome (ARDS), followed by bronchopleural fistula (BPF) and empyema, cardiac events and cerebrovascular accidents.

Reduction of Complications and Mortality

A number of recent advances in thoracic surgery have led to a reduction in the number of complications and mortality.

Video Assisted Thoracic Surgery (VATS)

Lobectomy remains the most commonly carried out lung resection procedure but there is a definite shift in the surgical approach towards minimal access (VATS) surgery. Provisional figures for 2013–2014 in the UK show 30% of lobectomies for lung cancer were carried out using a VATS approach (increasing from 23% in 2012–2013). The adoption of VATS techniques in thoracic surgery has driven improved patient outcomes including survival, reduced complications and a shorter recovery. However, as a result, increasingly complex surgical procedures are now being performed on older and sicker patients.

Pleural Drainage

Advances in chest drain technology and the understanding of the management of pleural spaces has greatly advanced. There has been an introduction of chest drains with digital quantification of leaks and pleural pressures, the use of miniature dry suction chambers with one-way valves which have improved safety and allow easy early mobilisation with a shoulder strap. The avoidance of suction and early removal have allowed earlier discharge. In the case of prolonged air leaks, discharge with a chest drain in situ, reviewed 2–4 weeks later, has decreased length of stay and reoperation rate.

Following pneumonectomy, the space within the pneumonectomised hemithorax gradually fills with fluid over a period of days to weeks (see Figure 43.1). In the immediate postoperative period close clinical and radiological monitoring is required for signs of accumulation of blood or air and for mediastinal shift, i.e. movement of the mediastinal contents from their midline position as a result of changes in intrathoracic pressure. This cavity can be managed with:

- No drainage
- Underwater seal drain clamped and released intermittently to allow assessment of blood loss and release any trapped air
- Balanced pleural drainage (injection/aspiration of air to limit mediastinal shift).

The use of balanced pleural drainage may be associated with a lower incidence of mediastinal shift and postoperative ARDS. This may be because limitation of movement of the heart and pulmonary vessels from their usual position reduces changes in transpulmonary vascular pressures in the remaining lung and so decreases the propensity for the development of pulmonary oedema. Or it may be that maintenance of the mediastinal contents in their midline position reduces the mechanical stresses on the residual lung caused by over-distension or compression.

Enhanced Recovery

The adoption of enhanced recovery programmes for thoracic surgery has served to increase throughput and decrease hospital length of stay. The enhanced recovery programme aims to institute a number of evidence-based interventions in order to assess and optimise the patients preoperatively, reduce the stress associated with the surgery and promote recovery and restoration of normal function. These programmes have led to a decrease in complications and ICU admissions, as well as a reduction in hospital length of stay. The enhanced recovery programme recommendations for thoracic surgery are listed in Table 43.1.

Within the enhanced recovery programme, the aim of preoperative assessment and optimisation is to identify patients at risk of complications and where possible take measures to prevent such complications from arising. Specific risk factors have been identified in the development of postoperative complications:

- Age >75
- Male sex
- Smoker or ex-smoker
- COPD
- Interstitial lung disease
- Concurrent cardiac disease
- Lung function FEV1 <60%, TLCO <50%.

Analgesia

Thoracotomy ranks amongst the most painful of surgical procedures. The constant motion of respiration and coughing compounds the pain from muscles that have been transected or overstretched and torn, and ribs that have been partially excised or fractured during thoracotomy. The surgical technique can be modified to reduce the severity of pain, for example by avoiding rib fracture or resection or performing the procedure by VATS rather than thoracotomy.

Pain relief after thoracic procedures can be achieved in many ways, including systemic analgesics, epidural analgesia, paravertebral or intercostal blocks, intrapleural regional anaesthesia or cryoanalgesia. Ineffective analgesia often results in poor chest expansion and expectoration, leading to atelectasis and chest infection. Multimodal analgesia combining systemic non-opioid and opioid analgesics together with some form of nerve block is regarded as the most effective means of rendering the patient comfortable, but without over-sedation.

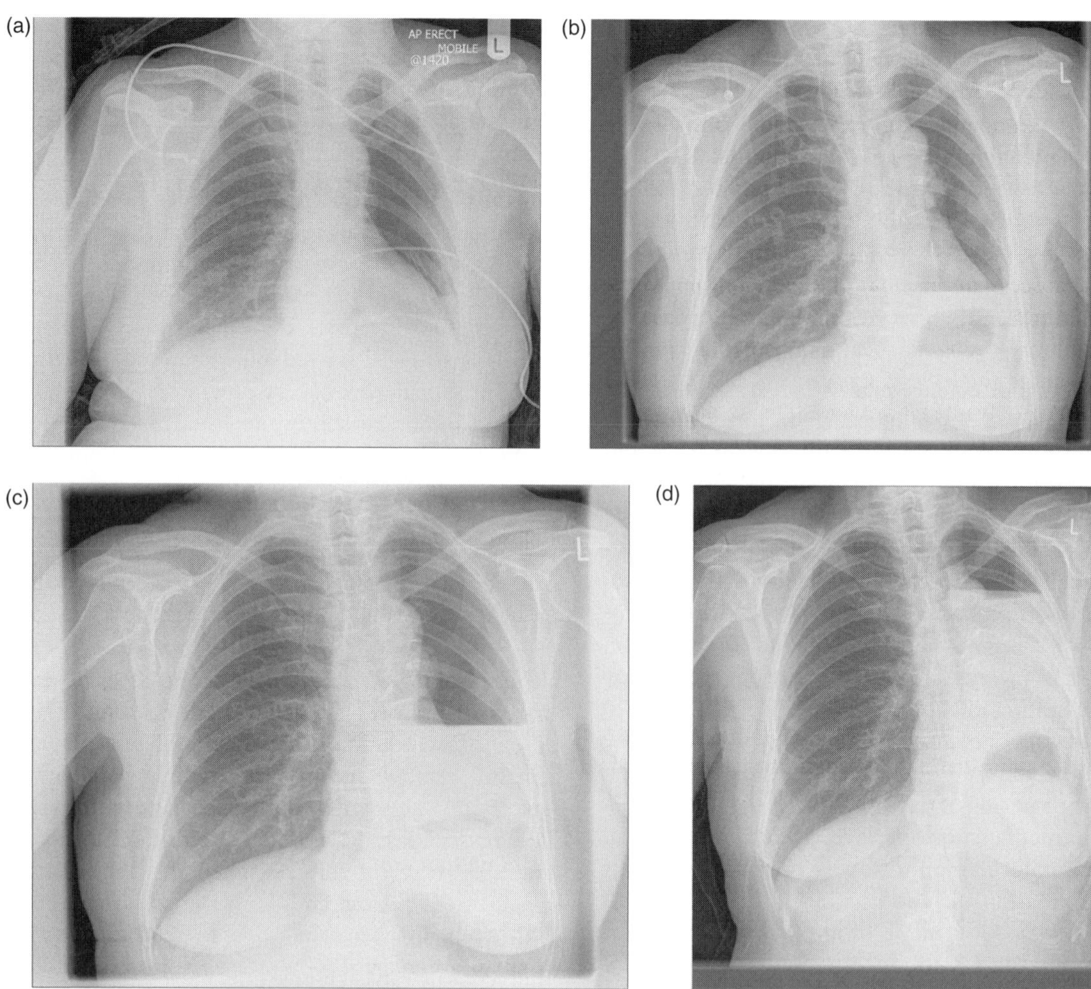

Figure 43.1 Sequential chest X-rays from a post-pneumonectomy patient demonstrating normal filling of the left hemithorax. (a) Day of surgery, (b) day 1, (c) day 4, (d) day 8.

Table 43.1 Enhanced recovery recommendations

Preoperative	Admission	Anaesthesia	Surgery	Postoperative
Identify and treat anaemia	Same day admission	Appropriate antibiotic prophylaxis	VATS if possible	DVT prophylaxis
Nutrition support	Avoid premedication	Short acting agents	Single chest drain if possible	Avoid drain suction
Smoking cessation	Minimise fasting	Protective ventilation		Early drain removal
Medical therapy optimisation	DVT prophylaxis	Avoid fluid overload		Early mobilisation
Physiotherapy prehabilitation	Consider AF prophylaxis	Paravertebral analgesia preferred to epidural		Physiotherapy
Risk calculation		Early extubation		
Education regarding stay, recovery and discharge				

Thoracic epidural analgesia has been the mainstay of thoracic anaesthetic practice for many years and provides arguably the best postoperative pain relief. Although epidural infusions have been shown to reduce the incidence of chest infection, large numbers of complications have been attributed to epidural insertion and to the management of epidural infusions. Serious complications include nerve injury, epidural abscess and haematoma – the routine use of low molecular weight heparin for thromboprophylaxis and burgeoning use of novel oral anticoagulant agents making the latter a significant concern. Other significant disadvantages are hypotension due to concomitant sympathetic block, requiring the use of intravenous fluids or vasopressors, and delay in patient mobility and, therefore, recovery and discharge.

These factors have led to the search for alternative safer techniques of regional block. The most commonly used techniques today are paravertebral block, or intercostal nerve block. The analgesic efficacy of these techniques may often not be as great as that provided by an epidural infusion, but complications are certainly reduced and the patient is able to mobilise quicker and can be discharged sooner. Paravertebral blocks can be placed either as single shot blocks at multiple levels or via placement of a catheter with an infusion of local anaesthetic for longer or more complex procedures. Paravertebral catheters may be placed by the anaesthetist at the beginning of the procedure, or placed directly by the surgeon at the end of the procedure. Multilevel intercostal nerve blocks are also commonly utilised and are effective at controlling acute pain, but usually are only effective for up to 4–6 hours.

Thromboprophylaxis

Evaluation of venous thromboembolic risk in all patients and the routine use of pharmacological and non-pharmacological prevention has significantly decreased the incidence of morbidity and death from thromboembolic disease in thoracic surgical patients.

Complications Post Thoracic Surgery

Common complications post thoracic surgery include:

- ARDS
- Air leak and pneumothorax
- Sputum retention and atelectasis
- Arrhythmias
- Cardiac dysfunction
- Pulmonary embolism
- Bleeding
- Bronchopleural fistula.

ARDS Post Lung Resection

Pulmonary complications are a major cause of mortality and morbidity following thoracic surgery, with ARDS the leading cause of death. The incidence and severity of ARDS is related to the extent of pulmonary resection, with pneumonectomy posing a risk of 3–10% while a lesser resection poses a risk of only 2–5%. Mortality in those who develop ARDS is as high as 25–60%.

One-lung ventilation is non-physiological and will result in some degree of lung injury. Over-hydration and high tidal volumes were traditionally thought to be the cause of the damage; however, it is now known that the mechanism is more complex and multifactorial and occurs in both the ventilated and collapsed lung for different reasons.

In the ventilated lung, damage occurs from ventilator induced lung injury with high pulmonary pressures and tidal volumes along with loss of functional residual capacity and hyperperfusion. The collapsed lung is affected by surgical manipulation and resection along with ischaemia-reperfusion injury and sheer forces from lung re-expansion. The resultant reactive oxygen species and cytokines released into the circulation then act to cause injury in both lungs. This cumulates in damage to the endothelial glycocalyx with vascular leakage and cell migration.

There is no single pre-emptive measure that has shown to be beneficial in preventing the development of ARDS. Studies indicate, however, that lower tidal volumes (4–5 ml/kg), the addition of a moderate amount of PEEP (5–10 cmH_2O), avoiding hyperoxia and the use of recruitment manoeuvres can help to reduce atelectasis, acute lung injury, ICU admission and hospital length of stay. PEEP may, however, exacerbate and delay spontaneous resolution of air leaks from the lung surface and PEEP should be applied judiciously if air leak is observed from pleural drains during positive pressure ventilation.

Surgical factors predisposing to the development of ARDS include:

- Extent and duration of surgery
- Pneumonectomy (R>L, carinal>non-carinal)
- Intraoperative and postoperative fluid load
- Volume of blood loss

- Administration of blood products
- Non-balanced hemithorax drainage post-pneumonectomy.

Post-extubation, non-invasive ventilation (NIV) and high flow nasal oxygen therapy have been shown to improve lung mechanics and oxygenation and are beneficial in those at high risk of respiratory complications.

The treatment strategies for ARDS post thoracic surgery are similar to those in general:

- Consider NIV
- Invasive ventilation should comprise low tidal volume, low peak airway pressure, PEEP applied at a level commensurate with minimising persistent air leak via pleural drains
- Permissive hypercapnoea
- Avoid hyperoxia
- Balanced pleural drainage, for prevention of mediastinal shift following pneumonectomy
- Appropriate antibiotic use
- Conservative fluid management
- Avoid blood products due to risk of transfusion related lung injury (TRALI)
- Use of ICU care bundles, for example DVT prophylaxis, sedation breaks, CVP line care.

Air Leak and Pneumothorax

Air leak is a common problem after thoracic surgery. Following lung resection, the residual tissue usually expands and fills the pleural space. However, if there are damaged areas on the lung surface these can communicate with the pleura, causing air leak via the chest drain or a pneumothorax in the absence of an effective patent drain. The air leak can be either an alveolar-pleural fistula, due to an open communication with lung parenchyma, or a bronchopleural fistula, due to a communication between a bronchus and pleura.

Management is usually conservative. The alveolar-pleural fistulae often seal over the first few days. This is aided by spontaneous ventilation and application of negative pressure suction to chest drains. If suction is applied too vigorously, however, it may perpetuate the air leak and in some cases cause respiratory compromise as a result of loss of tidal volume. Prolonged air leak after lung resection is associated with an increased complication rate and prolonged hospital stay.

Bronchopleural Fistula

A bronchopleural fistula (BPF) is a significant cause of morbidity and mortality following thoracic surgery. It is a persistent communication between the bronchial stump and the pleura, resulting in a persistent air leak. The incidence is approximately 0.5% after lobectomy and 4.5–20% after pneumonectomy, more commonly following right pneumonectomy. It is most often diagnosed at day 7–15 postoperatively.

The fluid filled pleural space may become infected and aspirated into the airway, leading to sepsis and respiratory compromise. Onset of breathlessness, exacerbated in the supine position, a low grade pyrexia and blood stained expectoration are the classical presentation, although it may present as a tension pneumothorax and cardiorespiratory collapse. The typical radiological finding is an air-fluid level within the pneumonectomised hemithorax, with repeat chest radiographs showing a falling fluid level (see Figure 43.2) and CT scan may demonstrate a hydropneumothorax, pneumomediastinum and in a few cases the actual fistulous communication (see Figure 43.3).

Emergency surgical treatment is often required with repair of the stump with an omental or muscle patch. More recently, the uses of tissue glue, fibrin or valves applied bronchoscopically to seal the defect have been advocated. Thoracoplasty to occlude the pneumonectomy space may also be considered.

Intubation and positive pressure ventilation may be required to manage respiratory distress accompanying sepsis or for surgical closure of the fistula. Induction and intubation in this situation can be challenging, as the patients may be hypoxic, haemodynamically unstable and distressed. In the absence of a chest drain, there is a risk of tension pneumothorax during positive pressure ventilation; furthermore, the application of positive pressure may fail to produce adequate ventilation if large volumes of inspired gas are lost through the fistula and may also exacerbate spill-over of the infected pleural fluid into the bronchial tree as gas is forced into the pleural cavity displacing fluid.

Inhalational induction and subsequent lung isolation with a double lumen endobronchial tube in the semi-erect position offer good protection against lung soiling with infected fluid and avoid positive pressure ventilation to the bronchial stump. However, inhalational induction to the depth of anaesthesia required

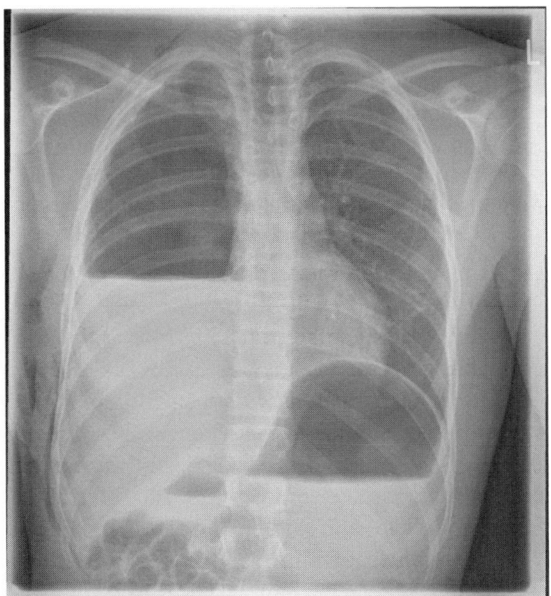

Figure 43.2 Chest X-ray demonstrating a drop in the air-fluid level in the absence of a chest drain.

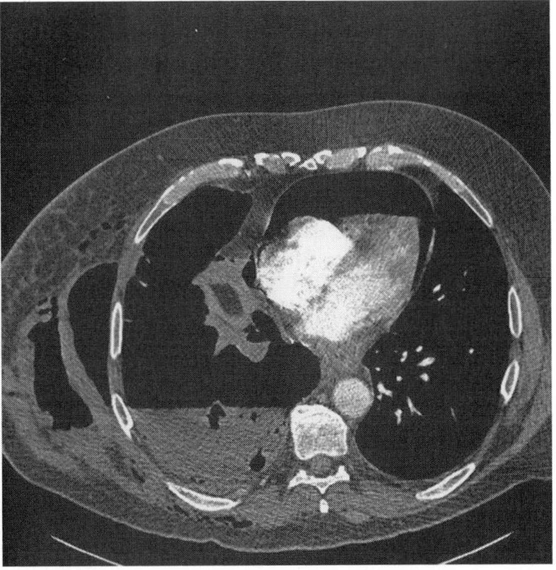

Figure 43.3 CT scan demonstrating a bronchopleural fistula post right pneumonectomy. Note the right-sided hydropneumothorax with air extending into the mediastinum creating a pneumoperitoneum and decompressing into the subcutaneous tissues.

for passage of an endobronchial tube can be accompanied by cardiovascular compromise, particularly in septic, unstable patients, and can be difficult to safely achieve in practice. The use of rapid sequence induction and intubation has been advocated as offering a more rapid means of securing the airway. Awake fibreoptic endobronchial intubation has also been described in this situation.

Medical management involves dependent drainage, appropriate antibiotics, low pressure ventilatory support to promote healing without compromising gas exchange, physiotherapy and good nutrition.

Sputum Retention, Atelectasis and Chest Infection

Poor respiratory reserve, combined with inadequate analgesia and infrequent physiotherapy, often leads to atelectasis and respiratory tract infection (see Figure 43.4). The incidence of pneumonia after thoracic surgery is 5–25%, and carries a mortality of around 20%. The preoperative predictors include old age, chronic obstructive pulmonary disease, significantly reduced forced expiratory volume and prolonged/extensive surgery. Common pathogens are *Haemophilus*, *Streptococcus*, and *Pseudomonas*. The best treatment is probably prevention, but once established the infective complications should be treated promptly with appropriate antibiotics after culture, effective analgesia and physiotherapy.

Cardiac Dysfunction

Arrhythmias

The commonest arrhythmia following lung resection is atrial fibrillation (AF). The incidence of AF ranges from 12 to 44%. Patients who develop AF are more likely to develop other complications and it is associated with a longer hospital stay and higher mortality. Risk factors for the development of AF include:

- Male sex
- Older age
- Extent of surgery (higher incidence following pneumonectomy)
- Pre-existing cardiac disease, in particular congestive cardiac failure and previous AF
- Length of procedure
- Pericardial involvement or inflammation.

In one-third of the patients who develop AF, the onset is associated with chest infection or sepsis. It is most prevalent on the second and third postoperative day.

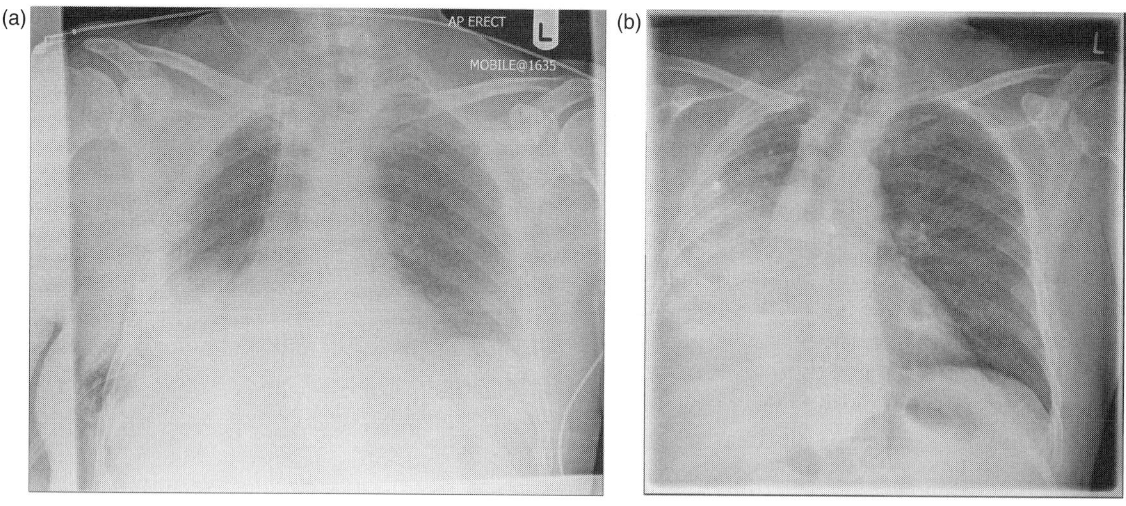

Figure 43.4 Sequential chest X-rays of a patient post left lower lobectomy who developed sputum retention and collapse/consolidation of remaining right lower lobe postoperatively. (a) Day of surgery, (b) day 2.

The Society of Thoracic Surgeons published recommendations on the prophylaxis and treatment of AF related to general thoracic surgery. Due to the high morbidity and mortality and costs related to AF, prophylaxis should be considered in higher risk patients. Beta-blockers and diltiazem are the drugs of choice for prophylaxis. There is some evidence that amiodarone may be beneficial prophylactically, but should be avoided in pneumonectomy patients because of the pulmonary side effects associated with amiodarone. Magnesium is useful as an adjunctive measure for the short-term management of acute atrial fibrillation and ensuring that plasma magnesium and potassium levels are within normal ranges may reduce the risk of developing AF. There is no evidence that prophylactic digitalisation is of benefit and so it should not be used.

The treatment of AF, once it has occurred, can be pharmacological rate or rhythm control or synchronised direct current (DC) cardioversion. The choice depends on haemodynamic stability and symptoms. In the haemodynamically unstable patient, DC cardioversion is recommended. In the haemodynamically stable patient, if symptoms are intolerable, pharmacological cardioversion should be considered with amiodarone or flecainide. If symptoms are tolerable, rate control with beta-blockers, or diltiazem if beta blockade is contraindicated due to COPD or bronchospasm, should be first line treatment in the first 24 hours together with optimisation of electrolyte status (magnesium, potassium and acid–base balance). Digoxin should not be used as a primary agent for rate control, but can be used in combination if other rate control measures fail.

Prophylactic anticoagulation with low molecular weight heparin is recommended as an early measure during the acute phase postoperatively to prevent the development of thrombus in the left atrial appendage if the patient has two or more risk factors for stroke. This should be converted to warfarin in the longer term if AF persists. If the patient is at low risk of stroke, aspirin is recommended.

Myocardial Ischaemia

Perioperative myocardial ischaemia and infarction, a commonly feared complication, is rarely reported in the literature and there is a scarcity of data on the current incidence. In a large historical study of postoperative thoracotomy patients, the incidence of ECG changes indicative of myocardial ischaemia was reported as 3.8% and myocardial infarction 1.2%. The perioperative factors most strongly predictive of ischaemic events were poor preoperative exercise tolerance and intraoperative hypotension.

Thoracic surgical patients often have concomitant cardiac risk factors or overt cardiac disease and rigorous preoperative assessment and selection can limit the incidence of postoperative morbidity and mortality ascribable to myocardial ischaemia and infarction. The American College of Cardiology and American Heart Association guidelines for perioperative evaluation and management for non-cardiac surgery is a useful resource, thoracic surgery being classified as high risk in the context of that guidance. Coronary angiography should be performed in the presence of major clinical predictors, i.e. unstable angina, heart failure, arrhythmias or valvular disease. In patients requiring preoperative stenting, surgery should be postponed for 2–4 weeks. Patients who are considered at risk of myocardial ischaemia should ideally be invasively monitored intraoperatively and postoperatively. Appropriate measures should be taken to maintain cardiac filling pressures and arterial blood pressure at optimum levels and consideration given to the use of inotropes, vasopressors or vasodilators to prevent or limit the sequelae of ischaemic myocardial dysfunction.

Right Heart Failure

Theoretically the strain on the right ventricle should increase with the increase in afterload following lung and pulmonary artery resection. However, the right ventricular end-diastolic pressure in fact remains stable in the first few hours postoperatively, and only increases significantly on the first and second day. As concomitant cardiac disease is not uncommon in patients undergoing lung resection, postoperative cardiac failure is a possibility and preventative measures such as careful monitoring of fluid balance need to be taken.

Pulmonary embolism and heart herniation are rare causes of RV decompensation but carry very high mortality following lung resection. Heart herniation may occur if the pericardium is opened intraoperatively and not adequately closed.

Bleeding

Bleeding is a rare complication after thoracic procedures with an incidence of 0.1–3% of thoracotomies and 2% of VATS cases, with re-exploration rates for haemostasis in less than 1.9% and 1% respectively. Most bleeding is secondary to technical problems, although patient comorbidities and medication may be predisposing factors. Meticulous attention to intraoperative haemostasis and correction of coagulopathy are thus essential.

Bleeding is usually from the lung parenchyma, bronchial vessels or intercostal arteries. It is usually detected from the effluent chest drainage, but chest drains may become blocked and in the presence of hypotension and tachycardia a chest radiograph may be informative. The indications for re-thoracotomy are rapid blood loss, a large intrathoracic collection or persistent hypoxia due to compression of the lung or pulmonary veins.

Learning Points

- Postoperative thoracic surgical patients should not be admitted routinely to the ICU; only those patients who require organ support as an emergency measure should be considered for ICU admission.
- Morbidity and mortality following thoracic surgery has significantly improved over the last few years with the increase in minimal access surgery, advances in equipment and drainage systems, development of enhanced recovery programmes, thromboprophylactic protocols and improvement in analgesic strategies.
- ARDS remains the leading cause of death following thoracic surgery and protective lung strategies should be routine in patients undergoing one-lung mechanical ventilation. PEEP should be applied judiciously during positive pressure ventilation at a level commensurate with minimising persistent air leak via pleural drains.
- Patients with a bronchopleural fistula may present as an emergency due to a tension pneumothorax or due to respiratory compromise or sepsis. They can present a considerable challenge for induction and intubation.
- AF post thoracic surgery is common and is associated with a higher morbidity, mortality and hospital length of stay. High-risk patients should be considered for prophylaxis.

Further Reading

De Decker K, Jorens PG, Van Schil P. Cardiac complications after noncardiac thoracic surgery: an evidence-based current review. *Annals of Thoracic Surgery*. 2003; 75: 1340–1348.

Fernando H, et al. The Society of Thoracic Surgeons Practice Guideline on the prophylaxis and management of atrial fibrillation associated with general thoracic surgery: executive summary. *Annals of Thoracic Surgery*. 2011; 92: 1144–1152.

Jones NL, Edmonds L, Ghosh S, Klein AA. A review of enhanced recovery for thoracic anaesthesia and surgery. *Anaesthesia*. 2013; 68: 179–189.

Lohser J, Slinger P. Lung injury after one lung ventilation: a review of the pathophysiologic mechanisms affecting the ventilated and collapsed lung. *Anaesthesia & Analgesia*. 2015; 121: 302–318.

The SCTS Thoracic Surgery Audit Group. The Thoracic Surgery Registry Brief Report: Audit Years 2011–12 to 2013–14. Society for Cardiothoracic Surgery in Great Britain and Ireland.

MCQs

1. **Following lung resection, which of the following are common complications?**
   (a) Air leak via pleural drains
   (b) Atrial fibrillation
   (c) Acute lung injury
   (d) Sputum retention and atelectasis
   (e) All of the above

2. **Risk factors for post lung resection complications include which of the following?**
   (a) Age
   (b) Concurrent cardiac disease
   (c) On lung function tests: FEV1 > 60%, TLCO > 50%
   (d) Extent of lung resection
   (e) (a), (b) and (d)

3. **Which of the following are beneficial in managing ALI/ARDS?**
   (a) IPPV with tidal volumes of 9–10 ml/kg and PEEP of 5 cmH_2O
   (b) IPPV with tidal volumes of 4–5 ml/kg and PEEP of 8–10 cmH_2O
   (c) Permissive hyperoxia
   (d) Conservative fluid management regimens
   (e) Low tidal volumes and conservative fluid management

4. **Regarding bronchopleural fistulae (BPF) which of the following are true?**
   (a) BPF most commonly occurs after left lung lobectomy
   (b) BPF is usually diagnosed within the first 24 hours postoperatively
   (c) Symptoms include a high temperature
   (d) Breathlessness and expectoration of blood tinged sputum are exacerbated when sitting upright
   (e) None of the above

5. **Recommendations for the management of atrial fibrillation (AF) in thoracic surgical patients include:**
   (a) Prophylaxis with digoxin in high risk patients
   (b) Amiodarone for pharmacological cardioversion
   (c) Rate control with either beta-blockers or diltiazem
   (d) The use of aspirin in all patients who develop AF to reduce the risk of stroke

Exercise answers are available on p.469. Alternatively, take the test online at www.cambridge.org/CardiothoracicMCQ

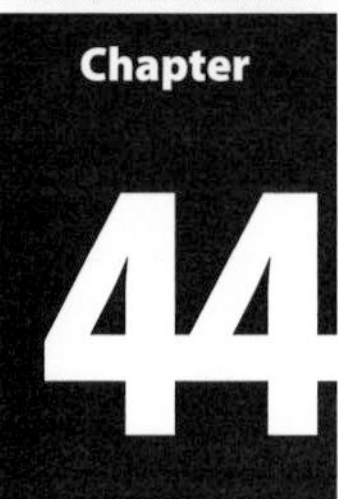

Respiratory Disorders: Acute Respiratory Distress Syndrome

Alastair Proudfoot and Charlotte Summers

Definitions and Epidemiology

Acute respiratory distress syndrome (ARDS) is characterised by acute inflammation affecting the gas exchange surface of the lung, presenting clinically with acute hypoxaemia, in the presence of bilateral pulmonary infiltrates on chest radiography.

It has to be made clear from the outset that ARDS is not a disease. It is a state of dramatically diminished lung function of variable aetiology. A working definition of ARDS was established in 1994 by the American-European Consensus Conference. A more recent report recommends use of definitions of mild, moderate and severe ARDS, based on the degree of hypoxaemia (Table 44.1). Additionally, the exclusion of pulmonary oedema secondary to cardiac failure is now not mandated, positive end expiratory pressure (PEEP) is accounted for as an indicator of severity, and a known ARDS risk factor must be present within 7 days of onset.

ARDS develops after exposure to a wide variety of insults, and given the nature of the diagnostic criteria, should be considered a syndrome rather than a disease. Initiating insults can be divided into two groups: direct (e.g. pneumonia) or indirect (e.g. sepsis) as outlined in Table 44.2. Risk of progression to ARDS varies according to the type, number and severity of predisposing conditions, as well as the genetics and other patient characteristics including gender, body mass index, smoking status, and alcohol usage. Diagnosing and treating conditions that mimic, or are associated with, ARDS is the first principle of successful management; prediction scores such as the Lung Injury Protection Score (LIPS) are intended to facilitate early recognition and treatment.

Incidence and Outcomes

Data from the late 1990s determined that the age adjusted incidence of ARDS was 86.2 per 100,000 person-years, with an in-hospital mortality rate of 38.5%. Other data suggest that the incidence of ARDS may have declined since the 1990s. The decline in incidence has been attributed to improvements in healthcare delivery and process, including adherence to low tidal volume ventilation, and early recognition and management of sepsis. More recent data bring the reported declines into question, and suggest that ARDS occurs in 10.4% of all ICU admissions, with a hospital mortality of 34.9–46.1%, although these data are not without controversy.

Once treatment of the precipitating condition has commenced, prognostic factors relate to the patient's response to therapy. Severe arterial hypoxaemia ($PaO_2/FiO_2 < 100$ mmHg) and an increase in the pulmonary dead-space fraction (>0.60) are associated with increased mortality. Mortality also correlates with the number of organ system failures, increasing to 83% when three or more are present. Complications appearing during the course of ARDS, including circulatory shock, acute renal failure and liver dysfunction, allied with age over 60 years, are associated with a higher mortality. Lung function in most survivors returns to normal over 6–12 months, although the majority have persistent, abnormal exercise endurance, and neuromuscular and neurocognitive morbidity significantly impairs longer term health related quality of life.

Pathobiology

Alveolar Epithelial Injury

The alveolar epithelium is composed of approximately equal numbers of flat type I cells (hAT1) and cuboidal type II cells (hAT2). hAT2 have several critical functions, including surfactant production, ion transport and functioning as progenitor cells for the

Table 44.1 Berlin definition of ARDS

	Mild ARDS	Moderate ARDS	Severe ARDS
Timing	Within 1 week of a known clinical insult or new or worsening respiratory symptoms		
PaO_2:FiO_2	201–300 mmHg	≤200 mmHg	≤100 mmHg
PEEP	PEEP ≥ 5 cmH_20	PEEP ≥ 5 cmH_20	PEEP ≥ 10 cmH_20
Chest X-ray	Bilateral opacities	Bilateral opacities	Bilateral opacities

PaO_2/FiO_2 arterial partial pressure of oxygen/inspired oxygen fraction.
PEEP positive end expiratory pressure.

Table 44.2 Hallmarks of indirect versus direct ARDS

	Indirect ARDS	Direct ARDS
Causes	Severe sepsis Trauma Blood product transfusion Pancreatitis Cardiopulmonary bypass Burns	Pneumonia Aspiration Smoke inhalation Pulmonary contusion Reperfusion injury
Clinicopathological hallmarks	Neutrophilic alveolitis Hyaline membranes Microthrombi Predominance of endothelial injury Imaging/plasma evidence of (non-pulmonary) pathology, e.g. pancreatitis	Neutrophilic alveolitis Hyaline membranes Microthrombi Predominance of alveolar epithelial injury Thoracic imaging evidence of initiating pulmonary pathology, e.g. lung contusion

regeneration of hAT1 cells after injury. Typical histological appearances of ARDS include extensive necrosis of hAT1 and the formation of protein-rich hyaline membranes on a denuded basement membrane. The extent of alveolar epithelial damage is a predictor of outcome.

Alveolar fluid clearance by hAT2 is primarily driven through sodium uptake on the apical membrane, followed by extrusion of sodium on the basolateral surface by Na^+K^+-ATPase. Loss of alveolar epithelial integrity and down regulation of sodium and chloride transporters results in the accumulation of protein-rich and highly cellular oedema fluid in the interstitium and alveoli. Loss of surfactant producing hAT2, allied with the effect of plasma proteins in the airspace, contributes to ARDS through atelectasis, increased oedema formation and impairment of local host defence. Clinically this presents with collapse of lung units and reduced pulmonary compliance. Epithelial cells also play key roles in regulating the inflammatory response through production of injury-driven pro-inflammatory cytokines and chemokines, the expression of leucocyte adhesion molecules, and cell–cell interactions with resident lung cells, particularly alveolar macrophages.

Endothelial Activation and Injury

The pulmonary endothelium forms a continuous barrier of endothelial cells, which regulate fluid permeability as well as modulating host inflammation, vascular tone, angiogenesis and interactions with blood-borne cells. Loss of barrier integrity, characterised by the formation of reversible intercellular gaps between endothelial cells, is accepted as the ultrastructural basis for the pulmonary oedema observed in ARDS. Gap formation is induced by the binding of mediators, including thrombin and tumour necrosis factor-alpha (TNF), which induce cytoskeletal rearrangement and endothelial barrier disruption.

Similar to the alveolar epithelium, the lung endothelium orchestrates and propagates the inflammatory response. Endothelial cells release cytokines and chemokines, up regulate the expression of adhesion molecules, and shift from an antithrombotic to a pro-thrombotic activated state, resulting in capillary thrombosis and extravascular fibrin deposition, potentiating pulmonary inflammation and contributing to the increased dead-space fraction observed in ARDS. Inflammation in the vascular space also counteracts hypoxic pulmonary vasoconstriction, partly by causing dysregulation of the production of vasoactive mediators including prostanoids, endothelins and nitric oxide.

Role of Circulating Cells

The recruitment of circulating inflammatory cells into the lung has long been recognised in ARDS. Neutrophils are central to the initiation and propagation of the inflammation observed, and neutrophilic alveolitis is a histological hallmark of ARDS (see Figure 44.1). The extent of neutrophilia present within the bronchoalveolar lavage fluid (BALF) of patients with ARDS has been reported to correlate with clinical outcome. However, the presence of neutrophils per se is not damaging, rather the priming/activation status of these cells is the major determinant of their subsequent injury-inducing behaviour. Recent data have shown that the healthy human pulmonary endothelium plays a role in host defence by trapping primed/activated neutrophils, facilitating their depriming, and later releasing them back into the systemic circulation in a quiescent state. Failure of this homeostatic depriming mechanism was observed in patients with ARDS.

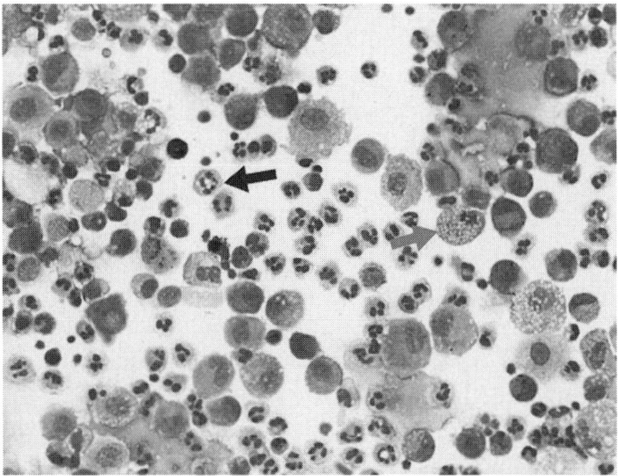

Figure 44.1 Bronchoalveolar lavage fluid from a patient with ARDS. Photomicrograph of modified Wright's stained cytospin. The white arrow denotes a hypersegmented neutrophil; the black arrow denotes a neutrophil which has been efferocytosed by a macrophage. (A black and white version of this figure will appear in some formats. For the colour version, please refer to the plate section.)

Monocytes appear to play a role in regulating neutrophil influx to the lung. However, whilst direct depletion of monocytes in mice consistently reduced LPS-induced blood and alveolar neutrophilia, as well as lung injury, peripheral mononuclear cell depletion in humans was unsuccessful in preventing the recruitment of neutrophils into the alveolar space.

Ventilator Associated Lung Injury

The application of mechanical ventilation exacerbates ARDS in a process called ventilator-associated lung injury (VALI). Mechanical forces applied during ventilation cause physical disruption of the alveolar-capillary membrane leading to pulmonary oedema, whilst cyclical stretch induces activation of cell-signalling pathways in epithelial, endothelial and inflammatory cells. In the context of the already injured lung, this results in pro-inflammatory and/or pro-fibrotic responses both locally *and* in the systemic circulation. Thus, in addition to local injury, VALI can drive systemic inflammation and extrapulmonary organ damage. This is reflected in the observation that the majority of patients with ARDS die from multisystem organ failure, rather than hypoxaemic respiratory failure.

Resolution of Inflammation and Repair of the Injured Lung

Most patients gradually recover normal physiology and lung function. In the alveolar epithelium, hAT2 cells proliferate in response to stimulation by epithelial growth factors. hAT2 cells are thought to act as progenitor cells for both daughter type II cells and type I cells. Local and bone marrow derived stem cells may also contribute to repair. Resolution of inflammation is macrophage and T-cell driven. Collectively, these mechanisms combine to reconstitute the epithelial barrier and restore lung function.

If epithelial injury is severe, or repair is impaired, a fibroproliferative phase of ARDS can ensue either following, or in parallel with, epithelial injury. During this phase, mesenchymal cells proliferate, neovascularisation occurs, and the alveolar space becomes filled with activated fibroblasts and myofibroblasts that synthesise excessive collagenous extracellular matrix. A small proportion of patients progress to a chronic phase of respiratory insufficiency characterised by widespread pulmonary fibrosis, with disordered lung architecture.

Clinical Investigations

The main clinical priority is identification and treatment of the initiating pathology and any complications that may have ensued. It may be necessary, particularly in the immune compromised host, to undertake invasive diagnostic procedures, such as bronchoscopy, to establish a diagnosis. Further, it has been shown that intercurrent pulmonary infection occurs in up to 70% of patients with ARDS, necessitating vigilance for the subsequent development of infection.

Ventilator Management

Protective Ventilation

The magnitude of the clinical burden of VALI was demonstrated by the ARDS Network study, in which patients with ARDS were randomised to receive either a high tidal volume (12 ml/kg predicted body weight (PBW)) with end inspiratory pressure limited to a plateau pressure $P_{plat} \leq 50$ cmH_2O, or a low tidal volume (6 ml/kg PBW) and $P_{plat} \leq 30$ cmH_2O. A PEEP ladder was used to determine the PEEP level administered, according to the fraction of inspired oxygen and the respiratory rate. The low tidal volume cohort demonstrated a 9% absolute reduction in mortality (40% to 31%). Accordingly, low tidal volume ventilation has become the standard of care in ARDS, and the goal of mechanical ventilation has shifted from normalisation of gas exchange parameters to minimising VALI with pragmatic acceptance of modest biochemical derangement.

High PEEP and Recruitment Manoeuvres

The application of PEEP has been used to mitigate the pulmonary oedema and atelectasis of ARDS. Several studies have failed to show clinical benefit of higher PEEP levels; nonetheless, a meta-analysis demonstrated improved survival in those with most severe physiological derangements (PaO_2:FiO_2 < 200 mmHg). Despite these data, consensus for this approach is lacking, particularly as response is heterogeneous and may be associated with lung hyperinflation and haemodynamic compromise. Determination of 'optimal PEEP' levels has thus far been elusive; calculation of driving pressure, estimation of transpulmonary pressures using an oesophageal probe and imaging techniques have shown promise but none have been assessed in prospective trials and cannot be recommended routinely.

Recruitment manoeuvres involving a transient increase in transpulmonary pressure are designed to promote reinflation of collapsed alveoli. A variety of techniques have been proposed, including graded incremental pressure increases, and a sustained high inflation pressure manoeuvre followed by a decremental reduction to an optimal PEEP level determined by dynamic analysis of flow-volume relationships, as well as image guided strategies. Whilst data support improvements in oxygenation, such manoeuvres are associated with complications, in particular haemodynamic compromise, barotrauma and exacerbation of existing air leaks; these appear to relate to the frequency of applied manoeuvres.

Ventilatory Modes

Despite inverse ratio ventilation (IRV) demonstrating no clear benefit when compared with conventional ventilator modes, the application of airway pressure release ventilation (APRV) in ARDS has been advocated by some centres. APRV utilises inverse ratio, pressure controlled, intermittent mandatory ventilation in patients with unrestricted spontaneous breathing to maintain alveolar recruitment and improve oxygenation, whilst limiting inflation pressures and sedation. Unlike IRV, APRV does not mandate paralysis and hence is an attractive mode. Nonetheless, APRV risks tidal hyper-inflation, increased transpulmonary pressures, and has shown no clear benefit over conventional modes. The use of high-frequency oscillatory ventilation (HFOV) to deliver small tidal volumes at high frequency with high mean airway pressures has been similarly tempered by two large multicentre trials demonstrating no benefit in one and increased mortality in the other. Accordingly, despite the theoretical mitigation of VALI, HFOV can no longer be recommended in ARDS, and conventional ventilator modes should suffice for the majority of patients. Where conventional modes fail to facilitate low tidal volume ventilation and acceptable physiology, extracorporeal gas exchange techniques should be considered in appropriate patients.

Extracorporeal Gas Exchange

Extracorporeal gas exchange (ECGE) is technology whereby blood is drained from a major vein, pumped through an artificial membrane to facilitate gas exchange, and returned to the venous or arterial system, depending on the physiological needs of the patient. Various extracorporeal circuit arrangements are available and are discussed in Chapter 24.

Non-ventilator Therapies

General Supportive Measures

Prompt administration of appropriate antibiotics in sepsis, a reduction in iatrogenic injury through use of reduced tidal volume ventilation and stewardship for hospital-acquired aspiration/ventilator-associated pneumonia, coupled with lower blood transfusion thresholds and the removal of females from the plasma donor pool have combined to limit hospital-acquired ARDS. The use of sedation holds, spontaneous breathing trials and early mobilisation/rehabilitation programmes, where appropriate, are also likely to have contributed.

Non-hydrostatic pulmonary oedema in the context of increased pulmonary vascular permeability is pathogonomic of ARDS. Limitation of fluid administration is therefore an attractive strategy. Studies have shown an association between a persistent positive fluid balance and poor outcome in ARDS. The latter hypothesis is supported by a study assessing the safety and efficacy of 'conservative' versus 'liberal' fluid management strategies. Although the primary endpoint (death at 60 days) did not differ between strategies, benefits in ventilator free and organ failure free days were observed in the 'conservative' group, without an increase in renal dysfunction.

Wherever possible, supplemental feeding should be administered via the enteral route. The use of prokinetic drugs where needed, and the avoidance of agents that delay gastric emptying, may limit the risk of aspiration pneumonitis.

Pharmacotherapy

The anti-inflammatory and antifibrotic properties of steroids present a rational therapy to dampen the dysregulated inflammation which propagates ARDS. Numerous studies have failed to demonstrate clinical benefit from a short course of high dose steroids for the prevention, or treatment, of early ARDS (within 72 hours of onset), with some suggesting steroids may be harmful. The role of steroid therapy in late or unresolving ARDS, i.e. ≥7 days, remains controversial, with data suggesting improvements in both mortality and liberation from mechanical ventilation, but post hoc analysis indicating an increased mortality in patients treated after day 13. In addition, a significant proportion of patients required re-ventilation following steroid weaning, and concerns persist about the relationship between steroid therapy and ICU-acquired weakness.

Inhaled vasodilators, including nitric oxide, prostacyclin and prostaglandin E_1, improve ventilation-perfusion matching and pulmonary hypertension by inducing selective vasodilation in well-ventilated lung. Transient improvements in oxygenation are well established, but inhaled vasodilators are expensive, challenging to administer and associated with adverse events without concomitant mortality benefit. Their use should therefore be limited to those patients with refractory hypoxaemia, either as a bridge to extracorporeal oxygenation, or to provide time for ancillary therapies to take effect, or for those patients with reversible pulmonary hypertension in the setting of ARDS.

Neuromuscular blockade is used in over half of ARDS patients to prevent ventilator dysynchrony. A recent randomised controlled trial found the early use (<48 hours of ARDS onset) of cisatracurium improved 90-day survival in those patients with a PaO_2:FiO_2 ≤ 150 mmHg. Of note, neuromuscular weakness was not more prevalent in the cisatracurium group. Further trials are required to clarify whether these effects are reproducible and to clarify the mechanisms of benefit.

Despite promising experimental data, recent large trials of a range of therapies, the majority of which were designed to reduce cellular and mediator driven inflammation, have failed to demonstrate improvements in clinical outcomes. Statins, beta-2-agonists, ketoconazole, vitamin D supplementation and antioxidants were all found not to confer benefit. This has highlighted the need to limit the heterogeneity of subjects recruited into clinical trials through improved understanding of the pathobiology.

Cell Therapies

Several clinical trials of mesenchymal stem cells (MSCs) for the treatment of ARDS are currently underway (ClinicalTrials.gov: NCT01775774, NCT02444455, NCT02215811, NCT02611609). However, engraftment within the lung does not seem to be the major therapeutic effect of MSCs, rather the effect derives from their capacity to secrete paracrine factors that modulate immune responses and alter the host responses to injury.

Pre-clinical work has shown that cryopreserved allogeneic human MSCs are therapeutic in a human ex vivo lung model, but the antimicrobial effects of the MSCs could be largely duplicated by keratinocyte growth factor (KGF), a major paracrine product of MSCs. A clinical trial investigating the efficacy and safety of KGF in ARDS has been completed, but the results have not as yet been reported (ISRCTN95690673).

Prone Positioning

Mechanical ventilation in the prone position is frequently used in the management of refractory hypoxaemia in ARDS. Approximately 60% of patients demonstrate improvements in oxygenation, which are often sustained on return to the supine position. Proposed mechanisms of benefit include more homogenous distribution of ventilation, better ventilation-perfusion matching and a reduction in VALI. Recently, proning, combined with a protective ventilatory strategy, for at least 16 hours a day in patients with severe ARDS ($PaO_2/FiO_2 < 150$ mmHg with PEEP of at least 5 mmHg and FiO_2 of ≥ 0.6) demonstrated a significant reduction in both 28-day and 90-day mortality. Whilst proning confers a risk of pressure ulcers, facial oedema and endotracheal tube obstruction/displacement, favourable haemodynamic effects have been observed with increasing cardiac index in those patients with preload reserve.

Learning Points

- ARDS is a heterogeneous syndrome rather than a single disease, hence a variety of supportive and therapeutic approaches may be required for optimal management.
- The mainstay of ARDS management is the identification and treatment of the predisposing condition, along with supportive care, which includes lung-protective ventilation.
- Fluid restriction, after patients are appropriately resuscitated.
- The early, and short-term, use of cisatracurium in more severe ARDS cases may improve outcome over and above lung-protective ventilation.
- There are currently no licensed pharmacological therapies for ARDS.

Further Reading

Bellani G, Laffey JG, Pham T, et al. Epidemiology, patterns of care, and mortality for patients with acute respiratory distress syndrome in intensive care units in 50 countries. *Journal of the American Medical Association*. 2016; 315: 788–800.

Bernard GR, Artigas A, Brigham KL, et al. The American–European Consensus Conference on ARDS: definitions, relevant outcomes, and clinical trial coordination. *American Journal of Respiratory and Critical Care Medicine*. 1994; 149: 818–824.

Boyle AJ, MacSweeney R, McAuley DF. Pharmacological treatments in ARDS: a state-of-the-art update. *BMC Medicine*. 2013; 11: 166.

Ferguson ND, Cook DJ, Guyatt GH, et al. High-frequency oscillation in early acute respiratory distress syndrome. *New England Journal of Medicine*. 2013; 368: 795–805.

Guérin C, Reignier J, Richard J-C, et al. Prone positioning in severe acute respiratory distress syndrome. *New England Journal of Medicine*. 2013; 368: 2159–2168.

Herridge MS, Tansey CM, Matte A, et al. Functional disability 5 years after acute respiratory distress syndrome. *New England Journal of Medicine*. 2011; 364: 1293–1304.

Lee JW, Krasnodembskaya A, McKenna DH, et al. Therapeutic effects of human mesenchymal stem cells in ex vivo human lungs injured with live bacteria. *American Journal of Respiratory and Critical Care Medicine*. 2013; 187: 751–760.

Marshall RP, Webb S, Hill MR, et al. Genetic polymorphisms associated with susceptibility and outcome in ARDS. *Chest*. 2002; 121: 68S-69S.

Miller F, Summers C, Griffiths M, et al. The pulmonary endothelium in acute respiratory distress syndrome: insights and therapeutic opportunities. *Thorax*. 2016; 71: 462–473.

National Heart Lung and Blood Institute (NHLBI) Acute Respiratory Distress Syndrome Clinical Trials Network. Comparison of two fluid-management strategies in acute lung injury. *New England Journal of Medicine*. 2006; 354: 2564–2575.

NHLBI Acute Respiratory Distress Syndrome Network. Ventilation with lower tidal volumes as compared with traditional tidal volumes for acute lung injury and the acute respiratory distress syndrome. *New England Journal of Medicine*. 2000; 342: 1301–1308.

Papazian L, Forel J-M, Gacouin A, et al. Neuromuscular blockers in early acute respiratory distress syndrome. *New England Journal of Medicine*. 2010; 363: 1107–1116.

Peek GJ, Mugford M, Tiruvoipati R, et al. Efficacy and economic assessment of conventional ventilatory supprt versus extracorporeal membrane oxygenation for severe adult respiratory failure (CESAR): a multicentre randomised controlled trial. *Lancet*. 2009; 374: 1351–1363.

Ranieri VM, Rubenfeld GD, Thompson BT, et al. Acute respiratory distress syndrome: the Berlin definition. *Journal of the American Medical Association*. 2012; 307: 2526–2533.

Summers C, Singh NR, White JF, et al. Pulmonary retention of primed neutrophils: a novel protective host response, which is impaired in the acute respiratory distress syndrome. *Thorax*. 2014; 69: 623–629.

Villar J, Schultz MJ, Kacmarek RM. The LUNG SAFE: a biased presentation of the prevalence of ARDS! *Critical Care*. 2016; 20: 108.

MCQs

1. **ARDS is defined by the following except:**
   (a) Arterial hypoxaemia
   (b) Hypercapnoea
   (c) Bilateral pulmonary infiltrates on chest radiograph
   (d) Progressive dyspnoea over 4 weeks
   (e) Histological evidence of diffuse alveolar damage

2. **The following have demonstrated a mortality benefit in ARDS:**
   (a) Inhaled nitric oxide
   (b) Cisatracurium
   (c) Ketoconazole
   (d) Surfactant therapy
   (e) Mesenchymal stem cell therapy

3. **ARDS management includes:**
   (a) Transfusion to >11 g/dl haemoglobin concentration to optimise tissue oxygen delivery
   (b) Administration of beta-2-agonists to improve alveolar fluid clearance
   (c) Early appropriate antibiotics in the management of sepsis related ARDS
   (d) Liberal administration of intravenous fluids to ensure adequate tissue perfusion
   (e) Daily recruitment manoeuvres

4. **Regarding ECMO:**
   (a) It has demonstrated a clear mortality benefit in multiple clinical trials in ARDS
   (b) Provides just oxygenation with no carbon dioxide removal
   (c) Has a complication rate <5%
   (d) Should be considered in patients who deteriorate despite optimal medical therapy and 4 weeks of supportive ventilation
   (e) Facilitates protective lung ventilator strategies

5. **Evidence-based mechanical ventilation in ARDS includes:**
   (a) Low tidal volume (6 ml/kg PBW) ventilation
   (b) High frequency oscillatory ventilation (HFOV)
   (c) Airway pressure release ventilation (APRV)
   (d) Inversed I:E ratio ventilation
   (e) Utilisation of PEEP >10 in all cases

Exercise answers are available on p.469. Alternatively, take the test online at www.cambridge.org/CardiothoracicMCQ

Cardiovascular Disorders: the Heart Failure Patient in the Intensive Care Unit

Anna Kydd and Jayan Parameshwar

Introduction

The combination of the aging of the population and improved survival after myocardial infarction has increased the prevalence of heart failure. Most patients with advanced heart failure are admitted to hospital as a result of acute decompensation but some patients with new onset heart failure may present acutely in extremis. Patients with impaired ventricular function who undergo surgery may also present with low output states in the ICU.

The clinical syndrome of heart failure can result from any structural or functional impairment of ventricular filling or ejection of blood. Coronary artery disease remains the most common cause of heart failure. In younger patients (such as the population referred for cardiac transplantation), dilated cardiomyopathy (often of unknown aetiology) is the commonest cause. The true incidence of acute myocarditis in patients with a short history of heart failure is not known because of the difficulty in confirming the diagnosis.

Clinical Presentation

Patients requiring admission to critical care because of severe heart failure usually have one of two clinical syndromes:

1. Pulmonary oedema accompanied by severe respiratory distress and low oxygen saturation (prior to treatment).
2. Cardiogenic shock: defined as tissue hypoperfusion induced by heart failure after correction of preload. It is usually characterised by hypotension (systolic BP <90 mmHg), oliguria (<0.5 ml/kg/hour) and evidence of end-organ dysfunction such as renal, hepatic and cognitive impairment, and elevated blood lactate level.

Bedside assessment may provide clues to the haemodynamic profile of a patient. It is important to distinguish between elevated and non-elevated cardiac filling pressures ('wet' or 'dry'), and adequate or severely impaired tissue perfusion ('warm' or 'cold') (see Figure 45.1).

Elevated filling pressure can be diagnosed clinically by orthopnoea or by elevated jugular venous pressure. Blood pressure is only a guide to tissue perfusion; proportional pulse pressure (pulse pressure/systolic pressure) less than 25% has been reported to correlate with a cardiac index less than 2.2 l/min/m^2 in the population of patients referred for cardiac transplantation.

Patients admitted to the critical care unit are most likely to have elevated filling pressures and inadequate end-organ perfusion (wet and cold). This group is associated with the highest mortality.

Cardiorenal Syndrome

Both an acute deterioration and chronic impairment of cardiac function can lead to a progressive decline in renal function. The umbrella term cardiorenal syndrome is used to describe this. The pathophysiology varies depending on specific clinical circumstances; however it involves transrenal perfusion pressure, intrarenal haemodynamics and systemic neurohormonal factors. Alterations in the balance of vasoconstrictor and vasodilator hormones adversely affect renal function, and the combination of increased central venous pressure with low systemic pressure may lead to a severe compromise of net renal perfusion pressure.

In the acute setting, worsening renal function (acute kidney injury) frequently complicates hospital admissions with acute decompensated heart failure. Patients with worsening renal function have a higher

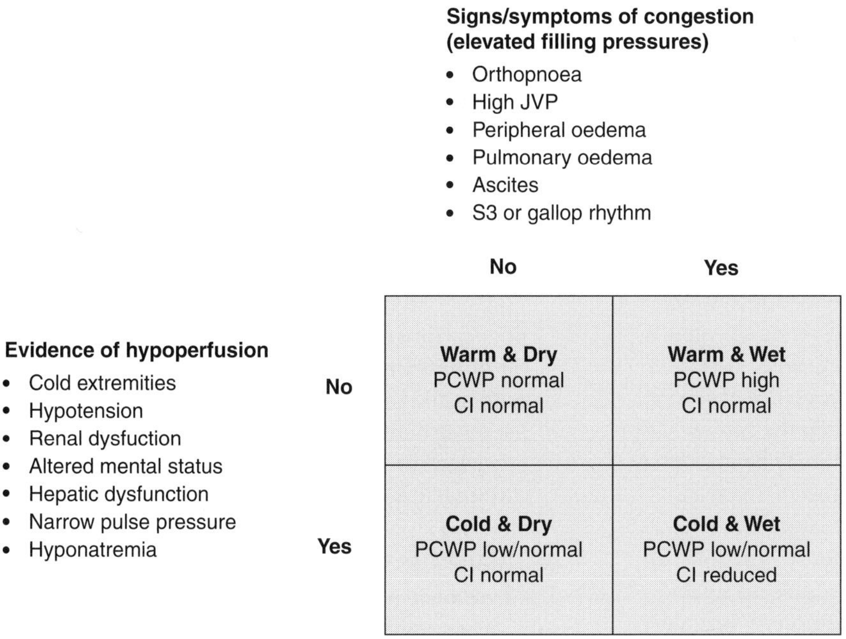

		No	Yes
		Signs/symptoms of congestion (elevated filling pressures) • Orthopnoea • High JVP • Peripheral oedema • Pulmonary oedema • Ascites • S3 or gallop rhythm	
Evidence of hypoperfusion • Cold extremities • Hypotension • Renal dysfuction • Altered mental status • Hepatic dysfunction • Narrow pulse pressure • Hyponatremia	No	**Warm & Dry** PCWP normal CI normal	**Warm & Wet** PCWP high CI normal
	Yes	**Cold & Dry** PCWP low/normal CI normal	**Cold & Wet** PCWP low/normal CI reduced

Figure 45.1 Assessment of haemodynamic profile using haemodynamic signs and symptoms of patients presenting with heart failure. JVP jugular venous pressure.

mortality and morbidity and increased duration of hospitalisation.

In the more chronic state, renal dysfunction develops in patients who have chronic volume overload, prior renal dysfunction, right ventricular dysfunction and high baseline diuretic requirements. When filling pressures are measured they exceed the optimal levels required to maintain cardiac output. A stable clinical state may be maintained in some patients with high serum urea and creatinine levels but the prognosis is poor. Inotropic infusions may relieve the congestion and improve renal function but the problem often recurs when inotropes are withdrawn.

Investigations

In addition to a detailed clinical history and physical examination a number of investigations are required:

1. Electrocardiogram to determine rhythm and aetiology of heart failure (e.g. acute coronary syndrome or myocarditis).
2. Chest radiograph for heart size, pulmonary congestion, lung consolidation or pleural effusions.
3. Echocardiography to assess regional and global left and right ventricular function, valve structure and function, pericardial effusion, and mechanical complications of myocardial infarction. The pulmonary artery systolic pressure may also be estimated from the tricuspid regurgitation jet and echocardiography.
4. Blood tests: full blood count, coagulation screen, C-reactive protein, creatinine and electrolytes, glucose and liver function tests in all patients. Troponin and plasma BNP (B-type natriuretic peptide) may also be indicated. For the assessment of a patient presenting with acute dyspnoea a low BNP has a high negative predictive value for heart failure as the aetiology. BNP may be less helpful in the critical care setting.
5. Coronary angiography if revascularisation is indicated.

Monitoring

1. Non-invasive monitoring – temperature, respiratory rate, blood pressure, continuous ECG monitoring and pulse oximetry are required for all patients.
2. Arterial line – essential in unstable patients for continuous arterial blood pressure monitoring and frequent analysis of blood gases.
3. Central venous line – monitoring right sided filling pressure is often essential in patients with advanced heart failure and a central venous line is required for the delivery of fluids and drugs.

Estimation of superior vena caval or right atrial oxygen saturation can be a useful marker of oxygen transport. Central venous pressure may be significantly affected by positive end-expiratory pressure ventilation.

- Pulmonary artery catheter (PAC) – PAC allows direct measurement of right atrial (RA), right ventricular (RV), pulmonary artery (PA), pulmonary capillary wedge pressure (PCWP) and calculation of pulmonary and systemic vascular resistance. Mixed venous oxygen saturation can also be monitored. This is particularly useful in the presence of severe tricuspid regurgitation when the cardiac output derived by thermodilution may be inaccurate.
- In patients with heart failure, right atrial pressure does not correlate well with left sided filling pressure. In many situations, an estimate of left atrial pressure is invaluable. In patients with a high pulmonary vascular resistance (PVR) associated with heart failure, direct measurement of pulmonary pressure is important. In patients requiring inotropic or vasoconstrictor drugs, monitoring of cardiac output and estimation of systemic vascular resistance facilitates therapy based on pathophysiological principles.
- Complications associated with the use of a PAC increase with duration of use and it should not be left in situ longer than necessary. In advanced heart failure, therapy tailored to haemodynamic goals as guided by PAC has been shown to result in sustained improvement in symptoms, stroke volume and cardiac output.
- Cardiac power output (CPO) describes the relationship between flow and pressure in the circulation and is a powerful predictor of prognosis in cardiogenic shock. It is calculated as the product of simultaneous mean arterial pressure (MAP) and cardiac output corrected for a constant and expressed as watts.
- Although PAC is the 'gold standard' there are a number of non-invasive cardiac output monitoring devices available that can derive haemodynamic data, but most have not been validated in low cardiac output states.

4. Echocardiography – there is an emerging role for both transthoracic and transoesophageal echocardiography in monitoring haemodynamics in critically ill patients; however, interpretation of data requires specific training and expertise.

Treatment

The treatment of chronic heart failure has been the subject of several large randomised clinical trials and evidence-based guidelines are available.

Critically ill patients with acute heart failure are a heterogeneous group with respect to aetiology, haemodynamic abnormalities and comorbidities, and are therefore difficult to subject to randomised trials. Treatment strategies should be based on the underlying pathophysiology with the aim of reversing haemodynamic abnormalities. If an underlying treatable cause is identified, clinical condition should be optimised so that definitive treatment can be carried out with the minimum of risk. Immediate therapy should focus on relieving symptoms. Reducing congestion is often the most effective way of achieving this (see Table 45.1).

General management involves a multidisciplinary team due to the complexity of the pathophysiology in the critically ill heart failure patient. In

Table 45.1 Treatment goals in advanced heart failure

Clinical	Elimination of peripheral and pulmonary oedema Systolic blood pressure >85 mmHg Stable or improving renal function Normal or improving liver function and coagulation parameters Adequate oxygenation
Haemodynamic	Central venous/right atrial pressure ≤8 mmHg Pulmonary capillary wedge pressure ≤16 mmHg Cardiac index >2 l/min/m^2 Mixed venous oxygen saturation >60% Systemic vascular resistance 800–1200 dyne s cm^{-5} (secondary goal to guide therapy)

addition to the specific treatments described below, management should include investigation and correction of anaemia, electrolyte abnormalities, thyroid and adrenal function and optimal glucose control. Infection is common; therefore standard infection control measures and evidence-based antimicrobial treatment are essential. Patients should receive appropriate nutrition, mobilisation and physiotherapy. Provision of psychological support and involvement of palliative care teams are also important considerations.

Oxygenation

Achieving an adequate level of oxygenation at the cellular level is important to prevent end-organ dysfunction. Treatment should aim to achieve optimal rather than supraphysiological arterial oxygenation, i.e. arterial oxygen saturation above 95%. Respiratory muscle fatigue often results from hypoxaemia and low cardiac output.

Non-invasive Ventilation

Either continuous positive airway pressure (CPAP) or non-invasive ventilation (NIV) can be used to reduce the work of breathing. Both CPAP and NIV result in pulmonary recruitment and an increase in functional residual capacity and a reduction in pulmonary oedema. Clinical trials comparing CPAP with standard therapy have shown a decreased need for endotracheal intubation.

Mechanical Ventilation with Endotracheal Intubation

If non-invasive ventilation does not reverse hypoxaemia or if there is compromise to airway patency, endotracheal intubation is indicated.

Drug Therapy

The major goals of medical therapy in the heart failure patient in the ICU are (i) reducing venous congestion (optimising preload), (ii) optimising afterload with vasodilators, in the absence of severe hypotension, and (iii) inotropic support.

Diuretics

The reduction of elevated filling pressures is the most effective way to relieve symptoms of heart failure. Patients with acute decompensation of chronic heart failure are likely to be on diuretic therapy when admitted. Data are lacking on the relative efficacy and tolerability of different diuretics. In the acute setting, a loop diuretic is administered intravenously with dose titration to produce optimal urine output. A large bolus of diuretic may also lead to reflex renal vasoconstriction and a higher risk of ototoxicity. An intravenous infusion of furosemide at 5–10 mg/hour is sufficient in most patients once steps have been taken to increase the cardiac output. Fluid restriction (usually to 1.5 l/day) is an important adjunct to diuretic therapy in severely fluid-overloaded patients. Using a 'fluid challenge' in such patients with obvious fluid retention is irrational and has no place in treatment of heart failure patients in the cardiothoracic ICU; inadequate urine output in these patients is usually related to a low cardiac output and treating this often requires inotropic therapy. Once filling pressures have been reduced to normal, the dose of diuretic should be reduced; the dose required to maintain euvolaemia is usually less than that required to achieve it.

The combination of a thiazide (e.g. metolazone or bendroflumethiazide) with a loop diuretic can augment the diuresis achieved in patients with chronic heart failure and is of use in the acute setting. Heart failure patients are often hyponatraemic in the ICU and care needs to be taken not to exacerbate this with combination diuretic therapy. Serum potassium should be monitored as hypokalaemia may predispose to arrhythmias. Combining loop diuretics with a mineralocorticoid receptor antagonist like spironolactone or eplerenone may be effective provided the serum potassium is <5 mmol/l and serum creatinine <200 μmol/l.

Vasodilators

In the absence of severe hypotension, vasodilators are indicated in most patients with acute heart failure. Decreasing preload relieves congestion and decreasing afterload is usually beneficial as most patients with heart failure are vasoconstricted (Table 45.2). When administering vasodilators or positive inotropic drugs, the following equation is useful in manipulating the circulation:

$$MAP - CVP = CO \times SVR$$

where MAP is the mean arterial pressure, CVP is the central venous pressure, CO is the cardiac output and SVR is the systemic vascular resistance.

Table 45.2 Typical doses of intravenous inotropes used in heart failure

Drug	Bolus	Dose
Dopamine	No	2–10 μg/kg/min
Dobutamine	No	2–20 μg/kg/min
Adrenaline	No	0.05–0.5 μg/kg/min
Noradrenaline	No	0.02–0.2 μg/kg/min
Enoximone	0.25–0.75 mg/kg	1.25–7.5 μg/kg/min
Milrinone	25–75 μg/kg	0.375–0.75 μg/kg/min
Levosimendan	12–24 μg/kg	0.05–0.2 μg/kg/min

Nitrates

In low doses, nitrates are venodilators but high doses can also cause arterial dilatation. They are particularly useful in acute coronary syndromes associated with heart failure. Oral nitrates in combination with hydralazine have been shown to be beneficial in chronic heart failure and at least two randomised controlled trials have shown that intravenous nitrate in combination with furosemide is superior to furosemide alone. Tolerance to nitrate can develop within 24 hours of commencing an infusion.

Nesiritide

Nesiritide (recombinant brain natriuretic peptide) is licensed in the USA for the treatment of acute heart failure. It relaxes smooth muscle leading to arterial and venous dilatation and leads to an increase in cardiac output without direct positive inotropic effect. Compared with nitroglycerin, nesiritide has been shown to produce faster relief of dyspnoea and a more pronounced decrease in pulmonary capillary wedge pressure. Nesiritide has both natriuretic and diuretic effects although up to half of patients with advanced heart failure are reported to be resistant to its natriuretic effect. There is no conclusive evidence that nesiritide improves renal function; clinical studies have not demonstrated better clinical outcomes and it may increase risk of adverse cardiovascular events. The role of nesiritide in the management of heart failure remains unclear.

Hydralazine

Hydralazine is a potent arteriolar vasodilator. A combination of hydralazine and nitrates has been shown to be beneficial in patients with chronic heart failure. In patients who cannot tolerate an angiotensin converting enzyme inhibitor (ACEI) because of hyperkalaemia or worsening renal function, it is reasonable to use this combination orally or intravenously.

Inotropic Support

Inotropic agents are indicated in the presence of tissue hypoperfusion and pump failure often manifested by worsening renal function or fluid retention (peripheral or pulmonary oedema) refractory to treatment with diuretics and vasodilators. A common clinical scenario is a volume-overloaded patient with hypotension, hyponatraemia, and a rising serum urea and creatinine on intravenous diuretic therapy. Continuing such therapy is likely to exacerbate metabolic abnormalities and is unlikely to induce a significant diuresis. Intravenous inotropic therapy may be necessary to improve the patient's haemodynamic state until some form of definitive therapy or long-term palliation can be considered.

Although inotropic agents in heart failure can result in short-term beneficial haemodynamic effects, they increase myocardial oxygen consumption and carry a risk of inducing life-threatening arrhythmia. Rational use of inotropic therapy in a critically ill population requires invasive haemodynamic monitoring. The lowest effective dose should be used; patients receiving beta-blockers may require higher doses. Very few trials have been conducted in patients with advanced heart failure and there is no definite evidence of the superiority of one agent compared to any other.

Dopamine

Dopamine has complex effects, which vary according to dose. Low doses of dopamine (<2 μg/kg/min) are thought to act predominantly on peripheral dopaminergic (D1) receptors leading to vasodilatation. Although controversial, low dose dopamine has been shown to increase renal blood flow. In addition it is possible that in some patients it may also have an inotropic effect.

A higher dose of dopamine (>5 μg/kg/min) has β-adrenergic effects increasing cardiac output and α-adrenergic effects increasing peripheral vascular resistance and arterial pressure.

Dobutamine

Dobutamine acts through stimulation of β1 and β2 receptors and is positively inotropic and chronotropic; it may also induce mild arterial vasodilatation. High doses of dobutamine (above 10 μg/kg/min)

cause vasoconstriction but the exact effect at any given dose varies between patients. Heart rate is generally thought to increase less than with other catecholamines, however atrioventricular conduction is facilitated. The commonly used dose range is 2 to 10 μg/kg/min.

Adrenaline

This drug has a high affinity for β1, β2 and α-receptors causing inotropy, chronotropy, dromotropy and splanchnic hypoperfusion. It is generally infused at a rate of 0.05–0.5 μg/kg/min.

Noradrenaline

This drug is used to increase systemic vascular resistance (SVR) because of its affinity for α-receptors. The lowest dose required to increase the SVR (and hence the blood pressure), and to maintain perfusion of vital organs, should be used. Septic shock is a common indication for its use; the occasional patient after acute myocardial infarction will present with a low SVR due to cytokine release and will benefit from noradrenaline. Excessive vasoconstriction is associated with a reduction in cardiac output.

Type III Phosphodiesterase (PDE) Inhibitors

PDE inhibitors block the breakdown of cyclic-AMP, which modulates intracellular calcium handling. Enoximone and milrinone are the two agents used in clinical practice. They cause marked peripheral vasodilatation and have positive inotropic effects and are therefore useful in patients with advanced heart failure who have an elevated SVR and a low cardiac output. Because of their powerful vasodilating effect, haemodynamic monitoring is recommended whenever they are used. Both agents have a long elimination half-life and tend to accumulate if the patient is oliguric. As their site of action is distal to the β-adrenergic receptor, PDE inhibitors maintain their effect in patients who have been treated with beta-blocking drugs. In patients with atrial fibrillation, they may increase ventricular rate less than dobutamine.

Levosimendan

This drug has two main mechanisms of action: Ca^{2+} ion sensitisation of the contractile proteins (positive inotropic effect) and smooth muscle K^{+} channel opening (peripheral vasodilating effect). There is also a suggestion that levosimendan has a PDE inhibiting effect. Intravenous infusions of levosimendan are usually maintained for 24 hours, but the haemodynamic effects persist beyond this, probably because of the long half-life of its metabolite. Levosimendan infusions in patients with heart failure have been associated with a dose-dependent increase in stroke volume and cardiac output, a decline in the pulmonary capillary wedge pressure, a decrease in SVR and PVR, a slight decrease in blood pressure and a slight increase in heart rate. An improvement in symptoms of dyspnoea and fatigue has been shown in trials comparing levosimendan with dobutamine. The haemodynamic effects were seen even in the presence of beta-blocker therapy. Tachycardia and hypotension are side effects associated with the use of levosimendan and it is not recommended in patients with a systolic blood pressure below ~85 mmHg.

Angiotensin Converting Enzyme (ACE) Inhibitors and Angiotensin Receptor Blockers (ARB)

ACE inhibitors were the first drug class shown to improve outcome in severe chronic heart failure. ARBs are used as alternatives in patients intolerant of ACEI. They have no role in the early management of unstable heart failure patients but should be introduced as soon as the patient is haemodynamically stable and has acceptable perfusion and renal function. ACE inhibitors decrease renal vascular resistance, increase renal blood flow and promote sodium and water excretion. However, in patients with a very low cardiac output, they may significantly decrease glomerular filtration rate. If patients with acute decompensation of chronic heart failure are admitted to the ICU, it may be necessary to discontinue them temporarily.

Beta-Blockers

The role of beta-blockers in the management of chronic heart failure is well established following several large trials involving many thousands of patients. In volume-overloaded patients, beta-blockers are likely to increase the severity of heart failure and are best avoided. There is no consensus on the management of a patient receiving beta-blockers for chronic heart failure admitted to hospital with acute decompensation. Most will require at least a decrease in the dose of the drug but in patients requiring (beta-agonist) inotropic therapy it is logical to discontinue beta-blockers altogether.

Anticoagulation

Patients should receive standard prophylaxis for prevention of venous thromboembolism and anticoagulation for established indications, for example acute coronary syndromes, pulmonary embolism and atrial fibrillation. Patients with evidence of ventricular thrombus on echocardiography should also receive anticoagulation. Care is needed as concomitant liver dysfunction may lead to a prolonged prothrombin time. In patients with a creatinine clearance below 30 ml/min, low molecular weight heparin in therapeutic doses should be used cautiously, probably with monitoring of factor Xa level.

Ultrafiltration

Patients with gross fluid retention and hyponatraemia present a difficult clinical problem. Diuretics often worsen hyponatraemia and sometimes features of the cardiorenal syndrome become apparent. Inotropic drugs may help in this situation but if therapy needs to be prolonged, the risk of arrhythmia needs to be considered. Continuous venovenous haemofiltration (CVVH) is effective in removing fluid and the rate of fluid removal can be tailored to the patient's needs. CVVH may also remove cytokines with myocardial depressant properties (e.g. tumour necrosis factor) as macromolecules up to 20,000 Da can pass through the ultrafiltration membrane. If necessary, large volumes of fluid can be removed in a relatively short time to get the patient ready for a definitive procedure (heart transplantation, mechanical circulatory support).

CVVH usually requires large-bore central venous access although there are devices to allow ultrafiltration via cannulae in peripheral arm veins. Although the maximum rate of fluid removal is less than that attainable by central CVVH, an adequate rate is achieved for the most common clinical situations.

Compared to high dose diuretic therapy, ultrafiltration has been reported to induce less neurohormonal activation and vasoconstriction.

Intra-aortic Balloon Pump (IABP)

IABP use may reduce afterload, thereby decreasing left ventricular stroke work and myocardial oxygen consumption, as well as augmenting diastolic blood flow in the coronary and systemic circulation. Functional mitral regurgitation, a common problem in a patient with a dilated left ventricle, decreases with the use of the IABP.

The IABP is extremely useful in critically ill patients with heart failure who can be stabilised until definitive therapy can be carried out. In patients requiring support beyond that provided by IABP, consideration should be given to the use of mechanical circulatory support. There is no evidence of improved survival with any form of short-term mechanical support, including IABP, in patients with cardiogenic shock. However these therapies may improve haemodynamics and get the patient fit for definitive treatment (implantable device or heart transplantation).

Conclusion

Advanced heart failure in patients on critical care units carries a high mortality. Optimal management requires close cooperation between a cardiologist with an interest in heart failure, an intensive care physician and a cardiac surgeon. With appropriate therapy, many critically ill patients can be resuscitated and returned to a productive life.

Learning Points

- Heart failure is most commonly secondary to coronary artery disease and carries a poor overall prognosis.
- Admission to critical care is usually due to pulmonary oedema or cardiogenic shock.
- The major goals of medical therapy for the heart failure patient in the ICU are (i) optimising preload, (ii) optimising afterload and (iii) increasing cardiac output with inotropic support when required.
- Aggressive diuresis may be needed, and renal replacement therapy may be necessary to remove an adequate amount of fluid.
- Inotropes are often started to enhance cardiac output, but may lead to other complications; close haemodynamic monitoring is essential to direct therapy.

Further Reading

Binanay C, Califf RM, Hasselblad V et al. Evaluation study of congestive heart failure and pulmonary artery catheterization effectiveness: the ESCAPE trial. *Journal of the American Medical Association*. 2005; 294: 1625–1633.

Elkayam U, Ng TM, Hatamizadeh P, Janmohamed M, Mehra A. Renal vasodilatory action of dopamine in patients with heart failure: magnitude of effect and site of action. *Circulation*. 2008; 117: 200–205.

Felker GM, Lee KL, Bull DA, et al. Diuretic strategies in patients with acute decompensated heart failure. *New England Journal of Medicine*. 2011; 364: 797–805.

Francis GS, Bartos JA, Adatya S. Inotropes. *Journal of the American College of Cardiology*. 2014; 63: 2069–2078.

Hochman JS, Sleeper LA, Webb JG, et al. Early revascularization in acute myocardial infarction complicated by cardiogenic shock. SHOCK Investigators. Should we emergently revascularize occluded coronaries for cardiogenic shock. *New England Journal of Medicine*. 1999; 341: 625–634.

McMurray JJ, Adamopoulos S, Anker SD, et al. ESC guidelines for the diagnosis and treatment of acute and chronic heart failure 2012: The Task Force for the Diagnosis and Treatment of Acute and Chronic Heart Failure 2012 of the European Society of Cardiology. Developed in collaboration with the Heart Failure Association (HFA) of the ESC. *European Journal of Heart Failure*. 2012; 14: 803–869.

Nohria A, Lewis E, Stevenson LW. Medical management of advanced heart failure. *Journal of the American Medical Association*. 2002; 287: 628–640.

Steimle AE, Stevenson LW, Chelimsky-Fallick C, et al. Sustained haemodynamic efficacy of therapy tailored to reduce filling pressures in survivors with advanced heart failure. *Circulation*. 1997; 96: 1165–1172.

Stevenson LW. Management of acute decompensation. In: Mann DL (Ed). *Heart Failure*, Belvoir Publication, 2004, pp. 579–594.

Thiele H, Schuler G, Neumann FJ, et al. Intraaortic balloon counterpulsation in acute myocardial infarction complicated by cardiogenic shock: design and rationale of the Intraaortic Balloon Pump in Cardiogenic Shock II (IABP-SHOCK II) trial. *American Heart Journal*. 2012; 163: 938–945.

Yancy CW, Jessup M, Bozkurt B, et al. 2013 ACCF/AHA guideline for the management of heart failure: executive summary: a report of the American College of Cardiology Foundation/American Heart Association Task Force on practice guidelines. *Circulation*. 2013; 128: 1810–1852.

MCQs

1. **Clinical presentation of acute heart failure may include the following symptoms and signs:**
   (a) Raised jugular venous pressure
   (b) Third heart sound
   (c) Peripheral oedema
   (d) Altered mental state
   (e) All of the above
2. **Investigations and monitoring for the patient with acute heart failure may include:**
   (a) Pulmonary artery catheter
   (b) Systemic vascular resistance
   (c) Mixed venous oxygen saturation
   (d) Echocardiography as a first line investigation
   (e) All of the above
3. **First line drug therapy in the treatment of chronic heart failure includes the following:**
   (a) Dobutamine
   (b) Calcium channel blockers
   (c) Angiotensin converting enzyme inhibitors
   (d) Digoxin
   (e) Hydralazine
4. **Regarding inotropic drugs used for the treatment of patients with acute heart failure:**
   (a) Can be used to improve renal perfusion
   (b) High doses of catecholamines can be arrhythmogenic
   (c) Levosimendan is better at improving the symptoms of dyspnoea than dobutamine
   (d) All of the above
   (e) Enoximone has a short half-life
5. **Regarding the use of an intra-aortic balloon pump which of the following statements is true?**
   (a) Both systolic and diastolic blood pressure are increased
   (b) Haemodynamic effects include an increase in after-load and increase in cardiac output
   (c) Severe mitral regurgitation is a contraindication
   (d) Aortic regurgitation is a contraindication
   (e) Compartment syndrome is an unlikely complication

Exercise answers are available on p.469. Alternatively, take the test online at www.cambridge.org/CardiothoracicMCQ

Section 7 **Disease Management in the Cardiothoracic Intensive Care Unit: Incidence; Aetiology; Diagnosis; Prognosis; Treatment**

Neurological Aspects of Cardiac Surgery

Max S Damian

Introduction

Cardiac surgery's profound intervention in systemic blood pressure and circulation carries a high potential to affect the brain in a way that may offset the benefits of successful cardiac procedures. Astonishing progress has been achieved in safety and effectiveness, which has enabled cardiac surgery to become feasible in ever older and sicker patients. However, these are at higher risk of stroke, which in turn increases mortality fivefold, and neurological complications prolong intensive care treatment and rehabilitation. Conditions treated by emergency cardiac surgery, such as aortic dissection and acute cardiac failure, carry a high risk of neurological complications even without surgery, which may only come to light in the postoperative period.

Cardiac surgeons closely monitor effectiveness and adverse effects, so the complications of cardiac surgery have been well identified. Prevention of neurological complications includes thorough preoperative screening and perioperative monitoring, and this has deepened our understanding of potential risks. This chapter will provide an overview of the most significant neurological problems encountered around cardiac surgery, their diagnosis and management, and an outline of preventive options.

Neurological Considerations in Patients Undergoing Cardiac Surgery

Changing patient characteristics indicate a growing potential for neurological complications: the age of patients in cardiac surgery has increased, and the case mix accepted for CABG has also changed through the advent of PCI as an alternative procedure. Competent preoperative neurological assessment including a detailed cerebrovascular history may help identify patients at risk of developing neurological complications. In CABG patients generally, the risk of severe carotid stenosis may be higher than in the general population, and carotid ultrasound before elective CABG benefits carefully selected patients the most.

Neurological Aspects of Cardiopulmonary Bypass and Extracorporeal Oxygenation

Cardiopulmonary bypass has been a prerequisite for modern cardiac surgery, and in the past 60 years this has become a safe, routine procedure. Venous blood from the systemic circulation is drained to a reservoir, then pumped through a filter and membrane oxygenator system to the ascending aorta, which is cannulated distal to the aortic cross-clamp. In a second venous-to-arterial circuit originating from the bypass, some of the blood is diverted back to the heart together with cardioplegia solution, and from the heart to the venous reservoir after being purified from embolic material in a cardiotomy reservoir.

Neurological complications related to the cardiac bypass are fortunately rare. One main source of problems is related to embolism, when during preparation of the cardiopulmonary bypass circuits, cross-clamping, and turbulent or high-velocity blood flow can dislodge atheromatous material from the aortic wall. In addition, bypass circulation requires heparinisation and, together with cardioplegia solution and other admixtures causing haemodilution, alters the flow and oxygenation qualities of the blood perfusing the brain. Furthermore, contact between the blood and non-biological filter membranes and bypass surfaces induces a systemic inflammatory response with potential neurological significance which is not yet well understood.

A number of technical modifications may help reduce the risk of neurological complications. Preoperative transoesophageal or intraoperative epi-aortic ultrasound may help identify patients particularly at risk for embolism related to aortic cross-clamp and potentially may allow modification of the surgical strategy. Most procedures with cardiopulmonary bypass are performed using mild hypothermia. The importance of temperature management for brain protection in hypoxic conditions has been long recognised, both for cardiac surgery and for treatment after cardiac arrest. However, a Cochrane review of studies comparing neurological outcomes after hypothermic and after normothermic bypass surgery did not establish a clear benefit.

Deep hypothermia is used to prolong toleration of hypoxia to the brain in surgery with prolonged cerebral circulatory arrest, for instance aortic arch surgery or pulmonary thromboendarterectomy. Although the neuroprotective effect of deep hypothermia is beyond doubt, the precise temperature required to achieve maximum benefit, the parameters to which hypothermia should be implemented and how rewarming should take place remain unclear. Rapid rewarming after therapeutic hypothermia can trigger epileptic seizures. Other potentially neuroprotective strategies include the use of anterograde or even retrograde selective brain perfusion. The neurological benefits have not been established, although some evidence suggests that selective anterograde perfusion may permit procedures to take place in moderate rather than deep hypothermia. The use of Alpha-stat metabolic management or pH stat management, in which CPB gas sweep rate is adjusted at lower temperatures to compensate for the hypothermic alkaline drift, remains controversial. Proponents of pH stat management believe that it improves oxygen delivery, increases cerebral blood flow and thus allows more effective cooling of the brain. Alpha-stat management allowing an alkaline pH during hypothermia, on the other hand, may improve enzyme activity and protein function, preserve cerebral autoregulation, and produce less risk of embolism through reduced cerebral blood flow. Which method is more beneficial may depend on multiple factors, including the age of the patient, but the topic remains controversial.

It still remains to be proven whether 'off-pump' procedures are significantly safer than conventional cardiac bypass. The risk of postoperative delirium, which may prolong intensive care, is also claimed to be lower. It is unclear which systemic blood pressure is optimal for brain protection during surgery. Trials comparing a mean arterial blood pressure of 50 mmHg with 70 mmHg failed to demonstrate a significant benefit for either approach. Either target would mean a cerebral perfusion pressure (CPP) lower than the CPP of 70 mmHg currently advised for brain protection in acute traumatic brain injury; whether this has clinical significance has so far not been investigated.

Acute Neurological Complications of Cardiac Surgery

Central Nervous System

Stroke is the commonest neurological complication after cardiac surgery, occurring through embolism or hypoperfusion. The incidence of clinically relevant stroke has decreased to under 2% after CABG and under 4% after single valve replacement, despite the demographic increase in the proportion of elderly at-risk patients. Postoperative diffusion-weighted MRI scans demonstrate clinically silent new lesions in up to 18%. Valve replacement and combined CABG and valvular surgery procedures carry a higher risk of causing embolic territorial and branch infarcts, whereas prolonged cardiopulmonary bypass increases the risk of watershed infarcts related to hypoperfusion. In most cases currently, there is no acute active treatment as major surgery is a contraindication for thrombolysis, but the increasing availability of emergency clot retrieval may change the situation. Stroke associated with left ventricular assist devices has recently been shown to benefit from endovascular treatment, if recognised early. One likely consequence will be that rapid diagnosis in patients evidencing a neurological focal deficit on awakening becomes necessary more often in the near future, increasing the need for imaging. Ischaemic and haemorrhagic stroke cannot be differentiated clinically, so the different management mandates CT scanning of the brain, if emergency MRI is not feasible. Specific locations of ischaemic stroke are associated with particular risks, such as 'malignant' complete MCA territory stroke with the risk of life-threatening hemispheric swelling, or cerebellar stroke with the risk of hydrocephalus and brain stem compression; both these forms of stroke have high fatality if diagnosed late, but often have good outcomes if treated with prompt surgical decompression.

Intracranial haemorrhage is infrequent in cardiac surgery, and is related to a combination of intentional treatment and effects of bypass on platelet function and clotting factors, especially in patients with previously unrecognised predisposing conditions (Figure 46.1). The location of haemorrhage can be intraparenchymal, subdural, epidural and subarachnoid, and is often atypical. Intracranial haemorrhage warrants neurosurgical consultation and some cases may need decompression.

Encephalopathy is an umbrella term for diffuse brain dysfunction that can be due to multiple differen

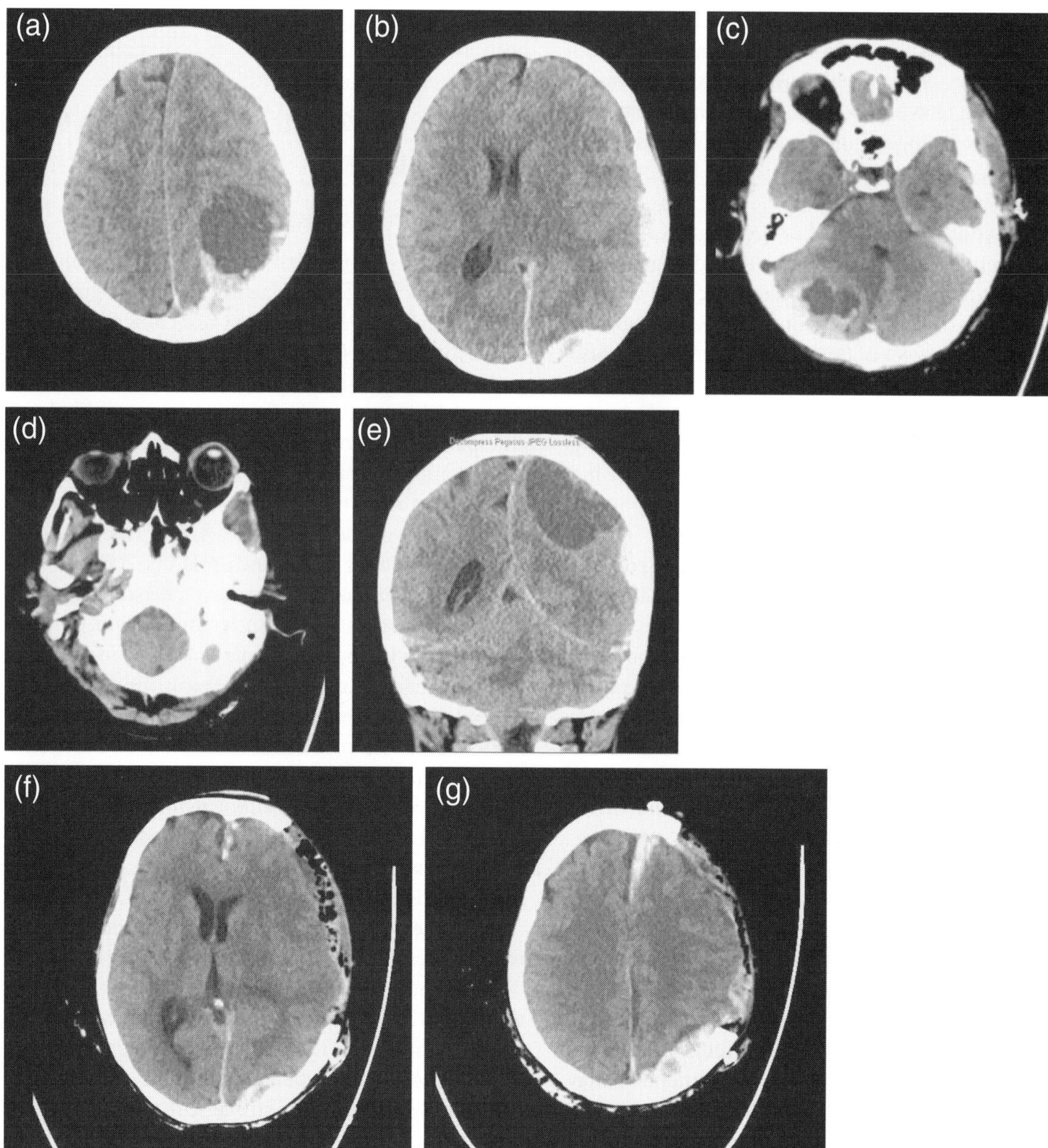

Figure 46.1 A 39 year old female admitted for redo pulmonary endarterectomy. Postoperatively she was heparinised, but also had low platelets (66×10^9). Failure to awaken, and right sided weakness prompted imaging. CT showed subdural haemorrhage and bleeding into two pre-existing, unrecognised arachnoid cysts. (a)–(e) Initial CT scans; (d) tonsillar herniation into the foramen magnum; (e) upward transtentorial herniation; (f), (g) CT post hemicraniectomy and cyst decompression shows improvement of midline shift.

aetiologies. In the acute phase after surgery, encephalopathy manifests as failure to awaken, and global hypoxia or ischaemia of the brain needs to be differentiated from sedative overhang. Elderly patients or those with cerebrovascular disease are at greater risk of encephalopathy. Patients scheduled for CABG are a population with risk factors for cerebrovascular disease, with a high prevalence of silent infarcts on preoperative MRI of the brain. A clinical diagnosis of global encephalopathy demands the absence of a focal neurological deficit, which makes a careful examination of oculomotor and other cranial nerve functions important. Dysconjugate eye movements imply the presence of a focal brain stem lesion, for instance stroke in the basilar distribution, which may go undetected in routine CT of the brain. Multiple simultaneous emboli can simulate global brain dysfunction, making imaging of the brain mandatory as well as extensive metabolic and infectious screening in prolonged encephalopathy. Negative CT but persistent failure to awaken will mean an indication for MRI of the brain and/or electrophysiological studies. Lumbar puncture may be needed after imaging, in the early postoperative period, to exclude subarachnoid haemorrhage, and in the later postoperative period to exclude infection.

Encephalopathic patients, when they awaken, may have persistent confusion or delirium, a fluctuating conscious state, or recurrent agitation and hallucinations. Repetitive movements such as tremor, asterixis, choreoathetosis or myoclonus are frequent, and are often suspected to be epileptic seizures. The clinical diagnosis or exclusion of epileptic seizures versus movement disorders, stereotypies or paroxysmal dysautonomia is notoriously unreliable. EEG is mostly needed to confirm the suspicion and make the indication for anticonvulsant drugs. Even in the absence of abnormal movements or stereotypes, a prolonged EEG may be necessary to exclude non-convulsive status epilepticus (NCSE). This condition has only recently been recognised and its incidence in cardiosurgical patients is unclear, but it has been shown to be prevalent in neurotrauma and in sepsis patients. A fluctuating dyscognitive state may be the only clinical sign of NCSE, and the features may be so unspecific that only EEG may differentiate it from other causes of delirium.

Posterior reversible encephalopathy is a syndrome of vasogenic oedema affecting predominantly white matter, more often the posterior region of the brain, and is diagnosed by MRI. It is occasionally seen in the immediate postoperative phase where it can occur as a form of 'reperfusion syndrome', for example after repair of aortic stenosis, after carotid endarterectomy or after transplantation when there is a rapid shift of arterial pressures. More often, in patients who have undergone transplantation, PRES is related to toxicity of calcineurin inhibitors, in particular tacrolimus, where a pronounced tremor is often a feature, or to many other drugs (Figure 46.2).

Optic neuropathies are uncommon but well-recognised complications of cardiac surgery. Infarction of the optic nerve results in permanent monocular loss of visual acuity and visual field defects, with optic disc swelling (anterior optic neuropathy) or without (posterior optic neuropathy). A monocular disturbance of vision needs to be differentiated from incongruous hemianopia due to infarction affecting the optic tracts, which does not affect the pupillary reaction and where the visual field defect in each eye differs in size. Infarction of the visual cortex causes homonymous hemianopia with an identical visual field defect in both eyes.

Peripheral Nervous System

Brachial plexus injury causes denervation in the distribution of multiple peripheral nerves, and after median sternotomy with sternal retraction a lower brachial plexus injury of varying severity occurs in up to 5% of patients. The majority are mild and transient, with sensory and motor symptoms resembling ulnar nerve injury, although findings on careful examination may show a Horner's syndrome, or sensory deficits and reflex abnormalities exceeding the distribution of a single peripheral nerve. Persistent and severe deficits warrant neurophysiological examination, which may help prognostication by estimating the degree of axonal injury versus demyelination. Intraoperative monitoring of sensory nerve conduction may help to avoid brachial plexus injury, and identify factors which make brachial plexus injury less likely, such as minimising the opening of the sternal retractor, caudal positioning of the retractor and reducing asymmetric traction. Transient injury to sympathetic fibres through ipsilateral jugular venous cannulation causing Horner's sign, but with no abnormalities in the arm, is a differential diagnosis to partial lower brachial plexopathy.

The **phrenic nerve** passes through the mediastinum adjacent to the pericardium and is therefore

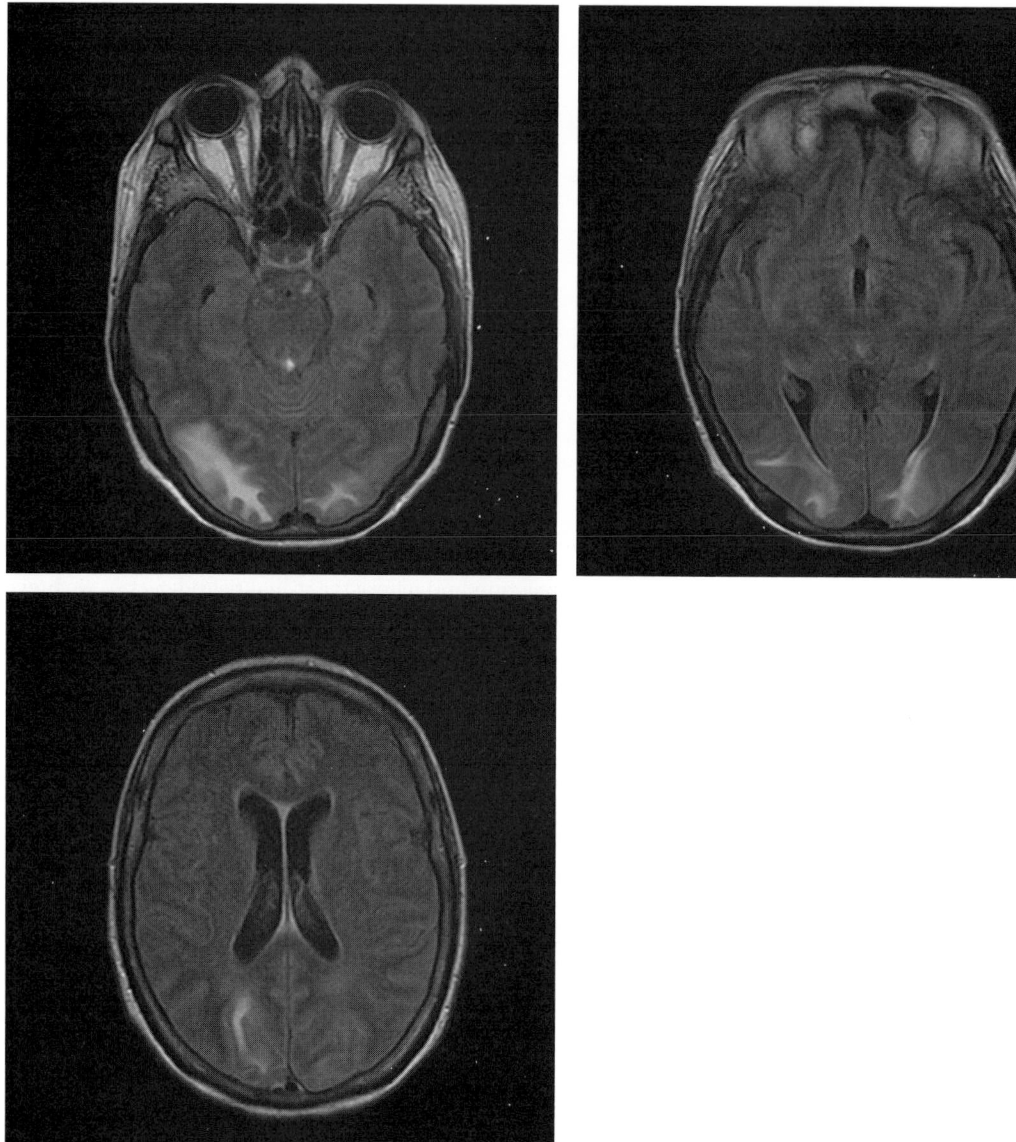

Figure 46.2 A 29 year old patient post double lung transplant. Agitation and visual hallucinations developed shortly after initialising the full dose of tacrolimus. CT scan was unremarkable. MRI shows PRES with symmetric high posterior white matter signal in FLAIR image sequence.

vulnerable to injury during surgery. The frequency of unilateral diaphragmatic weakness due to phrenic nerve injury may reach 10% after cardiac surgery. Diaphragmatic weakness causes weakness of inspiration and atelectasis, and predisposes to postoperative respiratory complications, especially in the presence of pre-existing pulmonary disease. Most cases recover within months, but weakness may persist if there is significant axonal degeneration, as with nerve transection. Rare bilateral phrenic nerve palsy causes failure to wean from the ventilator.

Unilateral **recurrent laryngeal nerve** injury causes dysphonia; the left side is more often affected due to its longer intrathoracic course. Bilateral laryngeal palsy leads to severe stridor and aspiration. Several mechanisms can be suspected, from central venous catheterisation to traction along the nerve's intrathoracic course, for instance traction on the oesophagus, subclavian arteries, or on the heart. Other mononeuropathies have been described related to nerve compression or trauma during prolonged surgery, including ulnar, radial, long thoracic, spinal accessory, peroneal, lateral femoral cutaneous, and facial nerves. Most of these are related to typical nerve compression sites, and are seldom persistent.

Intensive care unit acquired weakness (ICU-AW) is a complication which was originally named critical illness polyneuropathy, but is now recognised to affect primarily muscle at least as often, causing an acute or subacute myopathy. The exact causation remains unclear, but ICU-AW is most often associated with prolonged ventilation, sepsis and use of steroids and muscle relaxants. Muscle biopsy findings are variable, with some cases showing only Type 2 fibre atrophy, which is an unspecific abnormality, others showing necrotising myopathy or acute myosin loss. The clue to diagnosis is a patient who after prolonged ventilation is tetraplegic, fails to wean, but has relatively preserved eye and often facial movements. Nerve conduction studies are often normal, electromyography may be myopathic but is often unspecific, and muscle biopsy may be needed for confirmation. Crucially, CNS pathology, including spinal cord damage, has to be conclusively excluded.

Guillain–Barré syndrome (GBS), an autoimmune acquired demyelinating neuropathy, may rarely occur after cardiac or other surgery. In the chronic postoperative phase GBS has been described as a consequence of CMV reactivation after cardiac transplantation or as a symptom of graft-versus-host disease. Neuropathy after transplantation can be caused by tacrolimus toxicity, or by other commonly used neurotoxic medications such as amiodarone.

Delayed Neurological Complications

Cognitive Decline after Cardiac Surgery

Immediate postoperative neuropsychological impairment in the absence of a structural defect is common but reversible over the course of the days following surgery. A more persistent cognitive impairment, however, wears off over weeks or months; it is considered comparable to cognitive problems after non-cardiac surgery, possibly due to brain injury at a cellular level. Better cognitive performance is seen at 3 months after CABG surgery performed off pump compared with patients undergoing bypass, with a risk of cognitive decline reduced from 29% to 21%, but the difference becomes insignificant after 12 months (30.8% versus 33.6%) and currently no surgical technique has been shown to be protective.

Delayed cognitive decline occurring over the 5 years after CABG surgery has been described by various authors. However, comparative studies have demonstrated a similar change in patients treated with angioplasty and no difference between neuropsychological performance in patients treated with bypass CABG and with off-pump CABG. Therefore, the theory that the delayed decline is causally linked to CABG surgery remains unproven, although it seems that cognitive decline may be linked to an accumulation of vascular risk factors, and to the patients' preoperative conditions. The best preventative measure is therefore meticulous attention to the control of vascular risk factors postoperatively, and no decline has been demonstrated where this was the case. Microembolic brain injuries have been implicated in the genesis of delayed Alzheimer dementia after cardiac surgery, but there is currently no evidence that patients who undergo cardiac surgery are really at increased risk for dementia or Alzheimer's disease, and the significance of microemboli is not yet established.

Complications Specific to Cardiac and Heart and Lung Transplantation

The survival rate today of modern cardiac transplantation is impressive, exceeding 80% at 1 year, 70% at 5 years and 50% at 10 years. Neurological complications constitute a significant proportion of mortality and postoperative morbidity; whether modifications of the transplantation procedure such as preoperative use of ventricular assist devices, or of combining heart and lung transplantation, have an impact on morbidity is still under investigation. Interestingly, an increasing number of patients undergo cardiac transplantation with a known genetic neuromuscular disease causing cardiomyopathy, but also limb muscle weakness, and the outcomes for these patients are apparently no worse than for patients without underlying neurological disease.

Patients accepted for cardiac transplantation are likely to have heart failure and a high risk of embolism prior to surgery, and some may have needed prolonged preoperative treatment with ventricular assist devices or ECMO, which themselves carry a substantial risk of cerebral embolism (Figure 46.3). Until

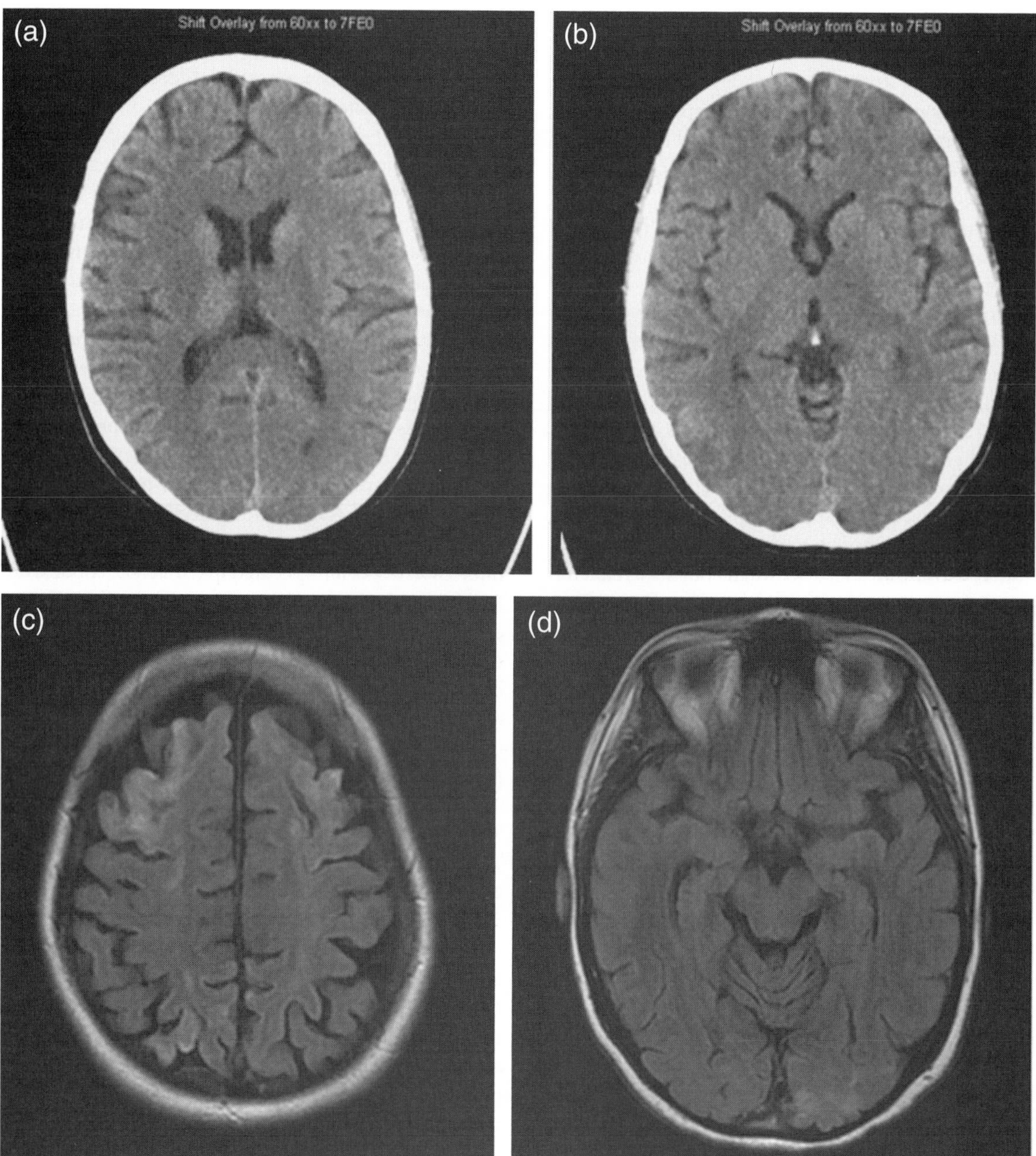

Figure 46.3 A 26 year old female after fulminant heart failure due to sarcoid cardiomyopathy, with emergency transfer under CPR for ECMO and ventricular assist device. Imaging took place after encephalopathy and agitation were noted. Initial CT shows a left basal ganglia infarct (a) and a right occipital cortical infarct (b). MRI shows both watershed infarcts (c) and a left occipital pole infarct (d). There was good functional recovery after cardiac transplant.

recently, the only treatment option for acute stroke was thrombolysis, unfeasible for patients who had just undergone heart surgery, but the situation may change with increasing availability of clot retrieval.

The early neurological complications related to transplantation surgery itself are similar to those found after other cardiac surgery, but they are more frequent. In one series, the frequency of perioperative

CNS complications in heart transplantation was 19.8% versus 3.1% in routine and 10.3% in emergency CABG surgery. The incidence varies widely between series. Perioperative neurological complications occurred in 23% in the Mayo Clinic series, and in other series early complications were even more frequent. Perioperative stroke occurs in up to 11%. Delirium and encephalopathy may occur in 10–20% of cases, including posterior reversible leucoencephalopathy.

Seizures are reported in 2% to 20% of patients, often as part of a generalised encephalopathy. Once embolic stroke has been excluded, the presumed aetiologies are rapid shifts of brain perfusion and drug effects, particularly of calcineurin inhibitors. As these patients are on multiple drugs, the possibility of unexpected interactions always needs to be considered. Levetiracetam is today the anticonvulsant of choice, due to its advantages of availability in intravenous preparation, lack of depression of conscious state and lack of enzyme induction or effects on cyclosporine, tacrolimus or warfarin levels. CSF studies are necessary in most cases, to exclude early onset of a CNS infection, although infections are more common beyond the immediate perioperative phase.

In this early period complications related to the peripheral nervous system are reported in between 4% and 11% of cases, and include both the nerve compression and nerve and plexus traction problems outlined earlier in this chapter, as well as immunological complications such as Guillain–Barré syndrome or early drug toxicity.

Later after transplantation, neurological complications include many conditions not seen in other types of cardiac surgery, broadening the spectrum of possible differential diagnoses, which emphasises the importance of early accurate identification. In the Mayo Clinic series reported by van den Beek and coworkers, the risk for neurological complications over a period of 18 years was 81%, including sleeping disorders in 32%, polyneuropathy in 26% and cumulative risk of stroke in 14%. The cause of death was neurological in 13%. Severe late complications are dominated by the effects of stroke and of problems related to immunosuppression, including direct side effects of immunosuppressive drugs, infection, transplant rejection, or post-transplantation lymphoproliferative disorder and other malignancies. Post-transplantation lymphoproliferative disorder (PCNS-PTLD) is an uncommon Epstein–Barr virus driven malignancy that may cause systemic uncontrolled B-cell proliferation affecting many organs, or primarily affecting the brain and central nervous system, according to a recent series, in 0.18% of heart and/or lung transplant recipients. It may regress with reduction of immunosuppressive treatment, or may require radiotherapy or chemotherapy.

Pharmacological side effects of immunosuppressive drugs are dominated by the effects of calcineurin inhibitors, and today in the first line by tacrolimus related side effects. These can be both direct toxic effects as well as immune reactions triggered by tacrolimus. Calcineurin toxicity affects both the CNS with tremor in early stages, and in more severe cases seizures, encephalopathy, cortical blindness and psychosis. Patients may have very variable MRI findings of the brain, and commonly posterior reversible encephalopathy syndrome (PRES) and vasogenic oedema, but imaging may be completely normal despite CNS symptoms. Calcineurin inhibitor toxicity may also affect the PNS, causing demyelinating neuropathy or inflammatory myopathy. Toxicity is not always closely related to the tacrolimus levels, but generally improves when the dose is reduced. Combination with other immunosuppressants (steroids, mycophenolate, sirolimus) may be helpful to minimise the dose, but newer immunosuppressants can demonstrate similar side effects. OKT3, another less frequently used immunosuppressant, has been seen to cause aseptic meningitis.

Infections of the CNS after cardiac transplantation occur in 2–3% of patients of recent larger series including some 600 patients, with a broad range of potential infectious agents; the incidence of any specific agent is too low to narrow the range of differential diagnoses. *Aspergillus* species, *Cryptococcus neoformans*, *Listeria monocytogenes*, *Herpes zoster* and JC virus occurred more than once. *Aspergillus* is a particular diagnostic concern. Other infectious agents that have been described include *Streptococcus pneumoniae*, West Nile Virus, HHV6, *Toxoplasma gondii*, *Nocardia* species, *Candida* species, *Cryptococcus*, *Balamuthia mandrillaris*, *Bipolaris spicifera*, *Tuberculosis*, *Acanthamoeba*, *Scedosporium* and syphilis. 'Acute flaccid paralysis' due to West Nile Virus has not been described after cardiac transplantation, but clearly, due to increasing prevalence, it needs to be included in the differential diagnosis of neuromuscular weakness.

Prevention and Risk Assessment in Cardiac Surgery

The best strategy to prevent neurological complications in cardiac surgery remains management of risk factors and thorough assessment of the patient's risk profile. The risk of stroke increases with age, reaching 5% in patients over 80, although results have improved in newer studies. Other characteristics elevating a patient's risk profile for stroke and neurological complications are the presence of hypertension, diabetes mellitus, smoking, a history of cerebrovascular disease, peripheral vascular disease and aortic atheroma, and the type of surgery required. Intraoperative factors associated with increased risk can be duration of the cardiopulmonary bypass and its haemodynamic performance. A postoperative risk factor for stroke is the presence of atrial fibrillation.

The 2011 ACC/AHA guidelines include recommendations on prevention of neurological complications. A number of potential strategies are aimed at reducing complications related to cardiopulmonary bypass. Shann et al. recommend the following evidence-based strategies:

1. Reducing emboli through arterial filtration, intraoperative aortic imaging, minimising direct reinfusion of pericardial suction blood, filtration of suction blood before reinfusion;
2. Minimising the prothrombotic response through reducing blood contact with non-biocompatible surfaces in CPB;
3. Ensuring perioperative normoglycaemia and avoidance of hyperglycaemia;
4. Avoiding low haematocrit and excessive haemodilution;
5. Managing rewarming rate and limiting arterial line temperature to 37 °C during rewarming;
6. Optimising metabolic management (pH stat versus alpha stat management remains a matter of controversy).

The ACC/AHA guidelines for CABG recommend perioperative administration of a beta-blocker drug to reduce the risk of atrial fibrillation, as well as perioperative statins and aspirin. Epiaortic ultrasound is advised to identify atherosclerosis of the aorta, and to enable measures to be taken that might help avoid embolism, such as choice of off-pump. Simultaneous carotid endarterectomy is recommended with CABG for symptomatic high grade (70–99%) internal carotid stenosis, because it can reduce the risk of embolism and stroke. The benefit of simultaneous CABG and CEA is not established in asymptomatic high grade stenosis, but the ACC/AHA guidelines and other authors suggest simultaneous endarterectomy and CABG in patients with high grade stenosis on one side, and severe stenosis or occlusion on the other.

How to Deal with the Patient Who Fails To Awaken?

Failure to awaken after cardiac surgery is a worrying neurological scenario encountered in the early postoperative phase, and may signify anything from transient encephalopathy to a catastrophic focal event. Patients may be systemically severely unwell, and ongoing procedures such as ECMO and pacing wires may limit the feasibility of standard neurological investigations. On the other hand, new treatment options such as clot retrieval increase the potential benefit of accurate early diagnosis.

In the comatose patient, diagnostic evaluation includes bedside clinical assessment, specialist review, appropriate use of neuromonitoring and neurophysiological techniques and timely choice of imaging. Any test is only as good as its availability at the right time, and a multimodal approach builds on good clinical evaluation.

Clinical assessment is primarily performed by the intensive care doctors and nursing staff, and their first responsibility is to recognise there is a potential neurological problem as early as possible, whether or not they have specialist neurological expertise. Standardised clinical scores are helpful, as long as their limitations are recognised and interpretation is consistent. The Glasgow Coma Score (GCS) is the most widespread tool, but it has significant limitations such as having inadequate validation in non-trauma patient groups, including largely irrelevant criteria such as the verbal response, and providing inadequate information on brain stem function or focal deficits. The clinical evaluation must reliably check for focal dysfunction and brain stem abnormalities, as either is unusual in generalised encephalopathy. The Full Outline of UnResponsiveness (FOUR) score provides better neurological information and in the author's experience more validity in serial examination. Performance in neurological scores informs a more comprehensive assessment by the neurocritical care specialist, as early as possible. This should ideally set the priorities for imaging and electrophysiological tests.

Neurophysiological investigations extend the clinical assessment; they are tailored to the clinical situation and are best done after clinical review. EEG is the only method to diagnose non-convulsive seizures. Routine bedside neuromonitoring promises to provide continuous assessment of brain function, but is still in its infancy. Continuous electroencephalography (CEEG) allows real time detection of seizures, and may alert to worsening encephalopathy or (less well) to evolving large focal lesions. It is gaining use in neurocritical care units, but the amount of data generated is difficult to handle, requiring experienced personnel with specialist knowledge and significant time. EEG trending with specialised analysis software may help overcome the problem but still requires 'raw' EEG for interpretation. Telemedicine-based EEG services today enable competent EEG assessment even in remote hospitals. Simplified EEG-based monitoring systems have not proved their value and are handicapped by the lack of spatial resolution offered by 2 to 4 channels. Somatosensory evoked potentials (SSEPs) are used intraoperatively, and in addition the evolution of serial SSEPs after hypoxia gives robust prognostic information. Monitoring of brain perfusion and oxygenation based on transcranial Doppler ultrasound and near infrared spectroscopy (NIRS) is under development, but their clinical value is not yet clear.

Neuroimaging is indicated if either clinical or neuromonitoring data suggest a focal or evolving lesion, as well as in persistent reduced conscious levels. Computerised tomography (CT) is rapid and sensitive in detecting haemorrhage and supratentorial stroke, and feasible in the presence of metal implants and electronic devices. Mobile bedside CT scanners allow imaging in the ICU. CT angiography is rapid and has largely superceded diagnostic catheter angiography, and CT perfusion studies can detect vasospasm. Magnetic resonance imaging (MRI) has exquisite sensitivity in the brain stem and cervical spinal cord, which are largely inaccessible to CT, but it is more cumbersome, slower and is not suitable for unstable patients undergoing ECMO. With the exception of magnetic material implants, however, most disadvantages can be overcome through using modern imaging sequences and some specialised equipment. MRI is much more sensitive for white matter lesions, and has much more capability to date lesion onset and provide biochemical and functional imaging than CT.

Conclusion

Cardiosurgical neurology is a unique field in which good cooperation between cardiac surgeons, cardiac intensivists and intensive care neurologists is significantly improving clinical outcomes. We now have powerful diagnostic tools applicable to the perioperative situation. There are still major obstacles to overcome, including improving neurological training in the CT ICU, improving neurologists' understanding of a complex field extending far beyond conventional neurology, and in making sophisticated neurological investigations available in a challenging environment within a very tight time frame. Currently, the capabilities of technology are still limited by personnel and training constraints, but the clear benefits they offer are rapidly driving change.

Learning Points

- Neurological complications are major determinants of outcome after cardiac surgery.
- Risk assessment prior to surgery takes into account age, cerebrovascular risk factors and comorbidity, type of surgery, and a detailed neurological assessment to identify patients at higher risk of neurological complications.
- The postoperative neurological assessment must screen for focal neurological deficits in order to diagnose vascular deficits early, in time to consider revascularisation in the brain.
- Focal neurological deficits in a patient with postoperative encephalopathy suggest a structural abnormality rather than drug effects of generalised hypoxia, and necessitate urgent brain imaging.
- A fluctuating impairment of the level of consciousness may suggest non-convulsive status epilepticus even if abnormal movements or stereotypies are absent.
- EEG is mandatory to diagnose and adequately treat status epilepticus.
- Lower brachial plexus injuries are the commonest mechanical peripheral nerve injuries after sternal retraction in cardiac surgery. Peripheral nerve injuries need to be clinically differentiated from complications related to the central nervous

system, as neurophysiological tests are often unrevealing in the acute phase.

- Calcineurin inhibitor (tacrolimus, cyclosporin A) toxicity can cause multiple peripheral and central neurological symptoms. Toxicity does not closely correlate with the individual's blood levels, but improves with dose reduction.
- The 2011 AHA/ACC guidelines recommend strategies to reduce the risk of neurological complications.

Further Reading

Al-Mufti F, Bauerschmidt A, Claassen J, et al. Neuroendovascular interventions for acute ischemic strokes in patients supported with left ventricular assist devices: a single-center case series and review of the literature. *World Neurosurgery*. 2016; 88: 199–204.

Hillis ID, Smith PK, Anderson J, et al. 2011 ACCF/AHA Guideline for coronary artery bypass graft surgery. *Circulation*. 2011; 124: e652–e735.

Mateen F, van den Beek D, Kremer WK, et al. Neuromuscular diseases after cardiac transplantation. *Journal of Heart and Lung Transplantation*. 2009; 28: 226.

Muñoz P, Valerio M, Palomo J, et al. Infectious and non-infectious neurologic complications in heart transplant recipients. *Medicine (Baltimore)*. 2010; 89(3): 166–175.

Pawliszak W, Kowalewski M, Raffa GM, et al. Cerebrovascular events after no-touch off-pump coronary artery bypass grafting, conventional side-clamp off-pump coronary artery bypass, and proximal anastomotic devices: a meta-analysis. *Journal of the American Heart Association*. 2016; 5: e002802.

Salazar JD, Wityk RJ, Grega MA, et al. Stroke after cardiac surgery: short- and long-term outcomes. *Annals of Thoracic Surgery*. 2001; 72: 1195–1201.

Shann KG, Likosky DS, Murkin JM, et al. An evidence-based review of the practice of cardiopulmonary bypass in adults: a focus on neurologic injury, glycemic control, hemodilution, and the inflammatory response. *Journal of Thoracic and Cardiovascular Surgery*. 2006; 132: 283–290.

van de Beek D, Kremers W, Daly RC, et al. Effect of neurologic complications on outcome after heart transplant. *Archives of Neurology*. 2008; 65: 226–231.

van de Beek D, Patel R, Daly RC, et al. Central nervous system infections in heart transplant recipients. *Archives of Neurology*. 2007; 64: 1715–1720.

Wijdicks EF, Bamlet WR, Maramattom BV, Manno EM, McClelland RL. Validation of a new coma scale: the FOUR score. *Annals of Neurology*. 2005; 58: 585–593.

MCQs

1. **The following factors are important for assessing the risk of neurological complications:**
   (a) Patient age
   (b) Premorbidity
   (c) In valvular surgery, which valve is to be replaced
   (d) Duration of cardiopulmonary bypass
   (e) Positioning for surgery
   (f) All of the above

2. **Which of the following is NOT associated with neurological problems and worse 1 year outcome after cardiac transplantation?**
   (a) Surgery performed in poor clinical status
   (b) Presence or absence of a pre-existing neuromuscular disorder
   (c) Choice of immunosuppressive agent
   (d) Duration of cardiopulmonary bypass
   (e) Need for ECMO or VADs

3. **Which following statement applying to postoperative epileptic seizures is accurate?**
   (a) EEG is seldom needed to identify the presence of epileptic seizures even with good clinical assessment
   (b) A neurologist can reliably exclude epileptic seizures on clinical grounds
   (c) EEG requires the neurophysiology laboratory and has little value in the ICU
   (d) A prolonged EEG has much higher value in identifying non-convulsive status epilepticus than a routine EEG
   (e) Phenytoin levels are needed to prove efficacy of anticonvulsant treatment

4. **Which of the following statements applies?**
   (a) Early diagnosis of postoperative stroke is important for prognostic reasons only
   (b) Patients cannot be thrombolised after major surgery, so early treatment is not available
   (c) Dysconjugate eye movements reliably indicate injury to the brain stem
   (d) A normal CT scan rules out significant hypoxic brain injury

Exercise answers are available on p.469. Alternatively, take the test online at www.cambridge.org/CardiothoracicMCQ

Chapter 47

Postoperative Delirium

Makeida B Koyi, Joseph G Hobelmann and Karin J Neufeld

Introduction

Delirium is a psychiatric syndrome produced by an underlying medical aetiology and it is a common complication in the postsurgical setting. It can be difficult to detect and is frequently missed by clinicians. It is important to recognise and prevent delirium, given its association with serious and costly negative outcomes. It is characterised by disturbances of awareness, attention and cognition including perception, thinking, memory, language and orientation. Psychomotor behaviour, emotion and sleep–wake cycle are also observed disturbances in delirium. Often abrupt in onset, delirium tends to fluctuate throughout the day and is variable in severity and duration. It can last from hours to days, and less commonly for weeks to months.

Negative clinical consequences associated with postoperative delirium include prolonged hospitalisation, loss of functional independence, reduced cognitive function, incomplete recovery, delayed rehabilitation and death. The duration of delirium in the intensive care unit setting is correlated with an increased cognitive impairment in ICU survivors, followed as outpatients up to 1 year after discharge. Delirium can also be associated with significant distress in patients and is frightening for family members who stand by and watch the pronounced and often perplexing changes in the behaviour of a loved one. In patients who undergo cardiac surgery, delirium is associated with postoperative complications including respiratory insufficiency and sternum instability. In the USA, the health care costs due to all episodes of delirium in hospitalised patients range from $38 to $153 billion annually, and among older hospitalised medical patients it has been shown to be preventable in up to 40% of cases.

Delirious patients are frequently overlooked or misdiagnosed and prevention strategies are not yet a part of routine care in most surgical units. The growing body of literature demonstrating the negative short-term and long-term impacts associated with delirium highlights the need to improve recognition, treatment and prevention of this syndrome. After describing the epidemiology, this chapter will review prevention strategies, and discuss detection and treatment of postoperative delirium in adult patients.

Delirium Epidemiology

Core Features of Delirium

Delirium presents as a sudden change in ability to think, resulting in faulty attention. Common findings in delirium include:

- Inability to attend and concentrate resulting in disrupted short-term recall and disorientation to time and place;
- Change in word finding ability and language usage – talk may seem confused and difficult to follow;
- Disrupted visuospatial abilities – clock drawing or copying interlocking pentagons;
- Changes in emotional tone – uncharacteristic mood lability and disinhibition;
- Change in level of arousal/sleep–wake cycle;
- Perceptual changes including hallucinations (usually visual);
- Unusual beliefs, which are often frightening and not uncommonly include misinterpreting the intensions of the medical staff.

A recognised feature of delirium is that the symptoms can fluctuate in severity throughout the day and night.

Delirium Subtypes

Three subtypes of delirium are distinguished by varying levels of psychomotor activity: hyperactive, hypoactive and mixed type.

The hyperactive subtype is associated with:

- Restlessness, psychomotor agitation and seemingly purposeless movement;
- Aggression on the part of the patient, often arising from fearfulness and misinterpretation of the intentions of the staff and/or disorientation to surroundings;
- Easy recognition that something is wrong with the patient;
- Agitated behaviour that may be misattributed to a primary psychiatric disturbance;
- Alcohol and benzodiazepine withdrawal states can be the underlying aetiology;
- Among trauma and surgical patients pure hyperactivity is rare compared to mixed or hypoactive subtypes, making up about 1% of delirium presentations.

The hypoactive subtype is associated with the following:

- Psychomotor slowing and somnolence – often misattributed to depression;
- Can be difficult to recognise – patients with hypoactive delirium do not demand much attention from staff;
- Easy to miss the cognitive changes with superficial interactions –such as asking patients only 'yes/no' questions;
- Generally associated with worse outcomes and more long-term cognitive effects;
- Most prevalent subtype (~88%) in surgical and trauma patients.

The mixed subtype is associated with the following:

- Alternating states of hypoactivity and agitation;
- Possibly resulting from the administration of sedating medications to a hyperactive delirious patient;
- About 11% of delirium presentations in surgical and trauma patients.

Incidence and Prevalence

Delirium is prevalent in all hospital settings and in the postoperative course ranges from 5 to 50% depending on the comorbidity and type of surgery. The incidence of delirium for the following surgeries is reported as:

- Hip fracture (35–65%);
- Coronary artery bypass grafting (37–52%);
- Peripheral vascular surgery (30–48%);
- Infrarenal abdominal aortic aneurysm repair (33–54%).

The risk of delirium increases with the degree of medical urgency. Emergency surgery is associated with much more delirium (both prior to and after surgery) compared with elective and outpatient surgeries. The highest risk ratings on the American Society Anesthesiology (ASA) scoring system are associated with a higher risk of postoperative delirium.

Risk Factors

The development of delirium is usually multifactorial involving the interaction of a vulnerable patient with one or more perioperative insults. However, delirium can develop in a young healthy patient if the insult is significant enough. Prediction models have been developed in both cardiac and non-cardiac surgery to help identify those patients most at risk for postoperative delirium.

The most important factors include:

- Advanced age; and
- Baseline cognitive impairment.

Other additional factors include:

- Impaired physical function;
- Preoperative depressive symptoms;
- Preoperative stroke or transient ischaemic attacks;
- Abnormal laboratory values such as low albumin;
- History of alcohol and other substance abuse;
- Invasiveness and length of the surgery.

Other predisposing factors, such as atrial fibrillation and peripheral vascular disease, and precipitating factors, such as transfusion of aged red blood cells and the use of an intra-aortic balloon pump (IAPB), have been described in other observational studies. Risk factors for the development of delirium can be divided into predisposing and precipitating, and are presented in a timeline related to surgical course in Figure 47.1.

Aetiological Mechanisms

Although the pathophysiology is not yet understood, neuroinflammation and neurotransmitter dysregulation have been implicated as possible mechanisms involved in delirium. More specifically, impaired cerebral oxidative metabolism resulting in increases

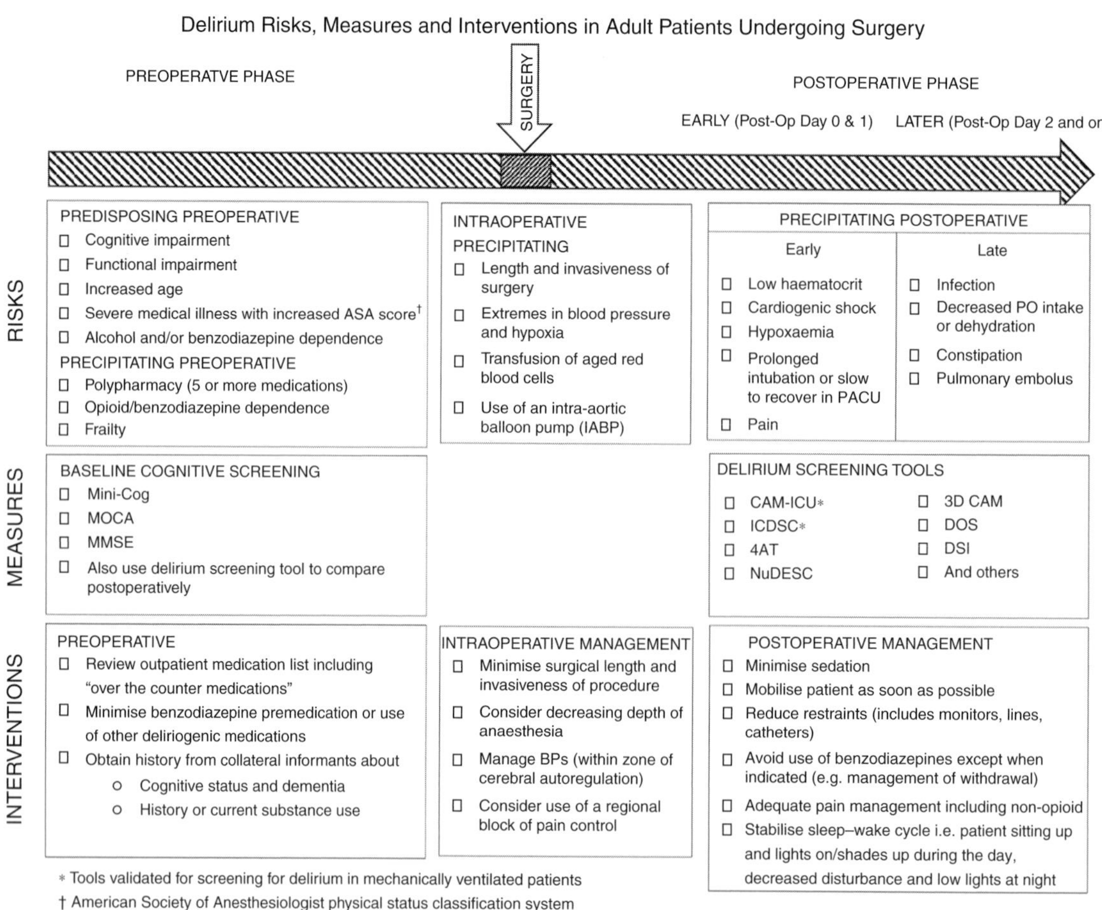

Figure 47.1 Delirium risks, measures and interventions in adult patients undergoing surgery.

in dopaminergic, noradrenergic, and glutamatergic activity and decreases in cholinergic activity in response to stress and inflammation of surgical procedures have been hypothesised to contribute to delirium.

Postoperative Delirium Prevention Strategies

Preoperative Cognitive and Functional Status Screening

Given that pre-existing cognitive impairment is the most common independent risk factor across studies, assessing for baseline cognitive impairment is beneficial for two reasons:

- It identifies those patients at highest risk for the development of delirium.
- It documents a baseline to which postoperative performance can be compared, aiding in the detection of delirium.

Standardised screening tests are the most efficient way to test cognition. Many brief tests are available. Casual conversation with a patient is not sufficient to assess for preoperative cognitive deficits. The American College of Surgeons' National Surgical Quality Improvement Program suggests using the Mini-Cog as a cognitive screen of the preoperative geriatric surgical patient to establish a cognitive baseline and identify high risk patients. Other tools can also be used and are listed in Table 47.1. Preoperative functional status is also an independent risk factor for the development of delirium. Assessing the functional status of a patient by using a screening tool assessing activities of daily living and frailty can provide risk stratification for delirium and can also provide information about the expected course of recovery postoperatively.

Table 47.1 Screening tools for non-intubated patients

Cognitive screening tools	Delirium screening tools
Abbreviated Mental Test (AMT) includes 10-item, 6-item and 4-item versions	4AT www.the4at.com 3D Confusion Assessment Method (CAM)
Clinical Dementia Rating (CDR)	Bedside Confusion Scale
Clock drawing test	Clinical Assessment of Confusion (CAC)
Days of the week backwards	Confusion Assessment Method (CAM), short form
Digit cancellation test	Confusion Assessment Method-ICU version (CAM-ICU)*
Digit span – forward and backward	Confusion Rating Scale (CRS)
Mini-Cog	Delirium Observation Screening (DOS)
Months of the year backward	Delirium Symptom Interview (DSI)
Montreal Cognitive Assessment (MOCA)	Intensive Care Delirium Screening Checklist (ICDSC)*
Trailmaking Test A	Nursing Delirium Screening Scale (Nu-DESC)
Trailmaking Test B	Single Question in Delirium (SQiD)

*Tools best used for mechanically ventilated, critically ill patients.
Adapted from AGS 2014.

Preoperative Screening for Comorbid Disease and Substance Use

Abnormal laboratory values, including glucose, sodium, potassium and albumin, which represent underlying disease or organ system dysfunction, are risk factors for delirium:

- Hypoalbuminaemia appears to be of particular importance due to its association with fluid management, drug binding and malnutrition;
- A blood urea nitrogen (BUN) to creatinine ratio of greater than or equal to 18 (index of dehydration).

Delirium is associated with preoperative alcohol, benzodiazepine and other substance abuse such as opioids, and prior stroke or transient ischaemic attack. In general, collection of historical information from the patient or collateral informant is sufficient and routine cerebral imaging is not required for complete assessment of delirium risk.

Depression has been identified as a risk factor for postoperative delirium in several studies and has been associated with incomplete recovery to independent functioning after surgery. The pathophysiology of this relationship has not been determined. There are many available tools that can be used to screen for depression. Assessment of depression may also help predict the patient's motivation for recovery and can help in postoperative planning.

Perioperative Interventions

In addition to baseline patient vulnerability, perioperative insults contribute to the development of delirium and several interventions to reduce the risk have been described. These include pharmacological as well as procedural interventions. A recent meta-analysis indicated that several interventions might reduce postoperative delirium.

- Light sedation versus deep sedation may reduce the prevalence of postoperative delirium, particularly in patients receiving spinal anaesthesia for hip replacements.
- Although deeper levels of sedation are associated with increased delirium, use of an electroencephalographic (EEG) monitor to measure depth of sedation is not yet routinely recommended.
- Type of general anaesthetic agent does not appear to affect the development of delirium but administering additional ketamine during anaesthesia induction may result in less postoperative delirium.
- Regional anaesthesia, specifically femoral block and fascia iliaca block, for lower extremity procedures has been shown to reduce postoperative delirium in the elderly.
- Additional areas of inquiry for delirium reduction and improved postoperative outcomes in cardiac surgery include personalised management

of blood pressure within the zone of cerebral autoregulation, as predicted through near infrared spectroscopy (NIRS) and Doppler monitoring.

Postoperative Interventions

Medications probably contribute to the complex pathophysiology of delirium through opioid and gamma-aminobutyric acid (GABA) receptor agonism. Moderate quality evidence suggests that opioid medication use is associated with delirium in medical and surgical patients. It is important to weigh the risks of opioid use with the benefits of treating acute severe pain, particularly since uncontrolled pain is also cited as a risk factor for delirium. It is best to use the lowest effective dose for pain control.

Evidence also suggests that benzodiazepine medication use increases delirium in a mixed surgical group of patients. This was demonstrated with higher doses of benzodiazepines over a 24 hour period and with longer acting agents. Studies investigating the risk of delirium with antihistamine medications such as diphenhydramine noted a trend toward increased delirium as well.

Adequate postoperative analgesia has been associated with decreased delirium incidence. Increased levels of pain in the postoperative period have been independently associated with the development of delirium. Non-opioid medications should be considered when possible: gabapentin and non-steroidal anti-inflammatory drugs are associated in some studies with reduced incidence and severity of postoperative delirium.

Preoperative and postoperative sedation regimens may have an impact on incidence of delirium. Significantly longer time to recovery in the PACU with more cognitive dysfunction following anaesthesia has been demonstrated in 1062 patients less than 70 years of age, receiving a premedication of lorazepam (2.5 mg) compared to placebo. This suggests that such premedication is best avoided in older more vulnerable patients. Dexmedetomidine has been shown in some studies to be more effective than other sedatives (benzodiazepines and propofol) in preventing postoperative delirium, but the results have been mixed. Benzodiazepine use is independently associated with delirium in the cardiac ICU and the Society for Critical Care Medicine (SCCM) Guidelines suggest that sedation reduction and discontinuation should be the goal for the management of the critically ill patient.

Some studies suggest that the prophylactic use of typical and atypical antipsychotics can reduce postoperative delirium; however the trials have been small, heterogeneous and of variable quality. At least one study bears replication in larger trials: a randomised controlled trial of on-pump cardiac surgery patients with subsyndromal delirium upon immediate recovery following surgery, treated with risperidone versus placebo, demonstrated a significant decrease in incident postoperative delirium. While there is more research to be done, the recommendations arising from a recent meta-analysis suggest that there is no clear evidence for routine prophylactic use of antipsychotics for delirium prevention at this time.

Several other interventions have not demonstrated a reduction in the prevalence or duration of postoperative delirium. These include:

- Intraoperative controlled hypotension;
- Neuraxial versus general anaesthesia;
- Long acting morphine postoperatively;
- Postoperative sedation using alpha-2 adrenoreceptor;
- Use of acetylcholinesterase inhibitors;
- Use of anticonvulsants;
- Use of histamine (H2) blockers.

General Non-pharmacological Interventions

Up to one third of cases of delirium have been shown to be preventable among medically hospitalised elderly patients through a bundled approach of non-pharmacological interventions. The bundle consists of the following:

- Enhancing the patient's ability to see and hear with the use of glasses and hearing aids;
- Encouraging increased mobility including ambulating at least twice per day;
- Pain control with non-narcotic agents;
- Cognitive stimulation through interaction and games and activities;
- Regular re-orientation through calendars and verbal interaction with the patient;
- Sleep enhancement (i.e. non-pharmacological sleep protocol and sleep hygiene);
- Nutrition and fluid repletion;

- Appropriate medication usage;
- Adequate oxygenation;
- Prevention of constipation.

Medications may be the sole precipitant in up to 39% of all cases of delirium. The risk of postoperative delirium increases significantly with polypharmacy (defined as the use of five or more medications at the same time). Anticholinergics, sedatives-hypnotics and meperidine contribute to postoperative delirium. For example, ranitidine and famotidine, histamine (H2) antagonists, are commonly used postoperatively for stress ulcer prophylaxis. Due to anticholinergic activity these agents may have an increased delirium risk compared to proton pump inhibitors (PPI) and consideration should be given to using the latter. Similarly benzodiazepines and antihistamines should not be prescribed routinely for sleep in high risk patients; however if benzodiazepines are part of the patient's longstanding medical regimen prior to surgery, it would be best to continue these as an inpatient given the likelihood of physiological dependence.

Screening for Detection of Delirium

American Geriatrics Society (AGS) and SCCM guidelines recommend screening all patients for the presence of delirium daily in the ICU setting in an effort to initiate delirium treatment as early as possible; daily postoperative screening for older patients at high risk for developing delirium is advised and should be conducted by a health care professional trained in the assessment of delirium using a validated delirium screening instrument. Two validated bedside screening tools with good sensitivity and adapted specificity for critically ill mechanically ventilated patients are:

- The Confusion Assessment Method for the ICU (CAM-ICU);
- Intensive Care Delirium Screening Checklist (ICDSC).

Screening for delirium should begin as soon as the patient is recovered from anaesthesia in the PACU, or is stabilised in the intensive care unit. Following general anaesthesia nearly one half of patients, considered stable for transfer, were found to be delirious when assessed by a psychiatrist or research nurse; of these patients, one half were still delirious on the next postoperative day. Once extubated and on the regular inpatient postsurgical services, screening for delirium is indicated at least among high risk patients (over the age of 65 years, history of cognitive impairment or brain injury). See Table 47.1 for a list of delirium screening tools that have been used on inpatient units in non-intubated patients.

The Richmond Agitation Sedation Scale (RASS) or other scales that document arousal may prove to be a very good way of screening for delirium. In a study using the RASS in 2000 elderly hospitalised patients, any rating other than that described as 'awake and alert' was an independent predictor of adverse clinical outcomes resulting in longer hospitalisations and discharge to a skilled nursing facility. The 'sleepy' patient may be the first clue to a sick patient.

Diagnosis

Getting a History

The diagnosis of delirium is based upon a complete medical evaluation, consisting of a thorough history and examination. Collateral informants often provide the best information regarding the onset, fluctuation and duration of a patient's symptoms. Family members are able to describe how a patient's current presentation differs from the presurgical baseline. Information from nurses, rehabilitation therapists and other clinical staff can be helpful given their time spent interacting with the patient. Patients who are initially cooperative with the plan and recommendations of the treatment team but who postoperatively present with decreased participation or refusal may be exhibiting one of the first signs of delirium. Altered social behaviour is a common, early presentation and it is often misconstrued as a symptom of a primary psychiatric illness. The patient's mood may be labile, or quickly changing, and can be accompanied with symptoms of apathy, anxiety, paranoia, fear, anger, irritability or even rarely, euphoria. Differentiating between symptoms of delirium and an exacerbation of a primary psychiatric illness can be difficult; however, delirium is most likely if the symptoms in question are abrupt in onset, fluctuate in severity over a 24 hour period and were not present prior to the surgery. A high index of suspicion is required to detect delirium as it is easily missed. Other prodromal symptoms of delirium include:

- Insomnia;
- Vivid nightmares or dreams;
- Hypersensitivity to sounds or light;
- Anxiety;

- Irritability or restlessness;
- Distractibility;
- 'A subjective sense of difficulty in marshalling one's thoughts.'

Examining the Patient

Testing of cognition is central to examination of the patient and comparison of performance to presurgical baseline will help make the diagnosis. The central cognitive deficit in the syndrome of delirium includes difficulty in sustaining and shifting attention. Test for attention by asking the patient to try the following:

- Saying the months of the year in reverse order (Pass is getting 7 months in a row without redirection or hints from the examiner);
- Saying the days of the week backwards correctly;
- Spelling the word 'world' or the patient's name backward;
- Counting backwards from 100.

In speaking with the delirious patient, one may note:

- Difficulty maintaining a conversation or following commands;
- Disorganised thinking – rambling and irrelevant conversation or incoherent speech;
- Fleeting illusions (misinterpreting a stimulus);
- Hallucinations (perception without a stimulus).

Altered perception is reported by up to 30% of patients and can be frightening. As described with the delirium subtypes, altered physical function may be displayed with marked agitation, restlessness or vigilance in hyperactive delirium or marked lethargy, decreased mobility, reduced movement or reduced appetite in hypoactive delirium.

Particular attention should be paid to the neurological examination, observing any abnormal movements with the presence of tremor suggesting a possible aetiology such as alcohol or benzodiazepine withdrawal, or serotonin syndrome. Asterixis may signal hepatic or renal failure resulting in metabolic derangements, and a focal neurological exam may suggest the presence of a stroke or TIA. Every effort should be made to mobilise the patient and examine truncal stability and gait. Thiamine deficiency resulting in Wernicke's syndrome rarely presents with the complete triad of ophthalmoplegia, gait instability and delirium, and so repletion of high dose intravenous thiamine should be readily implemented in a patient vulnerable to deficiency (i.e. malnutrition and recent heavy alcohol use or absorption defects).

General physical exam should focus on identifying any sources of infection such as respiratory, digestive and urinary tract, and should include examination of the oral cavity for dental infections and abscesses and pressure sores/ulcers on the skin. Severity and localisation of any complaints of pain may also be important clues to understanding the cause of delirium.

Clinical Investigations, Review of Records and Consultations

Medical record and medication administration review can point to a cause of delirium. Nursing notes may reveal changes in a patient's behaviour over the course of a few days suggestive of an incipient delirium. Noting the timing of a patient's onset of symptoms in relation to the initiation of a new medication or the sudden discontinuation of home medications (such as prescribed benzodiazepines) can point to a possible aetiology. Any history of substance abuse, or the regular use of alcohol or sedative hypnotics, should be noted.

In addition to reviewing the vital signs, including pulse oximetry as part of the physical examination, routine investigations should include:

- Urinalysis and toxicology;
- Full blood count;
- Metabolic panel including renal profile;
- Liver function tests including ammonia.

Depending on the findings of the history and examination, additional laboratory tests include thyroid function tests, cortisol, and B12, folate, syphilis serology, ANA, HIV, heavy metal screen, urine porphyrins and paraneoplastic antibodies such as anti-Hu, anti-Ma and anti-Ta. If CNS aetiology is suspected or neurological focal exam is demonstrated, CT/MRI of the head and lumbar puncture are indicated. An EEG is an important study to consider especially if one's differential includes delirium, non-convulsive seizures or delirium due to alcohol withdrawal. An EEG of a delirious patient due to systemic illness or metabolic disturbance will generally show diffuse abnormality with slowed background rhythms over the occiput. This is in contrast to the EEG of a patient who is delirious from alcohol withdrawal as that EEG is either normal or might show fast dysrhythmia or occasional seizure discharges. The EEG of a patient with non-convulsive status epilepticus will be diagnostic with evidence of seizure discharges throughout.

Finally, a consult from an expert in delirium such as a psychiatrist, geriatrician or neurologist may help determine the cause of the delirium and differentiate the symptoms of delirium from those of a primary psychiatric disorder. Symptoms found in hyperactive, hypoactive and mixed delirium can mimic symptoms seen in schizophrenia, depression or bipolar disorder. Providers should be wary of attributing any new onset psychiatric symptoms or new psychiatric diagnosis to an actively delirious patient in the postoperative setting.

Treatment

The most important approach to treatment of delirium lies in detecting and correcting the underlying aetiology. The management of the behavioural agitation that accompanies hyperactive and mixed delirium is often difficult. There is insufficient evidence for the prophylactic use of antipsychotics such as haloperidol in preventing or decreasing delirium severity once it occurs. AGS guidelines suggest that benzodiazepines should not be used in the management of agitation except if specifically indicated (i.e. substance withdrawal or serotonin syndrome) and that the lowest doses of either a typical or atypical antipsychotic should be used only if the patient is at significant risk of harming themselves or others or is distressed by hallucinations and delusions. One of the harms of antipsychotic prescribing in the course of a delirium is that patients are given these medications indefinitely. Long-term use of antipsychotics can result in CNS effects such as extrapyramidal symptoms and tardive dyskinaesia, cardiac abnormalities such as prolongation of the QTc interval with increased risk of Torsade de Pointes, and stroke and premature death especially in the cognitively impaired geriatric population. These agents should be used sparingly and on an as needed basis and discontinued at the earliest opportunity.

Multicomponent non-pharmacological interventions have proven highly effective in decreasing the occurrence of delirium and should be employed in delirious patients as well.

- Early mobilisation of the patient with the supervision of medical staff or family is one of the most helpful non-pharmacological measures and results in a shorter duration of delirium and better functional outcomes at hospital discharge.
- In patients unable to walk, physical therapy or occupational therapy should be engaged to carry out an active range of motion exercises or exercises to be done in bed.
- Getting an agitated patient out of bed and helping them walk around the unit, or to use the toilet, can be a successful way to calm them and avoid the use of sedative or antipsychotic medication.
- Protecting, improving or restoring the patient's sleep–wake cycle by keeping the patient upright in a quiet, well-lit room during the day, and a dimmed light and low stimulation environment at night, is best.
- Delirious patients may misinterpret sensory stimuli and incorporate them into symptoms of delirium such as fear, anxiety and delusions. It is best to decrease unnecessary stimuli such as the TV, unless the patient specifically requests to watch it.
- Ensure that the patient has eyeglasses and hearing aids. Examine for and remove earwax to help improve hearing.
- Reorient the patient regularly and provide accurate and updated wall clocks and calendars.
- Patients benefit from family or care provider visits and having family members in the room at night can provide significant reassurance to a distressed, disoriented person. A bedside sitter may be needed when no family is present, especially for delirious patients with agitation, as this patient will need frequent redirection.

Learning Points

- Delirium is a clinical syndrome with disturbances in awareness, attention, cognition, psychomotor behaviour, emotion and sleep–wake cycle with the hypoactive subtype most common in the postoperative surgical population.
- Delirium is a common postoperative complication that is associated with significantly poor short-term and long-term outcomes including increased morbidity and mortality.
- Patients with increased age and with pre-existing cognitive impairment are at highest risk of developing postoperative delirium.
- Prevention of delirium requires the identification of patients at increased risk by routinely screening for cognitive impairment prior to surgery and

implementing non-pharmacological strategies in the care of surgical patients.

- High risk patients should be screened for delirium postoperatively to identify delirium early in the course and correct modifiable causes.
- The prevention, detection and management of delirium are paramount to reduce its impact and improve postoperative outcomes among the most vulnerable patients.

Further Reading

American Geriatrics Society. Clinical Practice Guideline for Postoperative Delirium in Older Adults, 2014. Available at: http://geriatricscareonline.org/toc/american-geriatrics-society-clinical-practice-guideline-for-postoperative-delirium-in-older-adults/CL018.

Barr J, Fraser GL, Puntillo K, et al. Clinical practice guidelines for the management of pain, agitation, and delirium in adult patients in the intensive care unit. *Critical Care Medicine*. 2013; 41: 263–306.

Fleet J, Ernst T. Clinical Guideline: The Prevention, Recognition and Management of Delirium in Adult In-Patients. Guys and St. Thomas' National Health Service (NHS) Foundation Trust, 2011. DTC reference 11055i.

Gusmao-Flores D, Martins JC, Amorin D, Quarantini LC. Tools for diagnosing delirium in the critically ill: is calibration needed for the less sedated patient? *Intensive Care Medicine*. 2014; 40: 137–138.

Hshieh TT, Yue J, Oh E, et al. Effectiveness of multicomponent nonpharmacological delirium interventions: a meta-analysis. *Journal of the American Medical Association Internal Medicine*. 2015; 175: 512–520.

ICU Delirium and Cognitive Impairment Study Group. ABCDEFs of Prevention and Safety, 2013. Available at: www.icudelirium.org

Inouye SK, Westendorp RG, Saczynski JS. Delirium in elderly people. *Lancet*. 2014; 383: 911–922.

Johns Hopkins Medicine. Outcomes After Critical Illness and Surgery (OACIS), 2015. Available at: www.hopkinsmedicine.org/pulmonary/research/outcomes_after_critical_illness_surgery/.

Neto AS, Nassar (Jr) AP, Cardoso SO, et al. Delirium screening in critically ill patients: a systematic review and meta-analysis. Critical Care Medicine. 2012; 40: 1946–1951.

Pandharipande PP, Girard TD, Jackson JC, et al. Long-term cognitive impairment after critical illness. *New England Journal of Medicine*. 2013; 369: 1306–1316.

MCQs

1. **Which of the following factors has the best evidence of being associated with an increased incidence of delirium?**

   (a) Epilepsy

   (b) Premorbid cognitive impairment

   (c) Hypertension

   (d) Incontinence

   (e) Pre-existing psychiatric illness

2. **Which of the following outcomes has been associated with delirium?**

   (a) Cognitive impairment at 1 year of follow-up among ICU survivors

   (b) Increased institutionalisation following discharge from hospital

   (c) Increased healthcare costs

   (d) Increased risk of death

   (e) All of the above

3. **Important features of delirium include disturbances in:**

   (a) Ability to focus attention

   (b) Sleep–wake cycle

   (c) Psychomotor behaviour

   (d) All of the above

   (e) None of the above

4. **Which of the following is the best delirium screening tool to use in mechanically ventilated patients?**

   (a) MOCA

   (b) MMSE

   (c) CAM-ICU

   (d) 4AT

   (e) CAC

5. **Which one of the following interventions is recommended by the American Geriatrics Society Guidelines to prevent postoperative delirium?**
   (a) Preoperative administration of intravenous haloperidol
   (b) Pre-medication prior to surgery with 2.5 mg of lorazepam
   (c) Use of a non-pharmacological bundle of interventions postoperatively
   (d) Maintaining the patient on bedrest immediately after surgery to reduce fall risk
   (e) Intraoperative EEG monitoring of depth of sedation

Exercise answers are available on p.469. Alternatively, take the test online at www.cambridge.org/CardiothoracicMCQ

Haematological Disorders and Cardiothoracic Intensive Care

Jerrold H Levy, Kamrouz Ghadimi and Ian Welsby

Introduction

Cardiac surgical patients are at great risk for bleeding due to multiple factors. Many of these patients have underlying disease states that potentially may add to the risk for impaired haemostasis. Pharmacological therapy for cardiovascular disease, specifically anticoagulants and antiplatelet agents, can significantly contribute to these acquired causes of impaired haemostasis and bleeding. The additional effects of high-dose heparin anticoagulation for extracorporeal circulation, fibrinolysis, platelet activation associated with cardiopulmonary bypass, hypothermia and dilutional changes are some of the multiple factors that contribute to an acquired coagulopathy. Although pre-existing haematological diseases can further contribute to bleeding in cardiac surgical patients, most of the acquired haemostatic disorders are relatively uncommon. One of the critical haematological issues that significantly influences perioperative management in cardiac surgical patients includes heparin-induced thrombocytopenia (HIT). Other major issues related to hypercoagulability are also a potential issue that will be covered in understanding HIT and have been reviewed elsewhere.

Congenital Bleeding Disorders

Acquired haemostatic disorders due to pharmacological therapy are more common in cardiac surgical patients. A small percentage of patients (approximately 1%) may present with one or more of the common congenital bleeding disorders, most often haemophilia, von Willebrand's disease (vWD) and/or inherited qualitative platelet defects. Although other disorders may exist in patients, focus will be on these common congenital haemostatic defects. Critical to patient management is the evolution of purified and recombinant replacement factors. The haemostatic factors administered for managing cardiac surgical patients with haemophilia undergoing surgery are recombinant or plasma-derived factor VIII for haemophilia A or factor IX for haemophilia B, von Willebrand factor (vWF) concentrates for patients with von Willebrand's disease, and different therapies for patients with platelet defects including platelet transfusions.

Haemophilia

Haemophilia is an inherited X-linked recessive disorder, with an incidence of ~1 in 5000 male births for haemophilia A (factor VIII deficiency) and 1 in 25,000 male births for haemophilia B (factor IX deficiency). Haemophilia patients develop bleeding into their joints, probably due to the extensive presence of glycosaminoglycans in the synovial surfaces and the lack of tissue factor. Both forms of haemophilia are characterised by low levels of factors VIII or IX. Patients with haemophilia routinely require orthopaedic surgery because of repeated bleeding into their joints. They may also undergo cardiac surgery. There are specific guidelines developed in the haemophilia literature, and haematological management should include consultations with a consultant haematologist for specific timing and maintenance of factor replacement therapy. Depending on the factor levels, factor concentrate replacements should be administered within 10–20 minutes of starting a procedure and levels followed perioperatively to further determine specific factor replacement requirements for maintaining levels in the first few perioperative days.

Von Willebrand's Disease

A critical haemostatic protein is vWF, which is present in the circulation as a multimeric macromolecule. Its haemostatic function facilitates platelet adhesion to damaged blood vessels, and has critical importance facilitating platelet aggregation. The macromolecule functions as a carrier protein to factor VIII, and circulates complex to this coagulation factor. The actual von Willebrand's disease occurs in an estimated 1% of patients. The most common form of the disease is type 1, where vWF levels are 10% to 40%. Type 2 is a more complex qualitative vWF defect where the molecule has a decreased ability to bind factor VIII (type 2N), or increased (type 2B) or decreased (types 2A and 2M) ability to facilitate platelet-dependent vWF functions. Type 3 is the most severe form of the disease where vWF levels are <10% and factor VIII levels are also low. In addition, patients with severe aortic stenosis and ventricular assist devices develop an acquired form of the disease due to mechanical injury and disruption of the larger multimeric form. In patients with type 1 disease, desmopressin ~0.3 μg/kg is usually administered intravenously. However, in type 2 and type 3 vWD patients, vWF concentrates are the therapy of choice but should be administered after separation from cardiopulmonary bypass (CPB).

Although few clinical data are available, Bhave et al. reported one of the larger series of 17 patients undergoing cardiac surgery with CPB that included 13 patients with haemophilia A, one symptomatic haemophilia A carrier, one with haemophilia B and two with vWD. The cardiac surgical procedures included ten coronary revascularisations, two aortic valve replacements, two mitral valve repairs, two aortic root replacements, and one combined aortic valve replacement and coronary revascularisation. All procedures were managed by factor repletion to maintain normal levels. Two patients were re-explored for bleeding at 1 and 20 days postoperatively.

Other Less Common Inherited Bleeding Disorders

There is a paucity of information beyond case reports available for managing many of the other less common coagulation factor deficiencies. However, purified factor concentrates are available for most of the additional rare factor deficiency states. For many of these patients, fresh frozen plasma/plasma and other factors including factor concentrates may be important during management. Fortunately, many of these patients come previously diagnosed with their specific coagulation deficiency. Factor XII deficiency has important implications for cardiac surgery because patients present with a markedly prolonged partial thromboplastin time and activated clotting time, and can complicate managing anticoagulation with heparin for CPB. In patients with factor XII deficiency, fixed dose heparin should be administered based on time and/or duration of CPB and/or heparin monitoring using heparin-protamine titrations if available.

Inherited Platelet Disorders

Beyond the common problem of acquired platelet dysfunction due to the use of P2Y12 receptor antagonists (e.g. clopidogrel, prasugrel and ticagrelor), rare forms of congenital platelet dysfunction include Glanzmann's thrombasthenia and Bernard Soulier disease. Fortunately, most patients with this disease have a long history of easy bruisability, bleeding and/or family history. There are reports of these patients undergoing cardiac surgery. In patients with Glanzmann's thrombasthenia, there is a defect on the platelet surface for the fibrinogen receptor GPIIb/IIIa that prevents platelet aggregation, which is a critical component of clot formation. Fortunately, patients may have a long history of bruising, mucosal bleeding and other soft-tissue bleeding which should make the clinician suspicious of such a disorder. Of note is that recombinant factor VIIa is approved for treating bleeding in this patient population. Another rare aforementioned syndrome is Bernard Soulier disease, where patients have thrombocytopenia and a reduced ability of the platelets to adhere to the damaged blood vessel owing to abnormality of the GPIb/V/IX receptor on the platelets, therefore preventing appropriate vWF binding, which is another critical step in platelet adhesion and activation. Other additional platelet abnormalities include storage pool disorders that may manifest in variable ways and are another rare cause of platelet dysfunction. Again, acquired platelet dysfunction due to the use of antiplatelet agents is a far greater issue in cardiac surgical patients.

Procoagulant Disorders

Heparin Resistance

'Adequate anticoagulation' for CPB is traditionally determined by the activated clotting time (ACT), a whole blood haemostatic activation test that is influenced by multiple causes. Heparin resistance has been frequently reported in the literature, often due to a variety of causes. The definition commonly used for heparin resistance is ACT <480 seconds following addition of 500 U/kg of heparin. Unfortunately, the terminology we use for heparin resistance is a misnomer, because actual resistance does not occur; rather there is an alteration in heparin dose responsiveness and an alteration of the slope of the heparin response curve. The ACT actually increases following heparin administration, but not in a linear fashion.

Multiple factors are responsible for producing altered heparin dose responses, in addition to antithrombin, including preoperative heparin use, high and low platelet counts (both thrombocytosis and thrombocytopenia), altered platelet function and use of other anticoagulants. The association between decreased preoperative antithrombin and heparin resistance is complicated by multiple factors that affect the ACT in addition to antithrombin levels. Ranucci et al. suggested a 10% predictive chance of a patient developing altered heparin dose responsiveness/heparin resistance. Antithrombin (also called antithrombin III) is a serine protease inhibitor that circulates in the plasma at 80–110% assuming normal levels, approximately 2.4 μmol. Antithrombin is associated with altered heparin responsiveness due to the fact that heparin requires the cofactor of antithrombin to inhibit factors Xa and thrombin (IIa). Antithrombin is activated by binding to heparin via the pentasaccharide sequence of heparin; the relative chain length of the sequence controls the binding selectively to factor Xa and/or IIa. Multiple investigators have noted that previous heparin administration decreases antithrombin levels, and produces alterations in heparin dose responsiveness.

Multiple reports note that antithrombin improves intraoperative anticoagulation, improves perioperative haemostasis and reduces biochemical markers of coagulation. Antithrombin administration to correct decreased levels of antithrombin would potentially be of benefit to all patients, as antithrombin levels fall to <50% during CPB. Although Linden et al. suggest therapeutic antithrombin is not of added benefit in heparin resistance because patients do not exhibit decreased antithrombin concentration compared with heparin responsive patients, this is not the case. Antithrombin administration will consistently increase ACT responsiveness in vitro and in vivo as previously reported.

Heparin-Induced Thrombocytopenia

Heparin-induced thrombocytopenia (HIT) is a prothrombotic disease where an anticoagulant has the potential to produce a procoagulant effect. The pathophysiology is due to an antibody that develops following heparin administration to a specific alpha granule protein released from platelets called platelet factor 4 (PF4). When PF4 is released, it fuses with the platelet membrane to form a new epitope/antigen, and as a result immunoglobulin (Ig) G develops that binds to PF4 complexes on platelets, causing activation, sequestration and microparticle formation, all of which have profound prothrombotic effects. Patients following cardiac surgery and CPB are at an increased risk of producing the antibodies which may occur in up to 50% of patients although potentially at low levels. The presence and the level of the antibodies are associated with an increased risk for adverse events, and occur in approximately 1–5% of patients who receive unfractionated heparin, although cardiac transplant patients may be at an even higher risk for HIT (~11%).

Diagnosis

HIT should be suspected if the platelet count drops by 50%, or new thrombosis occurs in a patient 5 to 14 days after the start of heparin therapy. The 4T score (thrombocytopenia, timing of platelet count fall, thrombosis or other sequelae, and other causes for thrombocytopenia) has also been used to determine the probability of HIT and is thought to correlate well with antibody formation. However, in cardiac surgical patients in the perioperative setting, thrombocytopenia is a common problem and is due to multiple causes including dilutional changes post CPB, intra-aortic balloon pump presence and mechanical destruction, sepsis or other drug-induced causes, especially IIb/IIIa inhibitors. Following cardiac surgery and CPB, HIT may present in a biphasic pattern. Several days postoperatively, the platelet count begins to normalise after CPB-related thrombocytopenia, followed by a decreasing platelet count >4 days postoperatively. Following heparin administration intraoperatively, an acute hypersensitivity response may occur due to pre-existing IgG levels, with hypotension, other systemic responses and acute thrombocytopenia. HIT can also occur weeks after heparin exposure and is termed 'delayed-onset HIT' but this is less common.

Laboratory Testing

Although suspicion of HIT is of critical importance to stop use of heparin and facilitate another anticoagulant, laboratory testing is an important adjunct to making the correct diagnosis. The standard testing includes antibody determination for screening and functional assay for definitive diagnosis. Antibody testing includes a standard enzyme-linked immunosorbent assay (ELISA) that detects either polyclonal antibodies or IgG specific antibodies to complexes of PF4 and heparin. ELISA results are commonly reported to clinicians as either positive or negative; specific information regarding optical density (OD) should also be obtained to facilitate clinical decisions regarding management and/or further workup. Based on the time of sampling, 'high-titer negative' ELISA results have the potential to become positive several days later if retested. More importantly, higher optical density results are associated with increased probability for true HIT, based on published data that will be discussed later. The serotonin release assay (SRA) and platelet aggregation testing are functional assays that are only undertaken in specialised laboratories.

Warkentin et al. reported a study that is important for clinical management and is based on antibody testing. In this study, the magnitude of positive ELISA results, as determined by optical density (OD) units, was correlated with functional platelet serotonin-release assay (SRA) results, the gold standard for determining whether a patient is indeed HIT positive. They reported that if the results were weakly positive, 0.40–1.00 OD units, the ELISA had a low probability of 5% or less for a positive SRA. However, the risk increased to ~90% with an OD of ≥2.00 units. Their study evaluated 1553 patient sera and reported that for every increase of 0.50 OD units in the ELISA-IgG, the risk of a positive SRA increased by OR = 6.39, and for every increase of 1.00 OD units in the EIA-IgG, the risk increased by OR = 40.81.

Treatment

Postoperatively, in patients with clinical suspicion of HIT or confirmed HIT, stopping heparin and starting an alternative anticoagulant, most commonly the direct thrombin inhibitor bivalirudin or argatroban, are mainstays of therapy. The alternative danaparoid is not available in most countries. Management for CPB will be considered separately. As previously mentioned, the 4T score has been suggested to determine the relative risk of true HIT. Low molecular weight heparin should not be used because of potential cross-reactivity with antibodies. Anticoagulation with warfarin should be avoided based on guidelines until platelet count recovers. Heparin should be avoided, if possible, at least as long as heparin-PF4 antibody testing is positive.

For patients requiring cardiac surgery and CPB, although alternative anticoagulants can be used, heparin is still the best agent due to its acute reversibility. For patients with current HIT who require cardiac surgery, if elective, the surgery should be delayed until heparin-PF4 antibodies are negative. Alternatively, plasmapheresis has been recommended and used successfully to manage patients. However, alternative anticoagulation for CPB is best performed with bivalirudin, based on all of the reported data.

Managing HIT Patients for Cardiovascular Surgery

Antibody Positive

If the SRA is negative, then heparin can be used for CPB but avoiding heparin re-exposure postoperatively should be considered. If the patient is HIT positive and SRA is either positive and/or not available and cardiac surgery cannot be delayed, either plasmapheresis or the use of an alternative anticoagulant (specifically bivalirudin) should be considered, based on ACCP guidelines. The most extensive practical clinical and reported experience with an alternative non-heparin anticoagulant is with the direct thrombin inhibitor bivalirudin. Although dosing guidelines have been reported for the use of argatroban for CPB, based on retrospective analysis of 21 adult cases, there is far more extensive experience with bivalirudin. Argatroban for postoperative anticoagulation in the intensive care unit, however, is a potential heparin alternative.

Bivalirudin

The most extensive experience with an alternative anticoagulant for CPB or off-pump cardiac surgery is with bivalirudin as previously mentioned. One of the initial series for coronary artery bypass grafting using CPB and bivalirudin anticoagulation used a 1.5 mg/kg loading dose before cannulation and continuous 2.5 mg/kg/hour infusion during CPB. Anticoagulation was monitored using a target ACT of 2- to 2.5-fold over baseline (approximately 300–350 seconds), but with the prolonged half-life and lack of reversibility, caution should be considered targetting normal ACT values. Anticoagulation during CPB was effective, and total operating times were acceptable. One patient experienced excessive postoperative bleeding. Prospective studies have evaluated bivalirudin (versus heparin) in non-HIT patients undergoing cardiac surgery using CPB or undergoing coronary artery bypass grafting without CPB. Across the studies, bivalirudin was administered to 206 patients and provided effective anticoagulation with a safety profile similar to that of heparin. Bivalirudin dosing in surgery without CPB is similar to that used in PCI.

Surgical techniques that allow blood to stay stagnant should be avoided when using bivalirudin, which is metabolised by enzymes present in blood exposed to wound or foreign surfaces. Therefore, direct retransfusion of shed pericardial/mediastinal blood into the cardiotomy container should be avoided during bivalirudin administration in order to avoid systemic activation and circulation of thromboemboli. Alternatively, shed pericardial blood can be processed via cell salvage systems when using bivalirudin.

Managing HIT Patients in the ICU

Standardised criteria such as the 4Ts clinical scoring system and platelet profiles can be used to appropriately send for PF4/heparin antibody testing and immediately initiate argatroban. Often clinicians delay initial anticoagulation therapy on clinical suspicion of HIT due to safety concerns about bleeding. The lack of increased risk for adverse events with argatroban in the cardiothoracic ICU after surgery suggests early therapy with argatroban as a DTI should be considered. Other DTIs currently available for use include the parenteral agents lepirudin, desirudin and bivalirudin, and the direct oral anticoagulant, dabigatran. The results from our study support argatroban use upon immediate clinical suspicion of HIT as detected by an otherwise unexplained drop in platelet count of >50% at approximately 5–10 days after surgery. In addition, argatroban use is endorsed in thrombotic complications for all patients after cardiothoracic surgery, and prior to confirmation of laboratory results. Additional prospective, randomised studies are needed to support our findings, and to determine the relative safety of argatroban and other DTIs.

Learning Points

- Most congenital bleeding disorders for cardiac surgical patients are relatively rare; however these patients can also develop cardiac disease and require cardiac surgery.
- Factor repletion is the mainstay of therapy for patients with factor deficiency states such as haemophilia or von Willebrand's disease.
- Heparin-induced thrombocytopenia (HIT) is another important immunological haemostatic disorder characterised by prothrombotic potential after heparin administration.
- Management of HIT patients includes recognition, monitoring and avoidance of heparin as an anticoagulant.
- For management of cardiac surgical patients undergoing cardiopulmonary bypass (CPB) who have been diagnosed with HIT, bivalirudin as an alternative anticoagulant is a mainstay of therapy. Argatroban is another direct thrombin inhibitor which can also be used for postoperative anticoagulation but there are far less data for its use during CPB.

Further Reading

Bhave P, McGiffin D, Shaw J, et al. Guide to performing cardiac surgery in patients with hereditary bleeding disorders. *Journal of Cardiac Surgery*. 2015; 30: 61–69.

Despotis GJ, Avidan MS, Hogue (Jr) CW. Mechanisms and attenuation of hemostatic activation during extracorporeal circulation. *Annals of Thoracic Surgery*. 2001; 72: S1821–S1831.

Dyke CM, Smedira NG, Koster A, et al. A comparison of bivalirudin to heparin with protamine reversal in patients undergoing cardiac surgery with cardiopulmonary bypass: the EVOLUTION-ON study. *Journal of Thoracic and Cardiovascular Surgery*. 2006; 131: 533–539.

Levy JH. Heparin resistance and antithrombin: should it still be called heparin resistance?[comment]. *Journal of Cardiothoracic and Vascular Anesthesia*. 2004; 18: 129–130.

Levy JH, Despotis GJ, Szlam F, Olson P, Meeker D, Weisinger A. Recombinant human transgenic antithrombin in cardiac surgery: a dose-finding study. *Anesthesiology*. 2002; 96: 1095–1102.

Levy JH, Faraoni D, Spring JL, Douketis JD, Samama CM. Managing new oral anticoagulants in the perioperative and intensive care unit setting. *Anesthesiology*. 2013; 118: 1466–1474.

Levy JH, Key NS, Azran MS. Novel oral anticoagulants: implications in the perioperative setting. *Anesthesiology*. 2010; 113: 726–745.

Levy JH, Montes F, Szlam F, Hillyer CD. The in vitro effects of antithrombin III on the activated coagulation time in patients on heparin therapy. *Anesthesia & Analgesia.* 2000; 90: 1076–1079.

Levy JH, Weisinger A, Ziomek CA, Echelard Y. Recombinant antithrombin: production and role in cardiovascular disorder. *Seminars in Thrombosis and Hemostasis.* 2001; 27: 405–416.

Mannucci PM. Treatment of von Willebrand's disease. *New England Journal of Medicine.* 2004; 351: 683–694.

Sniecinski RM, Chandler WL. Activation of the hemostatic system during cardiopulmonary bypass. *Anesthesia & Analgesia.* 2011; 113: 1319–1333.

Sniecinski RM, Hursting MJ, Paidas MJ, Levy JH. Etiology and assessment of hypercoagulability with lessons from heparin-induced thrombocytopenia. *Anesthesia & Analgesia.* 2010; 112: 46–58.

Warkentin TE, Sheppard JI, Moore JC, Sigouin CS, Kelton JG. Quantitative interpretation of optical density measurements using PF4-dependent enzyme-immunoassays. *Journal of Thrombosis and Haemostasis.* 2008; 6: 1304–1312.

MCQs

True or False

1. **Common congenital bleeding disorders include:**
   (a) Haemophilia
   (b) Protein C/S deficiency
   (c) von Willebrand's disease
   (d) Bernard Soulier disease
   (e) Heparin-induced thrombocytopenia

2. **Von Willebrand's:**
   (a) Factor inhibits platelet adhesion to damaged blood vessels
   (b) Factor is a carrier protein to factor IX
   (c) Disease occurs in an estimated 1% of patients
   (d) Disease can occur as an acquired form
   (e) Disease may be due to qualitative or quantitative defects in VWF

3. **Heparin resistance:**
   (a) Is defined as ACT < 280 seconds following addition of 500 U/kg of heparin
   (b) Is due to an alteration in heparin dose responsiveness
   (c) Is less common in patients who have been on heparin preoperatively
   (d) Is associated with high antithrombin levels
   (e) Can be treated by administration of antithrombin

4. **Heparin-induced thrombocytopenia (HIT):**
   (a) Is a prothrombotic disease
   (b) Is antibody mediated
   (c) Is associated with complexes between PF8 and heparin
   (d) Should be suspected if the platelet count increases by 50%
   (e) Diagnosis is confirmed by the 4T score

5. **Treatment for HIT includes:**
   (a) Platelet transfusion
   (b) Argatroban
   (c) Plasmapheresis
   (d) Bivalirudin
   (e) Low molecular weight heparin

Exercise answers are available on p.470. Alternatively, take the test online at www.cambridge.org/CardiothoracicMCQ

Pregnancy and Cardiovascular Disorders

Kiran Salaunkey

Introduction

There is an increasing prevalence of cardiovascular disease (CVD) in women of child bearing age. It is estimated that about 0.2–4% of all pregnancies in the developed world have cardiovascular complications despite no known prior disease. CVD is a major cause of non-obstetric death amongst expectant and new mothers in the UK. Hypertensive disorders are the most frequent CVD during pregnancy, occurring in 6–8% of all pregnancies.

The improved longevity following successful medical and surgical treatment of congenital heart diseases has led to an increased number of women becoming pregnant with treated congenital heart disease, with an increased predominance of shunt lesions.

In the developing world the burden of valvular heart disease among pregnant women persists, but these issues are also seen in the developing world amongst immigrant populations.

Increased prevalence of risk factors for atherosclerotic disease along with an increased maternal age has led to an increased incidence of coronary artery disease.

Cardiomyopathies, though rare, cause significant morbidity. Peripartum cardiomyopathy (PPCM) is the most common cause of severe complications.

CVD in pregnancy poses a challenging scenario due to changes in the maternal physiology adversely affecting the suboptimal cardiovascular system. The responsibility of the treating physician in these cases ranges from prenatal counselling, antenatal and postnatal care of the mother and also potentially extends to the care of the unborn foetus. Considering the difficulties of conducting research in this area, it is not surprising that robust prospective randomised studies are lacking.

Cardiovascular Physiological Changes in Pregnancy

Though there are widespread metabolic changes in the pregnant female, for the purposes of this chapter we will confine our discussion to the cardiovascular changes that occur during pregnancy

Pregnancy has a profound effect on the circulatory system to meet the additional metabolic demands of the mother and the foetus.

The placenta invades maternal uterine tissue early in pregnancy and releases an array of hormones and other factors. These hormones create physiological changes in the mother, which favour nutrient and oxygen delivery to the growing foetus.

There is an increase in red cell mass and increase in blood volume, causing increased preload. However, there is dilutional anaemia due to a disproportionate increase of the plasma component of blood as compared to its cellular component.

Further increases in cardiac output by about 20–50% are achieved by an increase in stroke volume of about 15–30% in early pregnancy and an increase of heart rate by about 15–30%, mainly towards the latter stages as caval compression prevents further increases in stroke volume.

There is a decrease in total vascular resistance by about 30% due to increased flow into the uteroplacental circulation, coupled with secretion of vasodilatory substances from the placenta such as nitric oxide and prostaglandins. The systolic blood pressure for the most part remains unchanged but the mean arterial pressure is reduced initially but increases towards the end of pregnancy.

The cardiac performance improves with progressive LV remodelling during pregnancy. There is dilatation of the heart by about 30% with eccentric hypertrophy. These changes tend to resolve within 2 weeks of postpartum state.

By the second trimester the enlarging uterus will cause a degree of aortocaval compression, reducing the amount of venous return in the supine position.

A series of haemostatic changes, such as increased platelet adhesiveness and increased concentration of coagulation factors, leads to a hypercoaguable state; this, coupled with stasis due to caval compression described above, can increase the risk of deep vein thrombosis.

Further during labour, pain, anxiety and uterine contractions cause increased cardiovascular stress. Efforts to mitigate pain with neuraxial anaesthesia or intercurrent haemorrhage during delivery affect cardiovascular performance.

Post delivery, the phenomenon of autotransfusion, resorption of oedema and uterine involution places a significant stress on the cardiovascular system.

There is a reduction in cardiac output in the postpartum period.

Diagnosis of Cardiovascular Diseases

History and Clinical Examination

A thorough history, specifically looking to elicit familial history of cardiomyopathies, Marfan syndrome, long QT syndromes and sudden deaths, should be sought. Assessment of progression of ongoing breathlessness is a good prognostic tool to predict heart failure. History should include baseline functional status and previous cardiac events as these are strong predictors of peripartum cardiac events.

The strongest predictors are:

- Any prior cardiac event;
- Cyanosis or poor functional status;
- Left sided obstruction;
- Ventricular dysfunction.

Examination is directed towards looking for signs of heart failure; if new signs or murmurs are found, this mandates further investigations. Blood pressure is measured either at home or in the clinic in the left lateral recumbent position.

Urinalysis for glucose and proteinuria should be performed.

Electrocardiography

A standard 12 lead ECG, which is a safe and inexpensive screening tool, should be used. The normal ECG of pregnancy sometimes manifests as left axis deviation, increased R wave amplitude in V1 and V2, T wave inversion in V2, small Q wave in lead II, III and aVF, and inverted T wave in lead III, V1–V3.

There is an increase in the rate of maternal arrhythmias during pregnancy.

Further analysis of rhythm disturbances may warrant exercise ECG, tilt table testing and electrophysiological studies.

Echocardiography

This is the preferred mode of cardiac imaging due to its non-invasive nature, safety profile and reproducibility. The transthoracic route is preferred to the transoesophageal (TOE) route.

In cases where TOE is used, care must be taken regarding aspects such as gastric stasis, reflux and sedation needs, which might impact on foetal well being, necessitating foetal monitoring.

Exercise Testing

This provides an objective quantification of cardiopulmonary function especially in patients being followed up for grown-up congenital heart disease (GUCH) and valvular heart disease. It should preferably be performed in the prenatal period to help with risk assessment and prenatal counseling.

The European Society of Cardiology (ESC) recommends that in asymptomatic patients it is advisable to use exercise testing to attain 80% of maximal capacity during pregnancy. The safety of exercise testing during pregnancy has not been established, but there is no evidence that it increases the risk of spontaneous abortion.

Magnetic Resonance Imaging

This is a useful modality that will provide information for diagnosis and therapy. It is probably safe in the second and third trimesters. It can also be used to diagnose foetal neurological defects identified by ultrasound.

Gadolinium ions are known to cross the placental barrier; the safety of gadolinium is not known in a developing foetus and should be avoided.

Cardiac Catheterisation

If needed in a pregnant patient, this should preferably be undertaken by the radial route, limiting the radiation exposure time and shielding the foetus from direct radiation.

Electrophysiological studies or ablation if needed should use an electroanatomical mapping system in conjunction with MRI to reduce radiation dose.

Chest X-rays and CT Scans

A single diagnostic investigation requiring radiation exposure is not sufficient to threaten the well being of the developing foetus. However, frequency of exposure, and accumulated dose of radiation, do result in adverse foetal effects such as foetal cell death, teratogenesis, carcinogenesis and mutations in germ cells in the foetus.

A radiation dose below 50 mGy to the pregnant mother is the accepted level of radiation below which there is no evidence of increased foetal risk.

If ionising radiation is used, its dose should be documented in the record and the principle of ALARA 'as low as reasonably achievable' should be used.

The foetus as a rule is protected by the mother's abdomen and the exposure to radiation is far below the level of exposure of the mother.

Table 49.1 gives the amount of radiation exposure for common radiological procedures.

Common Cardiovascular Disorders

Hypertensive Disorders of Pregnancy

Definitions

Gestational hypertension is a clinical diagnosis defined by the new onset of hypertension (systolic blood pressure ≥140 mmHg and/or diastolic blood pressure ≥90 mmHg) at ≥20 weeks of gestation in the absence of proteinuria or new signs of end-organ dysfunction. The blood pressure readings should be documented on at least two occasions at least 4 hours apart. Gestational hypertension is severe when systolic blood pressure is ≥160 mmHg and/or diastolic blood pressure is ≥110 mmHg on two consecutive blood pressure measurements at least 4 hours apart.

Gestational hypertension is a temporary diagnosis for hypertensive pregnant women who do not meet the criteria for pre-eclampsia (see Table 49.2) or chronic hypertension (hypertension first detected before the twentieth week of pregnancy). The diagnosis is changed to:

- Pre-eclampsia, if proteinuria or new signs of end-organ dysfunction develop;
- Chronic (primary or secondary) hypertension, if blood pressure elevation persists ≥12 weeks post partum;
- Transient hypertension of pregnancy, if blood pressure returns to normal by 12 weeks post partum.

Thus, reassessment up to 12 weeks post partum is necessary to establish a final diagnosis.

Gestational hypertension occurs in 6–17% of healthy nulliparous women and 2–4% of multiparous women. Previous history of pre-eclampsia, multifoetal pregnancies and raised body mass index are the significant risk factors.

Diagnosis

Blood pressure monitoring is the cornerstone on which the diagnosis is made; home blood pressure monitoring is useful to differentiate white coat hypertension. It is important to differentiate gestational hypertension from pre-eclampsia and pre-eclampsia from severe pre-eclampsia.

Table 49.1 Estimated foetal and maternal effective doses for various diagnostic and interventional radiology procedures

Procedure	Foetal exposure	Risk of childhood cancer
Chest radiograph (PA and lateral)	0.001–0.01 mGy	<1:100,000
CT chest (including CTPA)	0.01–0.1 mGy	<1:100,000
Lung perfusion scan	0.1–1 mGy	1:100,000 to 1:10,000
CT chest abdomen pelvis	10 mGy	1:10,000 to 1:1000
Coronary angiography	1.5 mGy	1:10,000 to 1:1000
PCI or radiofrequency catheter ablation	3 mGy	1:10,000 to 1:1000

CT computed tomography; PCI percutaneous coronary intervention; PA posteroanterior.
Natural childhood cancer risk 1:500.

Table 49.2 Diagnosis of pre-eclampsia

Systolic blood pressure ≥140 mmHg or diastolic blood pressure ≥90 mmHg on two occasions at least 4 hours apart after 20 weeks of gestation in a previously normotensive patient. If systolic blood pressure is ≥160 mmHg or diastolic blood pressure is ≥110 mmHg, confirmation within minutes is sufficient	
AND	
Proteinuria ≥0.3 g in a 24-hour urine specimen or protein (mg/dl)/creatinine (mg/dl) ratio ≥0.3	
Dipstick ≥1+ if a quantitative measurement is unavailable	
In patients with new-onset hypertension without proteinuria, the new onset of any of the following is diagnostic of pre-eclampsia:	
Platelet count <100,000/μl	Liver transaminases raised to twice normal limits
Serum creatinine > 100 μmol/l OR doubling of serum creatinine in the absence of renal disease	
Cerebral or visual symptoms	Pulmonary oedema

Table 49.3 Diagnostic features of severe pre-eclampsia

Symptoms of nervous system dysfunction New onset cerebral or visual disturbance, such as: • Photopsia, scotomata, cortical blindness, retinal vasospasm • Severe headache (i.e. incapacitating, 'the worst headache I've ever had') or headache that persists and progresses despite analgesic therapy • Altered mental status	
Hepatic abnormality: Severe persistent right upper quadrant or epigastric pain unresponsive to medication and not accounted for by an alternative diagnosis or serum transaminase concentration ≥ twice normal, or both	
Severe blood pressure elevation: Systolic blood pressure ≥160 mmHg or diastolic blood pressure ≥110 mmHg on two occasions at least 4 hours apart while the patient is on bed-rest (unless the patient is on anti-hypertensive therapy)	
Renal abnormality: Progressive renal insufficiency (serum creatinine >100 μmol/l or doubling of serum creatinine concentration in the absence of other renal disease)	
Thrombocytopenia: <100,000 platelets/μl	Pulmonary oedema

Table 49.3 gives the diagnosis of severe pre-eclampsia.

Foetal well being should be evaluated with estimation of foetal weight; umbilical artery Doppler is helpful for foetuses with intrauterine growth restriction. An abnormal Doppler profile is highly specific for severe pre-eclampsia.

HELLP syndrome represents a severe form of preeclampsia. It is characterised by:

- Haemolysis with a microangiopathic picture on blood smear;
- Elevated liver enzymes; and a
- Low platelet count.

Patients with HELLP have a high risk of developing serious hepatic injury due to infarction, haemorrhage and hepatic rupture.

Management

Delivery minimises the risk of development of serious maternal and foetal complications due to pre-eclampsia. The management decision is a trade-off between:

- The foetal benefits from expectant management (i.e. further growth and maturation);
- The maternal and foetal benefits from early intervention (i.e. avoidance of complications from progression of hypertensive disease over the remainder of pregnancy); and
- The maternal and foetal risks from expectant management (i.e. progression of hypertensive disease and possible sequelae, including stillbirth or asphyxia).

An overview of management of gestational hypertension is beyond the scope of this chapter; however we will focus on the management of severe eclampsia in patients likely to need intensive care.

For the common scenarios where intensive care intervention is required, parenteral drug therapy for acute management of severe hypertension is possible.

Labetolol intravenously is recommended for first line therapy because it is effective, has a rapid onset of action and a good safety profile. Suggested regime: begin with 20 mg intravenously over 2 minutes followed at 10 minute intervals by doses of 20 to 80 mg up to a maximum total cumulative dose of 300 mg, or an intravenous infusion of 1–2 mg/minute.

Hydralazine administered intravenously is a good alternative to labetolol. Suggested regime: begin with 5 mg intravenously over 1 to 2 minutes, repeat as required waiting for a response that usually takes up to 15–20 minutes to manifest. The maximum bolus dose is 20 mg. If a total dose of 30 mg does not achieve optimal blood pressure control, another agent should be used.

Calcium channel blockers, sustained release nifedipine (30 mg) and immediate release nicardipine, are other options. Nicardipine can be given intravenously. Experience with these drugs in pregnancy is limited. Immediate release oral or sublingual nifedipine is best avoided as it can cause precipitous hypotension resulting in uteroplacental insufficiency.

Nitroglycerin (glyceryl trinitrate) is a good option for treatment of hypertension associated with pulmonary oedema. It is given as an intravenous infusion of 5 μg/minute and gradually increased every 3 to 5 minutes to a maximum dose of 100 μg/minute.

Antenatal corticosteroids may also be administered. Neonatal respiratory distress is very common in premature neonates of pre-eclamptic mothers. Betamethasone should be administered to mothers <34 week' gestation to promote foetal lung maturation as the risk of these patients developing severe pre-eclampsia is high.

A 'restrictive' fluid strategy is advocated as patients with severe disease can develop pulmonary oedema. Oliguria should be managed by modest trials of fluid boluses and if it does not respond it should be tolerated or renal replacement therapy considered if indicated. Pulmonary oedema might warrant use of loop diuretics.

For seizure prophylaxis, magnesium sulphate is the drug of choice and should be administered for all patients with severe pre-eclampsia. Suggested regime: a loading dose of 4 to 6 g intravenously and maintenance dose of 1 to 3 g/hour. Intramuscular regimes have been described but they are associated with pain at the injection site and fluctuating drug levels. Magnesium sulphate is continued for 24 hours post partum. Therapeutic levels between 2.0 and 3.5 mmol/l are to be maintained. Dose reduction might be needed in patients with renal failure. Clinical monitoring for signs of hypermagnesaemia, such as reduced patellar reflexes and respiratory depression, should be monitored and the dose reduced if signs of toxicity appear (Table 49.4).

Table 49.4 Signs of magnesium toxicity

Serum magnesium level (mmol/l)	Corresponding clinical features
3.5–5	Loss of deep tendon reflexes
5.0–6.5	Respiratory paralysis
>7.5	Cardiac conduction disturbances
>12.5	Cardiac arrest

Magnesium toxicity can be counteracted by administration of intravenous calcium chloride 10 mmol slowly over 15–30 minutes.

Magnesium has a central effect in increasing seizure threshold. The probable mechanisms of anticonvulsant action proposed are:

- NMDA receptor antagonism;
- Non-specific calcium channel blockade, resulting in reduced release of acetyl choline at the postsynaptic motor nerve terminals;
- Improved cerebral circulation by direct antagonism of calcium mediated vasospasm.

Invasive haemodynamic monitoring is useful in managing these patients on the intensive care unit to help monitor blood pressure, central venous pressure and fluid status optimisation. The risk of bleeding due to thrombocytopenia should be considered whilst placing these devices in patients.

Postpartum Care

A slow intravenous infusion of oxytocin (<2 U/min), which avoids systemic hypotension, is administered after placental delivery to prevent maternal haemorrhage. Prostaglandin F analogues are useful to treat postpartum haemorrhage, unless an increase in pulmonary artery pressure (PAP) is undesirable. Methyl-ergometrine is contraindicated because of the risk (>10%) of vasoconstriction and hypertension.

Meticulous leg care, elastic support stockings and early ambulation are important to reduce the risk of thromboembolism. Delivery is associated with important haemodynamic changes and fluid shifts, particularly in the first 12–24 hours, which may precipitate heart failure, hence haemodynamic monitoring should therefore be continued for at least 24 hours after delivery.

Amniotic Fluid Embolism

Amniotic fluid embolism (AFE) is an extremely rare but catastrophic event resulting in severe haemodynamic collapse with disseminated intravascular coagulation. It occurs when foetal cells, amniotic fluid and foetal hair enter the maternal circulation and incite an inflammatory reaction similar to anaphylaxis.

Induction of labour, uterine rupture and polyhydroamnios are known risk factors. Most cases occur around the time of delivery, either vaginally or during caesarean sections (Table 49.5).

Successful outcomes depend on early recognition, aggressive resuscitation and prompt delivery of the baby within 5 minutes of commencing resuscitation. Hysterectomy should be performed early if needed to prevent major obstetric haemorrhage.

Suspected cases should be reported to UKOSS (www.npeu.ox.ac.uk).

Cardiomyopathy

Peripartum Cardiomyopathy

Peripartum cardiomyopathy is defined as the development of heart failure in the last month of pregnancy or in the first 5 months after delivery without any identifiable aetiology and with objective assessment of left ventricular dysfunction. Risk factors associated with peripartum cardiomyopathy are maternal age older than 30 years, gestational hypertension and twin pregnancies. The aetiology is commonly a myocarditis or an autoimmune mechanism due to the presence of high serum titres of autoantibodies against human cardiac tissue proteins. Ischaemic heart disease should be considered.

Conventional heart failure management principles should be followed; however ACEI and angiotensin receptor blockers are contraindicated prior to delivery due to risk of impacting foetal growth. Amlodipine is particularly beneficial in peripartum cardiomyopathy due to its anti-inflammatory nature.

Mortality has reduced from approximately 7% to 2% with increased awareness and active management. Unlike traditional cardiomyopathies, cardiac function normalises within 6 months post delivery in over 50% of patients suffering from the disease.

Subsequent pregnancies should be discouraged due to the high risk of recurrence, and if it occurs should be managed at specialist obstetric units.

Table 49.5 Diagnostic criteria for amniotic fluid embolism

Absence of a clear cause of acute maternal collapse with:	
Acute foetal compromise	Cardiac arrest
Rhythm disturbances	Coagulopathy
Hypotension	Maternal haemorrhage
Seizure	Shortness of breath
Excluding women with maternal haemorrhage as the first presenting feature in whom there was no evidence of early coagulopathy or cardiorespiratory compromise	
OR	
Women in whom the diagnosis was made at post mortem examination with the finding of foetal squames or hair in the lungs	

Hypertrophic Cardiomyopathy

Hypertrophic cardiomyopathy (HCM) is relatively rare. Clinical deterioration during pregnancy is uncommon and it is determined by the degree of outflow tract obstruction. Baseline functional status is a significant predictor of outcome.

Management of HCM in pregnancy should focus on preventing blood loss and avoiding vasodilatation. Beta-blockers, diuretics and calcium channel blockers are preferred to manage symptoms. Implantation of an automatic defibrillator should be considered in patients with syncope or increased arrhythmogenicity.

Oxytocin is preferred over prostaglandins for induction of labour. Vaginal delivery is preferred with active management of second stage.

Congenital Heart Disease

The physiological changes of increased intravascular volume, decreased systemic vascular resistance and demand for increased cardiac output pose challenges for patients with structural heart disease. These, along with the rapid fluid shifts during labour and delivery, can precipitate heart failure.

Maternal Risk Stratification

The modified WHO risk classification for maternal risk assessment has four classes:

Class I: Conditions with no detectable increase in risk of maternal mortality and no/mild increase in morbidity. For example, small patent ductus arteriosus, mild pulmonic stenosis, mitral valve prolapse.

Class II: Small increase in risk of maternal mortality or moderate increase in morbidity. For example unrepaired ventricular septal defect, repaired tetralogy of Fallot, most arrhythmias.

Class III: Conditions are associated with significantly increased risk of maternal mortality or severe morbidity. For example mechanical valve, systemic right ventricle, Fontan circulation, bicuspid aortic valve with an enlarged ascending aorta <50 mm and Marfan's syndrome with an ascending aorta <45 mm.

Class IV: Conditions are associated with extremely high risk of maternal mortality or severe morbidity; pregnancy is contraindicated. For example severe mitral stenosis, symptomatic severe aortic stenosis, bicuspid aortic valve with ascending aorta diameter >50 mm, Marfan's syndrome with aorta dilated >45 mm, severe systemic ventricular systolic dysfunction (left ventricular ejection fraction <30%, New York Heart Association [NYHA] III to IV), native severe coarctation and significant pulmonary arterial hypertension of any cause (i.e. pulmonary artery systolic pressure >25 mmHg at rest or >30 mmHg with exercise).

Individual Risk Factors

The following are risks and predictors for maternal or foetal complications in women with congenital heart disease during pregnancy:

- Pulmonary hypertension (pulmonary vascular disease);
- Maternal cyanosis;
- Poor maternal functional class;
- History of arrhythmia;
- Maternal anticoagulants.

Pulmonary hypertension The most serious risk to the mother is pulmonary hypertension, particularly Eisenmenger syndrome, which includes the additional risk of maternal cyanosis. Pulmonary hypertension limits appropriate adaptive responses to the circulatory changes of pregnancy and to the volatile changes during labour, delivery and the postpartum period. These patients are also particularly susceptible to pregnancy related complications such as pre-eclampsia, postpartum haemorrhage and preterm delivery resulting in an extremely high mortality rate in the first postpartum week.

If deemed necessary for a patient with class III or IV disease, the option of termination of pregnancy should be discussed and if the patient is willing this should be performed in the first trimester of pregnancy with a multidisciplinary team with surgical techniques. If medical techniques are to be used, mifoprostol (PGE1) is preferred. PGE2 and PGF should be avoided.

Management of Labour

Supplemental oxygen therapy is always beneficial. Oxytocin and mechanical methods (i.e. rupture of membranes) is the preferred technique to induce labour. The parturient is nursed in the left lateral position to relieve aortocaval compression. Pushing during labour should not be encouraged as the raised intrathoracic pressure causes worsening of right to left shunt. The second stage should be assisted either with forceps or vacuum extraction.

Preterm labour is a major concern because immature foetuses are unlikely to be viable. Management of this scenario includes use of tocolytics such as salbutamol, which causes tachycardia and can precipitate heart failure. Nifedepine and indomethacin are preferred agents to arrest preterm labour.

Caesarean delivery is reserved preferably for obstetric indications, due to the additional risks of general anaesthesia, increased blood loss and postoperative infections.

Oxytocin is the preferred uterotonic drug for postpartum use.

Coronary Artery Disease in Pregnancy

Myocardial ischaemia in pregnancy is a relatively rare occurrence, but the risk is higher during pregnancy than in non-pregnant reproductive age women. Its incidence is expected to increase due to advancing maternal age and increased prevalence of risk factors for coronary artery disease in the population. The physiological changes of increased cholesterol, low density lipoprotein and triglycerides, and reduction in high density lipoproteins during pregnancy contribute. Diagnosis is established by conventional means of ECG and cardiac enzyme analysis.

Initial management consists of low dose aspirin and beta-blockade due to their safety profile. Nitrates and calcium channel blockers are to be used with caution to prevent maternal hypotension. Thrombolysis is a relative contraindication due to the risk of antepartum haemorrhage. Both percutaneous transluminal coronary angioplasty and coronary bypass graft surgery aiming to restore flow to the coronaries have favourable outcomes. Fluoroscopy and cineangiography times should be limited. The foetus should be shielded from direct radiation.

The final trimester poses the highest risk due to haemodynamic changes and the stress of labour. Delivery is preferably delayed by 2–3 weeks after an acute MI with active management of labour to prevent a prolonged second stage of labour.

Cardiac Surgery with Cardiopulmonary Bypass

There is a significant risk of miscarriage and foetal neurological impairment and foetal malformations with cardiopulmonary bypass, though maternal morbidity and mortality is similar to that of the non-pregnant population. The best period for surgery is between the thirteenth-twenty eighth week. Before surgery a full course (at least 24 hours) of corticosteroids should be administered to the mother to aid foetal lung maturation. During cardiopulmonary bypass, foetal heart rate and uterine tone should be monitored in addition to standard patient monitoring. Pump flow >2.5 l/min/m^2 and perfusion pressure >70 mmHg are mandatory to maintain adequate blood flow into the pressure passive uteroplacental bed. Maternal haematocrit >28% is recommended to optimise the oxygen delivery. Normothermic perfusion, when feasible, is advocated, and state of the art pH management is preferred to avoid hypocapnia responsible for uteroplacental vasoconstriction and foetal hypoxia. Cardiopulmonary bypass time should be minimised.

Arrhythmias in Pregnancy

Palpitation is a very common symptom during pregnancy especially in structurally abnormal hearts; about 50% of Holter monitoring recordings demonstrate an abnormal rhythm. Sinus tachycardia is commonest. The management of arrhythmia follows the general principles as for non-pregnant patients, but drug therapy has to consider effects on the foetus and breast feeding.

Table 49.6 gives a list of the common drugs used and their effects during pregnancy.

Deep Vein Thrombosis

Pregnancy is a prothrombotic state; due to stasis in the lower extremity caused by caval compression, there is an increase in vitamin K dependent clotting factors and a reduction in free protein S.

The impact of this thromboembolic state is higher in patients with heart disease due to prosthetic valves, atrial arrhythmias and congenital heart disease with cavopulmonary shunts.

Prophylactic anticoagulation with LMWH should be continued and bridging anticoagulation regimes with unfractionated heparin during labour or operative delivery should be commenced approximately 4–6 hours prior to procedural intervention.

Counselling and Genetic Testing

Mothers with heart disease should be educated about the risks of pregnancy so that they can make an informed decision. Patients with Eisemenger's syndrome should be counselled against pregnancy and if pregnant the option to terminate the pregnancy should be discussed.

Children born to mothers with CVD have a high risk of developing cardiovascular disease, hence genetic testing may be useful, especially in cardiomyopathies and channelopathies such as long QT syndrome. All women with congenital heart disease should be offered foetal echocardiography in the second trimester, and a chorionic villous biopsy around 12 weeks of gestation if indicated.

Learning Points

- Pregnancy causes complex alterations in cardiovascular physiology and the changes tend to persist for about 2 weeks into the postpartum period.
- A single diagnostic investigation requiring radiation exposure does not threaten the well being of the developing foetus.

Table 49.6 Antiarrhythmic drugs used in pregnancy

Drug	Safety in pregnancy	Safety in breastfeeding	Comments
Class I			
Quinidine	Safe	Safe	Can precipitate premature labour
Procainamide	Safe	Safe	Can cause lupus like syndrome, agranulocytosis
Lidocaine	Safe	Safe	Toxicity can cause foetal distress
Flecainide	Safe	Unknown	Has been used, no significant complications reported
Class II: Beta-blockers			
Atenolol	Unsafe	Safe	Avoid atenolol in first trimester as can cause IUGR
Class III			
Amiodarone	Safe	Unsafe	For short term emergency use Can cause IUGR, goitre, foetal hypo/hyperthyroidism
Class IV: Calcium channel blockers			
Verapamil	Safe	Safe	
Diltiazem	Unsafe	Unknown	IUGR, skeletal anomalies, foetal death
Adenosine	Safe	Safe	Lesser dose needed as degradation is slower in pregnancy
Digoxin	Safe	Safe	Can cause miscarriage and foetal death at toxic levels
Atropine	Unknown	Unknown	Used in resuscitation
All antiarrhythmic drugs cross the uteroplacental barrier			

- ECMO should be considered as an option to manage amniotic fluid embolism.
- Pulmonary hypertension is a serious risk factor in pregnancy as it limits the cardiovascular system to mount appropriate adaptive responses to pregnancy and labour with a very high rate of mortality in the first week of the peripartum period.
- All antiarrthymic drugs cross the uteroplacental barrier and careful consideration should be given to the effects on the foetus.

Further Reading

ACOG Committee. Opinion #299: Guidelines for diagnostic imaging during pregnancy. *Obstetrics & Gynecology*. 2004; 104(3).

Diller G-P, Dimopoulos K, Okonko D, et al. Exercise intolerance in adult congenital heart disease: comparative severity, correlates, and prognostic implication. *Circulation*. 2005; 112: 828–835.

Honigberg MC, Givertz MM. Arrhythmias in peripartum cardiomyopathy. *Cardiac Electrophysiology Clinics*. 2015; 7: 309–317.

Kealey AJ. Coronary artery disease and myocardial infarction in pregnancy: a review of epidemiology, diagnosis, and medical and surgical management. *Canadian Journal of Cardiology*. 2010; 26: e185–189.

Magee LA, Pels A, Helewa M, Canadian Hypertensive Disorders of Pregnancy (HDP) Working Group, et al. The hypertensive disorders of pregnancy (29.3). *Best Practice & Research: Clinical Obstetrics & Gynaecology*. 2015; 29: 643–657.

Regitz-Zagrosek V, Gohlke-Bärwolf C, Iung B, Pieper PG. Management of cardiovascular diseases during pregnancy. *Current Problems in Cardiology*. 2014; 39: 85–151.

Regitz-Zagrosek V, Lundqvist CB, Borghi C, et al. ESC Guidelines on the management of cardiovascular diseases during pregnancy. *European Heart Journal*. 2011; 32: 3147–3197.

Savu O, Jurcuţ R, Giuşcă S, et al. Morphological and functional adaptation of the maternal heart during pregnancy. *Circulation: Cardiovascular Imaging*. 2012; 5: 289–297.

Siu SC, Sermer M, Colman JM, et al. Prospective multicenter study of pregnancy outcomes in women with heart disease. *Circulation*. 2001; 104: 515–521.

Tuffnell D, Knight M, Plaat F. Amniotic fluid embolism – an update. *Anaesthesia*. 2011; 66: 3–6.

Weiss BM, von Segesser LK, Alon E, Seifert B, Turina MI. Outcome of cardiovascular surgery and pregnancy: a systematic review of the period 1984–1996. *American Journal of Obstetrics and Gynecology*. 1998; 179: 1643–1653.

MCQs

1. **Cardiovascular disease in pregnancy:**
   (a) Is increasing in prevalence
   (b) Valvular heart disease is commonest
   (c) Congenital heart disease has the highest prevalence in cardiovascular disorders in pregnancy
   (d) There are multiple large cohort trials guiding management of cardiovascular disease in pregnancy
   (e) Complex congenital heart disease in pregnancy is best managed in the community
2. **Cardiovascular physiology in pregnancy:**
   (a) Anaemia in pregnancy is a result of decreased red cell mass
   (b) Systemic vascular resistance increases
   (c) Systolic blood pressure decreases from early pregnancy
   (d) Aortocaval compression by the uterus can be seen from the second trimester
   (e) Cardiac output increases post partum
3. **Pre-eclampsia:**
   (a) Is diagnosed if systolic blood pressure is over 120 mmHg
   (b) Is diagnosed if proteinuria is present
   (c) Home blood pressure monitoring is not a diagnostic tool; it needs to be measured in hospital
   (d) Liberal fluid infusions are the mainstay of treatment for reduced urine output
   (e) Does not present post partum
4. **Peripartum cardiomyopathy:**
   (a) Is unlikely to be diagnosed post partum
   (b) Has a mortality of 30% at 1 year
   (c) Angiotensin converting enzyme inhibitors are the mainstay of treatment during pregnancy
   (d) Unlike pre-eclampsia, twin pregnancy is not a risk factor
   (e) Further pregnancies should be discouraged as there is a high incidence of recurrence
5. **Diagnostics of cardiovascular disease in pregnancy:**
   (a) A radiation dose below 50 mGy to the pregnant mother is the accepted level of radiation below which there is no evidence of increased foetal risk
   (b) Gadolinium ions are known to cross the placental barrier
   (c) Amniotic fluid embolism is an extremely rare but catastrophic event resulting in severe haemodynamic collapse with disseminated intravascular coagulation
   (d) Echocardiography is the preferred mode of imaging of the heart in pregnancy
   (e) All of the above

Exercise answers are available on p.470. Alternatively, take the test online at www.cambridge.org/CardiothoracicMCQ

Section 7

Disease Management in the Cardiothoracic Intensive Care Unit: Incidence; Aetiology; Diagnosis; Prognosis; Treatment

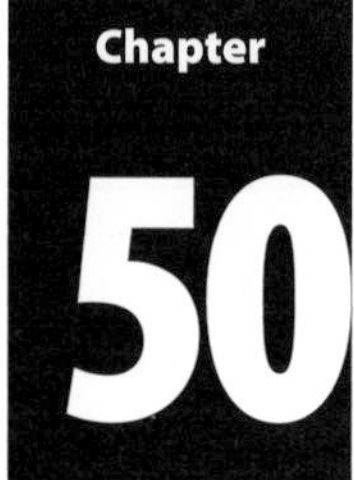

Paediatric Cardiac Intensive Care

Ajay Desai, Lidia Casanueva and Duncan Macrae

Introduction

Cardiovascular disorders are common in critically ill children, accounting for around 30% of the UK annual total of 20,000 paediatric critical care unit admissions. Of these children, over 60% were under 1 year of age and 83% under 5 years of age on admission.

Assessment of the Circulation in Children

Assessment of the circulation in children must include both a rapid 'ABC' safety assessment (Is the airway clear? Is the child breathing adequately? Is there a pulse?), and then a more detailed examination. A child's **appearance** is a good guide to their overall state of wellness. Are they moving normally for their age? Are they lethargic or lacking interest in parents or staff? Are they restless or inconsolable (cerebral hypoxia)? What do the parents think? Assessing **work of breathing (WOB)** is another important part of cardiorespiratory assessment, as it will be increased in the presence of pulmonary oedema which reduces lung compliance. The respiratory rate, the presence of grunting (indicating attempts to maintain lung recruitment), and the presence of intercostal and subcostal retractions, tracheal tug and head bobbing, which all indicate a child has significantly increased WOB, should be observed. **Skin perfusion** should be assessed by determining capillary refill time (<3 seconds after 5 seconds of pressure). Blood pressure, heart rate, respiratory rate and SpO_2 should always be measured as part of the child's initial admission assessment and at appropriate intervals thereafter, taking into account age related normal values (see Table 50.1) and in the case of SpO_2, the expected saturation values for the child's pathology. Understanding the physiology of congenital heart disease is key to its successful management in critical care.

For neonates, as a rule of thumb, mean arterial blood pressure for term (40 weeks' gestation) is 40 mmHg, and proportionately lower with increased prematurity.

Congenital Heart Disease

The incidence of congenital heart disease (CHD) is widely stated to be 8 per 1000 live births. Although rates vary, from region to region, up to 60% of babies with a congenital heart problem are identified antenatally. This is important as an appropriate plan for the care of the newborn infant can be established before birth. In the absence of antenatal detection, many babies with CHD present either immediately after birth or within the first weeks of life. The mode of presentation depends greatly on the nature and severity of the heart defect, and a structured approach to the neonate with CHD is required.

Approach to the Neonate with Suspected CHD

Common Presentations

Cyanosis

Persisting cyanosis after initial resuscitation at birth must be rapidly assessed and managed. The evaluation should assess the infant for airway, pulmonary and circulatory causes of cyanosis, using a logical ABC algorithm (see Table 50.2).

In the absence of major airway or breathing problems, neonatal cyanosis is most likely to be due to CHD or persistent pulmonary hypertension of the

Table 50.1 Normal values for heart rate and blood pressure in children

	Age of child (years)				
	<1	1–2	2–5	5–12	>12
Respiratory rate	30–40	25–35	25–30	20–25	15–20
Heart rate	110–160	100–150	95–140	80–120	60–100
Systolic blood pressure	80–90	85–95	85–100	90–110	100–120

Table 50.2 Common causes of severe cyanosis in the neonate

Airway	Breathing	Circulation
Tracheal anomalies • Tracheal stenosis • Vascular compression	Pneumonia	CHD with decreased pulmonary blood flow • Pulmonary atresia • Tetralogy of Fallot • Tricuspid atresia • Ebstein's anomaly
Choanal atresia • Remember neonates are obligate nose breathers	Congenital lung anomalies • Diaphragmatic hernia • Pulmonary hypoplasia • Congenital lobar emphysema	CHD with diversion of blood • Transposition of the great arteries
Vocal cord paralysis	Phrenic nerve palsy	Persistent pulmonary hypertension of the newborn • May occur in isolation or in association with sepsis, meconium aspiration or other lung anomalies
	Central hypoventilation	

newborn (PPHN), which may occur with or without clear triggers.

At birth, important changes in cardiovascular and respiratory systems must occur for infants to adapt adequately to extrauterine life. In the foetus pulmonary blood flow remains low due to a high pulmonary vascular resistance. At birth as the lungs fill with air, pulmonary vascular resistance should fall rapidly with an 8- to 10-fold rise in pulmonary blood flow ensuring adaption to pulmonary oxygenation of blood. If factors such as meconium aspiration are present, pulmonary vascular resistance may not fall normally, a physiological state described as PPHN. Right to left shunting of blood then continues through foetal channels (the foramen ovale and arterial duct) resulting in systemic cyanosis.

Cyanosis due to congenital heart disease occurs in broad groups of anomalies: firstly those anomalies in which there is obstruction to blood flow to the lungs such as pulmonary atresia and critical pulmonary stenosis, and secondly conditions in which oxygenated blood does not reach the systemic circulation.

Immediate management of the neonate with suspected cyanotic CHD and adequate breathing includes oxygen therapy and the administration of alprostadil (prostaglandin E1) or dinoprostone (prostaglandin E2) to re-establish patency of the arterial duct, which permits flow of blood from the aorta to the pulmonary artery. This will not cause harm even if the cause of the cyanosis is PPHN. Urgent evaluation will include chest X-ray, ECG, and echocardiogram and a hyperoxia test.

If CHD with obstructed pulmonary blood flow is confirmed, prostaglandin infusion should continue until a more definitive pulmonary blood supply is established through surgical or cardiological intervention. Care should be taken to ensure that prostaglandins E1 and E2 are infused at the lowest effective dose, as dose related apnoeas are common at doses >10 ng/kg/minute. Usual starting doses are 5–10 ng/kg/minute; maximum recommended dose for both drugs is 100 ng/kg/minute.

Cardiogenic Shock

Neonates may also present at birth or in the early neonatal period with shock. The differential diagnosis includes sepsis, metabolic disorders, arrhythmias and structural cardiovascular disease. Common structural heart conditions presenting as shock soon after birth include critical aortic stenosis, aortic coarctation and hypoplastic left heart syndrome (HLHS), all of which result in circulatory decompensation when the arterial duct closes. Decompensated babies with aortic coarctation or interrupted aortic arch classically present in shock due to minimal descending aortic blood flow, with raised plasma lactate, weak or absent femoral pulses and right upper limb hypertension. A standard ABC approach to evaluation and resuscitation should be adopted and, as with cyanotic lesions, a prostaglandin E1 or E2 infusion should be started even if the definitive diagnosis has not been established. Care should be taken to minimise FiO_2 in babies with HLHS and other 'single ventricle' lesions, as inadvertent lowering of pulmonary vascular resistance by generous oxygen therapy risks diverting blood away from the systemic circulation (Qs) by increasing pulmonary blood flow (Qp).

Pulmonary Oedema

Neonates with obstructed total anomalous pulmonary venous drainage (TAPVD) may present with severe dyspnoea, hypoxia and circulatory collapse soon after birth. Chest X-ray will show severe pulmonary oedema. Non-cardiac causes of neonatal cardiorespiratory failure must be rapidly ruled out, and echocardiographic examination obtained urgently, although TAPVD can be challenging to diagnose, especially in critically ill ventilated babies.

Other congenital heart lesions also present with pulmonary oedema (see below), although the severity of pulmonary oedema is initially less, and the onset of milder symptoms is more gradual, starting at the age of several weeks or months, rather than at or within days of birth.

Heart Failure and Failure to Thrive

Infants with several common congenital heart lesions, such as ventriculoseptal defect (VSD), atrioventriculoseptal defect (AVSD), large atrial-septal defects (ASD) and rarer conditions such as truncus arteriosus and aortopulmonary window, gradually develop congestive cardiac failure as their pulmonary vascular resistance gradually falls over the first weeks of life. This often presents as tachypnoea, hepatomegaly and failure to thrive. The chest X-ray usually demonstrates cardiomegaly and signs of increased pulmonary blood flow. Echocardiographic examination is required to establish the definitive diagnosis.

Initial management of infants presenting with heart failure, following a rapid 'ABC' assessment, is to start diuretics (frusemide ± spironolactone) and possibly an ACE inhibitor (captopril). Oxygen therapy should be avoided unless the baby presents with cyanosis, as higher inspired oxygen fractions will further lower pulmonary vascular resistance and may worsen cardiac failure. Nasal or facial CPAP or BiPAP is effective in off-loading the left ventricle and is an effective adjunct to diuretics in the acutely decompensated babies with left or congestive heart failure.

Arrhythmia

Babies may develop arrhythmia in utero to the extent that they are compromised before, during and after birth. **Congenital complete heart block** may be relatively well tolerated, or may be associated with foetal hydrops, critically low cardiac output and multiorgan failure. Adrenaline or isoprenaline infusions may be used to increase heart rate temporarily until definitive cardiac pacing is established.

Tachyarrhythmias commonly presenting at birth include atrial flutter and supraventricular tachycardia. Neonates may be severely shocked as a result of fast rhythms and require urgent treatments including cardioversion (atrial flutter), intravenous bolus adenosine (converts or permits diagnosis by transient slowing of heart rate in SVT) and intravenous amiodarone (slows/facilitates return to sinus rhythm in a variety of supraventricular and ventricular tachycardias).

Postoperative Care of the Child Following Cardiac Surgery

Cardiopulmonary bypass in neonates and young children frequently results in a clinically important systemic inflammatory response causing important organ assistant dysfunctions including myocardial depression, acute kidney injury and a loss of capillary integrity leading to generalised extravascular fluid accumulation.

Low cardiac output frequently occurs following cardiac surgery. Common causes include hypovolaemia, myocardial depression and the effects of residual cardiac defects and arrhythmias. A structured approach to the management of low cardiac output is shown in Figure 50.1. As well as clinical and haemodynamic assessment including ECG, careful echocardiograph examination should be undertaken to assess the integrity of the cardiac repair, detect the presence

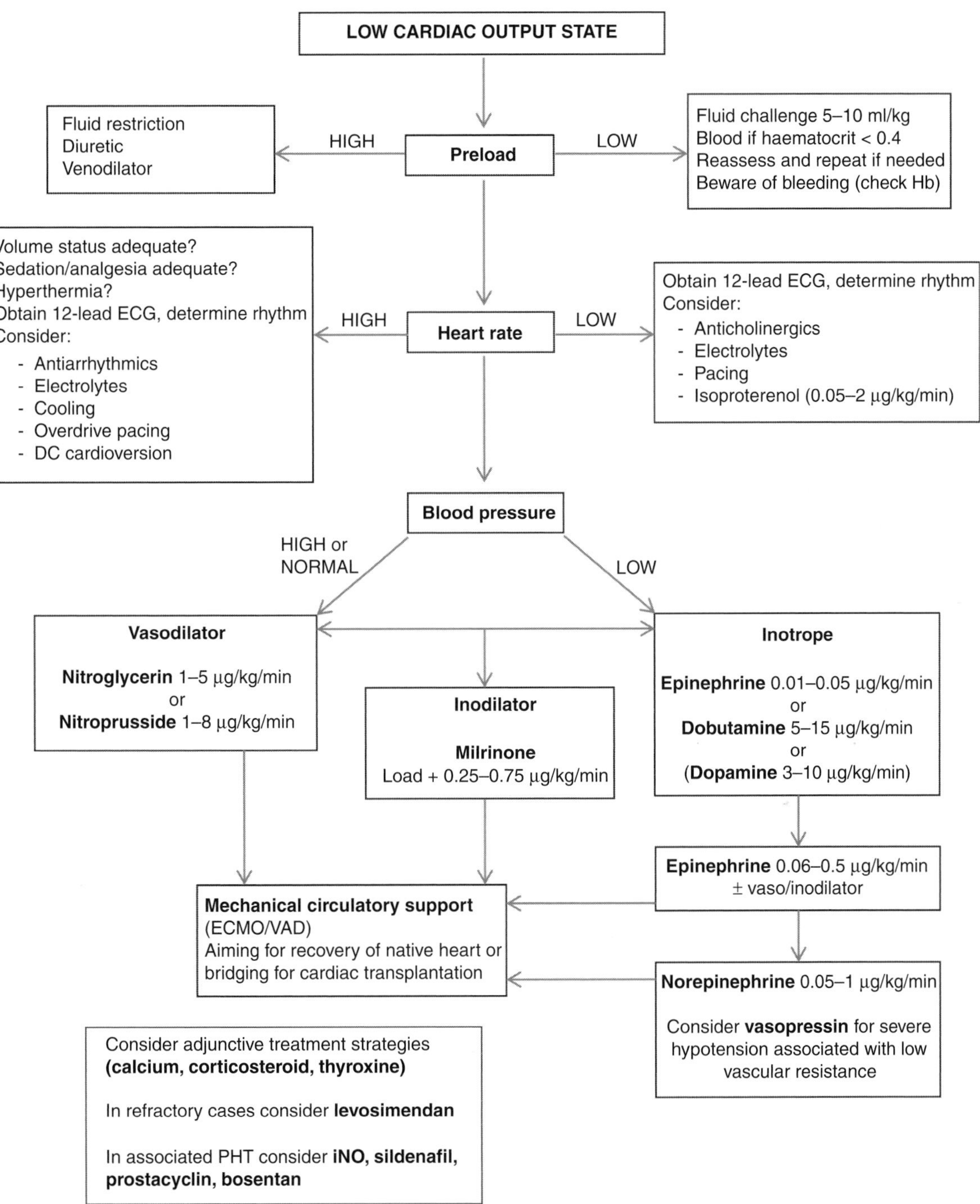

Figure 50.1 Management of a child with low cardiac output state.
Assess Airway, Breathing and Circulation:

- Consider underlying physiology – univentricular versus biventricular circulation
- Correct hypoxia, acidosis, hyperthermia and electrolyte imbalance
- Look for tamponade, residual or unsuspected anatomical or physiological abnormality – perform echocardiography
- Consider need for respiratory support – non-invasive or invasive – beware of vasodilatation and myocardial depression of anaesthesia drugs.

of any residual lesions, provide information on ventricular contractility to guide therapy, and to identify pericardial effusion as a cause of the low output state.

Tamponade and Delayed Sternal Closure

In children as in adults, haemorrhagic pericardial tamponade can cause major haemodynamic instability following cardiac surgery. Haemorrhagic tamponade must be actively prevented by careful surgical haemostasis and normalisation of coagulation. Tamponade must be actively excluded in patients who continue to bleed or who develop unexplained cardiovascular instability following surgery. In neonates and young children, tissue oedema resulting from the systemic inflammatory response may result in swelling of the intrathoracic organs and consequent pressure on the heart with similar effects to haemorrhagic tamponade. For this reason, many surgeons choose to delay sternal closure thereby decompressing the thorax and preventing this complication. The sternum can then be formally closed a few days following surgery once haemodynamic stability is achieved and tissue oedema has subsided.

Pulmonary Circulation and Pulmonary Hypertension

Understanding of the physiology and pharmacology of the right ventricle and pulmonary circulation are crucial to the good management of children with congenital heart disease. A low pulmonary vascular resistance (PVR) is necessary when congenital heart lesions require cavopulmonary connections (see below). Children with uncontrolled pulmonary blood flow from large left-to-right shunts, and those with obstructed pulmonary venous drainage or very high systemic atrial pressures are at risk of developing muscularisation of pulmonary arterioles, raised PVR and high pulmonary artery pressures (PAP). The inflammatory response to CPB may cause temporary elevations in PVR or increased pulmonary vascular reactivity requiring interventions to lower PVR and PAP, as failure to do so will result in acute right ventricle failure with secondary left ventricular failure and cardiovascular collapse.

Simple measures to ensure low PVR include careful pulmonary management. Maintaining lung recruitment, avoiding alveolar hypoxia whilst avoiding lung over-distension all act to minimise PVR. Acidosis, both metabolic and respiratory, and pain also cause PVR to rise. Whilst induced alkalosis is not recommended for the prevention of PHT, brief periods of hyperventilation to lower pCO_2 and raise pH, thereby lowering PVR, can be successful in controlling sudden dangerous rises in PAP/PVR. The aim should be to maintain normal pH and avoid acidosis and inadequate pain relief, which will act to raise PVR/PAP.

Inhaled nitric oxide (iNO) is a specific pulmonary vasodilator and can be extremely effective in lowering PAP/PVR in the postoperative period. Phosphodiesterase 5 inhibitors such as sildenafil may be used as an adjunct to iNO acutely, or for longer term pulmonary vasodilatation. Endothelin receptor blockers and prostacyclin are also effective pulmonary vasodilators most useful in longer term management.

Univentricular Circulations

Some congenital heart lesions are so severe that it is not possible to repair the heart to create two functioning ventricles. An extreme example of this is hypoplastic left heart syndrome (HLHS) in which all of the left heart structures, including the left ventricle, mitral valve, aortic valve and ascending aorta, are extremely small. If only one useful ventricle exists, or if the two ventricles cannot be partitioned, the ventricle(s) must be assigned to the systemic circulation and pulmonary blood flow secured initially with a systemic-pulmonary artery shunt (modified Blalock–Taussig shunt) or temporary ventricle-pulmonary artery conduit. The aim of this initial palliation is to enable the child to grow, and also allow time for the natural postnatal fall in pulmonary vascular resistance to occur, as low PVR is essential for progression down the 'univentricular' pathway.

Initial Palliation of the Univentricular Circuit

In neonates with systemic-pulmonary artery shunts, the pulmonary and systemic circulations are both fed by the systemic ventricle. The flow of blood to the lungs is limited by the resistance of the shunt, and also the pulmonary vascular resistance. The systemic blood flow is determined by any anatomical factors (e.g. residual aortic obstruction) and the systemic vascular resistance (SVR). The balance of these factors determines the balance of blood flow between the systemic and pulmonary circuits. If PVR is low and the Blalock shunt is large, pulmonary blood flow will be excessive at the expense of systemic blood flow. Postoperatively, intensivists may have to intervene, particularly with measures to raise the lower PVR or SVR to achieve the required balanced circulation. Measurement of the saturation of blood in the superior vena cava and the arterial blood enable a crude estimate of the Qp:Qs ratio to be determined, the aim being a ratio of 1:1 which, with normal cardiac output and oxygen extraction, typically results in a systemic saturation of 75–80%. High saturations (>85%) in shunted babies strongly suggest excessive Qp (Qp:Qs > 1). Babies with unexpectedly low saturations after shunt procedures may have high PVR and/or low cardiac output but must always be investigated for shunt patency and function: is the shunt blocked? Is the shunt too small or compromised in some way?

Superior Cavopulmonary Connection

At around 4–6 months of age, babies with palliated (i.e. shunted) univentricular circulations typically undergo a superior cavopulmonary connection or 'bi-directional Glenn' procedure. In this operation the SVC is disconnected from the atrium and anastomosed to a central pulmonary artery. SVC return now flows directly to the lungs without any cardiac assist. For this 'cavopulmonary' circulation to succeed, the baby must have a low PVR and the systemic ventricle must function well and specifically have a competent systemic AV valve, and low systemic atrial pressure. After a Glenn shunt, the SVC pressure is the upstream pulmonary artery pressure, whilst the systemic atrial pressure, directly measured or inferred from measurement of femoral vein pressure, gives the transpulmonary pressure gradient (TPG). A TPG gradient of <10 mmHg is entirely satisfactory, typically giving a PA/SVC pressure of 12–15 mmHg (TPG + systemic atrial pressure). Pulmonary blood flow is maximised by reducing the mean intrathoracic pressure generated by positive pressure ventilation. Spontaneous breathing improves venous return to the thorax and should be encouraged as early as possible in postoperative children with cavopulmonary circulations. Alkalosis, easily induced by injudicious hyperventilation, has been shown to reduce flow in the superior cavopulmonary shunt as a result of cerebral vasoconstriction. Positive pressure ventilation in children with superior cavopulmonary connections should therefore be carefully delivered to avoid excessive intrathoracic pressure and respiratory alkalosis, although in doing so loss of lung volume through failure to apply adequate PEEP must also be avoided. Hypovolaemia is poorly tolerated in cavopulmonary patients, as it is the hydraulic gradient across the lungs, which drives blood from the SVC to the systemic atrium. Arterial saturations after a Glenn shunt are usually in the 80–85% range. Saturations below 75% are inadequate and require careful investigation to determine the cause, which might include compromise of the surgical shunt or elevated PVR.

Total Cavopulmonary Connection

The final stage of palliation for 'single ventricle' circulations is the completion of the cavopulmonary pathway by connecting inferior vena caval blood to the pulmonary artery in what is often referred to as a 'Fontan completion' or total cavopulmonary connection' (TCPC) operation. This is typically done in early childhood and results in normal or near normal systemic oxygenation despite the presence of only one effective ventricle. Post procedure, Fontan patients tolerate hypovolaemia or factors raising PVR poorly, as blood must flow passively across the lungs driven by central venous/pulmonary artery pressure alone. Early postoperative hypotension in Fontan patients usually responds well to volume augmentation although care should also be taken to ensure that ventricular function is adequate, and the ventricle supported appropriately with inotropes if required.

Mechanical Circulatory Support in Children

Mechanical circulatory support, usually venoarterial ECMO, plays an important role in the management of children with very severe circulatory failure in the cardiac intensive care unit. Indications include:

- Failure to separate from intraoperative cardiopulmonary bypass;
- Severe postoperative low cardiac output syndrome;
- Cardiac arrest not responding promptly to standard resuscitation;
- Severe heart failure as a bridge to transplantation or recovery.

Several key factors are important in achieving good outcomes from paediatric cardiac ECMO support. ECMO is a complex and costly technique, and should only be considered when children are not responding adequately to conventional support measures. Its deployment must be timely, and not delayed beyond the point where recovery of the heart or other organs is no longer probable. Perioperative support should be considered in children with severe but potentially recoverable myocardial dysfunction, or where bridging to cardiac transplantation, perhaps with later implantation of a long-term ventricular assist device, is possible.

Several technical aspects are necessary to achieve excellent outcomes. Good ECMO cannula position is key to obtaining ECMO flows and therefore organ system support. Cardiac decompression lowers myocardial oxygen consumption, facilitating myocardial recovery, and decompresses the systemic atrium, preventing pulmonary oedema or haemorrhage, and must be assured at the initiation of ECMO. Left (or systemic) atrial decompression can be achieved in a number of ways including supplementary direct left atrial cannulation or percutaneous creation of an interatrial communication. Bleeding is particularly challenging during cardiac extracorporeal life support (ECLS) in postoperative children. Meticulous surgical haemostasis and cannulation, together with careful monitoring of heparin administration, and clotting parameters, must be ensured.

International figures show that approximately 40% of children receiving cardiac ECMO survive to ICU discharge. Acute fulminant myocarditis, once considered a fatal disease, is associated with 60–80% chance of myocardial recovery with ECMO support. Conversely, patients with single ventricle physiology, especially those supported after the Norwood procedure, have relatively poor outcomes, with 20–25% chance of survival to PICU discharge.

ELSO have published standards, training material and supported many publications to which interested readers are referred (www.elso.org).

Common Complications

Bleeding

The management of bleeding following cardiac surgery in children differs little from that in adults.

Cardiac Tamponade

The occurrence of and management of haemorrhagic pericardial tamponade is managed as in adults: timely detection on clinical suspicion, confirmed if possible by echocardiogram, and re-exploration of the chest to evacuate clot and secure haemostasis.

Cardiac tamponade can also occur in children, especially neonates and infants, who may develop a significant inflammatory response following CPB, resulting in swelling of tissues including the intrathoracic organs and tissues resulting in 'tissue tamponade'. To prevent tissue tamponade, surgeons can elect to delay sternal closure, stenting the two sides of the sternum apart, undertaking closure once the inflammatory response has ebbed and cardiovascular stability is assured.

Arrhythmia

Common arrhythmias following cardiac surgery in children include slow and fast rhythms.

Slow Rhythms

There is a higher risk of partial or complete AV block during surgery on or near the ventricular septum or AV node. Complete AV block requires AV sequential pacing at an appropriate rate via temporary atrial and ventricular wires. Sinus rhythm may return but, beyond 10 days, implantation of a permanent pacing system is indicated.

Fast Rhythms

Junctional ectopic tachycardia (JET or His bundle tachycardia) occurs relatively commonly in children following surgery near the conducting system. Typically this rhythm 'warms up', that is the heart rate gradually rises as P waves become indistinct. Classically, the ECG will show that the ventricular rate exceeds the atrial rate with AV dissociation. Cardiac output is usually compromised in fast rhythms, and measures to control the rate usually include: (i) inducing moderate hypothermia (34–35 °C) to slow the ventricular rate and/or intavenous amiodarone, (ii) atrial or AV sequential pacing once the ventricular rate has slowed sufficiently. JET resolves after several days. Long-term antiarrhythmic control is not usually required.

Atrial fibrillation and malignant ventricular rhythms, although seen occasionally, are far less common following cardiac surgery in children than in adults.

Residual Lesions

Despite the best efforts of cardiologists and surgeons, children may fail to progress smoothly following surgery due to residual lesions. Any child whose postoperative course deviates from the expected course must be urgently re-evaluated clinically, further imaging undertaken (echocardiography, cardiac CT, CMR) and where indicated cardiac catheterisation performed.

Acute Kidney Injury

Transient perturbation of renal function is relatively common in neonates and young infants following cardiac surgery on CPB, and in any sick child with critically low systemic perfusion. Peritoneal dialysis is very effective in providing renal replacement therapy (RRT) in this age group. Although rarely needed, RRT in older children is undertaken using continuous venovenous haemofiltration.

CNS

Transient seizures or brain imaging anomalies are surprisingly common in neonates and infants before and after cardiac surgery. Whilst their prognosis is generally good, children with minor problems require close neurodevelopmental follow-up, whilst children developing infarcts, hypoxic ischaemic encephalopathy or intracranial bleeds require multidisciplinary postoperative management and specialist follow-up.

Phrenic Nerve Injury and Diaphragmatic Paralysis

The phrenic nerves run across the pericardium and may be injured or transected during cardiac surgery resulting in temporary or permanent paralysis of the associated hemidiaphragm. Paralysis of one hemidiaphragm is well tolerated in most adults and in children over 2 years of age. Neonates and infants do not have a well-developed intercostal-rib inspiratory system, and often fail to separate from mechanical respiratory support in the presence of a paralysed hemidiaphragm. Undertaking plication of the hemidiaphragm stabilises the base of the thorax, preventing paradoxical displacement of the affected lung during inspiration, improving inspiratory efficiency to a sufficient degree to facilitate ventilator weaning.

Chylous Effusions and Chylothorax

Postoperative chylothorax in its 'pure' form results from damage to a major lymphatic vessel at surgery, resulting in chyle accumulating in the affected pleural space. More commonly what is termed 'chylothorax' results from accumulation of lymph-rich pleural effusions due to overspill as the lymphatic system is overloaded, or lymphatic drainage is impeded by high systemic venous pressures (often seen in cavopulmonary circulations) of venous thrombosis.

Chylothorax is managed by diagnosing that the effusion is indeed chylous (white cells of fluid >85% lymphocytes). A potential cause for the problem should be sought, and adverse factors corrected if possible, or reoperation is required if the loss is clearly surgical in origin. Medical management includes as a first step, a diet severely limiting long chain fatty acids, replacing these with medium chain fats which are not transported by the lymphatic system. Further steps to reduce chyle production include nil-by-mouth with total parenteral nutrition and low-dose vasopressin infusion. If chylous effusions persist long-term, consideration should be given to performing a surgical pleuradhesis.

Learning Points

- Immediate management of the neonate with suspected cyanotic CHD and adequate breathing includes oxygen therapy and the administration of prostaglandin E1 or E2. There are no absolute contraindications to initiate prostaglandin therapy, although it may worsen the pulmonary oedema associated with obstructed total anomalous pulmonary venous return.
- Low cardiac output syndrome (LCOS) affects up to 25% of neonates and young children after cardiac surgery. Residual cardiac lesions, even when minor, may also adversely impact the postoperative course.
- Postoperative complete atrioventricular block, if it persists beyond 10 days, indicates implantation of a permanent pacing system.
- Hypovolaemia is poorly tolerated in cavopulmonary patients. After a Glenn shunt, a transpulmonary pressure gradient (TPG) of <10 mmHg is satisfactory, typically giving a PA/SVC pressure of 12–15 mmHg.
- The ICU survival rates are approximately 40% for children receiving cardiac ECMO. Whilst the ICU survival rates are relatively poorer (20–25%) for single ventricle physiology patients supported on ECMO, the chances of myocardial recovery on ECMO support are better for patients with acute fulminant myocarditis (60–80%).

Further Reading

Barr FE, Macrae D. Inhaled nitric oxide and related therapies. *Pediatric Critical Care Medicine*. 2010; 11(2 Suppl): S30–S36.

Brunner N, de Jesus Perez VA, Richter A, et al. Perioperative pharmacological management of pulmonary hypertensive crisis during congenital heart surgery. *Pulmonary Circulation*. 2014; 4: 10–24.

Chaturvedi RR, Macrae D, Brown KL, et al. Cardiac ECMO for biventricular hearts after paediatric open heart surgery. *Heart*. 2004; 90: 545–551.

Friedman AH, Fahey JT. The transition from fetal to neonatal circulation: normal responses and implications for infants with heart disease. *Seminars in Perinatology*. 1993; 17: 106–121.

Hallidie-Smith KA. Prostaglandin E1 in suspected ductus dependent cardiac malformation. *Archives of Disease in Childhood*. 1984; 59: 1020–1026.

Hoskote A, Li J, Hickey C, Erickson S. The effects of carbon dioxide on oxygenation and systemic, cerebral, and pulmonary vascular hemodynamics after the bidirectional superior cavopulmonary anastomosis. *Journal of the American College of Cardiology*. 2004; 44: 1501–1509.

Li S, Krawczeski CD, Zappitelli M, for the TRIBE-AKI Consortium. Incidence, risk factors, and outcomes of acute kidney injury after pediatric cardiac surgery: a prospective multicenter study. *Critical Care Medicine*. 2011; 39: 1493–1499.

Panthongviriyakul C, Bines JE. Post-operative chylothorax in children: an evidence-based management algorithm. *Journal of Paediatrics and Child Health*. 2008; 44: 716–721.

Penny DJ, Shekerdemian LS. Management of the neonate with symptomatic congenital heart disease. *Archives of Disease in Childhood. Fetal and Neonatal Edition*. 2001; 84: 141–145.

Talwar S, Patel K, Juneja R, Choudhary SK, Airan B. Early postoperative arrhythmias after pediatric cardiac surgery. *Asian Cardiovascular and Thoracic Annals*. 2015; 23: 795–801.

Tibby SM, Brock G, Marsh MJ, et al. Haemodynamic monitoring in critically ill children. *Care of the Critically Ill*. 1997; 13: 86–89.

Wernovsky G, Wypij D, Jonas RA, et al. Postoperative course and hemodynamic profile after the arterial switch operation in neonates and infants: a comparison of low-flow cardiopulmonary bypass and circulatory arrest. *Circulation*. 1995; 92: 2226–2235.

MCQs

True or False

1. Suspected total anomalous pulmonary venous drainage (TAPVD) in a blue baby is a contraindication for starting prostaglandin E1 or E2 therapy.
2. Hyperoxia test reliably distinguishes between congenital cyanotic heart disease and PPHN.
3. Cardioversion is the treatment of choice for neonatal atrial flutter.
4. In a neonate following Norwood operation with a modified BT shunt, systemic saturations in the 90s is highly desirable.
5. Match the following drugs and their mechanisms of action in treating pulmonary hypertension:

(a) Inhaled nitric oxide	1. cAMP pathway mediated vasodilation
(b) Bosantan	2. Nitric oxide synthase (NOS) pathway
(c) Sildenafil	3. Phosphodiesterase 5 inhibitor
(d) Prostacyclin	4. Endothelin receptor antagonist
(e) Arginine	5. Phosphodiesterase 3 inhibitor

Exercise answers are available on p.470. Alternatively, take the test online at www.cambridge.org/CardiothoracicMCQ

Chapter 51

Grown-up Congenital Heart Disease (GUCH) Patients in the Cardiothoracic Intensive Care Unit

Susanna Price and Niki Walker

Introduction

The numbers of patients with congenital heart disease (CHD) surviving to adulthood are increasing due to advances in both surgical and interventional cardiological techniques. In the USA it is estimated that >10 × 10^6 adult patients have CHD (grown-up congenital heart disease, GUCH), and in the UK the number of adult patients with moderate-severe lesions is predicted to increase by approximately 1600 per annum. The commonest indication for reintervention in GUCH is for treatment of dysrhythmia; however, this only rarely directly demands intensive care admission.

Most GUCH patients requiring ongoing medical and critical care attention are at the more severe end of the disease spectrum, requiring repeated interventions to replace valves or conduits, and to address persistent/worsening haemodynamic compromise. Critical care of the adult GUCH patient can be extremely challenging, as the pathophysiology of the patient may be complex, and response to usual intensive care interventions unpredictable or even harmful. In such patients, morbidity and mortality have been shown to increase with increasing complexity of disease; therefore expert advice should be sought, particularly at the complex end of the spectrum. Although recommendations are that critically ill GUCH patients be managed in specialist centres, where they present with medical emergencies, there may be insufficient time to transfer for treatment. Thus all cardiothoracic intensivists should have the knowledge and skills to assess and manage these patients whilst seeking expert advice.

This chapter will outline the general principles involved in the care of the critically ill GUCH patient, particularly where they differ from those of the general population. In addition, some of the commonly occurring medical presentations that any intensivist may face will be addressed, together with management of the postoperative GUCH patient.

Principles of Management of the GUCH Patient on the ICU

General Principles

Patients are generally classified as having simple, moderately complex and complex congenital heart disease according to the Canadian Consensus definitions, with increasing complexity of disease associated with higher ICU interventions, morbidity and mortality. Approaching such patients when critically ill demands application of a number of basic principles. The first principle of GUCH ICU management is to understand the cardiopulmonary anatomy of the individual patient. This involves knowledge of the primary lesion, the type of any corrective/palliative surgery or intervention performed, and the presence of any residual haemodynamic lesions – either dynamic or fixed. Second, an understanding of the normal physiology of the patient is essential. This includes the normal haemoglobin, oxygen saturations, systemic and pulmonary blood pressure and surface electrocardiogram. Third, the ICU clinician must consider how the effects of any supportive and therapeutic interventions might affect the circulation. This is of particular importance in the univentricular heart, in the presence of systemic-pulmonary shunts and in the Fontan circulation. In GUCH patients (particularly where complex) performance of relatively simple investigations and interventions may differ from those in the non-GUCH population. In addition to the basic

Table 51.1 General considerations in the critically ill GUCH patient

Pulmonary/respiratory	Cardiovascular	Renal, GI, endocrine, fluids
Difficult intubation: multiple GUCH lesions associated with difficult intubation	Absent or abnormal connections expected, i.e. Fontan or TCPC, or unexpected, i.e. persistent LSVC	May have associated asplenia, GI or renal malformations
Associated congenital pulmonary disease: i.e. hypoplastic lung/lung tissue/ severe congenital V/Q mismatch	Multiple previous arterial/venous cannulations, difficult vascular access – ultrasound may be essential	Renal impairment is common, particularly in cyanotic patients, and is associated with increased mortality
Lung reperfusion injury: ARDS-like picture (unilateral/bilateral) may occur	Air filters on all lines in patients with potential for right-left shunting	Severe right heart failure may necessitate low rates of enteral feeding where cardiac output is borderline
Difficulty weaning: associated congenital musculoskeletal deformities	Cardiac output measurement • Output from the right and left heart may differ – shunt • May be no PA, or right sided connection – PA catheters unusable • Oesophageal Doppler – calibration depends upon aortic dimensions	Abnormal liver function is common, and associated with increased postoperative mortality post cardiac surgery
Previous cardiac surgery: possible phrenic nerve palsy	Transvenous pacing, may have no access to the heart from the venous circulation (e.g. Fontan circulation)	High incidence of abnormal thyroid function in GUCH patients – associated with increased ICU mortality
Difficult tracheostomy: presence of collaterals, abnormal neck/trachea	ECG, atrial re-entry tachycardia may mimic sinus tachycardia, comparison with previous ECGs essential	Tolerance of fluid loading varies depending on the underlying diagnosis, i.e. TV repair versus Fontan/TCPC
Pulmonary hypertension: may need treating, care where possibility to shunt bidirectionally	Differential effects of vasoactive drugs on pulmonary and systemic vasculature may have unpredictable effects on CO and saturations	Patients with preoperative erythrocytosis may require higher haemoglobin levels postoperatively than is generally accepted on the ICU

Abbrevations: TCPC total cavopulmonary connection; LSVC left superior vena cava; GI gastrointestinal; V/Q ventilation/perfusion; ARDS adult respiratory distress syndrome; PA pulmonary artery; ICU intensive care unit; ECG electrocardiogram; TV tricuspid valve.

anatomy and physiology, there are further aspects relevant to ICU care that must be considered in this patient population (Table 51.1).

In all patients, close liaison between specialists in GUCH, heart failure, congenital cardiac surgery and echocardiography is crucial as the management of such patients demands a multidisciplinary approach.

The Cyanotic Patient

Cyanotic congenital heart disease is not a contraindication to ICU admission as such patients may have a relatively good prognosis, with mortality generally related to the admission diagnosis. The cyanotic patient has adaptive mechanisms to increase oxygen delivery, including a rightward shift in the oxyhaemoglobin dissociation curve, an increase in cardiac output, and an increased haematocrit. The resultant erythrocytosis may result in the hyperviscosity syndrome; however routine venesection is not recommended, and iron deficiency in these patients is common. Haemostatic changes including abnormalities of prothrombin time, partial thromboplastin time, factors V, VII, VIIII, IX and thrombocytopenia have been documented, but will not usually require treatment. When assessing the cyanotic patient, citrate bottles adjusted for the haematocrit must be used.

Renal dysfunction is common and occurs due to the combination of hyperviscosity with arteriolar vasoconstriction, resulting in renal hypoperfusion and progressive glomerulosclerosis, manifesting as proteinuria, hyperuricaemia or varying degrees of renal failure. Where a cyanotic patient is admitted with abnormal neurology, headache or is postictal, a high index of suspicion should exist for intracerebral thrombosis, haemorrhage or abscess. Where intravenous contrast is used, the patient must be well hydrated, and the minimal amount of contrast used as possible, as there is the potential to develop marked hyperkalaemia following administration.

The Failing Morphological Right Ventricle

The morphological right ventricle (RV) may be subpulmonary, subaortic or be the only effective ventricle in the univentricular heart. Causes of right ventricular dysfunction include previous cardiac surgery, pulmonary hypertension, Ebstein's anomaly, a significant shunt, systemic RV and volume overload. The subpulmonary failing RV may be supported using standard inotropic agents whilst avoiding pulmonary vasoconstrictors. Cardiac output may be maintained or improved by minimising RV afterload: minimising ventilator pressures, drainage of pleural collections, bronchodilation, the use of pulmonary vasodilators and early extubation.

Where the morphological RV is systemic (congenitally corrected transposition of the great arteries (ccTGA) and transposition of the great arteries (TGA) with Mustard/Senning) and failing, treatment is challenging. Reversible causes (including arrhythmia and volume overload) should be aggressively sought and treated. Although systemic RV fibrosis is common, the coronary arteries are usually angiographically unobstructed. Standard management of the failing systemic ventricle should be used, including pharmacological and mechanical support, but these may not be effective. In some centres the use of multisite RV pacing has been used with good effect.

The Univentricular Heart

This presents many challenges, from prevention of air embolism, to the unpredictability of the effects of vasoactive agents and the adverse effects of positive pressure ventilation. It is important to know the current and most previously documented function of the single ventricle (morphologically right or left), as recent rapid deterioration is often due to development of an arrhythmia. Expert echocardiography is indicated. When considering the use of inotropic and vasoactive agents, the nature of the pulmonary connections must be considered. Where the pulmonary vasculature is protected by PA banding, the relative effects of pulmonary versus systemic constriction or dilatation may be different when compared with where there is an absent pulmonary connection with systemic-pulmonary collaterals/shunts. In the patient with absent pulmonary connection and systemic-pulmonary collaterals/shunts a small increase in PVR may result in a significant reduction in pulmonary blood flow and desaturation. In contrast, an increase in SVR and/or a fall in PVR may result in an increase in systemic-pulmonary shunting with fall in cardiac output. Attention should also be paid to oxygen administration, as this may also alter the balance between pulmonary and systemic circulation.

Medical Indications for ICU Admission in the GUCH Patient

Mortality in GUCH patients requiring ICU admission for medical indications (excluding arrhythmia) is high (36%) and accurately predicted by the APACHE II score. Where the indication for admission is non-cardiological, the principles of management of the admission diagnosis are the same as for the non-GUCH population.

Arrhythmia

The commonest indication for hospital admission in the GUCH population is arrhythmia, and on occasion this will require ICU admission, or input from the critical care team. The management of arrhythmia in the ACHD ICU population is complex; however some general principles should be considered. First, the diagnosis of an arrhythmia may be challenging; atrial tachycardia may mimic sinus tachycardia to the non-expert. Here, comparison with previous 12-lead ECGs is useful, and where a pacemaker is implanted, interrogation may be critical in making the diagnosis. Second, as there is a high incidence of thyroid dysfunction and amiodarone prescription in the GUCH population, thyroid function tests should be performed upon diagnosis of a tachycardia or bradycardia. Third, although patients with a univentricular circulation in atrial tachycardia may tolerate a tachyarrhythmia well initially, decompensation may be rapid, and cardioversion should be considered at the earliest opportunity. Such patients should be managed by the most senior clinician, as cardioversion to a malignant arrhythmia is not uncommon, and as there may be no venous access to the heart. Transcutaneous pacing must always be available.

Heart Failure

The causes of heart failure in the GUCH population include one or more of: impaired ventricular function (left or right), volume overload, arrhythmia, valve lesions or an excessive shunt. Once an arrhythmia has been excluded, echocardiography is required to make or confirm the diagnosis. Where indicated, urgent surgical or catheter intervention may be required. Pre-optimisation of cardiac output prior to surgery has not been shown to improve patient survival, but if possible pulmonary oedema and sepsis should be treated prior to any run on bypass. Once surgically or catheter-directed correctable causes have been excluded, management is directed to treating ventricular dysfunction.

Haemoptysis

Haemoptysis in this population – particularly those with pulmonary hypertension – should always be considered a serious event, and early transfer to high level care with advanced airway skills immediately available is important. Minor haemoptysis may herald a major bleed, and patients with major haemoptysis usually die due to their unprotected airway rather than blood loss. Haemoptysis in the GUCH population has been attributed to bronchitis, bleeding diathesis, pulmonary arterial rupture, pulmonary embolism, tracheoarterial fistula (in prolonged intubation or tracheostomy) and rupture of aortopulmonary collaterals. In patients with Eisenmenger physiology, haemoptysis accounts for 11–15% of deaths. Investigation will depend upon the skills available locally, but would normally include plain chest radiography, CT angiography and angiography, with a view to embolisation, where it may be life saving.

Endocarditis

The diagnosis of endocarditis requires physicians to have a high index of suspicion, the performance of multiple blood cultures, and expert echocardiography. Echocardiography to exclude evidence of infection in this patient population is particularly challenging as it may not be confined to intracardiac structures. On occasion nuclear medicine (PET CT) and/or cardiac magnetic resonance scanning may give further indication as to the site of infection. Multidisciplinary team working, including the endocarditis team, is essential at an early stage following diagnosis.

Surgical/Postoperative Admissions in GUCH

The majority of GUCH patients requiring ICU admission will be postoperative. Here the mortality relates to the complexity of the underlying disease; however, unlike in medical GUCH admissions, standard scoring systems do not reflect the severity of illness of the patients as they tend to overestimate mortality in those with more simple disease, and underestimate predicted mortality in those with more complex disease. In specialist centres perioperative mortality and morbidity is low, but increases significantly with increasing disease complexity, and in the presence of preoperative abnormalities in renal, liver or thyroid function. As in the paediatric population, haemodynamically significant residual lesions postoperatively are associated with a significantly increased ICU morbidity. Good postoperative management relies on a clear understanding of not only the underlying disease, but also the precise surgical procedure and outcome, and also the haemodynamic responses of the patient in the operating theatre. Close liaison with and detailed handover from the operating surgeon and cardiac anaesthetist are essential.

Simple Congenital Heart Disease

Atrial Septal Defect (ASD)

The treatment of choice for closure of ASDs is percutaneous device closure; however, some large or complex defects will require surgical closure. Although in the younger patient population the procedure is well tolerated, there is a high incidence of postoperative arrhythmia. Pulmonary hypertension recorded preoperatively may not resolve immediately, but in the presence of an adequate cardiac output may not require treatment. The more elderly patient may have restrictive ventricular disease, which limits cardiac output. Where diagnosed, pacing should be optimised using echocardiography and continuous cardiac output monitoring (usually avoiding right heart catheterisation) to optimise the cardiac output and may require heart rates of up to 130 beats per minute.

Moderately Complex Congenital Heart Disease

Atrioventricular Septal Defect (AVSD)

Complete AVSD repair is usually performed in childhood; however, some adults may present with partial defects requiring surgical repair. Here the most important determinant of outcome is a successful surgical repair – in particular ensuring the absence of left ventricular outflow tract obstruction (LVOTO).

Where a patient has inadequate cardiac output postoperatively, in addition to exclusion of the usual postoperative complications, LVOTO should specifically be excluded using echocardiography.

Tetralogy of Fallot (TOF)

Patients admitted postoperatively with a diagnosis of TOF will either have undergone redo-surgery (usually pulmonary valve replacement) or, less frequently, primary repair. Although primary repair in the adult population is associated with significant ICU morbidity, even redo-surgery for pulmonary valve replacement should not be regarded as 'routine'. Complications and morbidity are usually associated with right ventricular dysfunction. However, significant left ventricular dysfunction may coexist, particularly in the presence of coronary artery disease. In patients undergoing primary repair the increased pulmonary blood flow may result in pulmonary capillary hyperpermeability, presenting with an ARDS-like picture, and managed as is standard for acute lung injury post-bypass.

Ebstein's Anomaly

The postoperative course of these patients is determined by the amount and function of the postoperative RV, meticulous intraoperative management (surgical and anaesthetic), and the technical expertise of the surgeon. Where there is significant RV dysfunction, this should be managed in the standard way. Significant postoperative RV dysfunction is associated with a high incidence of renal, gastrointestinal and hepatic dysfunction, and a significant requirement for prolonged respiratory support. If the cardiac output is inadequate despite all measures and an intra-atrial communication does not exist, atrial fenestration may be considered in the absence of significant left ventricular disease. The postoperative Ebstein's patient has a high incidence of atrial arrhythmias and these should be managed in collaboration with an electrophysiologist.

Complex Congenital Heart Disease

Congenitally Corrected Transposition of the Great Arteries (ccTGA)

Surgery in this patient population usually relates to requirement for tricuspid valve replacement (the systemic atrioventricular valve) due to regurgitation. In such cases, the added burden of significant volume overload on the systemic morphologically RV may result in significant ventricular dysfunction postoperatively (The Failing Morphological Right Ventricle). Where required in the postoperative period, mechanical circulatory support may be considered whilst the RV recovers from the surgical insult. Where associated with a small left (subpulmonary) ventricle, either with or without a LV-PA conduit, care must be taken to avoid left LVOTO as a result of inotropic support required for the RV. Here, aortic balloon counterpulsation may be useful by providing systemic RV support and minimising the need for inotropic administration.

Transposition of the Great Arteries (TGA)

Patients admitted to the ICU following surgery for TGA will have undergone either a Rastelli procedure (physiologically normal communications), Mustard/Senning (systemic RV, subpulmonary LV) or arterial switch (normal connections). The postoperative management of these patients illustrates the importance of understanding the underlying anatomy, surgery and physiology of the ACHD patient.

In a Rastelli procedure, the normal ventriculoarterial connections are restored, and adult patients are generally admitted following redo-surgery for conduit replacement. In patients with previous Mustard/Senning procedures the systemic ventricle remains morphologically a RV – thus postoperatively these patients have a higher incidence of ventricular dysfunction and have a greater requirement for cardiorespiratory support. Where patients undergo surgery for systemic baffle revision for baffle obstruction, chronic venous hypertension results in hepatic and renal dysfunction, which does not resolve immediately, and is associated with significant postoperative morbidity in some cases. In an arterial switch procedure, the ventriculoarterial connections are anatomically normal; however, late complications in adulthood include requirement for aortic or pulmonary valve replacement, and ventricular dysfunction due to coronary disruption. In these patient populations, postoperative recovery is generally uneventful, and does not significantly differ from standard post-cardiac surgical care.

Systemic-Pulmonary Shunt

Patients with either central or Blalock–Taussig type aortopulmonary shunts rely on systemic arterial pressure to maintain pulmonary blood flow via the shunt. In such patients, pulmonary blood flow may be reduced by aggressive ventilatory manoeuvres but the major determinant of pulmonary blood flow remains systemic aortic pressure, and therefore desaturation may require the use of systemic vasoconstriction.

GUCH patients previously palliated with either classical or modified Blalock–Taussig shunts will exhibit reduced arterial pressure in the ipsilateral arm, ranging from slight under-reading compared to aortic pressure to almost impalpable arm pulses.

Fontan and Fontan-Type Circulations

Surgery undertaken in this patient population is usually elective, comprising conversion from atriopulmonary Fontan to total cavopulmonary circulation (TCPC). The physiological effects of a univentricular circulation together with systemic venous hypertension over years in these adult patients present challenges to the intensivist in their postoperative management. Having a prolonged univentricular circulation results in ventricular dysfunction that should be managed using standard supportive measures (inodilators, pacing, mechanical support). Arrhythmias are common, and may be difficult to diagnose, particularly when temporary epicardial pacing is undertaken postoperatively. Where there is any haemodynamic disturbance an ECG (including atrial leads) should be performed. Prevention of atrial arrhythmias is important, as they will significantly reduce cardiac output in these patients, with close attention to electrolytes, early administration of amiodarone and cardioversion where indicated.

The passive flow of blood from the systemic venous circulation to the pulmonary circulation depends upon adequate preload and avoidance of pulmonary hypertension. When the patient is mechanically ventilated, positive pressure significantly reduces cardiac output. Thus, in order to maximise cardiac output, pulmonary vascular resistance and intrathoracic pressure should be kept as low as possible, with aggressive drainage of pleural collections, avoidance of pulmonary vasoconstrictors, treatment of bronchoconstriction, pulmonary vasodilators, minimising ventilator pressure settings and extubation as early as the patient allows. Respiratory failure will, however, also adversely affect this patient population, and the benefits of early extubation need to be carefully balanced against the requirement for ventilatory support. Where the patient needs respiratory support and is intubated, ventilator settings and fluid balance may be titrated against venous return using echocardiography. In patients with a fenestrated circulation, the presence of hypoxia may represent V/Q mismatch or excessive right-left shunting through the fenestration. Differentiating between the two is important, as hypoxia resulting in pulmonary vasoconstriction will limit cardiac output. Here, echocardiography may also be useful.

The postoperative recovery of these patients is unpredictable, ranging from immediate extubation and ICU discharge to prolonged ICU admission with multisystem dysfunction, a high incidence of coagulopathy, renal dysfunction, hepatic dysfunction and requirement for ventilatory support, particularly where surgery is undertaken in the presence of a significantly obstructed Fontan circulation associated with a very low cardiac output state.

Conclusion

Management of the critically ill GUCH patient requires a highly trained multidisciplinary team approach, and although it is best carried out in specialist centres, with improving patient survival patients will inevitably increasingly present to their local hospitals. Although training all intensivists in this interesting and complex specialty is not realistic, knowledge of the basic principles of assessment and management of the critically ill GUCH patient is important. Early discussion with the specialist centre is vital.

Learning Points

- Investigation and management of the critically ill GUCH patient is complex and requires input from an appropriately trained multidisciplinary team.
- The key to good management involves understanding the cardiopulmonary anatomy and physiology of each individual patient.
- Standard ICU parameters in the non-GUCH population may not be applicable in the GUCH patient.
- The response to standard ICU therapies may be unpredictable.

Further Reading

British Cardiac Society Working Party. Grown-up congenital heart (GUCH) disease: current needs and provision of service for adolescents and adults with congenital heart disease in the UK. *Heart.* 2002; 88(Suppl 1): i1-i14.

Cheung AT, Pochettino A, Mc Garvey ML, et al. Strategies to manage paraplegia risk after endovascular stent repair of descending thoracic aortic aneurysms. *Annals of Thoracic Surgery.* 2005; 80: 1280–1288.

Child JS, Collins-Nakai RL, Alpert JS, et al. Bethesda Conference Report – Task Force 3: Workforce description and education requirements for the care of adults with congenital heart disease. *Journal of the American College of Cardiology.* 2001; 37: 1183–1187.

Coselli JS, Le Maine SA, Köksoy C, et al. Cerebrospinal fluid drainage reduces paraplegia after thoracoabdominal aortic aneurysm repair: results of a randomized clinical trial. *Journal of Vascular Surgery.* 2002; 35: 631–639.

Daliento L, Somerville J, Presbitero P, et al. Eisenmenger syndrome. Factors relating to deterioration and death. *European Heart Journal.* 1998; 19: 1845–1855.

O'Sullivan JJ, Wren C. Survival with congenital heart disease and need for follow-up into adult life. *Heart.* 2001; 85: 438–443.

Price S, Jaggar SI, Jordan S, et al. Adult congenital heart disease: intensive care management and outcome prediction. *Intensive Care Medicine.* 2007; 33: 652–659.

Warnes CA, Liberthson R, Danielson GK, et al. Bethesda Conference Report – Task Force 1: The changing profile of congenital heart disease in adult life. *Journal of the American College of Cardiology.* 2001; 37: 1170–1175.

MCQs

1. **In a GUCH patient with a significant shunt, which of the following are reliable indicators of cardiac output? (more than one answer may be correct)**
   (a) Oesophageal Doppler
   (b) Pulmonary artery catheter
   (c) PiCCO
   (d) LiDCO
   (e) Thoracic impedance

2. **Adaptive mechanisms in the cyanotic patient include:**
   (a) A leftward shift in the oxyhaemoglobin dissociation curve
   (b) A fall in cardiac output
   (c) Polycythaemia
   (d) Erythrocytosis

3. **In a patient with arrhythmia, which of the following require cardioversion as soon as possible, even if haemodynamically stable? (more than one answer may be correct)**
   (a) Congenitally corrected transposition of the great arteries
   (b) Transposition with an arterial switch
   (c) Severe pulmonary regurgitation
   (d) Fontan circulation
   (e) Ebstein's anomaly

4. **In a patient with univentricular circulation, what is the potential effect of giving an inodilator? (more than one answer may be true)**
   (a) Increase in pulmonary circulation due to reduced pulmonary vascular resistance
   (b) Increase in cardiac output due to reduced systemic vascular resistance
   (c) Increase in saturations associated with an increase in systemic blood flow
   (d) Fall in saturations associated with an increase in systemic blood flow
   (e) Increase in saturations associated with a fall in systemic blood flow

5. **A GUCH patient is admitted to the ICU following a laparotomy. You are told they have had a repair for Tetralogy of Fallot. Which of the following statements are true? (more than one answer may be true)**
   (a) A previous Blalock–Taussig shunt will mean ipsilateral blood pressure monitoring may be inaccurate
   (b) The potential for intracardiac shunting still exists
   (c) The morphological right ventricle is systemic
   (d) The patient is expected to be erythrocytotic
   (e) Echocardiography is indicated, even if haemodynamically stable

Exercise answers are available on p.470. Alternatively, take the test online at www.cambridge.org/CardiothoracicMCQ

Difficult to Wean from Mechanical Ventilation Patients in the Cardiothoracic Intensive Care Unit

Michael G Davies

Introduction

Weaning from invasive mechanical ventilation (IMV) may be classified as simple, difficult or prolonged. Each category presents its own distinct clinical management issue. More than 75% of patients achieve simple weaning, namely extubation at first attempt. For such patients, the aim is to identify the soonest opportunity to resume spontaneous breathing. Shorter durations of IMV can reduce morbidity and the duration of ICU admission, therefore providing benefit at both individual and institutional level. Difficult weaning is defined as requiring up to three spontaneous breathing trials or up to 7 days. Finding the cause of failed extubation is of paramount importance, since these patients are at a clinical threshold; some will proceed to a recovery that is free from further complication, whereas others will succumb to other complications and may deteriorate towards multiorgan failure. Finally, patients who experience prolonged weaning (more than 7 days) form a small minority, but are an important clinical problem. Despite surviving the acute problem(s), they remain in respiratory failure and continue to require IMV for prolonged periods. This has a disproportionate effect upon ICU bed occupancy due to long ICU admissions. The distinct multidisciplinary expertise required to make progress in this patient group may not be available in a standard cardiothoracic critical care unit. This chapter will review the clinical challenges provided by each weaning category, although it will focus upon the management of patients who have required prolonged IMV.

Simple Weaning

Following uncomplicated and successful surgery, rapid weaning is expected. Ideally, IMV should be stopped as soon as the reason for ventilation has resolved and the patient can breathe spontaneously and protect the airway. A two-step process is used to ensure that extubation may be considered. Firstly, safe clinical parameters need to be achieved (screening) followed by a weaning trial (spontaneous breathing trial).

Screening Parameters for Early Extubation

Clinical criteria for early extubation following elective, uncomplicated cardiac surgery include:

- haemodynamic stability (satisfactory rhythm, blood pressure and urine output),
- adequate rewarming, haemostasis and metabolic status,
- intact neurological function,
- satisfactory respiratory and upper airway function.

Using Protocols to Achieve Earlier Extubation

For low-risk patients returning to critical care after elective surgery, a significant part of clinical decision-making relates to the timing of extubation. We know from studies of unplanned extubations that a sizeable proportion of patients who self-extubate do not require reintubation. This indicates that the opportunity for earlier extubation for some patients may have been missed by the clinicians. Formal weaning protocols have emerged to reduce the delays in the pathway towards extubation. Following cardiac surgery, such strategies are associated with a reduced ICU length of stay and no increase in morbidity if compared to non-fast-track care. Protocols and even automated weaning may therefore improve the organisational efficiency of a critical care unit with a high throughput of elective surgery. These strategies are often packaged together with other aspects of care, focused on achieving early discharge from critical care for patients judged to be at low risk preoperatively. Reducing ICU length of stay by a small amount for a large number of patients may reduce ICU bed occupancy, resulting in increased opportunity for surgical activity.

Difficult Weaning

Difficult weaning is defined as failing a weaning trial and requiring up to three trials of spontaneous breathing or a period of up to 7 days to achieve extubation. For patients in cardiothoracic critical care, this cohort may be identified as those who experience 'extubation delay'.

Extubation Delay

A sequential audit of unselected adult cardiac surgery patients found that extubation was achieved within 6 hours of surgery for 39% of patients, within 24 hours for 89% and within 48 hours for 95%. An extubation delay >48 hours after CABG is associated with longer ICU and hospital stays, and increased mortality. Factors associated with extubation delay are summarised in Table 52.1.

As shown, patients who experience extubation delay are characterised by preoperative comorbidity and/or adverse perioperative and postoperative events. Whilst respiratory factors, such as COPD, may have a role, for many patients the rate-limiting problem is cardiac in nature. The spontaneous breathing trial is, in effect, a type of exercise and will increase cardiac output requirements. If cardiac reserve is limited, then the transition from supported to unsupported breathing may cause haemodynamic decompensation.

It is just as important to note that extubation delay identifies the individual patient as at high risk of new complications; in the presence of extubation delay, a cascade of additional problems are more likely, including multiple-organ failure and death.

Table 52.1 Factors associated with extubation delay in cardiothoracic critical care

	Variable
Preoperative	↑ Renal dysfunction
	↑ NYHA stage
	COPD (reduced FEV1)
	Emergency surgery
	Female gender
	↑ Age
Operative	↑ Perfusion time
	↑ Blood loss
Postoperative	↑ Blood loss
	↑ Inotrope requirement
	Arrhythmia

Role of Checklists and Prompts

Extubation is an important part of the process towards recovery of function and discharge from the ICU. Failure to extubate may delay other processes such as intravascular line and urinary catheter removal. With increasing duration of IMV, there are increased rates of nosocomial infections. Alongside efforts to optimise cardiorespiratory function in preparation for extubation, general clinical stability needs to be maintained. The development of an infection or other complication at this key time point can lead to a spiral of clinical deterioration leading to death or prolonged IMV.

Strategies to reduce ICU associated complications have been shown to improve patient outcomes. Given the complexity of critical care medicine, human errors of omission in decision-making are especially important and can further delay weaning from IMV. The introduction of checklists and prompting are synonymous with attempts to reduce human error. Checklists reduce the incidence of catheter-based bloodstream infection and urinary sepsis and, when combined with active prompts, ICU length of stay and mortality are reduced. In one study the most significant effect was seen for patients in the third quartile of predicted risk (i.e. neither low risk or at highest risk of death). For such 'medium-risk' patients, hospital mortality was 8% if active prompting was used, compared to 33% for those who received usual care. Of course, preventing nosocomial infection is important for all patients; however, these data suggest that medium-risk patients, as evidenced by extubation delay, represent a clinical threshold in which infection avoidance usually leads to rapid discharge from ICU, whereas the development of infection confers a more challenging prognosis.

Role of Non-invasive Ventilation (NIV)

Non-invasive ventilation (NIV) refers to the delivery of ventilatory support using a mask, rather than an endotracheal or tracheostomy tube. Increasing recognition of its role in preventing the need for intubation in deteriorating patients has led to its use following extubation in selected patients. NIV may be delivered prophylactically after extubation if the patient is considered to be at high risk of respiratory failure, or as rescue therapy in the event of unanticipated postextubation respiratory failure.

A Cochrane systematic review showed that NIV reduced the rate of reintubation and ICU length of stay for selected patients. Identifying suitable patients for NIV requires an understanding of its physiological action. NIV acts as an additional respiratory pump to improve alveolar ventilation and, as such, reduce hypercapnia. Patients most likely to benefit from NIV are those who demonstrate evidence of, or a predisposition towards, hypercapnia. Patients at risk include those with a pre-existing problem with their respiratory muscle pump, such as COPD or neuromuscular conditions, and those who develop a degree of hypercapnia during a spontaneous breathing trial. Trial data support this assertion, showing that NIV provides significantly greater mortality benefit in trials enrolling patients with COPD compared to trials that included mixed patient populations.

Whilst the use of NIV to permit earlier extubation and prevent reintubation is likely to evolve further, current data support its use for selected patients. The success of NIV is also reliant upon the expertise of the team who are delivering it. In some healthcare systems, such as the UK, NIV has evolved as a ward-based practice. If competence in applying NIV and troubleshooting are lacking, then treatment failure is more likely.

Prolonged IMV (Weaning Failure)

The NHS Modernisation Agency Weaning and Long Term Ventilation Group defined weaning failure as the need for IMV for 3 weeks or more, at least three previous failed weaning trials, and in the absence of any non-respiratory cause.

Impact of Prolonged IMV

Approximately 5–10% of ICU patients experience prolonged weaning failure and continue to require IMV for periods exceeding 3 weeks. Numerous factors contribute to prolonged IMV; advances in critical care have led to an increasing proportion of patients who survive the acute episode and also to an older and increasingly frail patient population accessing complex surgery and critical care. The concept of 'chronic critical illness' has emerged, namely patients who continue to require life-sustaining organ support following acute critical illness. Prolonged dependence on IMV, a key feature of chronic critical illness, has emerged as a significant public health challenge, with annual costs in the USA estimated to be $35 billion.

Patients who experience prolonged IMV have higher mortality and occupy a disproportionate number of ICU bed days, leading to increased health care costs. However, after IMV has continued for 15 days or more, fewer patients have multiple-organ failure and mortality rates start to plateau. Most surviving patients enter a state of limbo, achieving relative clinical stability but continuing to require ICU support for single-organ respiratory failure. Protocols or automated changes in ventilator settings, used with success in simple weaning, have little impact upon the patients who lack the capacity to breathe independently.

Role of the Specialised Weaning Unit

An international consensus document concluded that standard critical care units may lack the necessary focus and structure to manage patients with weaning failure. On any given day, competing demands for the critical care team include new admissions and existing patients with acute instability or complex multiple organ failure. In such circumstances, it may be easy to maintain the clinical stability of the patient with weaning failure, but more challenging to make progress.

A variety of organisational models have emerged. Long-term acute care hospitals (LTACHs) manage patients with persisting failure of a range of organ systems, including weaning from IMV, whereas specialised weaning units focus on weaning from IMV alone. Both service models use lower staff to patient ratios than critical care units and therefore offer an economic advantage. The recommended model of care in the UK is the specialised weaning unit.

Factors Associated with Weaning Failure

Successful respiration depends upon an adequate capacity to breathe (respiratory capacity). Respiratory capacity requires an adequate muscle pump that receives appropriate signals from an intact neurological system. The control of respiration (respiratory drive) is complex and regulated by a number of physiological mechanisms, some via the automatic system (e.g. chemoreceptors sensitive to hypercapnia and hypoxia) and some via voluntary control during wakefulness. In simple terms, weaning failure reflects an imbalance between the respiratory capacity and the opposing force of workload applied (respiratory load). Impaired respiratory drive is uncommon in this patient population, assuming that excessively high $PaCO_2$ levels are avoided.

When assessing the reasons for weaning failure, it is helpful to consider the relative impact of opposing forces of capacity and load. Identifying such factors leads to a clearer management plan, both with respect to weaning in the short term and also in considering the level of long-term respiratory support that may be needed. Common factors associated with weaning failure are summarised in Table 52.2.

Table 52.2 Common factors associated with weaning failure

Decreased respiratory capacity	
Neurological	Cerebrovascular
	Critical illness neuropathy
	Guillain–Barré syndrome
	Myaesthenia
	Comorbid condition (e.g. motor neurone disease)
Muscle weakness	Deconditioning
	Critical illness myopathy
	Nutritional imbalance
	Electrolyte imbalance
	Comorbid condition (e.g. muscular dystrophy)
Increased respiratory load	
Airway related	Inadequate tracheostomy (position, size)
	Excessive secretions
	Bronchospasm
Reduced lung compliance	Pneumonia
	Parenchymal problems (e.g. fibrosis)
	Bronchospasm
	Obesity
Decreased cardiac reserve	Reduced LVEF
	Arrhythmia
	Pericardial collection
Decreased respiratory drive	
	Neurological
	Metabolic
	Drug related

Approach to the Patient with Weaning Failure

There are limited data regarding the recommended management approach for patients who have experienced weaning failure. However, features that are common to published series from specialised weaning units include the following.

Ventilate to Normalise Gas Exchange before Weaning

Liberation from IMV is more likely to succeed if gas exchange is stable and satisfactory. Despite this, patients admitted to specialised weaning units typically demonstrate hypercapnia and an elevated plasma bicarbonate concentration. Several factors may contribute, including relative underventilation, electrolyte disturbance (hypochloraemia, hypokalaemia and hypophosphataemia), hypoalbuminaemia, and the prior use of diuretics and steroids. Chronic hypercapnia blunts the respiratory drive, whereas reducing $PaCO_2$ and bicarbonate concentrations towards the normal range leads to an improved minute ventilation response to $PaCO_2$. A decreased response to CO_2, as measured by hypercapnic drive and ventilatory response, is associated prolonged failure to wean from IMV.

Hence, ventilation should be optimised and increased if necessary. Reducing $PaCO_2$ causes a temporary respiratory alkalosis until renal compensation of bicarbonate occurs. Weaning should not commence until this acid-base imbalance has resolved. Clinical stability needs to be achieved via the ventilator, including satisfactory oxygenation (FiO_2 <40%).

Review the Diagnosis and Factors Associated with Weaning Failure

Identifying and minimising any factors contributing to weaning failure are vital if weaning is to be achieved. Transfer to a weaning unit provides a good opportunity for diagnostic review, but continual assessment of progress is essential regardless of the location of care. An 'airway, breathing, and circulation' approach may identify new, important clinical issues. For example, bronchoscopic evaluation may find excessive secretions or a poorly located tracheostomy tube. Tracheal stenosis is uncommon, but may be the main cause of weaning failure for up to 5% of patients. The underlying respiratory pathology should also be carefully considered and there should be a low threshold for thoracic CT. Retrospective series have shown that

CT scanning impacts management in up to 30% of patients with weaning failure.

Weaning is rarely achieved in the setting of persistent infection and hypoalbuminaemia. Subacute infections (respiratory or non-respiratory), usually characterised by a moderate elevation of inflammatory markers, should be actively pursued and treated aggressively. Pleural effusions are common and can be identified, analysed and drained via bedside ultrasound. Cardiac status should be reviewed, since disturbances in cardiac perfusion, rhythm or ventricular function may affect cardiorespiratory capacity to wean. Simple non-invasive assessments, such as ECGs at the beginning and end of a weaning period and routine transthoracic echocardiography, can identify abnormalities that are contributing to a failure to wean. In rare circumstances, an additional systemic pathology may be found, such as hypothyroidism or an inflammatory disease.

Normalise the Environment

Critical care unit design focuses on the ability to monitor patients closely and respond quickly in the event of acute problems. However, from a patient's perspective some of these measures may be perceived as hostile and stressful, for example excessive noise arising from early warning alarms (such as ventilator disconnection). Critically ill patients sleep poorly and this is due, at least in part, to the critical care environment itself.

Simple interventions such as ear plugs and eyemasks may improve subjective measures of sleep quality following cardiac surgery. Whilst data are limited in this area, it is logical that efforts to reduce excessive noise, sleep disruption, pain and social isolation should have a positive impact upon the recovery of function. In the same way, positive strategies that restore normality to circadian patterns of sleeping and eating (if safe) should be encouraged. Compared to the critical care environment, the patient in the specialised weaning unit may experience fewer adverse alarms and disruption. To address this, some critical care units place less critically ill patients in a less 'intensive' environment.

Wean via Trials of Unsupported Breathing

Once gas exchange on the ventilator is optimised and there is sufficient clinical stability, then weaning should commence. The patient needs to be able to participate in the process and requires confidence in the team. Initial trails of breathing require 1:1 input from a member of the team who is skilled in weaning from prolonged IMV. Weaning consists of daytime periods of unsupported spontaneous breathing, a weaning method that has been shown to be associated with shorter weaning times in this patient group, when compared to weaning via pressure support. When possible, the tracheostomy cuff is deflated and a speaking valve employed to encourage communication. Short initial periods of unsupported breathing, usually undertaken in the morning, can build confidence in the process. Daytime weaning can then progress according to the respiratory capacity of the patient. Clinical and objective measures of respiratory function should be monitored during the weaning period (e.g. continuous transcutaneous carbon dioxide analysis with blood gas measurement as necessary). On completion of a weaning trial, the patient should be congratulated and IMV recommenced. Here, the ventilator is not an additional method of weaning, rather it should provide adequate support of breathing (e.g. pressure control ventilation) to rest and prepare for the next period of weaning.

Use a Multidisciplinary Team Approach

The multidisciplinary team (MDT) plays a key role in the management of the patient with weaning failure. Progress is usually made on a gradual basis and the nursing team is best equipped to provide continuous, holistic assessment. A positive approach towards rehabilitation is required and is achieved by the input of a physiotherapist with expertise in the management of such patients. Nutritional management can be complex and benefits from specialist dietetic and speech therapy input. Within our unit, we hold weekly MDT meetings, attended by all senior members of the medical, nursing, physiotherapy and dietetic teams. Clinical progress is reviewed in detail and a forward plan is agreed.

Use NIV as Part of the Weaning Process

Decannulation of the tracheostomy can only be considered when IMV is no longer necessary. For some patients, there is a continued need for ventilatory assistance at least on a temporary basis overnight. For example, a patient with pre-existing COPD who develops critical illness myoneuropathy following cardiac surgery may now lack the respiratory capacity for 24-hour independence from the ventilator. NIV can be helpful as part of the weaning process to build up periods of the day in which IMV is not required. In addition, applying NIV overnight can reduce the necessity to revert to IMV. Use of NIV in such circumstances requires a tracheostomy tube to be capped off and deflated. The tube should be small enough to permit airflow around it; if a voice is not achieved via use of a speaking valve during the day, then it is less likely that NIV via mask will provide benefit overnight. In downsizing a tracheostomy, one must also keep in mind that a small change in tube diameter can cause a significant increase in the work of breathing if all breathing passes only through the tube. The aim is to provide a safe and successful transition to decannulation and any change in airway management must reflect this.

Weaning to the Most Appropriate Level of Long-Term Respiratory Support

Patients who experience weaning failure represent a self-selecting group of survivors who have not yielded to the acute episode or its complications, yet remain in single-organ respiratory failure. Weaning success in this situation is defined as liberation from IMV to either self-ventilation or nocturnal NIV. This recognises that long-term survival following prolonged IMV is enhanced if long-term NIV is used when it is indicated. In the UK at least, the specialised weaning service is typically based within a regional long-term ventilation unit that has particular expertise in the use of NIV.

Data from Clinical Studies

Numerous clinical studies have reported outcomes across a range of organisational approaches. A recent meta-analysis has compared outcomes for reported studies of patients who have required prolonged IMV. It has provided clear insights into which patients benefit from continued attempts to wean following prolonged IMV and the optimal organisational approach to deliver care, although further research is needed. The meta-analysis found somewhat sobering results, with fewer than 50% of patients alive at 1year. However, important differences according to the organisational approach were found; UK studies (regional weaning units) reported significantly better outcomes than achieved for US studies from post-acute care facilities. For example, 75% of patients transferred to a UK specialised weaning service achieved discharge to their own home, compared to only 22% of patients at meta-analysis. Whilst patient selection may explain this disparity in part, significant differences in the organisation of care and use of long-term NIV appear to be more relevant. Current data support a specialised approach for this patient group.

Conclusions

Weaning from IMV is an area of care in which a 'one size fits all' approach cannot succeed. For patients in a 'simple weaning' category, extubation will proceed without difficulty. The challenge for care is to achieve this as quickly and safely as possible. Protocols that permit earlier extubation by the bedside nurse are favoured. Small improvements in weaning time can improve unit efficiency, especially for ICUs with a high elective surgical activity, providing that earlier discharge from critical care is achieved. Patients who experience extubation delay and difficult weaning are an 'at risk' group. Medical input is required to identify the cause of failure alongside high levels of general vigilance to avoid new complications. Protocols and prompts designed to reduce the impact of errors of omission have been shown to improve outcomes. Prolonged weaning is an important clinical challenge. Whilst fewer than 10% of patients experience weaning failure, critical care costs are high due to bed occupancy rates. Successful long-term survival can be achieved via transfer to a specialised weaning unit. Such units provide the distinct expertise that is required to maximise rates of discharge home and long-term survival.

Learning Points

- Strategies to reduce ICU associated complications, such as applying checklists aimed at reducing infection, improve ICU outcomes. This is especially evident for patients who have experienced extubation delay.
- Use of non-invasive ventilation (NIV) may facilitate earlier extubation for patients who have, or are predisposed to, hypercapnia (e.g. patients with coexistent COPD).
- Uncontrolled hypercapnia should be avoided for patients who have experienced prolonged invasive ventilation. Attempts should be made to normalise gas exchange prior to weaning.
- A significant proportion of patients who experience prolonged weaning failure will

continue to require nocturnal NIV following decannulation.

- Due to the specialised nature of care, transfer to a dedicated weaning unit is associated with improved patient survival and discharge home rates.

Further Reading

Blackwood B, Burns KE, Cardwell CR, O'Halloran P. Protocolized versus non-protocolized weaning for reducing the duration of mechanical ventilation in critically ill adult patients. *Cochrane Database of Systematic Reviews.* 2014; 11: CD006904.

Boles JM, Bion J, Connors A, et al. Weaning from mechanical ventilation. *European Respiratory Journal.* 2007; 29: 1033–1056.

Burns KE, Meade MO, Premji A, Adhikari NK. Noninvasive ventilation as a weaning strategy for mechanical ventilation in adults with respiratory failure: a Cochrane systematic review. *Canadian Medical Association Journal.* 2014; 186: E112–E122.

Damuth E, Mitchell JA, Bartock JL, Roberts BW, Trzeciak S. Long-term survival of critically ill patients treated with prolonged mechanical ventilation: a systematic review and meta-analysis. *Lancet Respiratory Medicine.* 2015; 3: 544–553.

Davies MG, Quinnell TG, Oscroft NS, et al. Hospital outcomes and long-term survival after referral to a specialized weaning unit. *British Journal of Anaesthesia.* 2017; 118: 563–569.

Kahn JM, Le T, Angus DC, et al. The epidemiology of chronic critical illness in the United States. *Critical Care Medicine.* 2015; 43: 282–287.

Naughton C, Reilly N, Powroznyk A, et al. Factors determining the duration of tracheal intubation in cardiac surgery: a single-centre sequential patient audit. *European Journal of Anaesthesiology.* 2003; 20: 225–233.

Pilcher DV, Bailey MJ, Treacher DF, et al. Outcomes, cost and long term survival of patients referred to a regional weaning centre. *Thorax.* 2005; 60: 187–192.

Smith IE, Shneerson JM. A progressive care programme for prolonged ventilatory failure: analysis of outcome. *British Journal of Anaesthesia.* 1995; 75: 399–404.

Vasilyev S, Schaap RN, Mortensen JD. Hospital survival rates of patients with acute respiratory failure in modern respiratory intensive care units. An international, multicenter, prospective survey. *Chest.* 1995; 107: 1083–1088.

Weiss CH, Moazed F, McEvoy CA, et al. Prompting physicians to address a daily checklist and process of care and clinical outcomes: a single-site study. *American Journal of Respiratory and Critical Care Medicine.* 2011; 184: 680–686.

MCQs

True or False

1. **Factors associated with extubation delay following cardiac surgery include:**
   (a) Increasing age
   (b) Male gender
   (c) Anaemia
   (d) COPD
   (e) Preoperative renal dysfunction

2. **For patients who experience prolonged ventilation, factors that may be associated with an increased LOAD on the respiratory system include:**
   (a) Excessive airway secretions
   (b) Obesity
   (c) The tracheostomy
   (d) Critical illness myopathy
   (e) Sedation

3. **Patients who experience weaning failure:**
   (a) Are defined as requiring invasive mechanical ventilation for 3 weeks or more and following three or more failed weaning trials.
   (b) Account for fewer than 10% of patients treated in ICU, but represent more than 30% of ICU bed occupancy
   (c) Rarely survive more than 12 months out of hospital
   (d) Represent an important but decreasing number of ICU patients
   (e) Benefit from a stepwise reduction in pressure support

Exercise answers are available on p.470. Alternatively, take the test online at www.cambridge.org/CardiothoracicMCQ

Chapter 53

Cardiothoracic Critical Care Nursing, Outreach and Follow-up

Jo-anne Fowles

Introduction

Caring for the critically ill cardiothoracic patient requires a multidisciplinary approach with nursing roles being pivotal. Nursing the critically ill cardiothoracic patient requires advanced skills and competence as well as in-depth knowledge of nursing practice, anatomy, physiology and pathophysiology, technology and pharmacology used in critical care. Integral to the nurses' role is supporting patients and their families during and after critical illness.

Critical care areas are constantly adapting to the needs of the patient and now often extend beyond the physical unit itself. The concept of 'critical care without walls' is well established and ensures continuity of the patient pathway before, during and after the ICU admission. Many units now further defragment the care of the critically ill patient through advanced nurse practice, developing the role of the healthcare support worker, establishing new ways of working and offering nurse led services.

The Nursing Team

Education Team

Most critical care area nursing teams include a dedicated education team, their role being primarily to ensure access to all nurses to appropriate education and to support the senior nursing team in sharing best practice.

Critical care is a complex specialty with the new nurse having to acquire many skills and competencies. The education team provides both a framework and support to meet these needs. Technology within critical care is constantly evolving and the education team has a vital role in ensuring all new equipment is introduced with a robust training programme to ensure patient safety. It is important that all nurses are provided with the opportunity to develop throughout their careers. The education team is able to ensure all staff have access to appropriate educational opportunities.

Bedside Nurse

Integral to the care of the patient is the bedside nurse. Their roles vary in different cardiac intensive care units and countries, but they are the person who has the most contact with the critically ill patient. The roles of the bedside nurse are summarised in Table 53.1. In critical care this is a registered practitioner who enhances the delivery of comprehensive patient centred care, for acutely ill patients, often on a 1:1 basis. Structured handover at the start of each shift ensures accurate transfer of clinical information ensuring continuity of safe care.

The primary role of the bedside nurse is continuous vigilance of the patient's vital signs, recognising and assessing changes and responding immediately. This response includes communicating with the nurse in charge and the rest of the multidisciplinary team (MDT) where appropriate.

Many patients are invasively monitored. Setting up, calibration and appropriate alarm limits to ensure accuracy and safety of monitoring is the responsibility of the nurse. The critically ill cardiothoracic patient may also require advanced support ranging from continuous renal replacement therapy (CRRT) and intra-aortic balloon pump (IABP) to ventricular assist devices (VAD) or extracorporeal membrane oxygenation (ECMO). Monitoring of the patient on these devices is the responsibility of the bedside nurse. In addition to basic nurse education, critical care nurses have specialised training. This training includes setting up and ongoing management of monitoring equipment and advanced mechanical support to ensure patient safety.

Assessing the needs and delivering basic nursing care remains an essential component of the bedside

Table 53.1 Duties of the bedside nurse

The bedside nurse's plan of care on a daily basis will include the following

Basic needs:
- Assess all needs and provide general hygiene including eye care, mouth care, bathing
- Prevent self harm when patients are agitated
- Bowel care

Skin care:
- Regular repositioning to prevent pressure sore development
- Correct positioning of invasive devices to avoid skin damage
- Assessing skin integrity and use of appropriate dressings and creams
- Ensuring correct pressure relieving mattress utilised
- Cleanliness to avoid development of moisture lesions
- Assessing wounds and ensuring correct dressings used

Infection control:
- Ensure local infection control policies are adhered to
- Recognise early signs of infection

Psychological support:
- Allay patients' fears and concerns by ensuring they are comfortable, reassured and fully informed

Family care:
- Ensure good communication and support family members

Monitoring:
- Documenting and interpreting monitored parameters and communicating concerns early to prevent further deterioration

Medications:
- Administering all prescribed medications
- Titrate infusions within defined parameters (e.g. sedative infusions)

MDT:
- Participate in MDT discussions acting as the patient's advocate

Rehabilitation:
- Be involved in the planning of rehabilitation
- Assist with mobilising patients whenever possible

Advanced support:
- Assisting with intubation
- Regular bronchial toilet in ventilated patients
- Care of tracheostomies including decannulation
- Monitoring and managing CVVH, plasmapheresis, IABP
- Measuring cardiac output studies, documenting and interpreting results and communicating concerns
- Assisting with the insertion of invasive lines
- Monitoring the patients supported with ECMO and VADs

nurse role. This includes communication with and support of both the patient and their family. Although the primary focus is the allocated patient, the nurse is part of a team delivering care and responding to the changing demands of the unit. This includes responding to unexpected events to allowing rapid turnover of patients when necessary, whilst ensuring patient care is never compromised.

The role of the bedside nurse may vary between units but regardless of differing degrees of autonomy, central to the bedside nurse role is the ability to rapidly respond to potentially life threatening conditions.

Health Care Support Worker/Assistant Practitioners

The value of the health care support worker role within cardiothoracic critical care is well recognised. They are not registered, and when delivering patient care always work under supervision of the registered nurse. The role is evolving and expanding with foundation degree pathways providing training in skills essential to delivering care and basic assessment.

In addition to direct patient care they perform a variety of tasks essential to the smooth running of any unit. These include checking emergency equipment, ordering supplies and cleaning and tidying the clinical area.

Nursing Hierarchy

In the UK there are a variety of senior nurse roles within cardiothoracic critical care. These may include all or some of the following:

- Lead nurse;
- Matron;
- Advanced nurse specialist/practitioner;
- Shift leader.

One or more of these roles may be filled by one individual, for example the shift leader may also be an advanced nurse specialist or nurse consultant.

Nurse Manager/Lead Nurse/Matron

The critical care manager carries responsibility for service delivery, budgetary management, recruitment and retention. Although all units vary they are usually supported by senior clinical nurses or matrons.

The nurse manager's role is multifaceted covering management of staff, including appraisal and performance management, handling complaints and investigating untoward incidents, and ensuring any lessons learnt are shared with the entire team. They provide leadership, ensuring that the nursing service is continually evolving to provide the highest standards of patient care. This is achieved through working with the MDT supporting, developing and implementing policies. A strong commitment to education and training, and involvement in research and audit projects is also essential.

Shift Leader

The nursing team in the clinical area is led by a senior nurse or in larger units a team of senior nurses. The role of the senior nurse in the clinical area is to maintain an overview of all patients. At the onset of each shift, the senior nurse allocates nurses to patients, ensuring the most appropriate, safe and effective use of available skills. Consideration is also given to providing opportunities for nurses to develop skills with adequate support. The senior nurse remains visible and available to the MDT, patients and relatives throughout the shift. The senior nurse is involved in all MDT rounds.

The senior nurse role also includes the coordination of admission, transfer and discharge of patients. Integral to the role is an awareness of infection status of all patients, with excellent infection control practice being important in preventing hospital acquired infection.

Advanced Nursing Roles

Advances, developments and challenges in modern healthcare provision result in a constantly changing clinical environment. This is especially evident in the cardiothoracic critical care area as this heavily resourced setting continues to proactively respond to deliver high quality, safe patient care. As a result there is an ever changing face to critical care nursing.

Advanced nursing roles have developed in recent years to improve patient care by ensuring immediate response and a less fragmented approach. The roles encompass many job titles, such as clinical nurse specialists, advanced nurse practitioners and nurse consultants. All of these roles enable the nurse to work with increased autonomy within specific guidelines, following appropriate training and assessment. An example of this is that in many units management of the immediate postoperative cardiac surgical patient is nurse led with advanced nurse specialists managing ventilation, haemostasis, fluid and electrolyte balance and drug prescription within defined guidelines.

Outreach

The early identification of the deteriorating patient on the hospital ward is crucial in preventing admission or readmission to the critical care area. The nurse led outreach team works closely with the ward and ICU staff to ensure this happens. The outreach team is available 24 hours/day, 7 days/week.

The three essential objectives of an outreach team are as follows:

1. Prevent readmissions by recognising and treating the deteriorating patient, and if required, ensure admission to critical care happens in a timely manner.
2. Enable discharge from critical care by supporting ward staff in the monitoring and management of this group of patients.
3. Share critical care skills, including recognition of the deteriorating patient, with ward staff.

Excellent communication and teaching skills are as important to the outreach nurse as advanced clinical skills. Their role is to support and develop ward staff in identifying and managing the deteriorating patient. An effective outreach team will enjoy excellent teamwork with ward staff, thus ensuring safe and effective care post discharge from the critical care area.

Many hospitals utilise an early warning system, for example MEWs, to provide an early predictor of clinical deterioration. Such systems provide a trigger for ward staff to alert the outreach team of the deteriorating patient so ensuring early intervention and management.

Follow-up

It is well recognised that patients can experience long lasting side effects after recovery from critical illness. Patients and their families need to be given support in managing the psychological impact of their illness.

The support and follow-up needs of the cardiothoracic patient post ICU and hospital discharge has traditionally been met by the 'parent' team of cardiology, surgery or transplantation. This is now changing with many units providing follow-up immediately post ICU discharge and longer term.

The impact, not only of a critical possibly life threatening illness, but also the sensory overload in the ICU and polypharmacy, including opiates, may affect patients' psychological recovery. Patients may also suffer from sleep deprivation and periods of delirium whilst in the ICU, both of which may impair long term psychological recovery. Symptoms reported by patients following an ICU admission include memory loss and/or memory gaps and nightmares that may continue after hospital discharge.

In addition to clinics assessing psychological recovery and offering specialist support, many cardiothoracic critical care units are introducing patient diaries. The diary is completed on behalf of the patient giving a day to day record of the admission to the ICU and is a useful tool for helping fill in memory gaps and promoting psychological recovery.

Conclusion

Nurses have an integral role within the multidisciplinary team in providing skilled, advanced care of the patient in cardiothoracic critical care. The recognition that care of the critically ill patient extends beyond the boundaries of the intensive care unit has led to the development of nursing roles to ensure early detection and supportive follow-up of all patients.

Learning Points

- Communication and collaborative working are central to safe, effective patient care regardless of each unit's nursing strategy or patient pathway.
- A well-organised education team is required to ensure development and maintenance of essential skills.
- The development of advanced nurse specialist roles is required to ensure patients receive care and intervention in a timely manner.
- An outreach team with excellent communication skills is essential to ensure ongoing care post ICU discharge.
- Follow-up of patients by ICU teams is important in long term recovery.

Further Reading

Galley J, O'Riordan B. Guidance for Nurse Staffing in Critical Care. Royal College of Nursing (RCN). 2003. www.rcn.org.uk

Jones C, Griffiths R, Humphris G, Skirrow P. Memory, delusions and the development of acute post-traumatic stress disorder-related symptoms after intensive care. *Critical Care Medicine*. 2001; 29: 573–580.

Chapter 54

Systems and Processes in Cardiothoracic Critical Care

James Moore and Alain Vuylsteke

A cardiothoracic critical care unit is a highly complex environment requiring an interplay of multiple medical specialties and allied health professionals involved in the care of those patients recovering from the insult caused by cardiac surgery. Most of these units will treat patients suffering from any organ dysfunction that happens in addition to cardiorespiratory issues. In general, systems and processes will be similar to those used in any critical care unit.

There is very limited room for error in this highly dynamic environment. The complexity of the patients' needs has driven the development of standardised pathways and protocols to improve outcomes and maximise efficiency. This is supported by the increasing demand by the public and regulatory authorities to provide treatment and support in an environment that operates within a structured framework.

Guidelines and Protocols

The past 10 years has seen an explosion in the number of guidelines and protocols available to the critical care clinician to aid the management of the individual patient. This has been facilitated by how easy it is now to share electronic documents.

A clinical guideline is a systematically developed statement to assist practitioner and patient decisions about appropriate health care for specific circumstances. Protocols tend to be a more prescriptive set of instructions for the management of a specific condition.

The publication of Rivers' Early Goal Directed Therapy study in 1999 popularised the development of bundles in critical care. This study showed that the use of a specific bundle of care for the management of severe sepsis in a single centre significantly improved mortality. Although the study has been subsequently exposed to significant criticism, bundles began to be developed for a wide range of situations within critical care.

A bundle is defined by the Institute for Healthcare Improvement (IHI) as a structured way of improving the processes of care and patient outcomes: a small, straightforward set of evidence-based practices – generally three to five – that, when performed collectively and reliably, have been proven to improve patient outcomes.

Advantages and criticisms of care bundles are listed in Table 54.1.

Bundles have now been developed for a wide range of clinical scenarios in the critical care unit. An example of a widely adopted bundle of care is that developed for the prevention of central line associated bloodstream infections (CLABSI) promulgated by the IHI and is shown in Table 54.2. Implementation of the central line bundle in the state of Michigan, USA resulted in a 66% reduction in CLABSI over an 18 month period.

Bundles are designed to be adopted as a full package rather than being taken up as single points in a piecemeal approach. It is essential that they are regularly reviewed, as some elements of the bundle may be subject to new research findings – an example being intensive blood glucose control, which was included for a time in ICU care bundles, but has subsequently been shown to be associated with higher mortality than more liberal targets.

Multidisciplinary Team Input

The care of patients in the cardiothoracic critical care unit benefits from the input of multiple medical specialists and allied health professionals. Complex patients often suffer from multiple medical comorbidities, and complications following surgery can affect almost every organ system.

Table 54.1 Advantages and criticisms of care bundles

Advantages of care bundles	Criticisms of care bundles
Standardisation between patients	May not take into account individual patient
Evidence of improved patient outcomes when bundles are used	May limit individual clinician's autonomy or independence
Promote efficient use of resources by utilising proven and effective interventions	An unintended side effect of standardisation may be that it discourages excellent or exceptional clinical practice
Can potentially limit fringe practices which may be unproven or dangerous (and frequently expensive)	May be unduly influenced by external forces such as government or industry
	Some individual bundle elements may have limited evidence; and evidence may change with time
	Result in additional administrative burden for staff

Table 54.2 Example of care bundle

Central Line Bundle
Hand hygiene
Maximal barrier precautions
Chlorhexidine skin antisepsis
Optimal catheter site selection – avoidance of using the femoral vein for central venous access in adult patients
Daily review of line necessity with prompt removal of unnecessary lines

There has been extensive research in the general critical care setting into the relative merits of 'open' versus 'closed' units. 'Closed' units have the care directed by specialists in critical care medicine who call on other teams as required. 'Open' units allow the primary team to admit and direct the care with (or without) support from critical care specialists. Complex patients may benefit from a shared model of care; however conflict over management strategies and goals of care can easily emerge.

A close and constructive working relationship between all teams, with clear and open communication, are essential to ensure the system works well for the patient.

Most surgical patients admitted in cardiothoracic critical care will move from a very high to a low level of dependency within a few hours. Such patients can be managed in a nurse led unit according to predefined pathways with minimal medical input. However, complex patients require input from a wider multidisciplinary team.

Clinical Governance

Clinical governance encompasses a variety of measures designed to ensure that health organisations are accountable for continually improving the quality of their services and safeguarding high standards of care by creating an environment in which excellence in clinical care will flourish.

The cardiothoracic critical care unit requires a strong focus on clinical governance, to ensure patient safety, and continuous improvement in quality of care. The key elements of clinical governance as published by the National Health Service (NHS) in England can assist in ensuring a comprehensive programme of quality improvement is in place within individual units.

One approach to developing a robust structure of clinical governance is to consider the so-called 'pillars' of a clinical governance as shown in Figure 54.1.

Clinical Audit

Clinical Audit involves a systematic analysis of an area of practice to improve clinical care and/or health outcomes, or to confirm that current management is consistent with the available evidence or accepted guidelines. Audit has become a core skill expected of health professionals, and can act as an important tool to drive improvements in quality of care.

The 'audit cycle' describes a widely accepted approach to undertaking clinical audit activities. After first identifying a topic to audit, accepted standards are clearly defined. Current practice is then measured and compared to those standards. This is then communicated to the team, a plan for change designed and implemented, and finally re-audit should take place to examine how those changes have influenced practice.

Clinical Effectiveness

Critical care is now firmly in the era of evidence-based medicine, and there is a vast array of literature

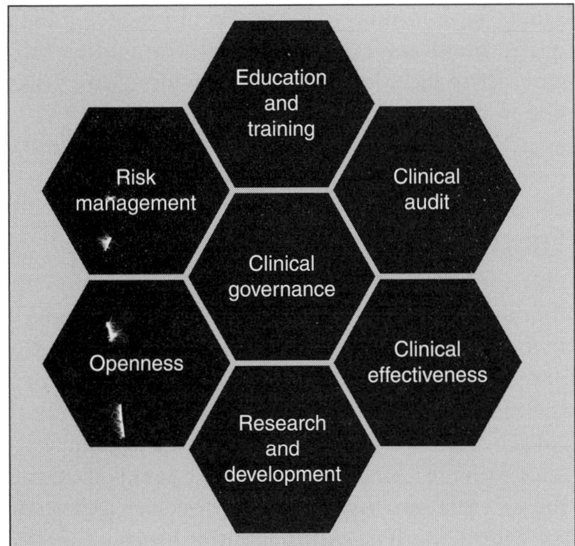

Figure 54.1 Pillars of clinical governance. Extracted from College of Intensive Care Medicine IC-8: Guidelines on Quality Improvement.

examining new concepts and re-examining established practices. Clinical effectiveness requires consideration of health economics and ensuring that best value for money is obtained.

The College of Intensive Care Medicine in Australia and New Zealand recommends examining three broad types of outcome measures as listed in Table 54.3.

Critical care units should participate in programmes that measure the effectiveness of the care they provide. A number of professional societies in intensive care around the world run audit and quality assurance programmes whereby individual units submit patient outcome data which are then analysed and compared to similar units. A number of outcome measures are able to be calculated, including the standardised mortality ratio (SMR), which compares actual mortality rates to those predicted by tools such as the APACHE-III (Acute Physiology and Chronic Health Evaluation III), and exponentially weighted moving average (EWMA) charts which may allow early identification of developing trends. These outcome measures will usually have a process for identifying poorly performing 'outlier' units, allowing investigation of cause and provision of support to improve quality of care.

Risk Management

An effective risk management system requires both proactive and reactive elements. Staff should be encouraged to identify and report risk (both clinical and non-clinical), and the department needs to have tools to manage and minimise this risk. Critical care remains a human endeavour and so errors will always be expected to occur – an effective risk management system understands this, but strives to prevent and minimise any harm that occurs as the result. When errors do occur, reporting needs to be strongly encouraged so that learning can take place, and systems examined to try and prevent similar events occurring in the future. Staff need to feel reassured that in reporting actual or potential ('near-miss') incidents, they will be supported – a 'no-blame' culture is essential for staff to feel safe to report. Equally, investigation of events should be undertaken in a structured, fair and open manner by trained staff. The aim of an accident investigation is not to assign blame, but to determine what can be done to prevent the event occurring again in the future. Regular mortality and morbidity review meetings are another important component of a system wide risk management programme. These meetings should ideally be multidisciplinary, including trainee involvement, and involve a thorough review and discussion of patient complications, adverse events and deaths. Action points should be minuted and progressed.

Risk management can frequently be seen as only examining negative events, but learning from good performance is equally important. Identifying and publicising examples of excellent practice can help to drive positive culture change as much as learning from negative events.

Openness

Learning from instances of both good and bad practice requires a culture of openness where these events can be discussed in a constructive and meaningful way.

Increasingly, the health system is moving to a culture of open public reporting of serious adverse events, as well as reporting outcomes and quality measures. Cardiothoracic surgery was one of the pioneering specialties in this field and has well-developed systems in place for public reporting of surgical outcomes.

'Dashboarding' is another developing area where key quality measures are made available in real time in an easy to follow graphical format. This can allow all members of the team to see the unit's achievements over a range of key performance indicators – the information can be made public, for example via a website.

Table 54.3 Three broad types of outcome measures recommended by the College of Intensive Care Medicine in Australia and New Zealand

1. Structural measures	**Examples:** Size of the ICU Whether the ICU is open or closed Type or amount of technology available Number and roles and responsibilities of ICU staff Clinical workload and case mix Levels of trainee supervision
2. Process measures	**Examples:** Rate of DVT prophylaxis Rate of stress ulcer prophylaxis Early enteral feeding Delayed discharge from ICU Appropriate transfusion threshold Blood glucose control Hand hygiene Time to administration of antibiotics Lung protective ventilation strategies End of life management
3. Outcome measures	**Examples** Severity adjusted mortality rate Health related quality of life Unplanned ICU readmission Serious adverse drug event rate Ventilator associated pneumonia rate Central line associated bloodstream infection rate Family satisfaction

Research and Development

Medical research is essential for the ongoing advancement of the specialty. This includes research into basic science, new innovations or technology, and re-examining traditional ideas and thinking (or medical dogma).

Research can drive improvements in quality and safety, such as the development of care bundles mentioned previously in this chapter. Medical research has traditionally been driven by individual researchers, but over the last 20 years a number of collaborative groups have formed with the aim of producing high quality multicentre clinical trials in critical care medicine. These include the Canadian Critical Care Trials Group, the Australia & New Zealand Intensive Care Society Clinical Trials Group and the UK Intensive Care Society, as well as many others.

Conclusion

Developing a safe and effective culture within cardiothoracic critical care requires multidisciplinary involvement in patient care, and the use of validated protocols and bundles of care, especially in the management of high risk conditions or technical procedures. The seven pillars of clinical governance provide an excellent structure for considering the essential elements of care, processes and quality within the ICU. Although often seen as 'background functions', these elements are essential to providing the highest quality of care to the individual patient.

Learning Points

- Cardiothoracic critical care is a highly complex environment requiring input from multiple health professionals.
- Standardised pathways and protocols have been developed to improve outcomes and maximise efficiency.
- Cardiothoracic critical care requires a strong focus on clinical governance to ensure patient safety and quality improvement.
- Risk must be actively managed and organisations should develop a culture which encourages the team to report when things have gone wrong.
- Learning from incidents should be incorporated into practice and clinical outcomes made available to the public so as to drive improvements in performance.

Further Reading

Scally G, Donaldson LJ. Clinical governance and the drive for quality improvement in the new NHS in England. *British Medical Journal.* 1998; 317: 61.

Chapter 55

Clinical Information Systems

Matthew Jones

Introduction

Critical care is a highly data intensive environment. It has been estimated that over the course of a 24 hour period nearly 1500 data items may be documented on a typical critical care patient and this volume of data is growing all the time. Historically, a subset of these data would have been transcribed into a paper-based record, which was not always legible, could sometimes go missing and was difficult to analyse. Under these circumstances the emergence of clinical information systems (CIS), computer-based systems that collect, store, manipulate and display clinical data, has been widely identified as offering significant benefits to healthcare delivery in critical care. While there is evidence that CIS can contribute to improvements in patient care, they also pose new challenges. A balanced appreciation of their capabilities and their effects on clinical work practices is therefore necessary.

The Components of a CIS

There is no universal model of a CIS and often the configuration in a specific critical care unit will reflect the particular combination of hardware and software installed locally. On the software side, early CIS in critical care tended to be bespoke developments, but now there is a wide range of commercial systems available, either as specialist modules of general hospital information systems, or standalone products designed specifically for intensive care settings. The former have the advantage of full integration with other specialisms, ensuring that critical care episodes are documented in a way that is consistent with practice elsewhere in the hospital, but may not be optimal for the particular requirements of critical care. The latter are likely to fit better with critical care practices, but may not exchange data seamlessly with other hospital systems. Hospital IT departments may also be reluctant to support more than one system.

Different systems vary too in the degree to which they can be customised to local requirements. Some offer relatively little flexibility and require adopting units to adapt themselves to the ways of working envisaged by the CIS designers. This simplifies CIS implementation and may therefore be attractive to hospital IT departments, but may provoke resistance from critical care staff who are required to adjust their work practices. At the other extreme, systems may be highly customisable, either by the vendor, or by the users. This is likely to make the system more attractive to clinical staff, for example, if displays can be made to appear similar to those of the paper or electronic systems the CIS replaces, but incurs additional costs and creates idiosyncratic systems, the integration of which with other services may be problematic. In practice, moreover, there will be limits to the extent to which systems can be customised and certain aspects of the CIS may be so deeply built into the design that changing them may be impractical. This can sometimes cause problems where CIS developed for one particular health system are imported to another. Nevertheless, even relatively superficial customisation, such as changing screen colours, adding a logo or presenting a familiar screen as the default may be significant in influencing user acceptance.

In terms of hardware, a CIS generally comprises a server, hosting the central database, and client computers, at the bedside or elsewhere, accessing the data over a network. Client computers may be desktops, laptops, tablets or other mobile devices. 'Thin' clients, which may run on relatively cheap and low powered devices, simply provide a view of data that are held and processed on the central server, while 'thick' clients, which require more powerful computers, carry out processing locally and only exchange data with the server. Thick clients may be more reliable than thin clients as they are not so vulnerable to network or server failures, but are more expensive to purchase and operate (Figure 55.1).

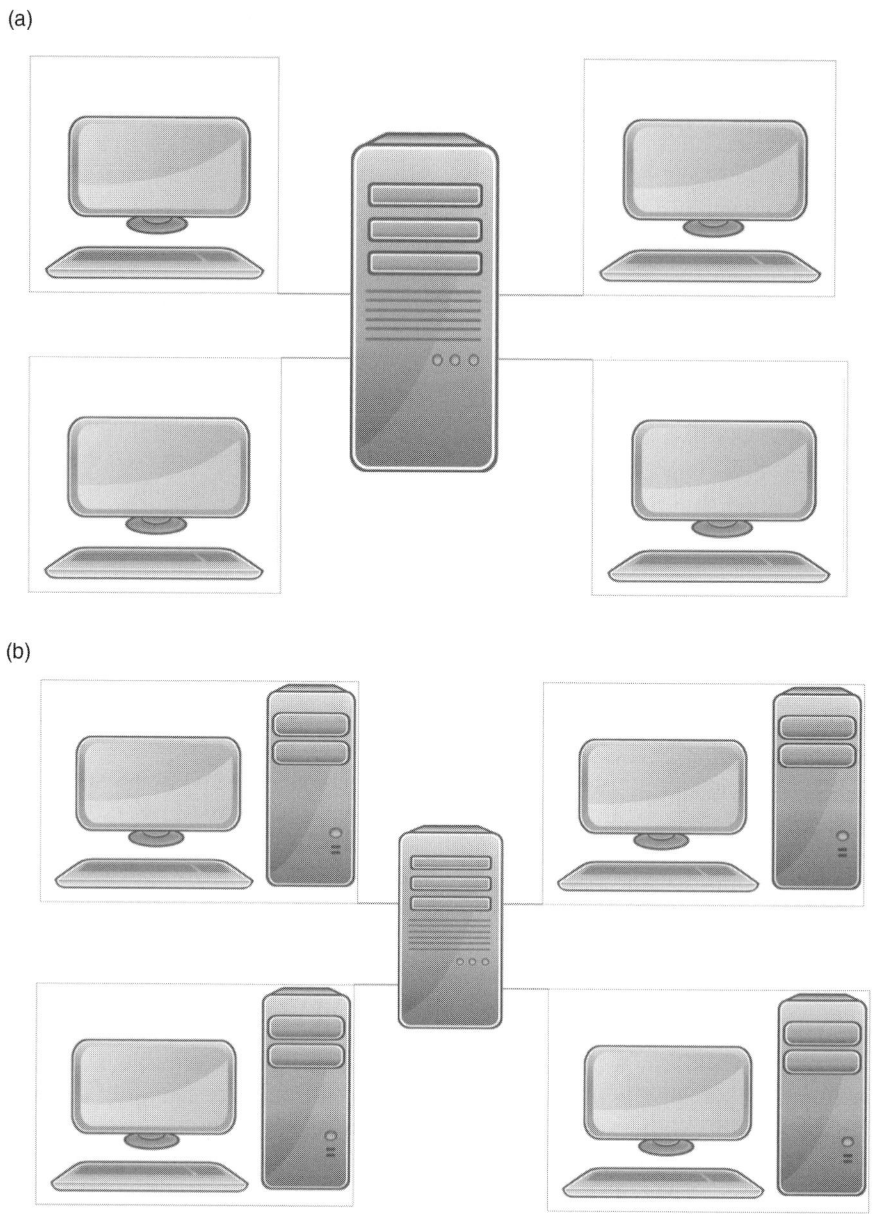

Figure 55.1 (a) Thin and (b) thick clients.

Although, in principle, a CIS integrates all patient data, in practice hardware constraints can mean that some elements of patient data may not always be incorporated. This may be due, for example, to the lack of compatible interfaces to enable critical care equipment to communicate with the CIS, or due to the resolution of screens being insufficient to display X-rays in sufficient detail. While the vision may be of a unified repository of all clinical data, therefore, this may not always be achieved. Nevertheless it is possible to identify a CIS as comprising a number of components that are present to a greater or lesser degree in most systems.

The core component of a CIS is an electronic medical record, a database containing a variety of forms of data about patients. Many of the data fields will be numeric, for example recording blood pressure or heart rate, and therefore readily capable of manipulation and analysis, but others may contain text, for example clinical notes, that are less easily analysed. There is a tendency for CIS to support numeric data entry in preference to free text, and thereby to promote a more systematic and standardised approach to recording clinical care. Textual data may be translated into numbers, for example by offering a pick list of common options to be selected from (option1, option2. … , option*n*), while perhaps retaining the possibility of free text entry for non-standard cases. Electronic records also avoid problems of legibility of text entries and identify unambiguously who has written them (as individuals need to log in to the CIS to be able to enter data).

With data transferred directly from medical equipment to the CIS, transcription errors (which may be of the order of 20%) are eliminated and recording is no longer dependent on staff availability (although it may be necessary for them to validate the data occasionally to ensure that erroneous data do not contaminate the record). Numerical calculations, for example of fluid balances, are also automated, thus avoiding another potential source of errors. Once in the database, moreover, the data are permanently stored and immediately retrievable, not just at the location where they were entered. Data should therefore no longer get lost, and may be accessed away from the bedside at any time by any authorised person. With suitable secure networks, this access may potentially be from locations distant from the patient, creating the opportunity for remote supervision and teleconsultation. Remote access may also encourage the use of 'sitting ward rounds' in which staff meet in an office to review the patients' CIS records rather than visit each bedside. Although this may allow for more focused discussion with fewer disruptions, it reduces interaction between clinicians and patients and bedside staff that may be significant for clinical decision making and patient welfare.

While the standardisation and centralisation of data and their easier availability may be a key feature of CIS, further advantages may be gained from functionality that makes use of the data. One area that has received particular attention is that of electronic prescribing (Figure 55.2), where the CIS may provide new functionality such as: presenting pre-filled order sets, for example of the drugs typically administered on postsurgery admission to critical care; restricting prescribed dosages within preset upper and lower bounds; or checking prescriptions against allergies or interactions with other medications. With remote access it is also possible for a pharmacist to review medication without needing to visit the bedside, or even the unit.

It is not just in prescribing that a CIS may support clinical practice. Some systems may include functionality to monitor the patient's condition and treatment and alert clinicians to potentially significant correlations, or remind them when actions have not been taken. Many also support checklists to guide and improve care. Such clinical decision support is not a necessary feature of a CIS, however, and may be perceived by some clinicians as intruding on their autonomy. Care is also needed to ensure that alerts are relevant and not so frequent that they are ignored.

Another potential contribution of CIS to clinical practice is in the display of data in new ways. Some individuals or professional groups, for example, may prefer to view data graphically, while others may prefer to focus on specific values. A CIS can enable multiple views of the same data, matched to individuals' preferences. The potential for immediate access to all a patient's data, not just, as was the case with paper records, those from the past 24 hours, also enables clinical staff both to view trends in particular values over any period and to zoom in on specific data points anywhere in that time series. The CIS thus provides both additional dimensionality and granularity to the data available for clinical decision making. Different CIS vary, however, in the flexibility they offer to users in the ways that data are presented. Some have a relatively limited menu of standard views, while others

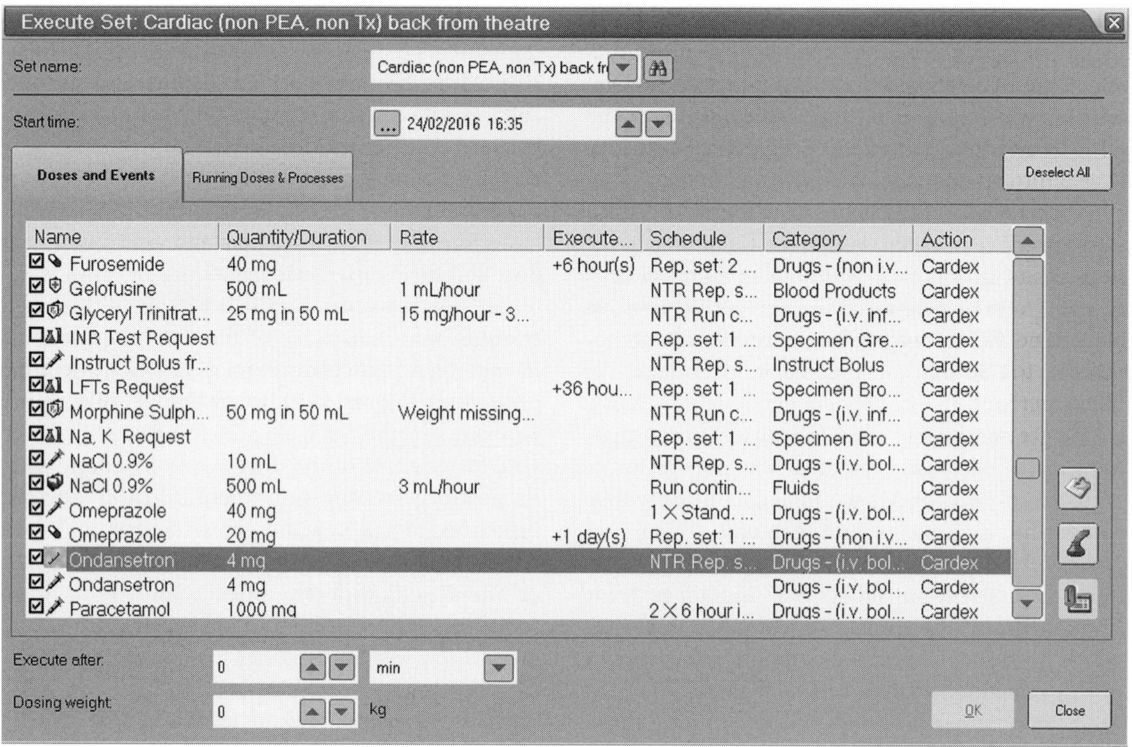

Figure 55.2 Electronic prescribing.

give users a high degree of control both on how data are presented and on what particular data items are displayed. More advanced CIS may support dynamic views, allowing health professionals to bring together different blocks of data on the same screen as relevant for each individual patient.

Over time, the accumulation of historical data in a CIS database can become a significant resource for care quality improvement, audit and research. The standard tools provided with many CIS, however, do not always make it easy to extract data and this resource is often underused as clinical staff lack the time and expertise to undertake the task. Reuse of data may also be discouraged by time and resources required to 'clean' and/or process the data before they can be analysed. Although offering great potential, the contribution of CIS to data led healthcare practice and policy may therefore be less than some current proponents of 'Big Data' envisage.

Costs and Benefits of a CIS

The direct expenditure on hardware and software constitutes only a small proportion of the cost of implementing a CIS. It is estimated, for example, that the five years cost of ownership of major computer systems can be five to eight times the initial outlay. Some of the more significant items contributing to this cost include: infrastructure, for example cabling and networks; interfaces (to enable the CIS to receive data from medical devices, perhaps requiring some of them to be updated); project management of the implementation process; customisation (to adapt the system to local practices); training (both the recruitment or secondment of staff to deliver the training and the time for staff to undertake it); and initial loss of staff productivity as they learn to use the CIS. Nor are costs restricted to the initial implementation – hardware maintenance and upgrading, software license fees and updates and ongoing training (of newly recruited staff and of existing staff if new functionality is added) mean that there is a continuing outlay.

Given these costs, there is likely to be, not unreasonably, an expectation that the CIS will deliver significant benefits. Some of these may be direct savings: through the elimination of tasks, such as processing of paper records, that the CIS makes redundant; through efficiency gains, for example staff being able to review the status of a patient without needing to visit the bedside; and through the elimination of costs (e.g. purchase, storage) associated with paper records. It is often assumed that an important benefit of a CIS will be in time saving, for example through the elimination of data transcription. In practice, however, while CIS use undoubtedly speeds up certain tasks, evidence suggests that CIS rarely frees up significant time overall as other tasks, such as data entry with a keyboard, take considerably longer than with pen and paper. What a CIS can provide, though, are better data to enable cost management.

It is perhaps the indirect benefits of a CIS that have the greatest impact on critical care. For example, although CIS may contribute to some new errors, such as selecting the wrong item from a pick list, in general, the legibility, availability and accountability of electronic records along with error checks and alerts contribute to a reduction in medication errors. Despite the difficulties that may be encountered in extracting data, moreover, CIS can enable fine-grained analysis of critical care practice to support service improvement, audit or research. Other indirect benefits may be less tangible, but successful adoption of a CIS can contribute to improvements in staff morale and unit reputation (with potentially positive effects on staff turnover). See Table 55.1 for a summary.

Table 55.1 Costs and benefits

Main costs associated with the implementation of a CIS	
Direct initial purchase costs	Hardware purchase and installation
	Software purchase/licence, customisation and installation
	Infrastructure purchase and installation
Indirect initial purchase costs	Replacement or upgrade of equipment to interface with the CIS
Direct recurrent costs	Hardware maintenance, repair and upgrade costs
	Software licence/upgrade costs
	Consumables
Direct initial staff costs	Project management
	Staff time for customisation
	Recruitment and employment of trainers
	Staff time during training
Direct recurrent staff costs	User support
	Ongoing training
	Ongoing customisation
	Data extraction
Indirect staff costs	Initial loss of productivity
	Management time
	Staff resistance/turnover

Main benefits associated with the implementation of a CIS	
Direct savings	Elimination of costs and tasks associated with paper records
	Efficiency gains in certain tasks
Indirect benefits	Improved legibility of records
	Improved availability of records
	Improved accountability for data
	Clinical decision support
	Data to support cost management, audit and research
	Improved staff morale
	Improved unit reputation

As may be evident, the adoption of CIS in critical care is not solely a technical exercise, but requires careful and effective leadership and management. It is generally recognised that this leadership needs to be clinical rather than managerial, both to ensure that the CIS is aligned with a clear clinical vision, but also to act as a credible 'champion' able to motivate and persuade others through what can sometimes be a trying process.

Effects of CIS on Clinical Practice

The objective of introducing a CIS in critical care is not to install yet more equipment, but to support and enhance clinical practice. The extent to which a CIS achieves this, however, will depend on its ability to support clinical workflows. Where a CIS is poorly aligned with the way in which staff carry out their tasks, for example by introducing additional stages to activities carried out under time pressure, they may be reluctant to use it, or, where use is mandated, may look for workarounds that will 'keep the CIS happy' with the minimum disruption to their work. This can lead to the persistence of unofficial, often paper-based work practices, discrepancies of which with the CIS record can be a potentially serious source of errors. It also means that the CIS record may be incomplete, inaccurate or out of date and that capabilities offered by the CIS are only partially utilised. A CIS that has been designed with significant user involvement to ensure that it facilitates rather than disrupts clinical workflows, however, is more likely to enable benefits to be effectively realised.

This is not to say, though, that some changes to clinical workflows may not be an intended and beneficial effect of CIS adoption. For example, where clinicians have developed unreflective routines that do not conform to emerging best practice, the CIS can be an opportunity to review these and to support the adoption of new protocols. Some staff may consider this as restricting their clinical autonomy, and it may be necessary to allow them to override system defaults to avoid resistance. If the new protocols are made easy to follow and can be shown to deliver benefits, however, then their use may become less contentious with time.

Another aspect of CIS that may provoke concern from clinicians is what is sometimes referred to as its 'Big Brother' effect. Because all actions taken with a CIS are time stamped and associated with a specific user name, this creates the possibility for retrospective review of any individual's practice. Even if this functionality is never used, some users may be uncomfortable with the prospect that their work may be subject to continuous surveillance. The association with a particular username depends, of course, on individuals only logging into the CIS under their own name. Even making this a mandatory requirement, with disciplinary consequences for non-compliance, may not be enough to prevent some, especially senior, users who consider that data entry is not a good use of their time or expertise, from finding ways to circumvent it, for example by getting colleagues to enter data for them, or sharing their login credentials. Notwithstanding such efforts, the clear accountability for actions that a CIS creates would seem a reasonable expectation of good clinical practice.

While it is not a necessary feature of a CIS that work practices are standardised (for example, systems can be designed to allow data entry in a variety of formats), a CIS can be perceived as promoting greater standardisation of care, for example by providing protocols and order sets that make it easy to follow best practice. This may be considered a good thing in many respects, ensuring that care tends to conform to a common evidence-based standard, but may be considered constraining by some clinicians. On the other hand, this standardisation may be welcomed by new, temporary and junior staff, for whom the cognitive load of learning a unit's distinctive practices is thereby reduced (although at the cost, some might argue, of excessive dependency on the CIS, which may cause problems if it ever goes down).

A further concern with use of a CIS may be data overload. The volume, detail and depth of data that may be accessed may be seen by some clinical staff as overwhelming, and may make it hard to distinguish the vital few data points from the less critical many. Studies also suggest that in most circumstances physicians are highly selective in the data to which they pay attention, for example considering perhaps only a handful of items on every occasion that a patient is admitted to critical care and never using a substantial portion of the available clinical data. To a degree, however, this is a problem that can be addressed through appropriate data display, ensuring that critical values are prominently visible, but having additional detail available when requested.

Looked at from another perspective, however, the volume of data accumulated with a CIS can be considered to offer a number of exciting new opportunities. It provides a more detailed, longitudinal and easily searchable record of a patient's stay in critical care than has previously been available. This can be used to enable systematic exploration of trends and relationships across a large population of patients, rather than just focusing on the immediate care of the individual. At the same time it may also be used to personalise care for an individual, based on their specific characteristics, rather than relying on standard values. Making best use of the opportunities provided by a CIS to support a data led approach to care that does not lose sight of the individual patient or of the importance of doctor–patient interaction, is not straightforward, but is potentially one of the more significant effects of CIS in critical care. Achieving this will require strong clinical leadership to ensure that opportunities are identified and that unit work practices and CIS design both support such an approach.

Conclusions

The volume of data that is documented on critical care patients would now seem beyond the capability of staff to record by hand, or of paper-based records to adequately represent in ways that can be used by clinicians. Deploying the power of modern computers to support this process would therefore seem a sensible move. It also offers a number of benefits over traditional paper-based records. Automating documentation, for example, can eliminate transcription errors. A repository of all data relating to a particular patient, and across the whole population of patients passing through critical care, can be built up and made continuously and immediately accessible at the point of care. These data can be analysed and displayed in a variety of ways according to clinicians' preferences. Data can be analysed automatically to alert clinical staff to significant interactions. Over time a data resource will be developed that can support audit and research. This process is not without its complexities and potential difficulties, but provided that these are handled sensitively, CIS can make a positive contribution to critical care.

Learning Points

- Critical care is a highly data intensive environment.
- CIS can support healthcare delivery in critical care.
- Benefits of CIS include ready access to legible patient records and electronic prescribing.
- CIS can however be costly to install and maintain.
- Over time CIS can provide a powerful data resource to support audit, quality improvement and research.

MCQs

1. **How many data items may be documented for an average critical care patient in 24 hours?**
   (a) 200
   (b) 1000
   (c) 1500
   (d) 10,000
2. **What is the core technical component of a CIS?**
   (a) A database
   (b) A bedside computer
   (c) The Internet
   (d) A power socket
3. **Which of the following is a generally recognised benefit of CIS?**
   (a) Time saving
   (b) Reduction in medical errors
   (c) Improved computer literacy of staff
   (d) Staff savings
4. **What proportion of the initial purchase cost of a major computer system does the five year cost of ownership amount to?**
   (a) 10–20%
   (b) 50–100%
   (c) 500–800%
   (d) 1000–2000%
5. **CIS adoption is more likely to be successful if led by:**
   (a) Hospital IT experts
   (b) The CIS vendor
   (c) External consultants
   (d) A senior clinician

Exercise answers are available on p.470. Alternatively, take the test online at www.cambridge.org/CardiothoracicMCQ

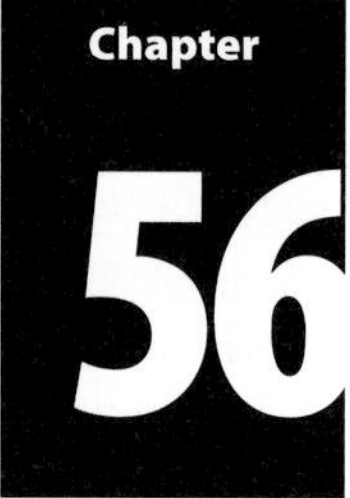

Medical Law and Ethics in the Cardiothoracic Intensive Care Unit

Oana Cole

The specialty of intensive care has evolved significantly since its inception, approximately 50 years ago. With further advances in the field and the development of subspecialist branches, the complexity of patients is increasing. A beautiful metaphor of the 'modern patient' is offered by the main character in Philip Roth's novel, *Everyman,* who contemplates '... time having transformed his own body into a storehouse for man-made contraptions designed to fend off collapse.' The flipside to that has been the increasing intricacy of medical law and ethics. In this chapter we propose to present some of the main issues briefly. The interested reader will find a short list of further reading material at the end of the chapter.

Ethics Principles

While there are a number of ethical models, which have been applied to medicine in general and to critical care in particular, the most commonly taught one is the Beauchamp and Childress approach. The four principles described act as a general guide to most aspects of patient care:

1. autonomy
2. beneficience
3. non-malfeasance
4. justice.

Autonomy

It can be argued that autonomy is the first among equals. The patient is owed the respect for his/her own decision making. It is intended to counter the old attitudes of medical paternalism and support the patient in their choices. There are two aspects that we must note here.

- It does not have any bearing on the wisdom of a decision; in other words, we cannot say that the patient's decision cannot be respected simply because it appears to be unwise.
- In order to make a decision, the patient needs to have the *capacity* to *consent* or not to the treatment proposed.

We have introduced two further concepts here, consent and capacity, which will be explained later.

Beneficience

All clinical actions taken must be to the benefit of the patient. In other words, if the patient cannot make a decision, the healthcare professionals must act in accordance to the *patient's best interests.*

Non-malfeasance

Also known as primum non nocere, it is probably the oldest and possibly the most controversial principle. Intensive care is characterised by very invasive, painful procedures, which sometimes carry substantial risks. Should we stop doing them altogether? Certainly not, but we should consider the harm versus benefit of each manoeuvre. In other words, we need to balance beneficience and non-malfeasance.

Justice

Most commonly this principle has been associated with the fair distribution of resources. While at organisational level this translates into resource allocation over a certain length of time, at individual patient level it is even more controversial. It underlies the issue of the last bed in the ICU or the long-term patient who is unlikely to get better but who is using up precious resources. In other words, cui prodest?

Consent and the Mental Capacity Act 2005

The Good Medical Practice Guide published by the GMC in 2013 stipulates that doctors should work in 'partnership with the patients, sharing with them information they will need to make decisions about their care'. This means that patients should consent to intensive care. But how do we define intensive care? Here are some of the aspects that may be important to consider:

- Intensive care is a process, rather than a geographical location;
- Various healthcare professionals are involved, each with a different impact on the patient's autonomy and dignity;
- The degree of 'burdensomeness' of the critical care process is individual to each patient;
- To date, there is not an accurate prognostic score for mortality or post-ICU morbidity; most of the scoring systems have been validated for populations, not individuals;
- There may be significant decrease in a person's quality of life following an intensive care admission; there are indications that the more prolonged and complex the critical care treatment, the more protracted the recovery to near premorbid condition.

Patients Who Have Capacity

Consent implies a two-way exchange of information between a doctor, or other healthcare professional, and the patient. The latter will have to demonstrate that they are capable of retaining and processing the information given and communicate their decision whether to accept or reject the treatment proposed, or even not to make the decision until a later date. This would demonstrate that they have capacity, as stipulated by the Mental Capacity Act, 2005.

Note that the Act stipulates that capacity is issue specific.

Consent is the legal counterpart of a patient's autonomy. If the patient is temporarily incapacitated, as most of the ICU patients are, then either the decision should be postponed until the patient recovers capacity, or other pathways of finding the best solution should be followed. Importantly, respect for the patient's autonomy should also be shown in the way the consent procedure is followed. What would the patient like and need to know about the treatment proposed? There are a few guiding principles.

- The Bolam test with the Bolitho amendment – the information provided should be what a 'reasonable' doctor would disclose towards a patient; the 'reasonable' doctor would be acting in accordance to the practice of a group of peers, provided there is a logical basis for the practice.
- The *Chester v. Ashfar* case moved the standard even higher, to explicitly offering information that a reasonable patient would want to know. The latter principle is usually explained as serious and common risks of a treatment or procedure. However, it is necessary to consider the individual patients as well – consenting a soprano or a chorister for intubation or tracheostomy is different to consenting an engineer to the same procedure.
- Following the case of *Montgomery v Lanarkshire Health Board*, doctors must now ensure that patients are aware of ***any*** 'material risks' involved in a proposed treatment, and of reasonable alternatives.

Patients Who Lack Capacity

The procedure for patients lacking capacity is more complex. There are several possible solutions.

1. The patient has an Advanced Directive (AD).
2. The patient does not have an AD; the healthcare professional should act in the patient's best interests.
3. There is disagreement amongst the multidisciplinary team members or between the medical team and the patient's family with regards to what constitutes the best interests:
   (a) for long-term ICU patients, a court decision should be sought;
   (b) for short-term and intermediate-term patients, an Independent Mental Capacity Advocate (IMCA) should be consulted.

The Mental Capacity Act has given more importance to the AD than previously. However, there is a plethora of cases in the medicolegal literature which prove that there are multiple ways in which an AD is not applicable in a particular situation, especially in critically ill patients.

Best Interests

The best interests test aims to canvass information regarding the patient's current and past views, as well as the views of the relatives and the next of kin's. For example, it can be fairly safely predicted that a member of the Jehova's Witnesses denomination would refuse a blood transfusion even if it were life saving. However, there have been cases where a former Jehova's Witness had been given a blood transfusion if proven that he/she were no longer an active member of the denomination. *HE v A Hospital NHS Trust (2003)* is a prime example of such a case.

Another important point is that should a patient choose to refuse treatment, his/her wishes should be respected; however, should they insist on a treatment, the doctor has the legal right to refuse based on clinical grounds.

Deprivation of Liberty

Article 5 of the Human Rights Act states that 'everyone has the right to liberty and security of person'. Persons, without capacity, who are under continuous supervision and not free to leave the place where they are being treated are deprived of their liberty. Every patient admitted to intensive care should be considered at risk of deprivation of liberty and those that are unable to consent should be referred for an urgent Deprivation of Liberty Safeguards (DoLS) authorisation. Once in place, the supervisory body will appoint a representative for the patient, and ensure regular review as to whether ongoing deprivation of liberty is required and remove the authorisation when it is no longer necessary. All deaths of patients which occur where a DoLS authorisation is in place should be reported to the coroner.

Withholding and Withdrawal of Treatment: Do Not Attempt Resuscitation (DNAR) Orders

- Withholding treatment – not initiating treatment due to no discernable benefit foreseen, usually in irreversible clinical situations, for example not offering vasoactive medication, intubation, renal replacement therapy.
- Withdrawing treatment – stopping ongoing treatment because of no benefit detectable, for example stopping inotropic support in refractory end-stage cardiogenic shock with end-organ dysfunction.
- Limitation of treatment (ceiling of treatment/no escalation) – occurs when the critical care team are reluctant to make recommendations either for withdrawal of treatment or for continuation of full support; in the words of SA Murray (2008), limitations of treatment are usually applied when 'we are hoping for the best but expecting the worst'.
- DNAR – an order usually put in by a senior clinician to not start cardiopulmonary resuscitation (CPR) on a patient in the event of cardiac arrest; most DNAR orders are initially in place for 48 or 72 hours and the critical care team are advised to revise the decision at the end of the specified time period. It is appropriate to make a DNAR when the patient's heart is not likely to restart, or when there is no benefit in doing so.

All the principles enumerated above have been subject to numerous ethical and legal debates and are likely to remain so, given the nature of the decisions involved. Importantly, following a landmark judgement in 2014 (*Tracey v Cambridge*) there is a presumption in favour of patient involvement in the DNAR decision making process and if they lack capacity, their family and carers. It should be remembered that whilst active treatment may be withheld, withdrawn, or a DNAR decision may be put in place, patient care is never withdrawn or withheld.

The Diagnosis of Death

There are many definitions of death. A layperson will have a certain concept of death, which will have a basis in the cultural and social characteristics of the group they belong to. In a multifaith society, as are now most of the Western countries, it would be disrespectful to try and define death according to a specific spiritual dogma. Moreover, when referring to death in a critically ill patient, other issues, such as organ donation, come to mind. The Academy of Medical Royal Colleges has produced a 'Code of practice for the diagnosis and confirmation of death' (2008).

Brain-Stem Death

The following are criteria for the diagnosis of death following irreversible cessation of brain-stem function.

Prerequisites:

- Known aetiology of brain damage
- Reversible causes of coma have been excluded
- No evidence of depressant drugs or residual muscle paralysis
- Temperature >34 °C
- Exclusion of reversible circulatory, metabolic or endocrine disturbances
- No reversible cause of apnoea.

Brain-stem death tests:

- No pupillary response to light
- No corneal reflex
- No vestibulo-ocular reflex
- Doll's eyes reflex
- No motor response to pain in the trigeminal nerve distribution
- No gag reflex and no cough reflex
- Apnoea despite $PaCO_2 > 6$ kPa with normal PaO_2, in the absence of bicarbonate administration or previous severe respiratory disease.

The test should be performed by at least two physicians who have been qualified more than 5 years and are competent to conduct and interpret the test. Each physician tests individually, and each set of tests is repeated twice. The time of death is the time of the first positive set of tests. There is no specific time interval that should be left between the tests, provided the acid-base balance and $PaCO_2$ have had time to normalise between examinations.

When appropriate or indicated, other investigations should be performed in order to ascertain irreversible cessation of brain-stem function. However, the details of these are beyond the scope of this chapter.

Cardiac Death

The following diagnostic procedure is common:

- Absence of mechanical cardiac function, as confirmed by absent heart sounds and absent central pulse on palpation for five minutes
- Fixed and dilated pupils
- Absent corneal reflexes
- Absent motor response to supra-orbital pressure.

In critical care these criteria may be supplemented by the following:

- Asystole on a continuous ECG display
- Still heart on echocardiography
- Absent pulsatile flow on intra-arterial pressure monitoring, provided the patient does not have a ventricular assist device or VA ECMO in place.

Organ Donation Framework in ICU – the UK Practice

Organ shortage is a growing issue all over the world and significant efforts have been made by all parties concerned, both nationally and internationally, to increase the donor pool. However, unlike countries such as Spain, where organ donation is opted out of rather than opted into, the UK does not have any such legislation at the time of writing this chapter. The UK Donation Ethics Committee has published several recommendations in 2014.

Donation after Brain Death (DBD)

This is organ donation which takes place after brain-stem death criteria have been met. It is also known as heart-beating donation. These donors have provided the majority of transplanted organs since the inception of transplant surgery in the 1950s. However, due to a multitude of factors, the numbers of DBD are decreasing. The consequence has been the rapid development of donations after circulatory death (DCD).

Donation after Circulatory Death (DCD)

This is organ donation which takes place after cardiorespiratory criteria of death have been met. It is also known as non-heart beating donation. Though there have been cases of organ retrieval after unanticipated death, such as patients presenting to the accident and emergency department, this practice is fraught with potential complications, not only ethical but also concerning organ viability. More frequent is organ donation following planned withdrawal of treatment in the ICU.

Whichever the pool of donors is considered, the guiding principles are the same.

- If donation is likely, the matter should be fully considered when caring for the patient.
- Once it has been established that further care is unlikely to benefit the patient and that, based on the patient's known beliefs and values, they would be supportive of organ donation, this consideration should become fully part of their care in the last days and hours of life; this includes invasive and pharmacological interventions that may benefit organs.

Special Considerations in Cardiothoracic Critical Care

Perhaps unlike other subspecialties of critical care, the cardiothoracic ICU landscape has changed dramatically in the last decade with the advent of extracorporeal life support. Both extracorporeal membrane oxygenation (ECMO) and ventricular assist devices have become relatively commonplace. It is also highly probable that the total artificial heart (TAH) technology will be perfected and will become accessible in the near future. There are a number of questions which arise.

1. What are the ethical implications of medical practice in these new categories of patients?
2. What is the legal framework governing the medical act?
3. (When) is the patient allowed to die?
4. How to diagnose death in the 'bionic man'?

Ethical and Legal Issues in ECMO Patients

ECMO patients are perhaps the prototype of cardiothoracic ICU patients that engender a flurry of discussions and ethical considerations given the limited nature of the support.

ECMO as a Bridge to Nowhere

This has become an unfortunately common encounter in the modern cardiothoracic ICU. The patient who has been on ECMO for days, or even weeks, and who has recovered function of most of the organs, including neurological integrity, poses a real ethical problem. They cannot survive without ECMO, but there is no way out, either because the patient is too debilitated to be a transplant candidate, or because of some other ongoing issue which was unbeknown at the time of initiation of therapy. The decision to withdraw life support and the discussions with the patient and their family put the whole critical care team under significant emotional stress.

Organ Retrieval from an ECMO Patient

The same principles governing the process of organ retrieval in the non-ECMO patient should be followed. However, if considering DBD, then consideration needs to be given as to how the apnoea test will be performed. Whilst there are no specific guidelines at present, several authors recommend reduction in the sweep gas flow.

ECPR

This involves placing the patient in cardiac arrest on VA ECMO while waiting for the heart function to recover, assuming that the dysfunction is mainly related to hibernation and stunning. The decision should be made in a timely fashion, before multiorgan failure sets in. Based on the evidence so far though, ECPR has not enjoyed the success anticipated. It is also accompanied by potentially prolonged suffering and, to some, is the harbinger of an undignified death. It is, therefore, a procedure that should be undertaken once extensive consultation amongst medical teams and with the patient's family has happened. Unfortunately, this is usually not physically possible within the timeframe, which may lead to very confusing and ultimately sad situations.

Medical Negligence

The doctor owes the patient a duty of care. The definition of a standard of care has the basis in the Bolam test, as well as the subsequent modifications to the law. In the last two decades there have been many published guidelines by the Royal Colleges, the National Institute for Clinical Excellence (NICE) and the Scottish Intercollegiate Guidelines Network (SIGN) amongst others. Since the guidelines are not and should not be anything else than a guide, the court of law and the GMC have been employing expert medical witnesses to advise on certain claims of negligence. An expert medical witness is an experienced, well-respected specialist in a particular field, who can inform and advise the jury on specific aspects of care.

As a result of the flurry of well-publicised medical scandals there has been the introduction of revalidation and relicensing for all practising doctors by the GMC. The aim is to ensure that all medical practitioners are up to date and fit to practise. The results of the revalidation process will probably be visible within the next 3 to 5 years, once all doctors have been through the process.

What to do if a doctor is accused of negligence?

Runciman et al. (2003) suggest a possible approach when dealing with accidental harm in healthcare.

Research in Critical Care

Research is necessary for the advancement of knowledge. But recent years have unfortunately also seen some medical research disasters. We refer the reader to the TGN 412 trial, which caused serious morbidity in six healthy volunteers, or to the experimental treatment with rGH in ventilator dependent ICU patients. The Declaration of Helsinki, adopted by the Medical Research Council, makes the distinction between:

- Clinical research – medical research combined with patient care; the patient must receive the

best care, or at least, not worse than conventional treatment;
- Non-clinical research – biomedical research, which is conducted on healthy volunteers.

Consent

The researcher has the obligation to obtain consent from the participants in the study; the language of the consent form must be clear enough to a 12 year old, and the participants in the trial or their next of kin must be aware that they can withdraw from the trail at any point, without any adverse consequence for their clinical care.

Publication Ethics

- Large trials are usually required to be registered with one of the international registries in order to avoid unnecessary duplication.
- Plagiarism – passing the work of others as one's own; this is a very serious offence, usually with significant repercussions from the GMC or other national and international bodies.
- Fabricated data – intentional use of selective or fictitious results of a trial; if the respective trial is included in a meta-analysis, it can skew the results significantly and ultimately impact on patient safety.
- Undisclosed conflicts of interest – recently, a number of significant, well-respected medical research figures have been employed by the medical industry as advisors on the development of new drugs or technology. Unfortunately, there have been cases where authors of significant trials in the recent past have failed to disclose the financial or other allegiances to the sponsoring company; this resulted in the publication of fabricated data and had severe consequences for all involved.

Most of those who have tried to initiate a medical research project will be familiar with the Research and Ethics Committees. Such a committee is appointed to examine the research proposal and determine whether it is ethical and whether it respects the standards of autonomy, beneficience, non-malfeasance and justice. For more details, the reader is referred to the Department of Health document on governance arrangements for research ethics committees.

Learning Points

- The most commonly used ethical framework in medicine is based on the four principles – autonomy, beneficience, non-malfeasance and justice.
- The Mental Capacity Act establishes the general guidelines with regards to obtaining consent or applying treatment to patients who lack capacity.
- Approximately a third of the patients who die in intensive care have their treatment withheld or withdrawn, or have been subject to a DNAR order.
- The diagnosis of death and the legal framework governing organ donation determine UK practice; they form the basis of transplant ethics.
- Medical research is subject to constraints laid by the Research and Ethics Committee and the Intellectual Property Law.

Further Reading

Academy of Medical Royal Colleges. *A Code of Practice for the Diagnosis and Confirmation of Death.* London: Academy of Medical Royal Colleges, 2010.

Danbury C, Newdick C, Lawson A, Waldmann C (Eds). *Law and Ethics in Intensive Care.* Oxford: Oxford University Press, 2010.

Department of Health. Governance Arrangements for Research Ethics Committees. 2012. Available from: www.gov.uk

Herring J. *Q&A Medical Law*, 3rd edition. London: Routledge, 2016.

Murray SA, Sheikh A. Palliative care beyond cancer: care for all at the end of life. *British Medical Journal.* 2008; 336: 958–959.

Roth P. *Everyman.* London: Jonathan Cape, 2006.

Runciman WB, Merry AF, Tito F. Error, blame, and the law in health care – an Antipodean perspective. *Annals of Internal Medicine.* 2003; 138: 974–979.

Chapter 57

Training in Cardiothoracic Intensive Care

Amy Needham and Chinmay Padvardthan

The hardest conviction to get into the mind of a beginner is that the education upon which he is engaged is not a medical course, but a life course, for which the work of a few years under teachers is but a preparation.

Sir William Osler The Student of Medicine

A Historical Perspective

From its nascence in the polio epidemic of Copenhagen in 1952 to the foundation of the Faculty of Intensive Care Medicine in 2010, intensive care medicine has made great strides to become one of the fastest growing specialties in hospital medicine. The past 60 years have brought great technological advances in medical devices and we now have better understanding of critical illness pathologies. We have improved the care processes in intensive care, implementing evidence based interventions such as low tidal volume ventilation, bundles of care and critical care outreach. We have introduced better predictors of risk and observed a reduction in mortality of the critically ill.

Developments and progress in anaesthesia and evolution of the concept of 'intensive care units' are inexorably linked with the progress of cardiac surgery. John H Gibbon Jr first successfully demonstrated the use of a cardiopulmonary bypass machine to perform open heart surgery in May 1953. Prior to this, cardiac surgery as we know today hardly existed. Surgeons were almost warned against operating on the heart. In the words of Theodor Billroth, the famous Viennese surgeon, 'Any surgeon who attempts operating on the heart should lose the respect of his colleagues'. Any cardiac surgery prior to Gibbon's bypass machine was mostly on cardiac trauma, and a few rheumatic mitral repairs. However, since 1953, great strides have been made in cardiac surgery and surgeons now routinely perform a plethora of complex procedures. Albert Starr was one of the early cardiac surgical pioneers who adopted a multidisciplinary team approach to postoperative care after cardiac surgery. He employed cardiologists, an anaesthesiologist, a haematologist, a neurologist, a nephrologist and a psychiatrist to look after his first postoperative case of mechanical aortic valve replacement in 1960. He can be credited as the trailblazer in the concept of cardiothoracic intensive care. The first purpose built, 12 bed cardiac surgery intensive care unit opened in 1964 at Broadgreen Hospital in Liverpool. The catalyst for growth of intensive care units was the growing demands of open heart surgery, which increasingly required specialised haemodynamic and metabolic monitoring.

Another important key change that influenced future cardiac intensive care was the development of coronary care units (CCU) in 1961, dedicated to looking after patients with myocardial infarction and addressing issues of arrhythmias and prompt resuscitation with closed chest compressions. In the late 1960s the second stage in the development of the CCU was ushered in by Bernard Lown and colleagues in Boston, Massachusetts. They described a shift from resuscitation at the time of an arrest to monitoring for early signs of clinical change and prevention of a cardiac arrest.

1978 saw recognition of cardiac anaesthesia as an anaesthetic subspecialty in its own right in North America with establishment of the Society of Cardiovascular Anesthesiologists. It was not until 1984 that the Association of Cardiac Anaesthetists (ACTA) came into existence in the UK. Dedicated cardiac anaesthetists became a vital part of the 'team' looking after cardiac surgical patients in the postoperative period. Over the past 40 years the post cardiac surgery care units evolved into the highly specialised cardiothoracic intensive care units of the twenty-first century.

From its humble beginnings, today's cardiothoracic intensive care unit (CTICU) is a highly complex behemoth. At its heart are the highly trained specialist intensivists, surgeons, cardiologists, specially trained nurses, pharmacists, dieticians, physiotherapists, perfusionists and technicians, all working together with input from almost every medical and surgical specialty in the hospital. The patient population has expanded from postsurgical patients, to include diverse pathologies such as advanced heart failure, severe pulmonary hypertension, mechanical circulatory support, extracorporeal membrane oxygenation (ECMO) support, transplant patients and post cardiac arrest patients. CTICUs now provide long term respiratory weaning, tracheostomy care, renal replacement therapies, plasma apheresis, bronchoscopies and every other form of therapeutic intervention offered on a general intensive care unit. Globally there has been a shift in patient demographics. Patient case mix in intensive care units is increasingly elderly, with multiple comorbidities such as diabetes mellitus, chronic airways disease, hypertension and renal failure. The falling incidence of fatal ST elevation myocardial infarction, on the other hand, has seen a rise in incidence of complications associated with non-ST elevation MI, and complications associated with mechanical support devices. These changes have altered the natural history of cardiovascular illnesses and these have started to resemble the natural history of critically ill patients on general intensive care units with a greater incidence of multiorgan dysfunction requiring organ support. The disease trajectory of a patient admitted after a cardiac complication now resembles that for any other critical illness, bringing with it the complications of prolonged immobility, critical illness neuropathy, resistant infections, renal failure requiring prolonged support, need for specialist nutrition, issues with vascular access, chronic sepsis etc. This means there is a significant effect on resources, bed allocation and availability and in particular need for specialist personnel training.

This need for specially trained medical staff to look after the complex needs of the critically ill patients was first recognised in the USA. The first critical care residency was established at the Presbyterian University Hospital, Pittsburgh in 1962 under the direction of Peter Safar. The residency was initially opened for anaesthesiologists. However, subsequently it became open to different hospital specialties like surgery, internal medicine, paediatrics and pulmonology. Each specialty introduced a different pathway to get into the specialty, with each stipulating their own specific requirements on training and experience. Training in the UK and Australasia, however, took a different pathway with intensive care medicine initially predominantly being the domain of anaesthetists.

Australia and New Zealand introduced a comprehensive subspecialty training programme in critical care in 1996 with the formation of the College of Intensive Care Medicine in 2008. In the UK the Faculty of Intensive Care Medicine was formally established in 2010. The General Medical Council approved the standalone subspecialty training programme for critical care medicine in 2012. The Canadians have a total training requirement which is similar to the rest of North America/Latin America (i.e. 5 years of specialty training); but all base specialties agreed to a 2 year critical care training programme following the primary subspecialty training with a single conjoint examination.

Spain and Latin American countries also went down the same route of requiring a minimum 5 years of base specialty training. The European Society of Intensive Care Medicine (ESICM) was established in 1984 in Geneva to promote education, training and standardisation across Europe in intensive care. ESICM offers a Diploma in Intensive Care Medicine (EDIC) to trainees from various specialties with 2 years of critical care experience.

Current Status of Intensive Care Medicine Training

Since 2010, the Faculty of Intensive Care Medicine has been responsible for regulation and organisation of training in the specialty. A separate curriculum was established for intensive care medicine training in 2011. Standalone intensive care medicine (ICM) specialty training received the approval of the General Medical Council in 2012.

Training in ICM in the UK is extensively modelled on the CoBaTriCE syllabus developed by the ESICM. The trainees are also expected to develop general professional knowledge, skills, attitudes and behaviours required of all doctors. These common competencies in the core aspects of medical practice are identified from the Academy of Medical Royal Colleges Common Competencies.

The single specialty CCT training programme in ICM lasts for 7 years; however in trainees in dual CCT, training may extend for 8.5 years or more. Prior to starting ICM training, trainees need to have completed a 2 year ICM core training programme. These include 'Common stem programme' in acute care common stem training (ACCS), which may include trainees from acute medicine, emergency medicine, common medical training (CMT) or core anaesthetic training. Trainees are required to have passed the relevant stage of examinations in their specialty (first part of the FRCA exam, full membership examination of the College of Emergency Medicine). Competitive entry into a national specialty training programme is at the specialist trainee year 3 (ST3) level. Training progresses through three stages. The first stage of higher specialist training lasts for 2 years and is aimed at developing core competencies in intensive care. For example, a trainee from an emergency medicine background would achieve competencies in anaesthesia. These competencies are detailed in the ICM curriculum.

The second stage of training lasts 2 years, and includes subspecialty training in various aspects of intensive care such as paediatric intensive care, cardiothoracic intensive care etc. The second stage also includes a 'specialist skills year' where trainees are able to pursue specialist interests such as echocardiography, pre-hospital medicine, medical education and importantly cardiac intensive care.

The final year (final stage) is a mandatory year in intensive care medicine, where a trainee is expected to absorb management and non-technical skills in the run up to becoming a consultant.

The dual CCT training programme is possible for trainees in acute medicine, respiratory medicine, renal medicine, anaesthesia and emergency medicine. This is again via a competitive recruitment process and extends the duration of training depending on the time taken for the competencies to be achieved. The Faculty of Intensive Care Medicine has laid out details of the competencies, practical skill sets and learning outcomes and assessment tools in its curriculum document. Australia and New Zealand have a similar structured specialty training programme in critical care medicine.

Opportunities for Training in Cardiothoracic Intensive Care

In the UK, currently training in cardiothoracic intensive care is provided as part of the standalone intensive care medicine training and anaesthesia. All intensive care medicine specialty trainees are currently expected to complete a mandatory 3 month block in a cardiothoracic intensive care unit during the second stage of their training. There are formal learning objectives that the trainees have to achieve by the end of the module. They are as follows:

- Be able to manage cardiac failure following an acute cardiac event;
- Be able to manage postoperative cardiac patients following both elective and emergency cardiac surgery;
- Be aware of the indications for discussion and transfer of critically ill patients to regional cardiothoracic units;
- Be able to stabilise and transfer patients with acute cardiorespiratory conditions requiring cardiothoracic intensive care.

In the final 3 months of the second stage of training, additional experience can be gained in cardiothoracic intensive care if a trainee wishes to do so.

In the second stage of training, a trainee who wishes to specialise in cardiothoracic intensive care may spend a year doing so. There also exists an opportunity to gain out of programme experience (OOPE) in the specialty. Thus a trainee coming out of a standalone ICM training programme may expect up to 18 months of training in cardiothoracic intensive care. But this programme does not allow the opportunity for an in depth experience in anaesthesia or cardiac anaesthesia unless trainees decide to dual accredit.

The Royal College of Anaesthetists (RCoA) is responsible for provision of specialist training in anaesthesia in the UK. The current specialty training programme in anaesthesia is a 7 year programme, which mandates a minimum 9 months of ICM training. In addition to this, the trainee in anaesthesia is expected to gain 9 months of 'spiral' learning in cardiac anaesthesia over the course of the programme at different stages, or 6 months of spiral learning and 12 months of specialist experience in the advance year (year 6 or 7), in cardiothoracic anaesthesia. During this time, the trainee is expected to gain knowledge, skills and experience of cardiothoracic anaesthesia, echocardiography skills and principles of cardiothoracic intensive care as required in the curriculum. The majority of the current cohort of cardiothoracic intensivists in the UK, to this date, have been trained via this route and only a few have a formal accreditation in intensive care medicine. Anecdotally, many anaesthetists pursue a further fellowship in cardiothoracic anaesthesia, which includes cardiothoracic intensive care built into it. This has traditionally been the training and service provision model in cardiothoracic intensive care in the UK. However, there is no separate curriculum in cardiothoracic intensive care other than the domains described in the CCT document.

Training in Echocardiography

Training and formal qualification in transoesophageal echocardiography (TOE) has for many years been a fundamental component of cardiothoracic anaesthesia and intensive care and has seen an exponential expansion in terms of clinical utility, supporting guidelines, literature, expertise and enthusiasts. This familiarity with the modality of ultrasound and echo and availability of resources has enabled cardiac anaesthetists and intensivists to rapidly adapt the technology and lead the way in terms of using ultrasound diagnostically in the intensive care unit. A working group composed of members from the Intensive Care Society (ICS) and the British Society of Echocardiography has developed a training scheme termed focused intensive care echo (FICE), which aims to equip intensivists with a practical basic competency platform from which to develop further echo skills. This training programme has been well supported by cardiac anaesthetists and intensivists. Based on this simple and practical model, lung ultrasound is also developing as a bedside investigation in the ICU with protocols such as BLUE (bedside lung ultrasound in emergency) and FALLS (fluid administration limited by lung sonography) being incorporated into daily clinical practice. Echocardiography remains a mainstay of cardiac perioperative care, and this unique concentrated exposure to echocardiography makes the CTICU a highly valuable training experience.

Future of Cardiothoracic Intensive Care Training

Recently, the Intensive Care Society and Faculty of Intensive Care Medicine (UK) published guidance on the provision of intensive care in the UK. On this background, in 2015 the Royal College of Anaesthetists have published guidance on the provision of cardiothoracic anaesthesia and intensive care which states that 'Consultant anaesthetists intending to undertake anaesthesia for cardiac or thoracic surgery should have received training to higher level in adult intensive care, adult cardiac and/or thoracic anaesthesia for a minimum of one year in recognised training centres as part of general training. Those providing intensive care for cardiac surgical patients should have received training to the minimum level as defined by the FICM special skills year in cardiothoracic ICM'.

As a consequence of these regulations, and the gradual arrival of specialist ICM trained consultants in cardiothoracic intensive care on the scene, the traditional service provision model is going to change. Already there is a lively debate in the medical literature on who is best placed to look after patients in cardiothoracic intensive care units. The European Society of Cardiology (ESC) Working Group for Acute Cardiac Care has recommended that intensive cardiac care units be directed by board certified cardiologists specially trained and accredited as acute cardiac care specialists, including training in the general intensive care unit. Recently, a leadership group within the American Board of Thoracic Surgery has recommended development of a cardiothoracic critical care certification pathway for the perioperative care of cardiothoracic surgery patients. The American Heart Association has also recognised the need for including intensive care medicine in training and developing training pathways for cardiologists to train in cardiothoracic intensive care medicine. The Society of Cardiovascular Anesthesiologists has sought approval from the Accreditation Council for Graduate Medical Education (ACGME) for accreditation of cardiothoracic anaesthesiology training as a new subspecialty.

There have been attempts at creating a comprehensive curriculum and described learning domains in cardiothoracic critical care training in the USA. Similar attempts have been made in the UK. A curriculum in cardiothoracic intensive care typically includes competencies in intensive care medicine, critically ill cardiology patients (advanced heart failure), specialist surgical skills (emergency sternotomy and management of postcardiac surgery cardiac arrest), echocardiography and ultrasound competencies, mechanical circulatory support, and extracorporeal membrane oxygenation support. Also included are competencies in end of life care, organ donation and provision of rehabilitation and support.

Cardiac Intensivists in ACTA (CIA)

A subgroup of the already well-established Association of Cardiothoracic Anaesthetists constituting elected consultant and trainee representatives was recently established in the UK with an aim of raising the profile of cardiac intensive care as a specialty and of developing excellence in clinical care through:

- Setting standards for education, training and clinical care provision;
- Sharing data for benchmarking;
- Sharing clinical guidelines and best practice;
- Sharing innovation;
- Involvement in guidelines produced by other affiliated societies, for example ICS, FICM and SCTS.

It is inevitable that as medicine continuously evolves, cardiothoracic critical care will become ever more complex. The expectations of patients and regulators, financial pressures, change of patient demographics and exponential increase in medical expertise will undoubtedly put pressure on current physician training programmes to deliver a comprehensive training in cardiothoracic intensive care. So new ways of training will have to be created. If current evolution of critical care medicine into an independent specialty has taught us anything, it is that it is only a matter of time! As the saying goes: All things are changing, and we are changing with them.

Exercise Answers

Chapter 2

1. (d), 2. (c), 3. (b), 4. (b), 5. (a)

Chapter 3

1. (a) True, (b) False, (c) False, (d) True, (e) False
2. (a) True, (b) False, (c) False, (d) False, (e) False
3. (a) False, (b) True, (c) True, (d) False, (e) True
4. (a) True, (b) True, (c) True, (d) True, (e) True
5. (a) True, (b) True, (c) False, (d) True, (e) True

Chapter 4

1. (d) Young patients at low risk do not need invasive coronary angiography.
2. (b) Saline prehydration is most useful at preventing CIN.
3. (d) Radial cases have longer screening times and higher radiation doses than femoral cases.
4. (c) Diagonal branches supply the anterolateral LV myocardium.
5. (b) Load with dual antiplatelet therapy so that ad hoc PCI can be performed if indicated. Intravenous fluid at 500 ml/hour may cause pulmonary oedema and make it difficult for the patient to lie flat for the procedure. Diuretics are usually omitted prior to angiography as are oral anticoagulants.

Chapter 5

1. (e) All of the above.
2. (c) Aspirin is not contraindicated in bronchoscopy.
3. (d) A double lumen tube has a maximum outer diameter of 4 mm which necessitates using a thin adult or paediatric bronchoscope.
4. (a) When scoping through a tracheostomy, the internal diameter (without inner tube) should be at least 2 mm greater than the bronchoscope outer diameter. Particular care should be taken when withdrawing the bronchoscope, especially in the case of fenestrated tubes, to avoid shearing damage to the scope.
5. (d) Endobronchial stents are deployed either via rigid bronchoscopy or using an over-a-guidewire insertion method using the fibreoptic scope to monitor deployment.

Chapter 6

1. False, 2. False, 3. True, 4. False, 5. False

Chapter 7

1. (a), 2. (d), 3. (b), 4. (a), 5. (d)

Chapter 8

1. (a) False, (b) True, (c) True, (d) False, (e) True
2. (a) False, (b) False, (c) False, (d) False
3. (a) True, (b) False, (c) True, (d) False, (e) True
4. (a) True, (b) True, (c) True, (d) True, (e) True
5. (a) True, (b) True, (c) False, (d) True, (e) False

Chapter 9

1. (e), 2. (a), 3. (a), 4. (d), 5. (c)

Chapter 10

1. (e), 2. (e), 3. (b), 4. (d), 5. (c)

Chapter 11

1. (c), 2. (d), 3. (c), 4. (a), 5. (a)

Chapter 12

1. (c) Tazocin and gentamicin would be the first choice in this hypothetical situation. In practice, we would give a combination of antibiotics to which the

patient responded clinically previously (e.g. ceftazidime + meropenem etc.). It may be worth considering nebulised colistin after discussing with the microbiologist. In case of severe sepsis, however, or known resistance to either of these antibiotics, meropenem would be a good second choice. All antibiotics, though, should be changed once cultures and sensitivities are back.

2. (c) Note: It is important to take at least two sets of blood cultures before giving antibiotics. Treatment should be reviewed with culture results (blood cultures and valve tissue if surgery is performed) and modified accordingly. In case of a culture-negative endocarditis, atypical serology should be done and 16/18S PCR considered.
3. (b)
4. (c) This patient is septic. Broad spectrum antibiotics should be started first, but take at least two sets of blood cultures first and a swab of pus if any, then review with cultures. Duration for LVAD endocarditis (as it is probably in this case) – 6 weeks but could be longer (e.g. until transplanted if surgery is imminent, if not, 6 weeks and stop, re-culture or give suppressive long-term treatment).
5. (a)

Chapter 13

1. (c), 2. (a), 3. (a), 4. (c), 5. (e)

Chapter 14

1. (c), 2. (b), 3. (a), 4. (c) no data support any of the other statements in cardiac ICU patients, 5. (b)

Chapter 15

1. (e), 2. (c), 3. (e), 4. (d), 5. (d)

Chapter 16

1. (c), 2. (a), 3. (e), 4. (d), 5. (b)

Chapter 17

1. (c), 2. (d), 3. (e), 4. (b), 5. (c)

Chapter 18

1. (d), 2. (b), 3. (a), 4. (e), 5. (a)

Chapter 19

1. (a) True, (b) False, (c) False

   Nutritional assessment of patients is best done by simple and cheap screening tools including physical examination and screening questionnaires.

2. (a) False, (b) False, (c) False

   Energy intake is notoriously under reported by diary entries. At energy balance, body weight will remain steady. BMR decreases with age as the body composition changes with a loss of lean tissue.

3. (a) False, (b) False, (c) True

   The critically ill patient has an increased protein turnover causing loss of lean body mass. There is no evidence that anti-inflammatory drugs improve protein metabolism in critically ill patients. Protein oxidation is often calculated from urinary nitrogen excretion.

4. (a) False, (b) False, (c) True

   Protein intake should exceed the recommended 0.8 g/kg/day for a healthy individual. A wide range of carbohydrate and fat should be administered at 2–6 and 0.5–1.5 g/kg/day, respectively. This would need adjustment for individual patient clinical requirements.

5. (a) True, (b) False, (c) False

   Nasograstric feeding should be commenced after 24–48 hours. There is no evidence suggesting gastric or postpyloric placement of the feeding tube is superior. The volume of gastric aspirates should be assessed when commencing nasogastric feeding.

Chapter 20

1. (e), 2. (c), 3. (e), 4. (c), 5. (d)

Chapter 21

1. (c), 2. (d), 3. (a), 4. (d), 5. (d)

Chapter 22

1. (c), 2. (a), 3. (d), 4. (d), 5. (a)

Chapter 23

1. (b), 2. (b), 3. (b), 4. (e), 5. (c)

Chapter 24
1. (c), 2. (b), 3. (c), 4. (d), 5. (a)

Chapter 25A
1. (e), 2. (d), 3. (c), 4. (b), 5. (d)

Chapter 25B
1. (c), 2. (d), 3. (b), 4. (c), 5. (c)

Chapter 26
1. (b), 2. (d), 3. (c), 4. (c), 5. (e)

Chapter 27
1. (b), 2. (e), 3. (c), 4. (c), 5. (c)

Chapter 28
1. (a), 2. (a), 3. (c), 4. (d), 5. (b)

Chapter 29
1. (c), 2. (e), 3. (d), 4. (b)

Chapter 30
1. (b), 2. (c), 3. (a), 4. (a), 5. (d)

Chapter 31
1. (e), 2. (e), 3. (e), 4. (b), 5. (d)

Chapter 32
1. (e), 2. (b), 3. (a), 4. (b), 5. (e)

Chapter 33
1. (c), 2. (c), 3. (c), 4. (a), 5. (d)

Chapter 34
1. (e), 2. (c), 3. (b), 4. (c), 5. (c)

Chapter 35
1. (a), 2. (d), 3. (e), 4. (b), 5. (a)

Chapter 36
1. (a) False, (b) False, (c) True, (d) False, (e) True
2. (a) False, (b) True, (c) True, (d) False, (e) True
3. (a) False, (b) False, (c) True, (d) False, (e) False
4. (a) False, (b) True, (c) True, (d) True, (e) False
5. (a) True, (b) False, (c) True, (d) False

Chapter 37
1. (c), 2. (a), 3. (c), 4. (d), 5. (d)

Chapter 38
1. (d), 2. (c), 3. (d), 4. (b), 5. (b)

Chapter 39
1. (c), 2. (b), 3. (d), 4. (d), 5. (a)

Chapter 40
1. (a), 2. (c), 3. (e), 4. (e), 5. (b)

Chapter 41
1. (b), 2. (b), 3. (b), 4. (e), 5. (c)

Chapter 42
1. (e), 2. (c), 3. (b), 4. (b), 5. (d)

Chapter 43
1. (e), 2. (e), 3. (e), 4. (e), 5. (b)

Chapter 44
1. (d), 2. (b), 3. (c), 4. (e), 5. (a)

Chapter 45
1. (e), 2. (e), 3. (c), 4. (d), 5. (d)

Chapter 46
1. (f), 2. (b), 3. (d), 4. (c)

Chapter 47
1. (b), 2. (e), 3. (d), 4. (c), 5. (c)

Chapter 48

1. (a) True, (b) False, (c) True, (d) True, (e) False
2. (a) False, (b) False, (c) True, (d) True, (e) True
3. (a) False, (b) True, (c) False, (d) False, (e) True
4. (a) True, (b) True, (c) False, (d) False, (e) False
5. (a) False, (b) True, (c) True, (d) True, (e) False

Chapter 49

1. (a), 2. (d), 3. (b), 4. (e), 5. (e)

Chapter 50

1. False, 2. False, 3. True, 4. False, 5. (a) 3, (b) 4, (c) 3, (d) 1, (e) 2 (both iNO and sildenafil act via phosphodiesterase 5 inhibition)

Chapter 51

1. (b), (c), (d), 2. (d), 3. (a), (d), 4. (a), (b), (d), 5. (a), (b), (e)

Chapter 52

1. (a) True, (b) False, (c) False, (d) True, (e) True
2. (a) True, (b) True, (c) True, (d) False, (e) False
3. (a) True, (b) True, (c) False, (d) False, (e) False

Chapter 55

1. (c), 2. (a), 3. (b), 4. (c), 5. (d)

Index